GORDON'S FUNCTIO

HEALTH PERCEPTION–HEALTH MANAGEMENT PATTERN

NUTRITIONAL–METABOLIC PATTERN

ELIMINATION PATTERN

ACTIVITY–EXERCISE PATTERN

*Modified by Marjory Gordon, 2012, with permission.

Nurse's Pocket Guide

Diagnoses, Prioritized Interventions, and Rationales

Marilynn E. Doenges, APRN, BC—Retired

Clinical Specialist—Adult Psychiatric/Mental Health Nursing
Retired Adjunct Faculty
Beth-El College of Nursing and Health Sciences, UCCS
Colorado Springs, Colorado

Mary Frances Moorhouse, RN, MSN, CRRN

Nurse Consultant
TNT-RN Enterprises
Adjunct Faculty
Pikes Peak Community College
Colorado Springs, Colorado

Alice C. Murr, BSN, RN—Retired

Nurse Consultant
Parkville, Missouri

FOURTEENTH EDITION

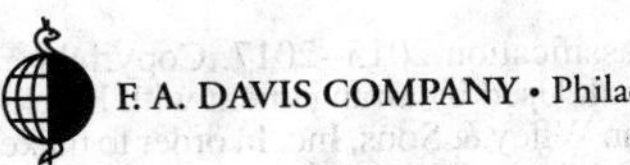

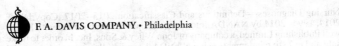

F. A. DAVIS COMPANY • Philadelphia

F. A. Davis Company
1915 Arch Street
Philadelphia, PA 19103
www.fadavis.com

Printed in the United States of America

Last digit indicates print number: 10 9 8 7 6 5 4 3 2 1
Publisher, Nursing: Megan Klim
Project Editor: Amy M. Romano
Design and Illustration Manager: Carolyn O'Brien

As new scientific information becomes available through basic and clinical research, recommended treatments and drug therapies undergo changes. The author(s) and publisher have done everything possible to make this book accurate, up to date, and in accordance with accepted standards at the time of publication. The author(s), editors, and publisher are not responsible for errors or omissions or for consequences from application of the book and make no warranty, expressed or implied, in regard to the contents of the book. Any practice described in this book should be applied by the reader in accordance with professional standards of care used in regard to the unique circumstances that may apply in each situation. The reader is advised always to check product information (package inserts) for changes and new information regarding dose and contraindications before administering any drug. Caution is especially urged when using new or infrequently ordered drugs.

Library of Congress Cataloging-in-Publication Data

Doenges, Marilynn E., 1922–
Nurse's pocket guide : diagnoses, prioritized interventions, and rationales / Doenges Marilynn E., Moorhouse Mary Frances, Murr Alice C.—Ed. 13
p. ; cm.
Includes bibliographical references and index.
ISBN-13: 978-0-8036-4475-5
ISBN-10: 0-8036-4475-2
I. Moorhouse, Mary Frances, 1947– II. Murr, Alice C., 1946– III. Title.
[DNLM: 1. Nursing Diagnosis—Handbooks. 2. Nursing Care—classification—Handbooks. 3. Patient Care Planning—Handbooks. WY 49]
616.07′5—dc23
2012036506

DEDICATION

This book is dedicated to:

Our families, who helped with the mundane activities of daily living that allowed us to write this book and who provide us with love and encouragement in all our endeavors.

Our friends, who support us in our writing, put up with our memory lapses, and love us still.

Bob Martone, former Publisher, Nursing, who germinated the idea for this project so long ago. Megan Klim and Amy Romano, who have taken on the challenge of providing direct support and keeping us focused. Robert Allen, who has guided us through the XML maze since the book went high tech and is a lifeline we greatly appreciate. The F. A. Davis production staff, who coordinated and expedited the project through the editing and printing processes, meeting unreal deadlines, and sending pages to us with bated breath.

Robert H. Craven, Jr., and the F. A. Davis family.

And last and most important:

The nurses we are writing for, to those who have found the previous editions of the *Pocket Guide* helpful, and to other nurses who are looking for help to provide quality nursing care in a period of transition and change, we say, "Nursing Diagnosis is the way."

CONTRIBUTORS

Sheila Marquez
Formerly Executive Director
Vice President/Chief Operating Officer
The Colorado SIDS Program, Inc.
Denver, Colorado

Cayrn F. Demaree, RN, BSN, IBCLC
Lactation Specialist
Denver Health Medical Center
Denver, Colorado

Research Assistant
Mary Katherine Blackwell
Mississippi State University
Columbus, Mississippi

ACKNOWLEDGMENTS

A special acknowledgment to Marilynn's friend, the late Diane Camillone, who provoked an awareness of the role of the patient and continues to influence our thoughts about the importance of quality nursing care, and to our late colleague, Mary Jeffries, who started us on this journey and introduced us to nursing diagnoses.

To our colleagues in NANDA International, who continue to formulate and refine nursing diagnoses to provide nursing with the tools to enhance and promote the growth of the profession.

Marilynn E. Doenges
Mary Frances Moorhouse
Alice C. Murr

CONTENTS

Health Conditions and Client Concerns with Associated Nursing Diagnoses appear on pages 947–1085.

HOW TO USE THE NURSE'S POCKET GUIDE

The American Nurses Association (ANA) *Social Policy Statement* of 1980 was the first to define nursing as the diagnosis and treatment of human responses to actual and potential health problems. This definition, when combined with the ANA *Standards of Practice*, provided impetus and support for the use of nursing diagnosis. Defining *nursing* and its effect on client care supports the growing awareness that nursing care is a key factor in client survival and in the maintenance, rehabilitative, and preventive aspects of healthcare. Changes and new developments in healthcare delivery in the past 30 years have given rise to the need for a common framework of communication to ensure continuity of care for the client moving between multiple healthcare settings and providers. Evaluation and documentation of care are important parts of this process.

This book is designed to aid the practitioner and student nurse in identifying interventions commonly associated with specific nursing diagnoses as proposed by NANDA International (NANDA-I). These interventions are the activities needed to implement and document care provided to the individual client and can be used in varied settings from acute to community/home care.

Chapter 1 presents a brief discussion of the nursing process, data collection, and care plan construction. Appendix 1 contains tools for choosing nursing diagnoses—an Adult Assessment Tool and the Diagnostic Divisions list. Appendix 2 puts theory into practice with a sample assessment database and a corresponding plan of care. A mind or concept map is also provided. For more in-depth information and inclusive plans of care related to specific medical or psychiatric conditions and maternal/newborn care (with rationale and the application of the diagnoses), the nurse is referred to the larger work, published by the F. A. Davis Company: *Nursing Care Plans: Guidelines for Individualizing Client Care Across the Life Span*, ed. 9 (Doenges, Moorhouse, & Murr, 2014) including access to psychiatric and maternal/newborn plans of care. For nursing diagnoses and interventions with evidence-based citations, refer to the more in-depth work published by the F. A. Davis Company: *Nursing Diagnosis Manual: Planning, Individualizing, and Documenting Client Care*, ed. 5 (Doenges, Moorhouse, & Murr, 2016).

Nursing diagnoses are listed alphabetically in Chapter 2 for ease of reference and include the diagnoses accepted for use by NANDA-I through 2015–2017. Each diagnosis approved for testing includes its definition and information divided into the NANDA-I categories of Related or Risk Factors and Defining Characteristics. Related/Risk Factors information reflects causative or contributing factors that can be useful for determining whether the diagnosis is applicable to a particular client. Defining Characteristics (signs and symptoms or cues) are listed as subjective and/or objective and are used to confirm problem diagnoses, aid in formulating outcomes, and provide additional data for choosing appropriate interventions. The authors have not deleted or altered NANDA-I's listings; however, on occasion, they have added to their definitions or suggested additional criteria to provide clarification and direction. These additions are denoted with brackets [ ].

The ANA, in conjunction with NANDA-I, proposed that specific nursing diagnoses currently approved and structured according to Taxonomy I Revised be included in the International Classification of Diseases (ICD) within the section "Family of Health-Related Classifications." Although the World Health Organization did not accept this initial proposal because of lack of documentation of the usefulness of nursing diagnoses at the international level, the NANDA-I list has been accepted by SNOMED (Systemized Nomenclature of Medicine) for inclusion in its international coding system and is included in the Unified Medical Language System of the National Library of Medicine. Today, nurse researchers from around the world have submitted new nursing diagnoses and are validating current diagnoses in support for resubmission and acceptance of the NANDA-I list in future editions of the ICD.

The authors have chosen to categorize the list of nursing diagnoses approved for clinical use and testing into Diagnostic Divisions, which is the framework for an assessment tool (Appendix 1) designed to assist the nurse to readily identify an appropriate nursing diagnosis from data collected during the assessment process. The Diagnostic Division label is listed under each nursing diagnosis heading.

Desired Outcomes/Evaluation Criteria are identified to assist the nurse in formulating individual client outcomes and to support the evaluation process.

Interventions in this pocket guide are primarily directed to adult care settings (although general age-span considerations are included) and are listed according to nursing priorities. Some interventions require collaborative or interdependent orders (e.g., medical, psychiatric), and the nurse will need to determine when this is necessary and take the appropriate action.

The inclusion of Documentation Focus suggestions is to remind the nurse of the importance and necessity of recording the steps of the nursing process.

Finally, in recognition of the ongoing work of numerous researchers over the past 30 years, the authors have referenced the

Nursing Interventions and Outcomes labels developed by the Iowa Intervention Projects (Bulechek, Butcher, & Dochterman; Moorhead, Johnson, Mass, & Swanson). These groups have been classifying nursing interventions and outcomes to predict resource requirements and measure outcomes, thereby meeting the needs of a standardized language that can be coded for computer and reimbursement purposes. As an introduction to this work in progress, sample NIC and NOC labels have been included under the heading Sample Nursing Interventions & Outcomes Classifications at the conclusion of each nursing diagnosis section. The reader is referred to the various publications by Joanne C. Dochterman and Marion Johnson for more in-depth information.

Chapter 3 presents 460 disorders/health conditions reflecting all specialty areas, with associated nursing diagnoses written as client diagnostic statements that include the "related to" and "evidenced by" components as appropriate. This section will facilitate and help validate the assessment and problem or need identification steps of the nursing process.

As noted, with few exceptions, we have presented NANDA-I's recommendations as formulated. We support the belief that practicing nurses and researchers need to study, use, and evaluate the diagnoses as presented. Nurses can be creative as they use the standardized language, redefining and sharing information as the diagnoses are used with individual clients. As new nursing diagnoses are developed, it is important that the data they encompass are added to assessment tools and current databases. As part of the process by clinicians, educators, and researchers across practice specialties and academic settings to define, test, and refine nursing diagnosis, nurses are encouraged to share insights and ideas with NANDA-I online at http://www.nanda.org or at the following address: NANDA International, PO Box 157, Kaukauna, WI 54130–0157.

NURSING DIAGNOSES ACCEPTED FOR USE AND RESEARCH (2015–2017)

Activity Intolerance [specify level]
Activity Intolerance, risk for
Activity Planning, ineffective
Activity Planning, risk for ineffective
*Adaptive Capacity, decreased intracranial
Airway Clearance, ineffective
Allergy Response, risk for
Anxiety [specify level]
Aspiration, risk for
Attachment, risk for impaired
Autonomic Dysreflexia
Autonomic Dysreflexia, risk for

Behavior, disorganized infant
Behavior, readiness for enhanced organized infant
Behavior, risk for disorganized infant
Bleeding, risk for
Blood Glucose Level, risk for unstable
Body Image, disturbed
Body Temperature, risk for imbalanced
Breast Milk, insufficient
Breastfeeding, ineffective
Breastfeeding, interrupted
Breastfeeding, readiness for enhanced
Breathing Pattern, ineffective

Cardiac Output, decreased
+Cardiac Output, decreased risk for
+Cardiovascular Function, risk for impaired
Childbearing Process, ineffective
Childbearing Process, readiness for enhanced
Childbearing Process, risk for ineffective
Comfort, impaired
Comfort, readiness for enhanced
Communication, impaired verbal
Communication, readiness for enhanced
Confusion, acute
Confusion, chronic
Confusion, risk for acute
Constipation
+Constipation, chronic functional

Constipation, perceived
Constipation, risk for
+Constipation, risk for chronic functional
Contamination
Contamination, risk for
Coping, compromised family
Coping, defensive
Coping, disabled family
Coping, ineffective
Coping, ineffective community
Coping, readiness for enhanced
Coping, readiness for enhanced community
Coping, readiness for enhanced family

Death Anxiety
Decision-Making, readiness for enhanced
Decisional Conflict
Denial, ineffective
Dentition, impaired
Development, risk for delayed
Diarrhea
Disuse Syndrome, risk for
Diversional Activity, deficient
Dry Eye, risk for
*Dysfunction, risk for peripheral neurovascular

Electrolyte Imbalance, risk for
*Elimination, impaired urinary
*Elimination, readiness for enhanced urinary
+Emancipated Decision-Making, impaired
+Emancipated Decision-Making, readiness for enhanced
+Emancipated Decision-Making, risk for impaired
+Emotional Control, labile

Falls, risk for
Family Processes, dysfunctional
Family Processes, interrupted
Family Processes, readiness for enhanced
Fatigue
Fear [specify focus]
Feeding Pattern, ineffective infant
Fluid Balance, readiness for enhanced
[Fluid Volume, deficient hyper-/hypotonic]
Fluid Volume, deficient [isotonic]
Fluid Volume, excess
Fluid Volume, risk for deficient
Fluid Volume, risk for imbalanced
+Frail Elderly Syndrome
+Frail Elderly Syndrome, risk for

Gas Exchange, impaired
Gastrointestinal Motility, dysfunctional
Gastrointestinal Motility, risk for dysfunctional
Gastrointestinal Perfusion, risk for ineffective
Grieving
Grieving, complicated
Grieving, risk for complicated
Growth, risk for disproportionate

Health, deficient community
Health Behavior, risk-prone
Health Maintenance, ineffective
*Health Management, ineffective
*Health Management, ineffective family
*Health Management, readiness for enhanced
Home Maintenance, impaired
Hope, readiness for enhanced
Hopelessness
Human Dignity, risk for compromised
Hyperthermia
Hypothermia
+Hypothermia, risk for
+Hypothermia, risk for perioperative

Impulse Control, ineffective
Incontinence, bowel
Incontinence, functional urinary
Incontinence, overflow urinary
Incontinence, reflex urinary
Incontinence, risk for urge urinary
Incontinence, stress urinary
Incontinence, urge urinary
Infection, risk for
Injury, risk for
+Injury, risk for corneal
+Injury, risk for urinary tract
Insomnia

Jaundice, neonatal
Jaundice, risk for neonatal

Knowledge, deficient [Learning Need (specify)]
Knowledge [specify], readiness for enhanced

Latex Allergy Response
Latex Allergy Response, risk for
Lifestyle, sedentary
Liver Function, risk for impaired
Loneliness, risk for

Maternal-Fetal Dyad, risk for disturbed
Memory, impaired
Mobility, impaired bed
Mobility, impaired physical
Mobility, impaired wheelchair
+Mood Regulation, impaired
Moral Distress
*Mucous Membrane, impaired oral
*Mucous Membrane, risk for impaired oral

Nausea
Noncompliance [ineffective Adherence] [specify]
Nutrition: less than body requirements, imbalanced
Nutrition, readiness for enhanced

+Obesity
+Overweight
+Overweight, risk for

Pain, acute
Pain, chronic
+Pain, labor
+Pain Syndrome, chronic
Parenting, impaired
Parenting, readiness for enhanced
Parenting, risk for impaired
Personal Identity, disturbed
Personal Identity, risk for disturbed
Poisoning, risk for
*Positioning Injury, risk for perioperative
Post-Trauma Syndrome [specify stage]
Post-Trauma Syndrome, risk for
Power, readiness for enhanced
Powerlessness [specify level]
Powerlessness, risk for
+Pressure Ulcer, risk for
Protection, ineffective

Rape-Trauma Syndrome
*Reaction to Iodinated Contrast Media, risk for adverse
Relationship, ineffective
Relationship, readiness for enhanced
Relationship, risk for ineffective
Religiosity, impaired
Religiosity, readiness for enhanced
Religiosity, risk for impaired
Relocation Stress Syndrome
Relocation Stress Syndrome, risk for
Renal Perfusion, risk for ineffective

Resilience, impaired
Resilience, readiness for enhanced
Resilience, risk for impaired
Role Conflict, parental
Role Performance, ineffective
*Role Strain, caregiver
*Role Strain, risk for caregiver

Self-Care, readiness for enhanced
Self-Care Deficit, bathing
Self-Care Deficit, dressing
Self-Care Deficit, feeding
Self-Care Deficit, toileting
Self-Concept, readiness for enhanced
Self-Esteem, chronic low
Self-Esteem, risk for chronic low
Self-Esteem, risk for situational low
Self-Esteem, situational low
Self-Mutilation
Self-Mutilation, risk for
Self-Neglect
[Sensory Perception, disturbed (specify: visual, auditory, kinesthetic, gustatory, tactile, olfactory)] (retired 2012)
Sexual Dysfunction
Sexuality Pattern, ineffective
Shock, risk for
+Sitting, impaired
Skin Integrity, impaired
Skin Integrity, risk for impaired
Sleep, readiness for enhanced
Sleep Deprivation
Sleep Pattern, disturbed
Social Interaction, impaired
Social Isolation
Sorrow, chronic
Spiritual Distress
Spiritual Distress, risk for
Spiritual Well-Being, readiness for enhanced
+Standing, impaired
Stress Overload
Sudden Infant Death Syndrome, risk for
Suffocation, risk for
Suicide, risk for
Surgical Recovery, delayed
+Surgical Recovery, risk for delayed
Swallowing, impaired

Thermal Injury, risk for
Thermoregulation, ineffective

Tissue Integrity, impaired
+Tissue Integrity, risk for impaired
Tissue Perfusion, ineffective peripheral
Tissue Perfusion, risk for decreased cardiac
Tissue Perfusion, risk for ineffective cerebral
Tissue Perfusion, risk for ineffective peripheral
Transfer Ability, impaired
Trauma, risk for
+Trauma, risk for vascular

Unilateral Neglect
Urinary Retention [acute/chronic]

Vascular Trauma, risk for
Ventilation, impaired spontaneous
Ventilatory Weaning Response, dysfunctional
Violence, risk for other-directed
Violence, risk for self-directed

Walking, impaired
Wandering [specify sporadic or continuous]

+New ND
*Change in alphabetical order reflecting NANDA-I's foci for the specific nursing diagnosis
Used with permission from Herdman, T.H. (2015). NANDA International: Definitions and Classification, 2015–2017. Oxford, UK: Wiley-Blackwell.
Information in brackets added by authors to clarify and enhance the use of the NDs.

CHAPTER 1

The Nursing Process and Planning Client Care

The Nursing Process

Nursing is both a science and an art concerned with the physical, psychological, sociological, cultural, and spiritual concerns of the individual receiving care. The science of nursing is based on a broad theoretical framework; its art depends on the caring skills and abilities of the individual nurse.

The nursing profession continues work to formally define what nurses do and what makes nursing unique, leading to a body of professional knowledge distinctive to nursing practice. A significant portion of defining the work of nursing has involved the establishment of a commonality of terminology or standardization of nursing language. Although several standardized nursing languages have been developed, the nursing diagnoses most commonly used today are the NANDA-I nursing diagnoses (see inside cover).

In 1980, the American Nurses Association (ANA) defined nursing as "the diagnosis and treatment of human responses to actual or potential health problems." As the nursing profession has evolved, the definition of nursing has been expanded to reflect that growth—"nursing is the protection, promotion, and optimization of health and abilities, prevention of illness and injury, alleviation of suffering through the diagnosis and treatment of human responses, and advocacy in the care of individuals, families, communities, and populations" (Nursing's Social Policy Statement, ANA, 2003, p. 6).

Nursing process is patterned after the scientific method of observing, measuring, gathering data, and analyzing findings. This process incorporates an interactive and interpersonal approach with a problem-solving and decision-making process (Peplau, 1952; King, 1971; Yura & Walsh, 1988). Shore (1988) described the nursing process as "combining the most desirable elements of the art of nursing with the most relevant elements of systems theory, using the scientific method." It can be applied in any healthcare or educational setting, in any theoretical or conceptual framework, and within the context of any nursing theory. Therefore, because nursing process is the basis of all nursing action, we believe that it is the essence of nursing.

The five steps of the nursing process are (1) assessment—systematically gathering data, sorting and organizing the collected data, and documenting the data in a retrievable format; (2) diagnosis—analyzing collected data to identify the client's needs or problems; (3) planning—setting priorities, establishing goals, identifying desired client outcomes, and determining specific nursing interventions; (4) implementation—putting the plan of care into action and performing the planned interventions; (5) evaluation—determining the client's progress toward attaining the identified outcomes and monitoring the client's response to and effectiveness of the selected nursing interventions.

Planning Care

The identification of client needs is the cornerstone for the plan of care. We support that healthcare providers have a responsibility for planning care along with the client with the goal toward the eventual outcome of an optimal state of wellness or a dignified death. Client-centered care engages the client in responsibility for his or her own care while helping to ensure that nursing interventions are timely and appropriate.

Creating a plan of care begins with the collection of data (assessment). The database consists of subjective and objective client information. Analysis of the collected data leads to the identification (diagnosis) of problems or areas of concern (including health promotion) specific to the client. These problems or needs are expressed as nursing diagnoses (NDs). To facilitate the diagnosis process, the authors have divided the NDs into Diagnostic Divisions (Appendix 1), and a sample assessment tool is also provided, designed to assist the nurse to identify appropriate NDs as the data are collected.

When the needs are identified, nursing diagnoses are categorized as (1) actual or *problem*-focused NDs; (2) potential or *risk for* NDs could develop due to specific vulnerabilities of the client; and (3) *health promotion* NDs reflect a client's desire to improve his or her well-being.

Setting goals and choosing appropriate nursing interventions are also essential to the construction of a plan of care and the delivery of quality nursing care. Desired outcomes are the incremental steps formulated to give direction to and evaluate effectiveness of the care provided in achieving broader goals. Interventions are those activities that the nurse, client, and/or significant others perform to promote the client's movement toward achieving the desired outcomes.

An individualized client diagnostic statement can be formulated using the problem, etiology, and signs and symptoms (PES) format by combining the ND label (problem) with the individual's specific related or risk factors (etiology) and defining characteristics (signs/symptoms) as appropriate. The resulting client diagnostic statement accurately represents the client's current situation providing direction for nursing care.

Once the plan of care is put into action, changes in client needs must be continually monitored because care is provided in a dynamic environment and flexibility is required to allow changing circumstances. Periodic review of the client's responses to nursing interventions and progress toward attaining desired outcomes helps determine effectiveness of the plan of care. Based on findings, the plan may need to be modified, referrals to other resources may be required, or the client may be ready for discharge from the care setting.

Properly written and applied plans of care can save time by providing direction for continuity of care and by facilitating communication among nurses and other caregivers. The format for recording the plan of care is determined by agency policy and may be handwritten or computer-generated and may utilize standardized forms as with clinical pathways.

Ongoing changes in healthcare delivery and computerization of client records require a commonality of communication across clinical settings. By way of example, whereas a medical diagnosis of diabetes mellitus is the same label used for all individuals with this condition, the nursing diagnostic statement is individualized to reflect a specific client need or response. We use the NANDA-I nursing diagnoses labels to define the client's responses to diabetes. For example, the diagnostic statement may read, "risk for unstable Blood Glucose Level as evidenced by risk factors inadequate blood glucose monitoring, ineffective medication management."

The plan of care is not only the end product of the nursing process, but it also documents client care in areas of accountability, quality assurance, and liability. It not only guides the nurse actively caring for the client (determining client's needs [NDs], goals/outcomes, and actions to be taken), but also substantiates the care provided for review by third-party payers, legal entities, and accreditation agencies. Therefore, the plan of care is a critical and permanent part of the client's healthcare record.

In Appendix 2, a sample scenario provides an opportunity to review a client assessment and the plan of care and Mind Map created based on the data collected.

CHAPTER 2

Nursing Diagnoses in Alphabetical Order

ACTIVITY INTOLERANCE and risk for ACTIVITY INTOLERANCE

[Diagnostic Division: Activity/Rest]

Definition: Activity Intolerance: Insufficient physiological or psychological energy to endure or complete required or desired daily activities.

Definition: risk for Activity Intolerance: Vulnerable to experiencing insufficient physiological or psychological energy to endure or complete required or desired daily activities, which may compromise health.

Related Factors (Activity Intolerance)—

Generalized weakness
Sedentary lifestyle
Bedrest/immobility
Imbalance between oxygen supply and demand

Risk Factors (risk for Activity Intolerance)

History of previous activity intolerance
Circulatory problem or respiratory condition; [dysrhythmias]
Physical deconditioning; [aging]
Inexperience with an activity

NOTE: A risk diagnosis is not evidenced by signs and symptoms as the problem has not yet occurred; rather, nursing interventions are directed at prevention.

Information that appears in brackets has been added by the authors to clarify and enhance the use of nursing diagnoses.

Defining Characteristics (Activity Intolerance)

Subjective

Fatigue, generalized weakness
Exertional discomfort; dyspnea

Objective

Abnormal heart rate or blood pressure response to activity
ECG change (e.g., arrhythmia, conduction abnormality, ischemia)

Functional Level Classification (Gordon, 2010):

Level I: Walk, regular pace, on level indefinitely; climb one flight or more but more short of breath than normal
Level II: Walk one city block [or] 500 ft on level; climb one flight slowly without stopping
Level III: Walk no more than 50 ft on level without stopping; unable to climb one flight of stairs without stopping
Level IV: Dyspnea and fatigue at rest

Desired Outcomes/Evaluation Criteria—Client Will (Activity Intolerance):

- Identify negative factors affecting activity tolerance and eliminate or reduce their effects when possible.
- Use identified techniques to enhance activity tolerance.
- Participate willingly in necessary/desired activities.
- Report measurable increase in activity tolerance.
- Demonstrate a decrease in physiological signs of intolerance (e.g., pulse, respirations, and blood pressure remain within client's normal range).

Desired Outcomes/Evaluation Criteria—Client Will (risk for Activity Intolerance):

- Verbalize understanding of potential loss of ability in relation to existing condition.
- Participate in conditioning/rehabilitation program to enhance ability to perform.
- Identify alternative ways to maintain desired activity level (e.g., walking in a shopping mall if weather is bad).
- Identify conditions or symptoms that require medical reevaluation.

Information that appears in brackets has been added by the authors to clarify and enhance the use of nursing diagnoses.

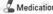

Actions/Interventions

Nursing Priority No. 1.

To identify causative/precipitating **or risk** factors:

- Note presence of acute or chronic illness, such as heart failure, pulmonary disorders, hypothyroidism, diabetes mellitus, AIDS, anemias, cancers, pregnancy-induced hypertension, and acute and chronic pain. **Many factors can cause or contribute to fatigue, having potential to interfere with client's ability to perform at a desired level of activity. However, the term "activity intolerance" implies that the client cannot endure or adapt to increased energy or oxygen demands caused by an activity.** (Refer to ND Fatigue.)
- Ask client/significant other (SO) about usual level of energy **to identify potential problems and/or client's/SO's perception of client's energy and ability to perform needed or desired activities.**
- Evaluate the client's actual and perceived limitations and severity of deficit in light of usual status. **This provides a comparative baseline and information about needed education or interventions regarding quality of life.**
- Identify factors, such as age, functional decline, client resistive to efforts, painful conditions, breathing problems, vision or hearing impairments, climate or weather, unsafe areas to exercise, and need for mobility assistance **that could block/affect the desired level of activity.**
- Note client reports of weakness, fatigue, pain, difficulty accomplishing tasks, and/or insomnia. **Symptoms may be a result of or contribute to intolerance of activity.**
- Assess cardiopulmonary response to physical activity, including vital signs, before, during, and after activity. Note accelerating fatigue. **Dramatic changes in heart rate and rhythm, changes in usual blood pressure, and progressively worsening fatigue result from an imbalance of oxygen supply and demand.**
- Ascertain the client's ability to stand and move about and the degree of assistance necessary or use of equipment **to determine current status and needs associated with participation in needed/desired activities.**
- Identify activity needs versus desires **to evaluate appropriateness (e.g., is barely able to walk upstairs but would like to play tennis).**
- Assess emotional and psychological factors affecting the current situation **(e.g., stress and/or depression may be increas-**

Information that appears in brackets has been added by the authors to clarify and enhance the use of nursing diagnoses.

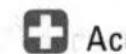  Acute Care 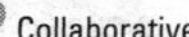  Collaborative 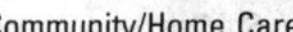 Community/Home Care 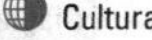 Cultural

ing the effects of an illness, or depression might be the result of forced inactivity).

- Note treatment-related factors, such as side effects and interactions of medications, **which can affect the nature and degree of activity intolerance.**
- Determine the client's current activity level and physical condition with observation, exercise-capacity testing, or use of a functional-level classification system (e.g., Gordon's), as appropriate. **This provides a baseline for comparison and an opportunity to track changes.**

Nursing Priority No. 2.

To assist client to deal with contributing factors and manage activities within individual limits (Activity Intolerance):

- Monitor vital and cognitive signs, watching for changes in blood pressure, heart, and respiratory rates; note skin pallor and/or cyanosis and presence of confusion.
- Reduce intensity level or discontinue activities that cause undesired physiological changes **to prevent overexertion.**
- Provide and monitor response to supplemental oxygen, medications, and changes in treatment regimen.
- Increase exercise/activity levels gradually; teach methods **to conserve energy,** such as stopping to rest for 3 min during a 10-min walk or sitting down to brush hair instead of standing.
- Plan care to carefully balance rest periods with activities **to reduce fatigue.**
- Provide positive atmosphere while acknowledging the difficulty of the situation for the client. **This helps to minimize frustration and rechannel energy.**
- Encourage expression of feelings contributing to or resulting from the condition.
- Involve client/SO(s) in planning activities as much as possible.
- Assist with activities and provide/monitor client's use of assistive devices (e.g., crutches, walker, wheelchair, or oxygen tank) **to protect client from injury.**
- Promote comfort measures and provide for relief of pain **to enhance ability to participate in activities.** (Refer to NDs acute Pain; chronic Pain.)
- Provide referral to other disciplines, such as exercise physiologist, psychological counseling/therapy, occupational/physical therapists, and recreation/leisure specialists, as indicated, **to develop individually appropriate therapeutic regimens.**

Information that appears in brackets has been added by the authors to clarify and enhance the use of nursing diagnoses.

Nursing Priority No. 3.

To develop alternative ways to remain active within the limits of the disabling condition/situation (risk for Activity Intolerance):

- Implement a physical therapy/exercise program in conjunction with the client and other team members (e.g., physical and/or occupational therapist, exercise/rehabilitation physiologist). **A collaborative program with short-term achievable goals enhances the likelihood of success and may motivate the client to adopt a lifestyle of physical exercise for the enhancement of health.**
- Promote and implement a conditioning program. Support inclusion in exercise and activity groups **to prevent/limit deterioration.**
- Instruct client in proper performance of unfamiliar activities and in alternate ways of doing familiar activities **to conserve energy and promote safety.**

Nursing Priority No. 4.

To promote wellness (Teaching/Discharge Considerations):

- Discuss with client/SO(s) the relationship between illness or debilitating condition and the ability to perform desired activities. **Understanding this relationship can help with acceptance of limitations or reveal opportunity for changes of practical value.**
- Assist client/SO(s) with planning for changes that may become necessary, such as use of supplemental oxygen **to improve the client's ability to participate in desired activities.**
- Plan for maximal activity within the client's ability. **This promotes the idea of normalcy of progressive abilities in this area.**
- Review expectations of client/SO(s)/providers **to establish individual goals.** Explore conflicts and differences **to reach agreement for the most effective plan.**
- Instruct client/SO(s) in monitoring response to activity and in recognizing signs/symptoms that **indicate need to alter activity level.**
- Plan for progressive increase of activity level/participation in exercise training, as tolerated by client. **Both activity tolerance and health status may improve with progressive training.**
- Give client information that provides evidence of daily/weekly progress **to sustain motivation.**
- Assist client in learning and demonstrating appropriate safety measures **to prevent injuries.**

Information that appears in brackets has been added by the authors to clarify and enhance the use of nursing diagnoses.

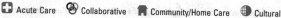

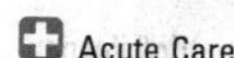

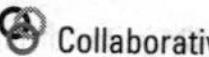

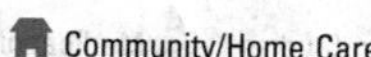

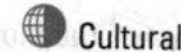

- Identify and discuss symptoms for which the client needs to seek medical assistance/evaluation, **providing for timely intervention.**
- Provide information about the effect of lifestyle on activity tolerance (e.g., nutrition, adequate fluid intake, getting sufficient rest and sleep, exercise, smoking cessation, and mental health status). **Many of these factors may be amenable to modification, thus reducing risk factors and promoting health.**
- Encourage client to maintain a positive attitude; suggest use of relaxation techniques, such as visualization or guided imagery, as appropriate, **to enhance sense of well-being.**
- Encourage participation in recreation, social activities, and hobbies appropriate for situation. (Refer to ND deficient Diversional Activity.)
- Refer to appropriate resources for assistance and/or equipment, as needed, **to sustain activity level.**

Documentation Focus

Assessment/Reassessment

- Level of activity as noted in Functional Level Classification
- Causative, precipitating; or risk factors
- Client reports of difficulty or change
- Vital signs before, during, and following activity

Planning

- Plan of care and who is involved in planning
- Treatment options, including physical therapy or exercise program, other assistive therapies and devices
- Lifestyle changes that are planned, who is to be responsible for each action, and monitoring methods

Implementation/Evaluation

- Response to interventions, teaching, and actions performed
- Implemented changes to plan of care based on assessment/reassessment findings
- Teaching plan and understanding of material presented
- Attainment or progress toward desired outcome(s)

Discharge Planning

- Referrals to other resources
- Long-term needs and who is responsible for actions

Information that appears in brackets has been added by the authors to clarify and enhance the use of nursing diagnoses.

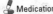

Sample Nursing Outcomes & Interventions Classifications (NOC/NIC)

NOC—Activity Tolerance
NIC—Energy Management

ineffective ACTIVITY PLANNING and risk for ineffective ACTIVITY PLANNING

[Diagnostic Division: Activity/Rest]

Definition: ineffective Activity Planning: Inability to prepare for a set of actions fixed in time and under certain conditions.

Definition: risk for ineffective Activity Planning: Vulnerable to an inability to prepare for a set of actions fixed in time and under certain conditions, which may compromise health.

Related and Risk Factors

Flight behavior when faced with proposed solution
Hedonism [motivated by pleasure and/or pain]
Insufficient social support
Insufficient information-processing ability
Unrealistic perception of event or personal abilities

Defining Characteristics (ineffective Activity Planning)

Subjective
Fear, worry, or excessive anxiety about a task to be undertaken

Objective
Absence of plan; insufficient resources (e.g., financial, social, knowledge)
Insufficient organizational skills
Pattern of failure, procrastination
Unmet goals for chosen activity

NOTE: A risk diagnosis is not evidenced by signs and symptoms, as the problem has not occurred; rather nursing interventions are directed at prevention.

Information that appears in brackets has been added by the authors to clarify and enhance the use of nursing diagnoses.

Desired Outcomes/Evaluation Criteria—Client Will: (Including Specific Time Frame)

- Acknowledge difficulty with follow-through of activity plan.
- Express awareness of negative factors or actions that are interfering, or could interfere, with planning.
- Establish mindfulness and relaxation activities to lessen anxiety.
- Develop a plan, including the time frame, for a task to be completed.
- Report lessened anxiety and fear toward planning.
- Be aware of and make plan to deal with procrastination.

Actions/Interventions

Nursing Priority No. 1.

To identify causative/precipitating **or risk** factors:

- Determine circumstances of client's situation that may impact participating in selective activities.
- Determine individual problems with planning and follow-through with activity plan. **Identifies individual difficulties (e.g., anxiety regarding what kind of activity to choose, lack of resources, lack of confidence in own ability).**
- Review the client's health history. **Underlying physical problems such as fatigue or medication side effects can affect the ability to engage in tasks.**
- Perform a complete physical examination. **The client may have underlying problems such as allergies, hypertension, or asthma that are contributing to fatigue and difficulty with undertaking a task.**
- Review medication regimen **for possible side effects affecting client's desire to become involved in any activity.**
- Note the client's ability to process information. **Compromised mental ability, low self-esteem, and anxiety can interfere with dealing with planning activities.**
- Assess mental status; use Beck's Depression Inventory as indicated.
- Identify client's personal values and perception of self including strengths and weaknesses.
- Determine client's need to be in control, fear of dependency on others (although may need assistance from others), or belief he or she cannot do the task. **This is indicative of external locus of control, where the client sees others as having the control and ability.**

Information that appears in brackets has been added by the authors to clarify and enhance the use of nursing diagnoses.

- Identify culture/religious issues **that may affect how individuals deal with issues of life or how they see their ability to make choices or manage their own life.**
- Discuss awareness of procrastination, need for perfection, and fear of failure. **Although the client may not acknowledge it as a problem, this may be a factor in his or her difficulty in planning for, choosing, and following through with activities that might be enjoyed.**
- Assess the client's ability to process information. **This may interfere with perception of the world and self.**
- Discuss the possibility that the client is motivated by pleasure to avoid pain (hedonism). **The individual may seek activities that bring pleasure to avoid painful experiences.**
- Note availability and use of resources.

Nursing Priority No. 2.

To assist client to recognize and deal with individual factors that do **or could** interfere with activities, and begin to plan appropriate activities:

- Encourage the expression of feelings contributing to/resulting from a situation. **Awareness of frustration and/or anxiety can help the client redirect energy into productive activities.** Maintain a positive atmosphere without seeming overly cheerful.
- Discuss the client's perception of self as worthless and not deserving of success and happiness. **This belief is common among individuals who struggle with feelings of low self-esteem and self-confidence. Sometimes the underlying feelings are those of wanting to be perfect, and it is difficult to finish the task because of the fear that it will not be perfect (perfectionism). They believe that anything they do is bound to fail, and feelings of anxiety and worry contribute to failure.**
- Help the client learn how to reframe negative thoughts about self into a positive view of what is happening.
- Encourage the client to recognize procrastinating behaviors and make a decision to change. **Procrastination is a learned behavior and serves many purposes for the individual.**
- Confront (in a gentle manner) the client's ambivalent, angry, or depressed feelings.
- Develop a plan with the client to deal with activities in small steps. **Learning to do this will help client to feel more organized and successful in completing the desired task.**

Information that appears in brackets has been added by the authors to clarify and enhance the use of nursing diagnoses.

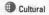

- Involve the client/SOs in planning an activity. **Having the support of family and the nurse will help promote success.**
- Direct the client to break down the desired activity into specific steps. **This makes the activity more manageable, and as each step is accomplished, the client feels more confident about his or her ability to finish the task.**
- Accompany the client to an activity of his or her own choosing, encouraging participation together if appropriate. **Support from the caregiver may enable the client to begin participating and gain confidence.**
- Assist the client in developing skills of relaxation, imagery/visualization, and mindfulness. **Using these techniques can help the client learn to overcome stress and be able to manage life's difficulties more effectively.**
- Assist the client to investigate the idea that seeking pleasure (hedonism) is interfering with the motivation to accomplish goals. **Some philosophers believe that pleasure is the only good for a person and that the individual does not see other aspects of life, which interferes with accomplishments.**

Nursing Priority No. 3.

To promote wellness (Teaching/Discharge Criteria):

- Assist the client in identifying life goals and priorities. **If the individual has never thought about setting goals, he/she may begin to think about the possibility of being successful.**
- Review treatment goals and expectations of client/SOs. **This helps clarify what has been discussed and decisions that have been made; it also provides an opportunity to change goals as needed.**
- Discuss progress in learning to relax and deal productively with anxieties and fears. **As the client sees that progress is being made, feelings of worthwhileness will be enhanced, and the individual will be encouraged to continue working toward goals.**
- Identify community resources such as social services, senior centers, or classes **to provide support and options for activities and change.**
- Refer for cognitive therapy as indicated. **This structured therapy can help the individual identify, evaluate, and modify any underlying assumptions and dysfunctional beliefs and begin the process of change. Learning to set one's**

Information that appears in brackets has been added by the authors to clarify and enhance the use of nursing diagnoses.

own schedule with reminders can also help a client to get tasks done in a timely manner.

Documentation Focus

Assessment/Reassessment
- Specific problems exhibited by client with causative or precipitating factors
- Individual risk factors identified
- Client concerns or difficulty making and following through with plans

Planning
- Plan of care and who is involved in planning
- Teaching plan

Implementation/Evaluation
- Response to interventions, teaching, and actions performed
- Attainment or progress toward desired outcome(s)

Discharge Planning
- Referrals to other resources
- Long-term needs and who is responsible for actions

Sample Nursing Outcomes & Interventions Classifications (NOC/NIC)

NOC—Motivation
NIC—Self-Awareness Enhancement
NIC—Self-Modification Assistance

decreased intracranial ADAPTIVE CAPACITY

[Diagnostic Division: Circulation]

Definition: Intracranial fluid dynamic mechanisms that normally compensate for increases in intracranial volume are compromised, resulting in repeated disproportionate increases in intracranial pressure (ICP) in response to a variety of noxious and non-noxious stimuli.

Related Factors

Brain injuries (e.g., cerebrovascular impairment, neurological illness, trauma, tumor)

Information that appears in brackets has been added by the authors to clarify and enhance the use of nursing diagnoses.

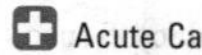

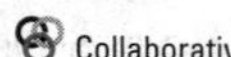

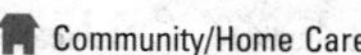

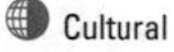

Sustained increase in intracranial pressure (ICP) of 10–15 mmHg
Decreased cerebral perfusion pressure ≥50–60 mmHg
Systemic hypotension with intracranial hypertension

Defining Characteristics

Objective

Repeated increase of ICP of ≥10 mm Hg for ≥5 minutes following external stimuli
Disproportionate increase in ICP following stimulus
Elevated P_2 ICP waveform
Volume-pressure response test variation (volume: pressure ratio of 2, pressure-volume index of less than 10)
Baseline ICP ≥10 mm Hg
Wide-amplitude ICP waveform

Desired Outcomes/Evaluation Criteria—Client Will:

- Demonstrate stable ICP as evidenced by normalization of pressure waveforms and appropriate response to stimuli.
- Display improved neurological signs.

Actions/Interventions

Nursing Priority No. 1.

To assess causative/contributing factors:

- Determine factors related to individual situation (e.g., cause of loss of consciousness or coma [such as fall, motor vehicle crash, gunshot wound], infection such as meningitis, or encephalitis, brain tumor) and potential for increased ICP.
- Monitor and document changes in ICP; monitor waveform and corresponding event (e.g., suctioning, position change, monitor alarms, family visit). **ICP monitoring may be done in a critically ill client with a Glasgow Coma Scale (GCS) score of 8 or less. The ICP offers data that supplement the neurological examination and can be crucial in client whose examination findings are affected by sedatives, paralytics, or other factors. Elevated pressure can be caused by the injury, environmental stimuli, or treatment modalities.**

Information that appears in brackets has been added by the authors to clarify and enhance the use of nursing diagnoses.

Nursing Priority No. 2.

To note degree of impairment:

- Assess and document client's eye opening, position, and movement; size, shape, equality, light reactivity of pupils; and consciousness and mental status via GCS **to determine client's baseline neurological status and monitor changes over time.**
- Note purposeful and nonpurposeful motor response (posturing, etc.), comparing right and left sides. **Posturing and abnormal flexion of extremities usually indicates diffuse cortical damage. Absence of spontaneous movement on one side indicates damage to the motor tracts in the opposite cerebral hemisphere.**
- Test for the presence of reflexes (e.g., blink, cough, gag, Babinski's reflex), nuchal rigidity. **Helps identify location of injury (e.g., loss of blink reflex suggests damage to the pons and medulla, absence of cough and gag reflexes reflects damage to medulla).**
- Monitor vital signs and cardiac rhythm before, during, after activity. **Helps determine parameters for "safe" activity. Mean arterial blood pressure should be maintained above 90 mm Hg to maintain cerebral perfusion pressure (CPP) greater than 70 mm Hg, which reflects adequate blood supply to the brain. Fever in brain injury can be associated with injury to the hypothalamus or bleeding, systemic infection (e.g., pneumonia), or drugs. Hyperthermia exacerbates cerebral ischemia. Irregular respiration patterns can suggest location of cerebral insult. Cardiac dysrhythmias can be due to brainstem injury and stimulation of the sympathetic nervous system. Bradycardia may occur with high ICP.**
- Review results of diagnostic imaging (e.g., computed tomography [CT] scans) **to note location, type, and severity of tissue injury.**

Nursing Priority No. 3.

To minimize/correct causative factors/maximize perfusion:

- Elevate head of bed, as individually appropriate. **Studies show that in most cases, 30 degrees elevation significantly decreases ICP while maintaining cerebral blood flow.**
- Maintain head and neck in neutral position, support with small towel rolls or pillows **to maximize venous return.** Avoid placing head on large pillow or causing hip flexion of 90 degrees or more.

Information that appears in brackets has been added by the authors to clarify and enhance the use of nursing diagnoses.

- Decrease extraneous stimuli and provide comfort measures (e.g., quiet environment, soft voice, tapes of familiar voices played through earphones, back massage, gentle touch as tolerated) **to reduce central nervous system stimulation and promote relaxation.**
- Limit painful procedures (e.g., venipunctures, redundant neurological evaluations) to those that are absolutely necessary.
- Provide rest periods between care activities and limit duration of procedures. Lower lighting and noise level, schedule and limit activities **to provide restful environment, reduce agitation, and limit spikes in ICP associated with noxious stimuli.**
- Limit or prevent activities that increase intrathoracic or abdominal pressures (e.g., coughing, vomiting, straining at stool). Avoid or limit use of restraints. **These factors markedly increase ICP.**
- Suction with caution—only when needed—to just beyond end of endotracheal tube without touching tracheal wall or carina. Administer lidocaine intratracheally per protocol **to reduce cough reflex,** and hyperoxygenate before suctioning, as appropriate, **to minimize hypoxia.**
- Maintain patency of urinary drainage system **to reduce risk of hypertension, increased ICP, and associated dysreflexia when a spinal cord injury is also present and spinal cord shock is past.** (Refer to ND Autonomic Dysreflexia.)
- Weigh, as indicated. Calculate fluid balance every shift or daily **to determine fluid needs, maintain hydration, and prevent fluid overload.**
- Administer or restrict fluid intake, as necessary. Administer IV fluids via pump or control device **to maintain circulating volume and cerebral perfusion pressure or to prevent inadvertent fluid bolus or vascular overload with potential cerebral edema and increased ICP.**
- Regulate environmental temperature; use cooling blanket as indicated **to decrease metabolic and O_2 needs when fever present or therapeutic hypothermia therapy is used.**
- Investigate increased restlessness **to determine causative factors and initiate corrective measures as early as possible.**
- Provide appropriate safety measures and initiate treatment for seizures **to prevent injury and increased ICP or hypoxia.**
- Administer supplemental oxygen, as indicated, **to prevent cerebral ischemia;** hyperventilate (as indicated per protocol) when on mechanical ventilation. **Therapeutic hyperventilation may be used ($PaCO_2$ of 30 to 35 mm) to reduce**

Information that appears in brackets has been added by the authors to clarify and enhance the use of nursing diagnoses.

intracranial hypertension for a short period of time, while other methods of ICP control are initiated.

- Administer medications (e.g., antihypertensives, diuretics, analgesics, sedatives, antipyretics, vasopressors, antiseizure drugs, neuromuscular blocking agents, and corticosteroids), as appropriate, **to maintain cerebral homeostasis and manage symptoms associated with neurological injury.**
- Administer enteral or parenteral nutrition **to achieve positive nitrogen balance, reducing effects of post–brain injury metabolic and catabolic states, which can lead to complications.**
- Prepare client for surgery, as indicated (e.g., evacuation of hematoma or space-occupying lesion), **to reduce ICP and enhance circulation.**

Nursing Priority No. 4.

To promote wellness (Teaching/Discharge Considerations):

- Discuss with caregivers specific situations (e.g., if client is choking or experiencing pain, needing to be repositioned, constipated, has blocked urinary flow) and review appropriate interventions **to prevent or limit episodic increases in ICP.**
- Identify signs/symptoms suggesting increased ICP (in client at risk without an ICP monitor), such as restlessness, deterioration in neurological responses.
- Review appropriate interventions.

Documentation Focus

Assessment/Reassessment

- Neurological findings noting right and left sides separately (such as pupils, motor response, reflexes, restlessness, nuchal rigidity); GCS
- Response to activities and events (e.g., changes in pressure waveforms or vital signs)
- Presence and characteristics of seizure activity

Planning

- Plan of care and who is involved in planning
- Teaching plan

Implementation/Evaluation

- Response to interventions and actions performed
- Attainment or progress toward desired outcome(s)
- Modifications to plan of care

Information that appears in brackets has been added by the authors to clarify and enhance the use of nursing diagnoses.

Discharge Planning

- Future needs, plan for meeting them, and determining who is responsible for actions
- Referrals as identified

Sample Nursing Outcomes & Interventions Classifications (NOC/NIC)

NOC—Tissue Perfusion: Cerebral
NIC—Cerebral Edema Management

ineffective AIRWAY CLEARANCE

[Diagnostic Division: Respiration]

Definition: Inability to clear secretions or obstructions from the respiratory tract to maintain a clear airway.

Related Factors

Environmental

Smoking; exposure to smoke; secondhand smoke

Obstructed Airway

Airway spasm
Chronic obstructive pulmonary disease [COPD]; hyperplasia of the bronchial walls
Excessive mucous; exudate in the alveoli; retained secretions
Foreign body in airway; presence of artificial airway

Physiological

Allergic airway; asthma
Infection
Neuromuscular impairment

Defining Characteristics

Subjective

Dyspnea

Objective

Absence of cough; ineffective cough
Diminished breath sounds; adventitious breath sounds [rales, crackles, rhonchi, or wheezes]

Information that appears in brackets has been added by the authors to clarify and enhance the use of nursing diagnoses.

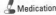

Excessive sputum
Alteration in respiratory rate or pattern
Difficulty verbalizing
Wide-eyed look; restlessness
Orthopnea
Cyanosis

Desired Outcomes/Evaluation Criteria—Client Will:

- Maintain airway patency.
- Expectorate/clear secretions readily.
- Demonstrate absence/reduction of congestion with breath sounding clear, noiseless respirations, and improved oxygen exchange (e.g., absence of cyanosis and arterial blood gas [ABG]/pulse oximetry results within client norms).
- Verbalize understanding of cause(s) and therapeutic management regimen.
- Demonstrate behaviors to improve or maintain clear airway.
- Identify potential complications and how to initiate appropriate preventive or corrective actions.

Actions/Interventions

Nursing Priority No. 1.

To maintain adequate, patent airway:

- Identify client populations at risk. **Persons with impaired ciliary function (e.g., cystic fibrosis or lung transplant recipients); those with excessive or abnormal mucus production (e.g., asthma, emphysema, pneumonia, dehydration, bronchiectasis, or mechanical ventilation); those with impaired cough function (e.g., neuromuscular diseases, such as muscular dystrophy; multiple sclerosis neuromotor conditions, such as cerebral palsy; or spinal cord injury); those with swallowing abnormalities (e.g., post-stroke, seizures, head/neck cancer, coma/sedation, tracheostomy, or facial burns/trauma/surgery); those who are immobile (e.g., sedated individual, frail elderly, developmentally delayed, institutionalized client with multiple high-risk conditions; infant/child (e.g., feeding intolerance, abdominal distention, and emotional stressors that may compromise airway) are all at risk for problems with the maintenance of open airways.**
- Assess level of consciousness/cognition and ability to protect own airway. **This information is essential for identifying**

Information that appears in brackets has been added by the authors to clarify and enhance the use of nursing diagnoses.

potential for airway problems, providing baseline level of care needed, and influencing choice of interventions.

- Monitor respirations and breath sounds, noting rate and sounds (e.g., tachypnea, stridor, crackles, or wheezes) **indicative of respiratory distress and/or accumulation of secretions.**
- Evaluate client's cough/gag reflex, amount and type of secretions, and swallowing ability **to determine ability to protect own airway.**
- Position head appropriate for age and condition **to open or maintain open airway in an at-rest or compromised individual.**
- Suction nose, mouth, and trachea prn **to clear airway when excessive or viscous secretions are blocking airway or client is unable to swallow or cough effectively.**
- Elevate head of bed, encourage early ambulation, or change client's position every 2 hr **to take advantage of gravity decreasing pressure on the diaphragm and enhancing drainage of/ventilation to different lung segments.**
- Monitor infant/child for feeding intolerance, abdominal distention, and emotional stressors **that may compromise airway.**
- Insert oral airway (using correct size for adult or child) when needed **to maintain anatomical position of tongue and natural airway, especially when tongue/laryngeal edema or thick secretions may block airway.**
- Assist with appropriate testing (e.g., pulmonary function or sleep studies) **to identify causative/precipitating factors.**
- Instruct in/review postoperative breathing exercises, effective coughing, and use of adjunct devices (e.g., intermittent positive pressure breathing or incentive spirometer) in preoperative teaching.
- Assist with procedures (e.g., bronchoscopy or tracheostomy) **to clear/maintain open airway.**
- Keep environment allergen free (e.g., dust, feather pillows, or smoke) according to individual situation.

Nursing Priority No. 2.

To mobilize secretions:

- Mobilize the client as soon as possible. **This reduces risk or effects of atelectasis, enhancing lung expansion and drainage of different lung segments.**

Information that appears in brackets has been added by the authors to clarify and enhance the use of nursing diagnoses.

- Encourage deep-breathing and coughing exercises or splint chest/incision **to maximize effort.**
- Administer analgesics **to improve cough when pain is inhibiting effort. (Caution: Overmedication can depress respirations and cough effort.)**
- Administer medications (e.g., expectorants, anti-inflammatory agents, bronchodilators, and mucolytic agents), as indicated, **to relax smooth respiratory musculature, reduce airway edema, and mobilize secretions.**
- Increase fluid intake to at least 2,000 mL/day within cardiac tolerance (may require IV in acutely ill, hospitalized client). Encourage/provide warm versus cold liquids as appropriate. Provide supplemental humidification, if needed (ultrasonic nebulizer or room humidifier). **Hydration can help prevent the accumulation of viscous secretions and improve secretion clearance.** Monitor for signs/symptoms of congestive heart failure (crackles, edema, or weight gain) when the client is at risk.
- Perform or assist the client in learning airway clearance techniques, such as postural drainage and percussion (chest physical therapy [CPT]), flutter devices, high-frequency chest compression with an inflatable vest, intrapulmonary percussive ventilation administered by a percussinator, and active cycle breathing (ACB). **Various therapies/modalities may be required to acquire and maintain adequate airways and improve respiratory function and gas exchange.** (Refer to NDs ineffective Breathing Pattern; impaired Gas Exchange; impaired spontaneous Ventilation.)
- Support reduction/cessation of smoking **to improve lung function.**
- Position appropriately (e.g., head of bed elevated, side lying) and discourage use of oil-based products around nose **to prevent vomiting with aspiration into lungs.** (Refer to NDs risk for Aspiration; impaired Swallowing.)

Nursing Priority No. 3.

To assess changes, note complications:

- Auscultate breath sounds and assess air movement **to ascertain current status and note effects of treatment in clearing airways.**
- Monitor vital signs, noting changes in blood pressure and heart rate.
- Observe for signs of respiratory distress (increased rate, restlessness/anxiety, or use of accessory muscles for breathing).

Information that appears in brackets has been added by the authors to clarify and enhance the use of nursing diagnoses.

- Evaluate changes in sleep pattern, noting insomnia or daytime somnolence, **which may be evidence of nighttime airway incompetence or sleep apnea.** (Refer to NDs Insomnia, Sleep Deprivation.)
- Document response to drug therapy and/or development of adverse side effects or interactions with antimicrobials, steroids, expectorants, and bronchodilators.
- Observe for signs/symptoms of infection (e.g., increased dyspnea with onset of fever or change in sputum color, amount, or character) **to identify the infectious process and promote timely intervention.**
- Obtain sputum specimen, preferably before antimicrobial therapy is initiated, **to verify appropriateness of therapy.**
- Monitor/document serial chest x-rays, ABGs, or pulse oximetry readings.

Nursing Priority No. 4.

To promote wellness (Teaching/Discharge Considerations):

- Assess client's/SO's knowledge of contributing causes, treatment plan, specific medications, and therapeutic procedures **to determine educational and support needs.**
- Provide information about the necessity of raising and expectorating secretions versus swallowing them **to report changes in color and amount in the event that medical intervention may be needed to prevent or treat infection.**
- Demonstrate/assist client/SO in performing specific airway clearance techniques (e.g., forced expiratory breathing [also called huffing] or respiratory muscle strength training, chest percussion, or use of a vest), as indicated.
- Encourage/provide opportunities for rest; limit activities to level of respiratory tolerance. **This prevents/reduces fatigue.**
- Refer to appropriate support groups (e.g., stop smoking clinic, COPD exercise group, weight reduction, the American Lung Association, the Cystic Fibrosis Foundation, or the Muscular Dystrophy Association).
- Determine that the client has equipment and is informed in the use of nocturnal continuous positive airway pressure (CPAP) **for the treatment of obstructive sleep apnea, when indicated.** (Refer to NDs Insomnia, Sleep Deprivation.)

Documentation Focus

Assessment/Reassessment

- Related factors for individual clients
- Breath sounds, presence and character of secretions, use of accessory muscles for breathing

Information that appears in brackets has been added by the authors to clarify and enhance the use of nursing diagnoses.

- Character of cough and sputum
- Respiratory rate, pulse oximetry/O_2 saturation, vital signs

Planning

- Plan of care and who is involved in planning
- Teaching plan

Implementation/Evaluation

- Client's response to interventions, teaching, and actions performed
- Use of respiratory devices/airway adjuncts
- Response to medications administered
- Attainment or progress toward desired outcome(s)
- Modifications to plan of care

Discharge Planning

- Long-term needs and who is responsible for actions to be taken
- Specific referrals made

Sample Nursing Outcomes & Interventions Classifications (NOC/NIC)

NOC—Respiratory Status: Airway Patency
NIC—Airway Management

risk for ALLERGY RESPONSE

[Diagnostic Division: Safety]

Definition: Vulnerable to an exaggerated immune response or reaction to substances, which may compromise health.

Risk Factors

Allergy to insect sting
Exposure to allergen (e.g., pharmaceutical agent)
Exposure to environmental allergen (e.g., dander, dust, mold, or pollen)
Exposure to toxic chemical
Food allergy (e.g., avocado, banana, shellfish, mushroom, or tropical fruit)

Information that appears in brackets has been added by the authors to clarify and enhance the use of nursing diagnoses.

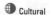

Repeated exposure to allergen-producing environmental substance

NOTE: A risk diagnosis is not evidenced by signs and symptoms, as the problem has not occurred; rather, nursing interventions are directed at prevention.

Desired Outcomes/Evaluation Criteria—Client Will:

- Be free of signs of hypersensitive response
- Verbalize understanding of individual risks and responsibilities in avoiding exposure
- Identify signs/symptoms requiring prompt response

Actions/Interventions

Nursing Priority No. 1.

To identify causative/precipitating factors related to risk:

- Question the client regarding known allergies upon admission to healthcare facility. **Basic safety information will help healthcare providers prepare a safe environment for the client while providing care.**
- Ascertain the type of allergy and usual symptoms if the client reports a history of allergies (e.g., seasonal rhinitis ["hay fever"], allergic dermatitis, conjunctavitis, environmental asthma, environmental substances [e.g., mold, dust, or pet dander], insect stings reactions, food intolerance, immunodeficiency such as Addison's disease, or drug or transfusion reaction). **Allergies can manifest as local reactions (as may occur in skin rashes) or may be systemic. The client/caregiver may be aware of some, but not all, allergies.**
- Obtain a written list of drug allergies upon first contact with the client. **This helps prevent adverse drug events while the client is in facility care.**
- Discuss the possibility of a latex allergy when entering facility care, especially when procedures are anticipated (e.g., laboratory, emergency department, operating room, wound care management, one-day surgery, or dental) **so that proper precautions can be taken by healthcare providers.** (Refer to ND Latex Allergy Response for related interventions.)
- Note the client's age. **Although allergies can occur at any time in a client's life span, there are some that can start**

Information that appears in brackets has been added by the authors to clarify and enhance the use of nursing diagnoses.

early in life. These include food allergies (e.g., peanuts) and respiratory ailments (e.g., asthma).

- Perform challenge or patch test, if appropriate, **to identify specific allergens in a client with known type IV hypersensitivity.**
- Note response to radioallergosorbent test (RAST) or enzyme-linked latex-specific IgE (ELISA), where available. **This is performed to measure the quantity of IgE antibodies in serum after exposure to specific antigens and has generally replaced skin tests and provocation tests. Note: These tests are useful in nonemergent evaluations.**

Nursing Priority No. 2.

To take measures to avoid exposure and reduce/limit allergic response:

- Discuss the client's current symptoms, noting reports of rash, hives, itching; teary eyes; localized swelling (e.g., of lips) or diarrhea; nausea; or a feeling of faintness. Ascertain if client/care provider associates these symptoms with certain food, substances, or environmental factors. **This may help isolate the cause for a reaction.**
- Provide an allergen-free environment (e.g., clean dust-free room or use air filters to reduce mold and pollens in the air) **to reduce client exposure to allergens.**
- Collaborate with all healthcare providers to administer medications and perform procedures with client's allergies in mind.
- Encourage the client to wear a medical ID bracelet/necklace **to alert providers to condition if the client is unresponsive or unable to relay information for any reason.**
- Refer to physician/allergy specialists as indicated **for interventions related to specific allergy conditions.**

Nursing Priority No. 3.

To promote wellness (Teaching/Discharge Criteria):

- Instruct/review with client and care provider(s) ways to prevent or limit client exposures. **They may need or desire information regarding ways to reduce allergens at home, school, or work; may desire information regarding potential exposures when traveling, or how to manage food allergies when eating in restaurants.**
- Instruct in signs of reaction and emergency treatment needs. **Allergic reactions range from skin irritation to anaphylaxis. Reaction may be gradual but progressive, affecting**

Information that appears in brackets has been added by the authors to clarify and enhance the use of nursing diagnoses.

multiple body systems, or may be sudden, requiring life-saving treatment.

- Emphasize the critical importance of taking immediate action for moderate to severe hypersensitivity reactions **to limit life-threatening symptoms.**
- Demonstrate equipment and injection procedure and recommend that the client carry auto-injectable epinephrine **to provide timely emergency treatment, as needed.**
- Emphasize the necessity of informing all new care providers of allergies.
- Provide educational resources and assistance numbers for emergencies. **When allergy is suspected or the potential for allergy exists, protection must begin with identification and removal of possible sources.**

Documentation Focus

Assessment/Reassessment

- Individual risk factors identified
- Client concerns or difficulty making and following through with plans

Planning

- Plan of care and who is involved in planning
- Teaching plan

Implementation/Evaluation

- Response to interventions, teaching, and actions performed
- Attainment or progress toward outcomes

Discharge Planning

- Referrals to other resources
- Long-term need and who is responsible for actions

Sample Nursing Outcomes & Interventions Classifications (NOC/NIC)

NOC—Allergy Response: Systemic
NIC—Allergy Management

Information that appears in brackets has been added by the authors to clarify and enhance the use of nursing diagnoses.

ANXIETY [specify level]

[Diagnostic Division: Ego Integrity]

Definition: Vague uneasy feeling of discomfort or dread accompanied by an autonomic response (the source is often nonspecific or unknown to the individual); a feeling of apprehension caused by anticipation of danger. It is an alerting sign that warns of impending danger and enables the individual to take measures to deal with that threat.

Related Factors

Conflict about life goals; unmet needs; value conflict
Exposure to toxin; substance abuse
Family history of anxiety; heredity
Interpersonal contagion/transmission
Major change (e.g., economic status, environment; health status, role function or status; threat to current status)
Maturational or situational crisis; stressors
Threat of death

Defining Characteristics

Subjective

Behavioral
Worried about change in life event; insomnia

Affective
Regretful; rattled; distressed; apprehensive; fearful; feeling inadequate; uncertain; worried; helpless

Cognitive
Fear; awareness of physiological symptoms

Physiological
Shakiness

Sympathetic
Dry mouth, heart palpitations, weakness, anorexia, diarrhea

Parasympathetic
Tingling in extremities, nausea, abdominal pain, diarrhea, urinary frequency/hesitancy/urgency, faintness, fatigue, alteration in sleep pattern

---

Information that appears in brackets has been added by the authors to clarify and enhance the use of nursing diagnoses.

Objective

Behavioral

Poor eye contact, glancing about, scanning behavior, hypervigilance, extraneous movement, fidgeting, restlessness, decrease in productivity

Affective

Increase in wariness, self-focused, irritability, jitteriness, overexcitement, anguish

Cognitive

Preoccupation; alteration in attention, concentration; forgetfulness; diminished ability to learn or problem solve; rumination; tendency to blame others; blocking of thoughts; confusion; decrease in perceptual field

Physiological

Voice quivering, trembling, hand tremors, increase in tension, facial tension, increase in perspiration

Sympathetic

Cardiovascular excitation; facial flushing; superficial vasoconstriction; increase in heart/respiratory rate, blood pressure; alteration in respiratory pattern; pupil dilation; twitching; brisk reflexes

Parasympathetic

Decrease in blood pressure or heart rate

Desired Outcomes/Evaluation Criteria—Client Will:

- Verbalize awareness of feelings of anxiety.
- Appear relaxed and report that anxiety is reduced to a manageable level.
- Identify healthy ways to deal with and express anxiety.
- Demonstrate problem-solving skills.
- Use resources/support systems effectively.

Actions/Interventions

Nursing Priority No. 1.

To assess level of anxiety:

- Review familial and physiological factors (e.g., genetic depressive factors), psychiatric illness, active medical conditions (e.g., thyroid problems, metabolic imbalances, cardiopulmonary disease, anemia, or dysrhythmias), and recent/

Information that appears in brackets has been added by the authors to clarify and enhance the use of nursing diagnoses.

ongoing stressors (e.g., family member illness or death, spousal conflict/abuse, or loss of job). **These factors can cause/exacerbate anxiety and anxiety disorders.**

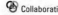

- Determine current prescribed medications and recent drug history of prescribed or over-the-counter (OTC) medications (e.g., steroids, thyroid preparations, weight loss pills, or caffeine). **These medications can heighten feelings and sense of anxiety.**
- Identify the client's perception of the threat represented by the situation.
- Note cultural factors that may influence anxiety. **Individual responses are influenced by cultural values and beliefs and culturally learned patterns of their family of origin.**
- Monitor vital signs (e.g., rapid or irregular pulse, rapid breathing/hyperventilation, changes in blood pressure, diaphoresis, tremors, or restlessness) **to identify physical responses associated with both medical and emotional conditions.**
- Observe behaviors **that can point to the client's level of anxiety:**

Mild

Alert, more aware of environment, attention focused on environment and immediate events

Restless; irritable; wakeful; reports of insomnia

Motivated to deal with existing problems in this state

Moderate

Perception narrower, concentration increased, able to ignore distractions in dealing with problem(s)

Voice quivers or changes pitch

Trembling, increased pulse/respirations

Severe

Range of perception is reduced, anxiety interferes with effective functioning

Preoccupied with feelings of discomfort, sense of impending doom

Increased pulse/respirations with reports of dizziness, tingling sensations, headaches, and so forth

Panic

The ability to concentrate is disrupted; behavior is disintegrated; and the client distorts the situation and does not have realistic perceptions of what is happening. The client may be expe-

Information that appears in brackets has been added by the authors to clarify and enhance the use of nursing diagnoses.

riencing terror or confusion or be unable to speak or move (paralyzed with fear).

- Note reports of insomnia or excessive sleeping, limited/avoidance of interactions with others, and use of alcohol or other drugs that can be abused, **which may be behavioral indicators of use of withdrawal to deal with problems.**
- Review results of diagnostic tests (e.g., drug screens, cardiac testing, complete blood count, and chemistry panel), **which may point to physiological sources of anxiety.**
- Be aware of defense mechanisms being used (e.g., denial or regression) **that interfere with ability to deal with problem.**
- Identify coping skills the individual is currently using, such as anger, daydreaming, forgetfulness, overeating, smoking, or lack of problem solving.
- Review coping skills used in the past **to determine those that might be helpful in current circumstances.**

Nursing Priority No. 2.

To assist client with identifying feelings and beginning to deal with problems:

- Establish a therapeutic relationship, conveying empathy and unconditional positive regard. **Note**: The nurse needs to be aware of his or her own feelings of anxiety or uneasiness, exercising care **to avoid the contagious effect or transmission of anxiety.**
- Be available to the client for listening and talking.
- Encourage the client to acknowledge and to express feelings, such as crying (sadness), laughing (fear or denial), or swearing (fear or anger).
- Assist the client in developing self-awareness of verbal and nonverbal behaviors.
- Clarify the meaning of feelings and actions by providing feedback and checking meaning with the client.
- Acknowledge anxiety/fear. Do not deny or reassure client that everything will be all right.
- Provide accurate information about the situation. **This helps the client identify what is reality based.**
- Be truthful, avoid bribing, and provide physical comfort (e.g., hugging or rocking) when dealing with a child **to soothe fears and provide assurance.**
- Provide comfort measures (e.g., calm/quiet environment, soft music, a warm bath, or a back rub).

Information that appears in brackets has been added by the authors to clarify and enhance the use of nursing diagnoses.

- Modify procedures as much as possible (e.g., substitute oral for intramuscular medications or combine blood draws/use finger stick method) **to limit the degree of stress and avoid overwhelming a child or anxious adult.**
- Manage environmental factors, such as harsh lighting and high traffic flow, which may be confusing and stressful to older individuals.
- Accept the client as is. **The client may need to be where he or she is at this point in time, such as in denial after receiving the diagnosis of a terminal illness.**
- Allow the behavior to belong to the client; do not respond personally. **The nurse may respond inappropriately, escalating the situation to a nontherapeutic interaction.**
- Assist the client to use anxiety for coping with the situation, if helpful. **Moderate anxiety heightens awareness and permits the client to focus on dealing with problems.**

Panic

- Stay with client, maintaining a calm, confident manner.
- Speak in brief statements using simple words.
- Provide for nonthreatening, consistent environment/atmosphere. Minimize stimuli. Monitor visitors and interactions **to lessen the effect of transmission of feelings.**
- Set limits on inappropriate behavior and help the client to develop acceptable ways of dealing with anxiety.

NOTE: The staff may need to provide safe controls and environment until the client regains control.

- Gradually increase activities/involvement with others as anxiety is decreased.
- Use cognitive therapy **to focus on or correct faulty catastrophic interpretations of physical symptoms.**
- Administer medications (anti-anxiety agents/sedatives), as ordered.

Nursing Priority No. 3.

To promote wellness (Teaching/Discharge Considerations):

- Assist the client in identifying precipitating factors and new methods of coping with disabling anxiety.
- Review happenings, thoughts, and feelings preceding the anxiety attack.

Information that appears in brackets has been added by the authors to clarify and enhance the use of nursing diagnoses.

- Identify actions and activities the client has previously used to cope successfully when feeling nervous/anxious.
- List helpful resources and people, including available "hot-line" or crisis managers **to provide ongoing/timely support.**
- Encourage the client to develop an exercise/activity program, **which may serve to reduce the level of anxiety by relieving tension.**
- Assist in developing skills (e.g., awareness of negative thoughts, saying "Stop," and substituting a positive thought) **to eliminate negative self-talk. Mild phobias tend to respond well to behavioral therapy.**
- Review strategies, such as role-playing, use of visualizations to practice anticipated events, and prayer/meditation. **This is useful for being prepared for/dealing with anxiety-provoking situations.**
- Review medication regimen and possible interactions, especially with OTC drugs, other prescription drugs, and alcohol. Discuss appropriate drug substitutions, changes in dosage, or time of dose **to minimize side effects.**
- Refer to the physician for drug management alteration of the prescription regimen. **Drugs that often cause symptoms of anxiety include aminophylline/theophylline, anticholinergics, dopamine, levodopa, salicylates, and steroids.**
- Refer to individual and/or group therapy, as appropriate, **to deal with chronic anxiety states.**

Documentation Focus

Assessment/Reassessment

- Level of anxiety and precipitating/aggravating factors
- Description of feelings (expressed and displayed)
- Awareness and ability to recognize and express feelings
- Related substance use, if present

Planning

- Treatment plan and individual responsibility for specific activities
- Teaching plan

Implementation/Evaluation

- Client involvement and response to interventions, teaching, and actions performed
- Attainment or progress toward desired outcome(s)
- Modifications to plan of care

Information that appears in brackets has been added by the authors to clarify and enhance the use of nursing diagnoses.

Discharge Planning

- Referrals and follow-up plan
- Specific referrals made

Sample Nursing Outcomes & Interventions Classifications (NOC/NIC)

NOC—Anxiety Level
NIC—Anxiety Reduction

risk for ASPIRATION

[Diagnostic Division: Respiration]

Definition: Vulnerable to entry of gastrointestinal secretions, oropharyngeal secretions, solids or fluids into the tracheobronchial passages, which may compromise health.

Risk Factors

Barrier to elevating upper body; facial surgery or trauma; neck surgery or trauma; oral surgery or trauma; wired jaw

Decrease in gastrointestinal motility; delayed gastric emptying; incompetent lower esophageal sphincter; increase in gastric residual; increase in intragastric pressure;

Decrease in level of consciousness; depressed gag reflex; impaired ability to swallow; ineffective cough;

Presence of oral/nasal tube (e.g., tracheal, feeding); enteral feedings

Treatment regimen

NOTE: A risk diagnosis is not evidenced by signs and symptoms, as the problem has not occurred; rather, nursing interventions are directed at prevention.

Desired Outcomes/Evaluation Criteria—Client/Caregiver Will:

- Experience no aspiration as evidenced by noiseless respirations; clear breath sounds; and clear, odorless secretions.
- Identify causative/risk factors.
- Demonstrate techniques to prevent and/or correct aspiration.

Information that appears in brackets has been added by the authors to clarify and enhance the use of nursing diagnoses.

Actions/Interventions

Nursing Priority No. 1.

To assess causative/contributing factors:

- Identify at-risk clients according to condition or disease process, as listed in Risk Factors, **to determine when observation and/or interventions may be required.**
- ∞ Assess for age-related risk factors potentiating risk of aspiration (e.g., premature infant, elderly infirm). **Aspiration pneumonia is more common in extremely young or old patients and commonly occurs in individuals with chronically impaired airway defense mechanisms.**
- Note the client's level of consciousness, awareness of surroundings, and cognitive function, **as impairments in these areas increase the client's risk of aspiration owing to the inability to cough or swallow well and/or the presence of an artificial airway, mechanical ventilation, and/or tube feedings.**
- Determine the presence of neuromuscular disorders, noting muscle groups involved, degree of impairment, and whether they are of an acute or progressive nature (e.g., stroke, Parkinson's disease, progressive supranuclear palsy, and similar disabling brain diseases; Guillain-Barré syndrome, or amyotrophic lateral sclerosis). **This may result in temporary or chronic, progressive impairment of protective muscle functions.**
- Assess the client's ability to swallow and cough; note quality of voice. **Sudden respiratory symptoms (such as severe coughing and cyanosis, or wet phlegmy voice quality) are indicative of potential aspiration. Also individuals with impaired or absent cough reflexes (such as may occur after a stroke, in Parkinson's disease, or during sedation) are at high risk for "silent" aspiration.**
- Observe for neck and facial edema. **A client with a head/neck surgery or a tracheal/bronchial injury (e.g., upper torso burns or inhalation/chemical injury) is at particular risk for airway obstruction and an inability to handle secretions.**
- Auscultate lung sounds periodically (especially in a client who is coughing frequently or not coughing at all; a client with artificial airways, endotracheal and tracheostomy tubes; or a ventilator client being tube-fed, immediately following extubation), and observe chest radiographs **to determine decreased breath sounds, rales, or dullness to percussion**

Information that appears in brackets has been added by the authors to clarify and enhance the use of nursing diagnoses.

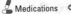

that could indicate the presence of aspirated secretions, and "silent aspiration" leading to aspiration pneumonia.

- Evaluate for/note presence of gastrointestinal (GI) pathology and motility disorders. **Nausea with vomiting (associated with metabolic disorders, or following surgery, and with certain medications) and gastroesophageal reflux disease (GERD) can cause inhalation of gastric contents.**
- Note the administration of enteral feedings, which may be initiated when oral nutrition is not possible. **The potential exists for regurgitation and aspiration with the use of nasogastric feeding tubes, even with proper tube placement.**
- Ascertain lifestyle habits (e.g., chronic use of alcohol and drugs, alcohol intoxication, tobacco, and other central nervous system [CNS] suppressant drugs). **These can affect awareness as well as impair gag and swallow mechanisms.**
- Assist with/review diagnostic studies (e.g., videofluoroscopy or fiberoptic endoscopy), **which may be done to assess for presence/degree of impairment.**

Nursing Priority No. 2.

To assist in correcting factors that can lead to aspiration:

- Elevate the client to the highest or best possible position (e.g., sitting upright in chair) for eating and drinking and during tube feedings. **Adults and children should be upright for meals to decrease the likelihood of drainage into the trachea and to reduce reflux and improve gastric emptying.**
- Encourage the client to cough, as able, to clear secretions. **The client may simply need to be reminded or encouraged to cough (such as might occur in an elderly person with delayed gag reflex or in a postoperative, sedated client).**
- Monitor the use of oxygen masks in clients at risk for vomiting. Refrain from using oxygen masks for comatose individuals.
- Keep wire cutters/scissors with the client at all times when jaws are wired/banded **to facilitate clearing the airway in emergency situations.**
- Maintain operational suction equipment at bedside/chairside.
- Suction (oral cavity, nose, and ET/tracheostomy tube), as needed, and avoid triggering the gag mechanism when performing suction or mouth care **to clear secretions while reducing the potential for aspiration of secretions.**

Information that appears in brackets has been added by the authors to clarify and enhance the use of nursing diagnoses.

- Avoid keeping the client supine/flat when on mechanical ventilation (especially when also receiving enteral feedings). **Supine positioning and enteral feedings have been shown to be independent risk factors for the development of aspiration pneumonia.**
- Perform scrupulous oral care **to prevent the accumulation of thickened secretions in the oral pharynx and to remove secretions that may interfere with the movement of air.**
- Provide a rest period prior to feeding time. **The rested client may have less difficulty with swallowing.**
- Feed slowly, using small bites, instructing the client to chew slowly and thoroughly.
- Vary the placement of food in the client's mouth according to type of swallowing deficit (e.g., place food in right side of mouth if facial weakness is present on the left side).
- Provide soft foods that stick together/form a bolus (e.g., casseroles, puddings, or stews) **to aid the swallowing effort.**
- Determine liquid viscosity best tolerated by client. Add thickening agent to liquids, as appropriate. **Some individuals may swallow thickened liquids better than thin liquids.**
- Offer very warm or very cold liquids. **This activates temperature receptors in the mouth that help to stimulate swallowing.**
- Avoid washing solids down with liquids.
- Ascertain that the feeding tube (when used) is in the correct position. **Placement may be done under fluoroscopy, and/or measurement of aspirate pH following placement of feeding tube may be indicated**. Ask the client about feeling of fullness and/or measure residuals (just prior to feeding and several hours after feeding), when appropriate, **to reduce risk of aspiration.**
- Determine the best resting position for infant/child (e.g., with the head of the bed elevated 30 degrees and the infant propped on the right side after feeding). **Upper airway patency is facilitated by an upright position, and turning to the right side decreases the likelihood of drainage into the trachea.**
- Provide oral medications in elixir form or crush, if appropriate.
- Minimize the use of sedatives/hypnotics whenever possible. **These agents can impair coughing and swallowing.**
- Refer to physician and/or speech/language therapist for medical or surgical interventions and/or exercises **to strengthen muscles and learn specific techniques to enhance swallowing/reduce potential aspiration.**

Information that appears in brackets has been added by the authors to clarify and enhance the use of nursing diagnoses.

Nursing Priority No. 3.

To promote wellness (Teaching/Discharge Considerations):

- Review with client/SO individual risk or potentiating factors.
- Provide information about the signs and effects of aspiration on the lungs. **Note: Severe coughing and cyanosis associated with eating or drinking or changes in vocal quality after swallowing indicate onset of respiratory symptoms associated with aspiration and require immediate intervention.**
- Instruct in safety concerns regarding oral or tube feeding. (Refer to ND impaired Swallowing.)
- Train the client how to self-suction or train family members in suction techniques (especially if the client has constant or copious oral secretions) **to enhance safety/self-sufficiency.**
- Instruct the individual/family member to avoid or limit activities after eating that increase intra-abdominal pressure (straining, strenuous exercise, or tight/constrictive clothing), **which may slow digestion/increase risk of regurgitation.**

Documentation Focus

Assessment/Reassessment

- Assessment findings, conditions that could lead to problems of aspiration
- Verification of tube placement, observations of physical findings

Planning

- Interventions to prevent aspiration or reduce risk factors and who is involved in the planning
- Teaching plan

Implementation/Evaluation

- Client's responses to interventions, teaching, and actions performed
- Foods/fluids client handles with ease or difficulty
- Amount and frequency of intake
- Attainment or progress toward desired outcome(s)
- Modifications to plan of care

Discharge Planning

- Long-term needs and who is responsible for actions to be taken

---

Information that appears in brackets has been added by the authors to clarify and enhance the use of nursing diagnoses.

 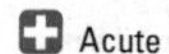 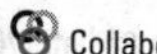 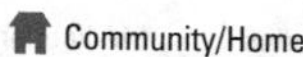 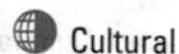

Sample Nursing Outcomes & Interventions Classifications (NOC/NIC)

NOC—Aspiration Prevention
NIC—Aspiration Precautions

risk for impaired ATTACHMENT

[Diagnostic Division: Social Interaction]

Definition: Vulnerable to disruption of the interactive process between parent/significant other and child that fosters the development of a protective and nurturing reciprocal relationship.

Risk Factors

Inability of parent to meet personal needs
Anxiety; [parents who themselves experienced impaired attachment]
Prematurity; child's illness prevents effective initiation of parental contact
Disorganized infant behavior; parental conflict resulting from disorganized behavioral organization
Parent-child separation, physical barrier (e.g., infant in isolette), insufficient privacy
Substance abuse
Difficult pregnancy and/or birth
Uncertainty of paternity, conception as a result of rape/sexual abuse

NOTE: A risk diagnosis is not evidenced by signs and symptoms, as the problem has not occurred; rather, nursing interventions are directed at prevention.

Desired Outcomes/Evaluation Criteria—Parent Will:

- Identify and prioritize family strengths and needs.
- Exhibit nurturing and protective behaviors toward child.
- Identify and use resources to meet needs of family members.
- Demonstrate techniques to enhance behavioral organization of the infant/child.
- Engage in mutually satisfying interactions with child.

Information that appears in brackets has been added by the authors to clarify and enhance the use of nursing diagnoses.

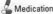

Actions/Interventions

Nursing Priority No. 1.

To identify causative/contributing factors:

- Interview parents, noting their perception of situation and individual concerns.
- Assess parent/child interactions.
- Ascertain availability and use of resources to include extended family, support groups, and financial resources.
- Evaluate parents' ability to provide protective environment and participate in a reciprocal relationship.

Nursing Priority No. 2.

To enhance behavioral organization of the child:

- Identify the infant's strengths and vulnerabilities. **Each child is born with his or her own temperament that affects interactions with caregivers.**
- Educate parents regarding child growth and development, addressing parental perceptions. **This helps to clarify realistic or unrealistic expectations.**
- Assist parents in modifying the environment **to provide appropriate stimulation.**
- Model care-giving techniques that best support behavioral organization.
- Respond consistently with nurturing to infant/child.

Nursing Priority No. 3.

To enhance best functioning of parents:

- Develop a therapeutic nurse-client relationship. Provide a consistently warm, nurturing, and nonjudgmental environment.
- Assist parents in identifying and prioritizing family strengths and needs. **This promotes a positive attitude by looking at what they already do well and using those skills to address needs.**
- Support and guide parents in the process of assessing resources.
- Involve parents in activities with the child that they can accomplish successfully. **This promotes a sense of confidence, thus enhancing self-concept.**
- Recognize and provide positive feedback for nurturing and protective parenting behaviors. **This reinforces the continuation of desired behaviors.**
- (Collaborative) Minimize the number of professionals on the team with whom parents must have contact **to foster trust in relationships.**

Information that appears in brackets has been added by the authors to clarify and enhance the use of nursing diagnoses.

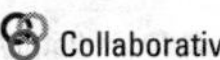

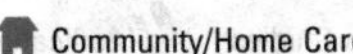

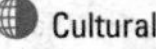

Nursing Priority No. 4.

To support parent/child attachment during separation:

- Provide parents with telephone contact, as appropriate. **Knowing there is someone they can call if they have problems provides a sense of security.**
- Establish a routine time for daily phone calls/initiate calls, as indicated. **This provides a sense of consistency and control and allows for the planning of other activities.**
- Minimize the number of professionals on the team with whom parents must have contact. **Foster a trust in these relationships, providing opportunities for modeling and learning.**
- Invite parents to use the Ronald McDonald House, or provide them with a listing of a variety of local accommodations and restaurants when child is hospitalized out of town.
- Arrange for the parents to receive photos and progress reports from the child.
- Suggest that the parents provide a photo and/or audiotape of themselves for the child.
- Consider the use of a contract with parents **to clearly communicate expectations of both family and staff.**
- Suggest that parents keep a journal of infant/child progress. **This serves as a reminder of the progress that is being made, especially when they become discouraged and believe the infant/child is "never" going to be better.**
- Provide "homelike" environment for situations requiring supervision of visits. **This supports the family as they work toward resolving conflicts and promotes a sense of hopefulness, enabling them to experience success when the family is involved with a legal situation.**

Nursing Priority No. 5.

To promote wellness (Teaching/Discharge Considerations):

- Refer to individual counseling, family therapies, or addiction counseling/treatment, as indicated. **Additional assistance may be needed when a situation is complicated by drug abuse (including alcohol), mental illness, disruptions in caregiving, parents who are burned out with caring for child with attachment or other difficulties.**
- Identify services for transportation, financial resources, housing, and so forth.
- Develop support systems appropriate to the situation (e.g., extended family, friends, or social worker). **Depending on individual situation, support from extended family, friends, social worker, or therapist can assist the family to deal with attachment disorders.**

Information that appears in brackets has been added by the authors to clarify and enhance the use of nursing diagnoses.

- Explore community resources (e.g., church affiliations, volunteer groups, or day/respite care). **Church affiliations, volunteer groups, or day or respite care can help parents who are overwhelmed with the care of a child with attachment or other disorder.**

Documentation Focus

Assessment/Reassessment

- Identified behaviors of both parents and child
- Specific risk factors, individual perceptions and concerns
- Interactions between parent and child

Planning

- Plan of care and who is involved in planning
- Teaching plan

Implementation/Evaluation

- Parents'/child's responses to interventions, teaching, and actions performed
- Attainment or progress toward desired outcomes
- Modifications to plan of care

Discharge Planning

- Long-term needs and who is responsible
- Plan for home visits to support parents and to ensure infant/child safety and well-being
- Specific referrals made

Sample Nursing Outcomes & Interventions Classifications (NOC/NIC)

NOC—Parent-Infant Attachment
NIC—Attachment Promotion

Information that appears in brackets has been added by the authors to clarify and enhance the use of nursing diagnoses.

AUTONOMIC DYSREFLEXIA and risk for AUTONOMIC DYSREFLEXIA

[Diagnostic Division: Circulation]

Definition: Autonomic Dysreflexia: Life-threatening, uninhibited sympathetic response of the nervous system to a noxious stimulus after a spinal cord injury at T7 or above.

Definition: risk for Autonomic Dysreflexia: Vulnerable to life-threatening, uninhibited response of the sympathetic nervous system postspinal shock, in an individual with a spinal cord injury [SCI] or lesion at T6 or above (it has been demonstrated in patients with injuries at T7 and T8), which may compromise health.

Related Factors (Autonomic Dysreflexia)

Bladder/bowel distention; [catheter insertion/obstruction; irrigation; constipation]
Skin irritation
Insufficient [client or] caregiver knowledge
[Sexual excitation; menstruation; pregnancy; labor and delivery]
[Environmental temperature extremes]

Defining Characteristics (Autonomic Dysreflexia)

Subjective

Headache (a diffuse pain in different portions of the head and not confined to any nerve distribution area)
Paresthesia; chilling; blurred vision; chest pain; metallic taste in mouth; nasal congestion

Objective

Paroxysmal hypertension [sudden periodic elevated blood pressure with systolic pressure > 140 mmHg and diastolic pressure > 90 mm Hg]
Bradycardia or tachycardia
Diaphoresis (above the injury), red splotches on skin (above the injury), or pallor (below the injury)
Horner's syndrome [contraction of the pupil, partial ptosis of the eyelid, enophthalmos, and sometimes loss of sweating over the affected side of the face]; conjunctival congestion
Pilomotor reflex

Information that appears in brackets has been added by the authors to clarify and enhance the use of nursing diagnoses.

Risk Factors (risk for Autonomic Dysreflexia)

Cardiopulmonary Stimuli

Deep vein thromobis
Pulmonary emboli

Gastrointestinal Stimuli

Bowel distention, constipation; difficult passage of feces; fecal impaction
Digital stimulation; enemas; suppositories
Gastrointestinal system pathology; esphogeal reflux disease; gallstones; hemorrhoids

Musculoskeletal-Integumentary Stimuli

Cutaneous stimulations (e.g., pressure ulcer, ingrown toenail, dressing, burns, rash); sunburn; wounds
Pressure over bony prominences/genitalia; range-of-motion exercises; spasm
Fracture; heterotrophic bone

Neurological Stimuli

Painful or irritating stimuli below the level of injury

Regulatory Stimuli

Temperature fluctuations; extremes of environmental temperatures

Reproductive Stimuli

Sexual intercourse; ejaculation; [vibrator overstimulation]
Menstruation; pregnancy; labor and delivery; ovarian cyst

Situational Stimuli

Constrictive clothing (e.g., straps, stockings, shoes)
Pharmaceutical agent [e.g., decongestants, sympathomimetics, vasoconstrictors]; substance withdrawal (e.g., narcotic/opiate)
Positioning; surgical [or diagnostic] procedure

Urological Stimuli

Bladder distention or spasm
Detrusor sphincter dyssynergia

Information that appears in brackets has been added by the authors to clarify and enhance the use of nursing diagnoses.

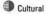

Urinary catheterization; instrumentation; surgery
Urinary tract infection; cystitis; urethritis; epididymitis; renal calculi

NOTE: A risk diagnosis is not evidenced by signs and symptoms as the problem has not occurred; rather, nursing interventions are directed at prevention.

Desired Outcomes/Evaluation Criteria—Client/Caregiver Will:

- Identify precipitating **or risk** factors.
- Recognize signs/symptoms of syndrome.
- Demonstrate corrective **or preventive** techniques.

Client Will:

- Experience no episodes of dysreflexia or seek medical intervention in a timely manner.

Actions/Interventions

Nursing Priority No. 1.

To assess for **risk** or precipitating factors:

- Monitor the client at home for potential precipitating factors, including urological (e.g., bladder distention, acute urinary tract infection, or kidney stones), GI (e.g., bowel overdistention, hemorrhoids, or digital stimulation), cutaneous (e.g., pressure ulcers, extreme external temperatures, or dressing changes), reproductive (e.g., sexual activity, menstruation, or pregnancy/delivery), and miscellaneous (e.g., pulmonary emboli, drug reaction, or deep vein thrombosis). **If problem is occurring, see more comprehensive listing of precipitating factors below.**
- Note the phase and specifics of injury. **Autonomic dysreflexia (AD) does not occur in the acute phase of spinal cord injury. However, some studies have identified factors that may point toward a client's likelihood of developing AD, perhaps early in recovery. These include higher levels of injury (e.g., cervical versus thoracic involvement) and more complete lesions.**
- Monitor for bladder distention, the presence of bladder spasms, stones, or infection. **The most common stimulus for AD is bladder irritation or overstretch associated with urinary retention or infection, blocked catheter, overfilled**

Information that appears in brackets has been added by the authors to clarify and enhance the use of nursing diagnoses.

collection bag, or noncompliance with intermittent catheterization.

- Assess for bowel distention, fecal impaction, or problems with bowel management program. **Bowel irritation or overstretch is associated with constipation or impaction; digital stimulation, suppository, or enema use during bowel program; hemorrhoids or fissures; and/or infection of the GI tract, such as might occur with ulcers or appendicitis.**
- Observe skin and tissue pressure areas, especially following prolonged sitting. **Skin and tissue irritants include direct pressure (e.g., object in chair or shoe, leg straps, abdominal support, or orthotics); wounds (e.g., bruise, abrasion, laceration, or pressure ulcer); ingrown toenails; tight clothing; sunburn or other burn.**
- Inquire about sexual activity and/or determine if reproductive issues are involved. **Overstimulation, vibration, sexual intercourse, ejaculation, scrotal compression, menstrual cramps, and/or pregnancy (especially labor and delivery) are known precipitants.**
- ∞ Note the onset of crying, irritability, or somnolence in an infant or child **who may present with nonspecific symptoms; he or she may not be able to verbalize discomforts.**
- Inform client/care providers of additional precipitators during the course of care. **The client is prone to numerous physical conditions or treatments (e.g., intolerance to temperature extremes; deep vein thrombosis; kidney stones; fractures/other trauma; or surgical, dental, and diagnostic procedures), any of which can precipitate AD.**

Nursing Priority No. 2.

To provide for **prevention** or early detection and immediate intervention:

- ∞ Monitor vital signs routinely, noting elevation in blood pressure, heart rate, and temperature, especially during times of physical stress, **to identify trends and intervene in a timely manner. Note: Baseline blood pressure in clients with spinal cord injuries (adults and children) is lower than in the general population; therefore, an elevation of 20 to 40 mm Hg above baseline may be indicative of AD.**
- Investigate associated complaints/symptoms (e.g., sudden severe headache, chest pains, blurred vision, facial flushing, nausea, or a metallic taste). **AD is a potentially life-threatening condition that requires immediate intervention.**

Information that appears in brackets has been added by the authors to clarify and enhance the use of nursing diagnoses.

- Eliminate causative stimulus immediately when possible, moving in a step-wise fashion. **Measures might include immediate catheterization, or restoration of urine flow if indwelling catheter is blocked; removing bowel impaction, or refraining from digital stimulation; reducing skin pressure by changing position or removing restrictive clothing; and protecting from temperature extremes.**
- Elevate the head of the bed as high as tolerated or place the client in a sitting position with legs dangling **to lower blood pressure.**
- Monitor vital signs frequently during an acute episode, **as blood pressure can fluctuate quickly due to impaired autonomic regulation.** Continue to monitor blood pressure at intervals after symptoms subside **to evaluate effectiveness of interventions.**
- Administer medications as required **to block excessive autonomic nerve transmission, normalize heart rate, and reduce hypertension.**
- Administer antihypertensive medications when an at-risk client is placed on a routine "maintenance dose," **as might occur when noxious stimuli cannot be removed (presence of chronic sacral pressure sore, fracture, or acute postoperative pain).**
- Know contraindications and cautions associated with antihypertensive medications; adjust dosage of antihypertensive medications carefully for children, the elderly, individuals with known heart disease, male client using sildenafil for sexual activity, or pregnant women. **This prevents complications such as untoward side effects, while maintaining blood pressure within the desired range.**

Nursing Priority No. 3.

To promote wellness (Teaching/Discharge Considerations):

- Discuss warning signs of AD with client/caregiver (i.e., sudden, severe pounding headache; flushed red face; increased blood pressure/acute hypertension; nasal congestion; anxiety; blurred vision; metallic taste in mouth; sweating and/or flushing above the level of SCI; goosebumps; bradycardia; or cardiac irregularities). **AD can develop rapidly (in minutes), requiring quick intervention. Knowledge can support adherence to preventive measures and promote prompt intervention when required.**
- Be aware of the client's communication abilities. **AD can occur at any age, from infants to the elderly, and the in-**

Information that appears in brackets has been added by the authors to clarify and enhance the use of nursing diagnoses.

dividual may not be able to verbalize a pounding headache, which is often the first symptom during onset of AD.

- Ascertain that the client/caregiver understands ways to avoid onset of the syndrome. Instruct and periodically reinforce teaching, as needed, regarding the following:
  - Keeping indwelling catheter free of kinks, keeping bag empty and situated below bladder level, and checking daily for deposits (bladder grit) inside catheter
  - Catheterizing as often as necessary **to prevent overfilling**
  - Monitoring voiding patterns for adequate frequency and amount
  - Performing a regular bowel evacuation program
  - Performing routine skin assessments
  - Monitoring all systems for signs/symptoms of infection and reporting promptly
- Instruct family member/caregiver in blood pressure monitoring, and client's usual blood pressure range; discuss plan for monitoring, reporting, and treatment of high blood pressure during acute episodes.
- Review proper use/administration of medication if indicated. **Client may have medication(s) both for emergent situations and/or prevention of AD.**
- Emphasize the importance of regularly scheduled medical evaluations **to monitor status and to identify developing problems.**
- Assist the client/family in identifying emergency referrals (e.g., physician, rehabilitation nurse, or home care supervisor). Place phone number(s) in a prominent place or program into the client's/caregiver's cell phone.
- Recommend wearing medical alert bracelet/necklace and carrying information card reviewing client's typical signs/symptoms and usual methods of treatment. **This provides vital information to care providers in an emergent situation.**
- Refer for advice or treatment of sexual and reproductive concerns as indicated. **The client requires information and monitoring regarding sexual issues that can precipitate AD, including vibration to achieve orgasm, use of erectile dysfunction medication, and labor and delivery.**

Documentation Focus

Assessment/Reassessment

- Individual risk factors or findings, noting previous episodes, precipitating factors, and individual signs/symptoms.

Information that appears in brackets has been added by the authors to clarify and enhance the use of nursing diagnoses.

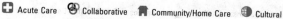

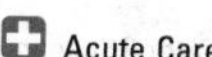

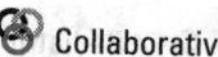

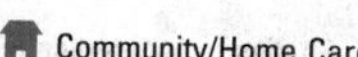

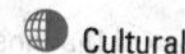

Planning

- Plan of care and who is involved in planning
- Teaching plan

Implementation/Evaluation

- Client's responses to interventions and actions performed, understanding of teaching
- Attainment or progress toward desired outcome(s)
- Modifications to plan of care

Discharge Planning

- Long-term needs and who is responsible for actions to be taken

Sample Nursing Outcomes & Interventions Classifications (NOC/NIC)

NOC—Risk Control
NOC—Neurological Status: Autonomic
NIC—Dysreflexia Management

disorganized infant BEHAVIOR and risk for disorganized infant BEHAVIOR

Taxonomy II: Coping/Stress Tolerance—Class 3 Neurobehavioral Stress (00116)

Definition: disorganized infant Behavior: Disintegrated physiological and neurobehavioral responses of an infant to the environment.

Definition: risk for disorganized infant Behavior: Vulnerable to alteration in integration and modulation of the physiological and behavioral systems of functioning (i.e., autonomic, motor, state-organization, self-regulatory, and attentional-interactional systems), which may compromise health.

Related Factors (disorganized infant Behavior)

Prenatal

Congenital or genetic disorders; exposure to teratogen

Information that appears in brackets has been added by the authors to clarify and enhance the use of nursing diagnoses.

Postnatal
Feeding intolerance; malnutrition
Impaired motor functioning; oral impairment
Invasive procedure; pain

Individual
Low postconceptual age; prematurity; immature neurological functioning
Illness; [hypoxia, birth asphyxia]

Environmental
Inadequate physical environment; insufficient containment within environment
Insufficient sensory stimulation, overstimulation, or deprivation

Caregiver
Cue misreading; insufficient knowledge of behavioral cues
Environmental overstimulation

Defining Characteristics (disorganized Infant Behavior)

Objective
Attention-interaction system: Impaired response to sensory stimuli (e.g., difficult to soothe, unable to sustain alert status)
Motor system:
Alteration in primitive reflexes; exaggerated startle response; jitteriness
Finger splay; fisting; hands to face; hyperextension of extremities
Impaired motor tone; tremor, twitching; uncoordinated movements
Physiological:
Abnormal skin color (e.g., pale, dusky, cyanosis)
Arrhythmia; bradycardia; tachycardia
Feeding intolerances
"Time-out signals" (e.g., gaze, grasp, hiccough, cough, sneeze, sigh, slack jaw, open mouth, tongue thrust)
Regulatory problems: Inability to inhibit startle reflex; irritability
State-organization system:
Active-awake (e.g., fussy, worried gaze); quiet-awake (e.g., staring, gaze aversion)

Information that appears in brackets has been added by the authors to clarify and enhance the use of nursing diagnoses.

Diffuse alpha EEG activity with eyes closed; state-oscillation
Irritable crying

Risk Factors (risk for disorganized infant Behavior)

Impaired motor functioning; oral impairment
Insufficient containment within environment; parent expresses desire to enhance environmental conditions
Prematurity [hypoxia and/or birth asphyxia]
Procedure or invasive procedure; pain

NOTE: A risk diagnosis is not evidenced by signs and symptoms, as the problem has not occurred; rather, nursing interventions are directed at prevention.

Desired Outcomes/Evaluation Criteria—Infant Will:

- Display signs/behaviors reflecting stable physiological state.
- Engage in some self-regulatory measures.

Parent/Caregiver Will:

- Identify cues reflecting infant's stress threshold and current status.
- Identify appropriate responses (including environmental modifications) to infant's cues.
- Develop or modify responses (including environment) to promote infant adaptation and development.
- Verbalize readiness to assume caregiving independently.

Actions/Interventions

Nursing Priority No. 1.

To assess causative/contributing **or risk** factors:

- Determine the infant's chronological and developmental age; note the length of gestation.
- Observe for cues suggesting the presence of situations that may result in pain/discomfort.
- Determine the adequacy of physiological support.
- Evaluate level and appropriateness of environmental stimuli.

Information that appears in brackets has been added by the authors to clarify and enhance the use of nursing diagnoses.

- Ascertain the parents' understanding of infant's needs and abilities.
- Listen to the parents' concerns about their capabilities to meet infant's needs.

Nursing Priority No. 2.

To assist parents in providing coregulation to the infant:

- Provide a calm, nurturing physical and emotional environment.
- Encourage parents to hold the infant, including skin-to-skin contact, using kangaroo care (KC) as appropriate. **Research suggests KC may have a positive effect on infant development by enhancing neurophysiological organization as well as an indirect effect by improving parental mood, perceptions, and interactive behavior.**
- Model gentle handling of baby and appropriate responses to infant behavior. **Provides cues to the parent.**
- Support and encourage parents to be with the infant and participate actively in all aspects of care. **The situation may be overwhelming, and support may enhance coping and strengthen attachment.**
- Encourage parents to refrain from social interaction during feedings, as appropriate. **The infant may have difficulty/lack necessary energy to manage feeding and social stimulation simultaneously.**
- Provide positive feedback for progressive parental involvement in the caregiving process. **Transfer of care from staff to parents progresses along a continuum as parents' confidence level increases and they are able to take on more complex care activities.**
- Discuss infant growth and development, pointing out current status and progressive expectations, as appropriate. **Augments parents' knowledge of coregulation.**
- Incorporate the parents' observations and suggestions into the plan of care. **This demonstrates valuing of parents' input and encourages continued involvement.**

Nursing Priority No. 3.

To deliver care within the infant's stress threshold:

- Provide a consistent caregiver. **This facilitates recognition of infant cues or changes in behavior.**
- Identify the infant's individual self-regulatory behaviors (e.g., sucking, mouthing, grasp, hand-to-mouth, face behaviors,

---

Information that appears in brackets has been added by the authors to clarify and enhance the use of nursing diagnoses.

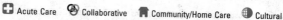

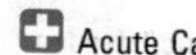 Acute Care 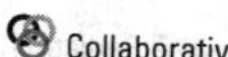 Collaborative 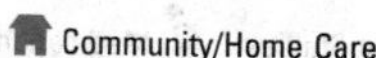 Community/Home Care 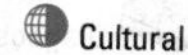 Cultural

foot clasp, brace, limb flexion, trunk tuck, or boundary seeking).

- Support hands to mouth and face; offer pacifier or nonnutritive sucking at the breast with gavage feedings. **This provides opportunities for the infant to suck.**
- Avoid aversive oral stimulation, such as routine oral suctioning; suction ET tube only when clinically indicated.
- Use Oxyhood large enough to cover the infant's chest so arms will be inside the hood. **This allows for hand-to-mouth activities during this therapy.**
- Provide opportunities for the infant to grasp.
- Provide boundaries and/or containment during all activities. Use swaddling, nesting, bunting, and caregiver's hands as indicated.
- Allow adequate time and opportunities to hold the infant. Handle the infant very gently, move the infant smoothly and slowly, and keep it contained, avoiding sudden or abrupt movements.
- Maintain normal alignment, position the infant with limbs softly flexed and with shoulders and hips adducted slightly. Use appropriate-sized diapers.
- Evaluate the chest for adequate expansion, placing rolls under the trunk if a prone position is indicated.
- Avoid restraints, including at IV sites. If IV board is necessary, secure to limb positioned in normal alignment.
- Provide a sheepskin, egg-crate mattress, water bed, and/or gel pillow or mattress for the infant who does not tolerate frequent position changes. **This minimizes tissue pressure and lessens the risk of tissue injury.**
- Assess color, respirations, activity, and invasive lines visually **to avoid disturbing the infant.** Assess with "hands on" every 4 hr as indicated and prn. **This allows for undisturbed rest and quiet periods.**
- Schedule care activities to allow time for rest and organization of sleep and wake states to maximize tolerance of the infant. Defer routine care to when the infant is in quiet sleep.
- Provide care with the baby in side-lying position. Begin by talking softly to the baby, then place hands in a containing hold on the baby, **which allows baby to prepare.** Proceed with least-invasive manipulations first.
- Respond promptly to infant's agitation or restlessness. Provide a "time out" when the infant shows early cues of overstimulation. Comfort and support the infant after stressful interventions.

Information that appears in brackets has been added by the authors to clarify and enhance the use of nursing diagnoses.

- Remain at the infant's bedside for several minutes after procedures and caregiving **to monitor the infant's response and provide necessary support.**
- Administer analgesics as individually appropriate.

Nursing Priority No. 4.

To modify the environment to provide appropriate stimulation:

- Introduce stimulation as a single mode and assess individual tolerance.

Light/Vision

- Reduce lighting perceived by the infant; introduce diurnal lighting (and activity) when infant achieves physiological stability. (Daylight levels of 20 to 30 candles and night light levels of less than 10 candles are suggested.) Change light levels gradually **to allow the infant time to adjust.**
- Protect the infant's eyes from bright illumination during examinations and procedures, as well as from indirect sources, such as neighboring phototherapy treatments, **to prevent retinal damage.**
- Deliver phototherapy (when required) with biliblanket devices, if available **(alleviates need for eye patches).**
- Provide caregiver face (preferably parent's) as visual stimulus when infant shows readiness (awake, attentive).
- Evaluate/readjust placement of pictures, stuffed animals, and so on, within the infant's immediate environment. **This promotes state maintenance and smooth transition by allowing the infant to look away easily when visual stimuli become stressful.**

Sound

- Identify sources of noise in the environment and eliminate/reduce them (e.g., speak in a low voice; reduce volume on alarms and telephones to quieter (but audible) levels; pad metal trash can lids; open paper packages, such as IV tubing and suction catheters slowly and at a distance from the bedside; conduct rounds or report away from bedside; place soft, thick fabric, such as blanket rolls and toys, near infant's head to absorb sound).
- Keep all incubator portholes closed, closing with two hands **to avoid a loud snap and associated startle response.**
- Refrain from playing musical toys or tape players inside the incubator.
- Avoid placing items on top of the incubator; if necessary to do so, pad the surface well.
- Conduct regular decibel (dB) checks of interior noise level in incubator (recommended not to exceed 60 dB).

Information that appears in brackets has been added by the authors to clarify and enhance the use of nursing diagnoses.

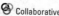

- Provide auditory stimulation **to console and support infant before and through handling or to reinforce restfulness.**

Olfactory

- Be cautious in exposing the infant to strong odors (e.g., alcohol, Betadine, perfumes), **as olfactory capability of the infant is very sensitive.**
- Place a cloth or gauze pad scented with milk near the infant's face during gavage feeding. **This enhances association of milk with act of feeding and gastric fullness.**
- Invite parents to leave near the infant a handkerchief that they have scented by wearing close to their body. **This strengthens infant recognition of parents.**

Vestibular

- Move and handle the infant slowly and gently. Do not restrict spontaneous movement.
- Provide vestibular stimulation **to console, stabilize breathing and heart rate, or enhance growth.** Use a water bed (with or without oscillation), a motorized or moving bed or cradle, or rocking in the arms of a caregiver.

Gustatory

- Dip pacifier in milk and offer to infant during gavage feeding **for sucking and to stimulate tasting.**

Tactile

- Maintain skin integrity and monitor closely. Limit the frequency of invasive procedures.
- Minimize the use of chemicals on the skin (e.g., alcohol, Betadine, solvents) and remove afterward with warm water, **because skin is very sensitive/fragile.**
- Limit the use of tape and adhesives directly on skin. Use DuoDerm under tape **to prevent dermal injury.**
- Touch the infant with a firm containing touch; avoid light stroking. Provide a sheepskin pad or soft linen. **Note: Tactile experience is the primary sensory mode of the infant.**
- Encourage frequent parental holding of the infant (including skin-to-skin). Supplement activity with extended family, staff, and volunteers.

Nursing Priority No. 5.

To promote wellness (Teaching/Discharge Considerations):

- Evaluate the home environment **to identify appropriate modifications.**
- Identify community resources (e.g., early stimulation programs, qualified childcare facilities, respite care, visiting nurse, home-care support, specialty organizations).

Information that appears in brackets has been added by the authors to clarify and enhance the use of nursing diagnoses.

- Determine sources for equipment and therapy needs.
- Refer to support or therapy groups, as indicated, **to provide role models, facilitate adjustment to new roles/ responsibilities, and enhance coping.**
- Provide contact number, as appropriate (e.g., primary nurse), **to support adjustment to home setting.**
- Refer to additional NDs, such as risk for impaired Attachment; compromised/disabled or readiness for enhanced family Coping; risk for disproportionate Growth; risk for delayed Development; risk for caregiver Role Strain.

Documentation Focus

Assessment/Reassessment

- Findings, including infant's cues of stress, self-regulation, and readiness for stimulation, and chronological and developmental age
- Parents' concerns/level of knowledge

Planning

- Plan of care and who is involved in the planning
- Teaching plan

Implementation/Evaluation

- Infant's responses to interventions and actions performed
- Parents' participation and response to interactions and teaching
- Attainment or progress toward desired outcome(s)
- Modifications of plan of care

Discharge Planning

- Long-term needs and who is responsible for actions to be taken
- Specific referrals made

Sample Nursing Outcomes & Interventions Classifications (NOC/NIC)

NOC—Preterm Infant Organization
NIC—Environmental Management

Information that appears in brackets has been added by the authors to clarify and enhance the use of nursing diagnoses.

readiness for enhanced organized infant BEHAVIOR

[Diagnostic Division: Neurosensory]

Definition: A pattern of modulation of the physiological and behavioral systems of functioning (i.e., autonomic, motor, state-organization, self-regulatory, and attentional-interactional systems) in an infant, which can be improved.

Defining Characteristics

Objective

The parent expresses a desire to enhance cue recognition.

The parent expresses a desire to enhance recognition of the infant's self-regulatory behaviors.

Desired Outcomes/Evaluation Criteria—Infant Will:

- Modulate physiological and behavioral systems of functioning.
- Achieve higher levels of integration in response to environmental stimuli.

Parent/Caregiver Will:

- Identify cues reflecting infant's stress threshold and current status.
- Develop or modify responses (including environment) to promote infant adaptation and development.

Actions/Interventions

Nursing Priority No. 1.

To assess infant status and parental skill level:

- Determine the infant's chronological and developmental age; note the length of gestation.
- Identify the infant's individual self-regulatory behaviors, such as suck, mouth, grasp, hand-to-mouth, face behaviors, foot clasp, brace, limb flexion, trunk tuck, and boundary seeking.
- Observe for cues suggesting the presence of situations that may result in pain/discomfort.
- Evaluate level and appropriateness of environmental stimuli.
- Ascertain the parents' understanding of the infant's needs and abilities.

Information that appears in brackets has been added by the authors to clarify and enhance the use of nursing diagnoses.

- Listen to the parents' perceptions of their capabilities to promote the infant's development.

Nursing Priority No. 2.

To assist parents to enhance infant's integration:

- Review infant growth and development, pointing out current status and progressive expectations.
- Identify cues reflecting infant stress.
- Discuss possible modifications of environmental stimuli, handling, activity schedule, sleep, and pain control needs based on the infant's behavioral cues. **Stimulation that is properly timed and appropriate in complexity and intensity allows the infant to maintain a stable balance of his/her subsystems and enhances development.**
- Provide positive feedback for parental involvement in the caregiving process. **The transfer of care from staff to parents progresses along a continuum as parents' confidence level increases and they are able to take on more responsibility.**
- Discuss use of skin-to-skin contact (kangaroo care [KC]), as appropriate. **Research suggests KC may have a positive effect on infant development by enhancing neurophysiological organization as well as an indirect effect by improving parental mood, perceptions, and interactive behavior.**
- Incorporate parents' observations and suggestions into the plan of care. **This demonstrates value of and regard for parents' input and enhances the sense of ability to deal with situations.**

Nursing Priority No. 3.

To promote wellness (Teaching/Learning Considerations):

- Identify community resources (e.g., visiting nurse, home-care support, and childcare).
- Refer to support group or individual role model **to facilitate adjustment to new roles/responsibilities.**
- Refer to additional NDs, such as readiness for enhanced family Coping.

Documentation Focus

Assessment/Reassessment

- Findings, including infant's self-regulation and readiness for stimulation; chronological and developmental age
- Parents' concerns/level of knowledge

Information that appears in brackets has been added by the authors to clarify and enhance the use of nursing diagnoses.

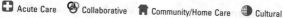

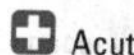
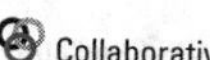
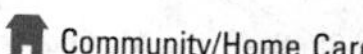
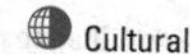

Planning

- Plan of care and who is involved in the planning
- Teaching plan

Implementation/Evaluation

- Infant's responses to interventions and actions performed
- Parents' participation and response to interactions and teaching
- Attainment or progress toward desired outcome(s)
- Modifications of plan of care

Discharge Planning

- Long-term needs and who is responsible for actions to be taken
- Specific referrals made

Sample Nursing Outcomes & Interventions Classifications (NOC/NIC)

NOC—Neurological Status
NIC—Developmental Enhancement: Infant

risk for BLEEDING

[Diagnostic Division: Circulation]

Definition: Vulnerable to decrease in blood volume, that may compromise health.

Risk Factors

Aneurysm; disseminated intravascular coaguloapathy; inherent coagulopathy (e.g., thrombocytopenia)
Gastrointestinal condition (e.g., ulcer, polyps, varices); impaired liver function (e.g., cirrhosis, hepatitis)
History of falls; trauma
Insufficient knowledge of bleeding precautions
Pregnancy complication (e.g., premature rupture of membranes, placenta previa/abruption, multiple gestation); postpartum complications (e.g., uterine atony, retained placenta)
Treatment regimen [e.g., surgery, medications, administration of platelet-deficient blood products, chemotherapy]; circumcision

Information that appears in brackets has been added by the authors to clarify and enhance the use of nursing diagnoses.

NOTE: A risk diagnosis is not evidenced by signs and symptoms, as the problem has not occurred; rather, nursing interventions are directed at prevention.

Desired Outcomes/Evaluation Criteria—Client Will:

- Be free of signs of active bleeding, such as hemoptysis, hematuria, hematemesis, or excessive blood loss, as evidenced by stable vital signs, skin and mucous membranes free of pallor, and usual mentation and urinary output.
- Display laboratory results for clotting times and factors within normal range for individual.
- Identify individual risks and engage in appropriate behaviors or lifestyle changes to prevent or reduce the frequency of bleeding episodes.

Actions/Interventions

Nursing Priority No. 1.

To assess risk factors:

- Assess client risk, noting possible medical diagnoses or disease processes that may lead to bleeding as listed in risk factors.
- Note the type of injury/injuries when the client presents with trauma. **The pattern and extent of injury and bleeding may or may not be readily determined. For example, unbroken skin can hide a significant injury where a large amount of blood is lost within soft tissues; or a crush injury resulting in interruption of the integrity of the pelvic ring can cause life-threatening bleeding from three sources: arterial, venous, and bone edge bleeding.**
- Determine the presence of hereditary factors, obtain a detailed history if a familial bleeding disorder is suspected, such as hereditary hemorrhagic telangiectasia (HHT), hemophilia, other factor deficiencies, or thrombocytopenia. **Hereditary bleeding or clotting disorders predispose the client to bleeding complications, necessitating specialized testing and/or referral to a hematologist.**
- ∞ Note the client's gender. **While bleeding disorders are common in both men and women, women are affected more owing to the increased risk of blood loss related to menstrual cycle and pregnancy complications/delivery procedures.**

Information that appears in brackets has been added by the authors to clarify and enhance the use of nursing diagnoses.

- Identify pregnancy-related factors, as indicated. **Many factors can occur, including overdistention of the uterus—pregnant with multiples, prolonged or rapid labor, lacerations occurring during vaginal delivery, or retained placenta that can place the mother at risk for postpartum bleeding.**
- Evaluate the client's medication regimen. **The use of medications, such as NSAIDs, anticoagulants, corticosteroids, and certain herbals (e.g., *Ginkgo biloba*), predispose client to bleeding.**

Nursing Priority No. 2.

To evaluate for potential bleeding:

- Monitor perineum and fundal height in a postpartum client, and wounds, dressings, or tubes in a client with trauma, surgery, or other invasive procedures **to identify active blood loss. Note: Hemorrhage may occur because of the inability to achieve hemostasis in the setting of injury or may result from the development of a coagulopathy.**
- Evaluate and mark boundaries of soft tissues in enclosed structures, such as a leg or abdomen, **to document expanding bruises or hematomas.**
- Assess vital signs, including blood pressure, pulse, and respirations. Measure blood pressure lying/sitting/standing as indicated to evaluate for orthostatic hypotension; monitor invasive hemodynamic parameters when present **to determine if an intravascular fluid deficit exists. Note: Fit, young patients may lose 40% of their blood volume before the systolic blood pressure drops below 100 mm Hg, whereas the elderly may become hypotensive with volume loss of as little as 10%.**
- Hematest all secretions and excretions for occult blood **to determine possible sources of bleeding.**
- Note client report of pain in specific areas, whether pain is increasing, diffuse, or localized. **This can help to identify bleeding into tissues, organs, or body cavities.**
- Assess skin color and moisture, urinary output, level of consciousness, or mentation. **Changes in these signs may be indicative of blood loss affecting systemic circulation or local organ function such as kidneys or brain.**
- Review laboratory data (e.g., complete blood count [CBC], platelet numbers and function, and other coagulation factors such as Factor I, Factor II, prothrombin time [PT], partial thromboplastin time [PTT], and fibrinogen) **to evaluate**

Information that appears in brackets has been added by the authors to clarify and enhance the use of nursing diagnoses.

bleeding risk. An abrupt drop in Hb of 2 g/dL can indicate active bleeding.

- Prepare the client for or assist with diagnostic studies such as x-rays, computed tomography (CT) or magnetic resonance imaging (MRI) scans, ultrasound, or colonoscopy **to determine the presence of injuries or disorders that could cause internal bleeding.**

Nursing Priority No. 3.

To prevent bleeding/correct potential causes of excessive blood loss:

- Apply direct pressure and cold pack to bleeding site, insert nasal packing, or perform fundal massage as appropriate.
- Restrict activity and encourage bedrest or chair rest until bleeding abates.
- Maintain the patency of vascular access **for fluid administration or blood replacement as indicated.**
- Assist with the treatment of underlying conditions causing or contributing to blood loss such as medical treatment of systemic infections or balloon tamponade of esophageal varices prior to sclerotherapy; use of proton pump inhibitor medications or antibiotics for gastric ulcer; or surgery for internal abdominal trauma or retained placenta.
- Provide special intervention for the at-risk client, such as an individual with bone marrow suppression, chemotherapy, or uremia, **to prevent bleeding associated with tissue injury:**

  Monitor closely for overt bleeding.

  Observe for diffuse oozing from tubes, wounds, or orifices with no observable clotting.

  Maintain direct pressure or pressure dressings as indicated for a longer period of time over arterial puncture sites **to prevent oozing or active bleeding.**

  Hematest secretions and excretions for occult blood **for early identification of internal bleeding.**

  Protect the client from trauma such as falls, accidental or intentional blows, or lacerations.

  Use soft toothbrush or toothettes for oral care **to reduce risk of injury to the oral mucosa.**
- Collaborate in evaluating the need for replacing blood loss or specific components and be prepared for emergency interventions.
- Be prepared to administer hemostatic agents, if needed **to promote clotting and diminish bleeding by increasing coagulation factors,** or medications to prevent bleeding such as

---

Information that appears in brackets has been added by the authors to clarify and enhance the use of nursing diagnoses.

proton pump inhibitors to reduce risk of gastrointestinal bleeding.

- Provide information to client/family about hereditary or familial problems that predispose to bleeding complications.

Nursing Priority No. 4.

To promote wellness (Teaching/Discharge Considerations):

- Provide information to the client/family about hereditary or familial problems that predispose to bleeding complications.
- Instruct at-risk client and family regarding:

Specific signs of bleeding requiring healthcare provider notification, such as active bright bleeding anywhere, prolonged epistaxis or trauma in a client with known factor bleeding tendencies, black tarry stools, weakness, vertigo, syncope, and so forth

Need to inform healthcare providers when taking aspirin and other anticoagulants (e.g., Coumadin, Plavix), especially when elective surgery or other invasive procedure is planned **(These agents will most likely be withheld for a period of time prior to elective procedures to reduce potential for excessive blood loss.)**

Importance of periodic review of client's medication regimen **to identify medications (prescriptions, OTC and herbals) that might cause or exacerbate bleeding problems**

Necessity of regular medical and laboratory follow-up when on anticoagulants **to determine needed dosage changes or client management issues requiring monitoring and/or modification**

Dietary measures to improve blood clotting, such as foods rich in vitamin K

Need to avoid alcohol in diagnosed liver disorders or seek treatment for alcoholism in the presence of alcoholic varices

Techniques for postpartum client to check her own fundus and perform fundal massage as indicated, and to contact physician for postdischarge bleeding that is bright red or dark red with large clots **(may prevent blood loss complications, especially if client is discharged early from hospital)**

Documentation Focus

Assessment/Reassessment

- Individual factors that may potentiate blood loss—type of injuries, obstetrical complications, and so on

Information that appears in brackets has been added by the authors to clarify and enhance the use of nursing diagnoses.

- Baseline vital signs, mentation, urinary output, and subsequent assessments
- Results of laboratory tests or diagnostic procedures

Planning
- Plan of care and who is involved in the planning
- Teaching plan

Implementation/Evaluation
- Responses to interventions, teaching, and actions performed
- Attainment or progress toward desired outcome(s)
- Modifications to plan of care

Discharge Planning
- Long-term needs, identifying who is responsible for actions to be taken
- Community resources or support for chronic problems
- Specific referrals made

Sample Nursing Outcomes & Interventions Classifications (NOC/NIC)

NOC—Blood Loss Severity
NIC—Bleeding Precautions

risk for unstable BLOOD GLUCOSE LEVEL

[Diagnostic Division: Food/Fluid]

Definition: Vulnerable to variation of blood glucose/sugar levels from the normal range, which may compromise health.

Risk Factors

Does not accept diagnosis; insufficient knowledge of diabetes management

Insufficient diabetes management or nonadherence to diabetes management plan; inadequate blood glucose monitoring; ineffective medication management

Insufficient dietary intake; excessive weight gain or loss; rapid growth period; pregnancy

Compromised physical health status

Average daily physical activity is less than recommended for gender and age

Information that appears in brackets has been added by the authors to clarify and enhance the use of nursing diagnoses.

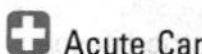

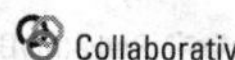

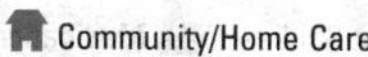

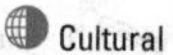

Excessive stress; alteration in mental status
Delay in cognitive development

NOTE: A risk diagnosis is not evidenced by signs and symptoms, as the problem has not occurred; rather, nursing interventions are directed at prevention.

Desired Outcomes/Evaluation Criteria—Client/Caregiver Will:

- Acknowledge factors that may lead to unstable glucose.
- Verbalize understanding of body and energy needs.
- Verbalize plan for modifying factors to prevent or minimize shifts in glucose level.
- Maintain glucose within satisfactory range.

Actions/Interventions

Nursing Priority No. 1.

To assess risk/contributing factors:

- Determine individual factors that may contribute to unstable glucose as listed in risk factors. **Client or family history of diabetes, known diabetic with poor glucose control, eating disorders (e.g., morbid obesity), poor exercise habits, or a failure to recognize changes in glucose needs or control due to adolescent growth spurts or pregnancy can result in problems with glucose stability.**
- Ascertain the client's/SO's knowledge and understanding of condition and treatment needs.
- Identify individual perceptions and expectations of treatment regimen.
- Note the influence of cultural, ethnic origin, socioeconomic, or religious factors impacting diabetes recognition and care, including how a person with diabetes is viewed by family and community; the seeking and receiving of healthcare; the management of factors such as dietary practices, weight, blood pressure, and lipids; and expectations of outcomes. **These factors influence a client's ability to manage his or her condition and must be considered when planning care.**
- Determine the client's awareness and ability to be responsible for dealing with the situation. **Age, maturity, current health status, and developmental stage all affect a client's ability to provide for his or her own safety.**
- Assess family/SO(s) support of the client. **The client may need assistance with lifestyle changes (e.g., food prepara-**

Information that appears in brackets has been added by the authors to clarify and enhance the use of nursing diagnoses.

tion or consumption, timing of intake and/or exercise, or administration of medications).

- Note the availability and use of resources.

Nursing Priority No. 2.

To assist client to develop preventive strategies to avoid glucose instability:

- Ascertain whether client/SOs are certain they are obtaining accurate readings on their glucose-monitoring device and are adept at using the device. **In addition to checking blood glucose more frequently when it is unstable, it is wise to ascertain that equipment is functioning properly and being used correctly. All available devices will provide accurate readings if properly used, maintained, and routinely calibrated. However, there are many other factors that may affect the accuracy of numbers, such as the size of blood drop with finger-sticking, forgetting a bolus from insulin pump, and injecting insulin into a lumpy subcutaneous site.**
- Provide information on balancing food intake, antidiabetic agents, and energy expenditure.
- Review medical necessity for regularly scheduled lab screening and monitoring tests for diabetes. **Screening tests may include fasting plasma glucose or oral glucose tolerance tests. In the known or sick diabetic, tests can include fasting and daily (or numerous times in a day) finger-stick glucose levels. Also, in diabetics, regular testing of hemoglobin (Hgb) A_1C and the estimated average glucose (eAG) helps determine glucose control over several months.**
- Discuss home glucose monitoring according to individual parameters (e.g., six times a day for a normal day and more frequently during times of stress) **to identify and manage glucose variations.**
- Review the client's common situations that could contribute to glucose instability on daily, occasional, or crisis bases. **Multiple factors can play a role at any time, such as missing meals, adolescent growth spurt, or infection or other illness.**
- Review the client's diet, especially carbohydrate intake. **Glucose balance is determined by the amount of carbohydrates consumed, which should be determined in needed grams per day.**
- Encourage the client to read labels and choose carbohydrates described as having a low glycemic index (GI), and foods with adequate protein, higher fiber, and low fat content. **These**

Information that appears in brackets has been added by the authors to clarify and enhance the use of nursing diagnoses.

foods produce a slower rise in blood glucose and more stable release of insulin.**

- Discuss how the client's antidiabetic medication(s) work. **Drugs and combinations of drugs work in varying ways with different blood glucose control and side effects. Understanding drug actions can help the client avoid or reduce the risk of potential for hypoglycemic reactions.**

For Client Receiving Insulin

- Emphasize the importance of checking expiration dates of medications, inspecting insulin for cloudiness if it is normally clear, and monitoring proper storage and preparation (when mixing required). **These factors affect insulin absorbability.**
- Review the type(s) of insulin used (e.g., rapid, short, intermediate, long-acting, or premixed) and delivery method (e.g., subcutaneous, intramuscular injection, prefilled pen, or pump). Note the times when short- and long-acting insulins are administered. Remind the client that only short-acting insulin is used in the pump. **This affects the timing of effects and provides clues to potential timing of glucose instability.**
- Check injection sites periodically. **Insulin absorption can vary from day to day in healthy sites and is less absorbable in lipohypertrophic (lumpy) tissues.**
- Ascertain that all injections are being given. **Children, adolescents, and elderly clients may forget injections or be unable to self-inject and may need reminders and supervision.**

Nursing Priority No. 3.

To promote wellness (Teaching/Discharge Considerations):

- Review individual risk factors and provide information to assist client in efforts to avoid complications, such as those caused by chronic hyperglycemia and acute hypoglycemia. **Note: Hyperglycemia is most commonly caused by alterations in nutrition needs, inactivity, and/or inadequate use of antidiabetic medications. Hypoglycemia is the most common complication of antidiabetic therapy, stress, and exercise.**
- Emphasize consequences of actions and choices—both immediate and long term. **Prevention and/or management of high blood pressure and blood lipids can go a long way toward reducing complications associated with diabetes. Research suggests that close control of glucose levels over**

Information that appears in brackets has been added by the authors to clarify and enhance the use of nursing diagnoses.

time may delay onset and reduce severity of complications, enhancing quality of life.

- Engage client/family/caregiver in formulating a plan to manage blood glucose level incorporating lifestyle, age and developmental level, and physical and psychological ability to manage the condition.
- Consult with the dietitian about specific dietary needs based on individual situation (e.g., growth spurt, pregnancy, or change in activity level following injury).
- Encourage the client to develop a system for self-monitoring to provide a sense of control and enable the client to follow his or her own progress and assist with making choices.
- Refer to appropriate community resources, diabetic educator, and/or support groups, as needed, **for lifestyle modification, medical management, referral for insulin pump or glucose monitor, financial assistance for supplies, and so forth.**

Documentation Focus

Assessment/Reassessment

- Findings related to individual situation, risk factors, current caloric intake, and dietary pattern; prescription medication use; monitoring of condition
- Client's/caregiver's understanding of individual risks and potential complications
- Results of laboratory tests and finger-stick testing

Planning

- Plan of care and who is involved in planning
- Teaching plan

Implementation/Evaluation

- Individual responses to interventions, teaching, and actions performed
- Specific actions and changes that are made
- Attainment or progress toward desired outcomes
- Modifications to plan of care

Discharge Planning

- Long-term plans for ongoing needs, monitoring and management of condition, and who is responsible for actions to be taken
- Sources for equipment/supplies
- Specific referrals made

Information that appears in brackets has been added by the authors to clarify and enhance the use of nursing diagnoses.

Sample Nursing Outcomes & Interventions Classifications (NOC/NIC)

NOC—Blood Glucose Level
NIC—Hyperglycemia Management

disturbed BODY IMAGE

[Diagnostic Division: Ego Integrity]

Definition: Confusion [and/or dissatisfaction] in mental picture of one's physical self.

Related Factors

Illness; trauma; injury; surgical procedure; treatment regimen
Alteration in body function (due to anomaly, disease, medication, pregnancy, radiation, surgery, trauma, etc.)
Cultural or spiritual incongruences
Alteration in self-perception, cognitive functioning
Impaired psychosocial functioning
Developmental transition
[Significance of body part or functioning with regard to age, gender, developmental level, or basic human needs]

Defining Characteristics

Subjective

Alteration in view of one's body (e.g., appearance, structure, or function)
Perceptions that reflect an altered view of one's body appearance
Fear of reaction by others
Focus on past strength, function, or appearance
Negative feeling about body
Preoccupation with change/loss
Refusal to verify actual change
Emphasis on remaining strengths
Personalization of body part/loss by name
Depersonalization of body part/loss by use of impersonal pronouns

Objective

Behaviors of: acknowledgment of one's body, monitoring one's body

Information that appears in brackets has been added by the authors to clarify and enhance the use of nursing diagnoses.

Nonverbal response to actual or perceived change in body (e.g., appearance, structure, or function)
Alteration in body structure or function; absence of body part
Avoids looking at or touching one's body
Trauma to nonfunctioning part
Change in ability to estimate spatial relationship of body to environment
Extension of body boundary (e.g., included external object)
Hiding or overexposure of body part
Change in lifestyle, social involvement
Heightened achievement
Aggression; low frustration tolerance level

Desired Outcomes/Evaluation Criteria—Client Will:

- Verbalize an understanding of body changes.
- Recognize and incorporate body image change into self-concept in an accurate manner without negating self-esteem.
- Verbalize the acceptance of self in a situation (e.g., chronic progressive disease, amputee, decreased independence, weight as is, effects of therapeutic regimen).
- Verbalize relief of anxiety and adaptation to actual/altered body image.
- Seek information and actively pursue growth.
- Acknowledge the self as an individual who has responsibility for self.
- Use adaptive devices/prosthesis appropriately.

Actions/Interventions

Nursing Priority No. 1.

To assess causative/contributing factors:

- Discuss pathophysiology present and/or situation affecting the individual and refer to additional NDs as appropriate. For example, when alteration in body image is related to neurological deficit (e.g., cerebrovascular accident—CVA), refer to ND Unilateral Neglect; in the presence of severe, ongoing pain, refer to ND chronic Pain; or in loss of sexual desire/ability, refer to ND Sexual Dysfunction.
- Determine whether the condition is permanent with no expectation for resolution (may be associated with other NDs, such as Self-Esteem [specify] or risk for impaired Attachment, when child is affected). **There is always something that can**

Information that appears in brackets has been added by the authors to clarify and enhance the use of nursing diagnoses.

be done to enhance acceptance, and it is important to hold out the possibility of living a good life with the disability.

- Assess mental and physical influence of illness or condition on the client's emotional state (e.g., diseases of the endocrine system or use of steroid therapy).
- Evaluate the level of the client's knowledge of and anxiety related to the situation. Observe emotional changes, **which may indicate acceptance or nonacceptance of the situation.**
- Recognize behavior indicative of overconcern with the body and its processes.
- Have the client describe self, noting what is positive and what is negative. Be aware of how the client believes others see self.
- Discuss the meaning of loss/change to the client. **A small (seemingly trivial) loss may have a big impact (such as the use of a urinary catheter or enema for continence). A change in function (such as immobility in elderly) may be more difficult for some to deal with than a change in appearance. Or the change could be devastating, such as permanent facial scarring of child.**
- Use developmentally appropriate communication techniques for determining exact expression of body image in a child (e.g., puppet play or constructive dialogue for toddler). **Developmental capacity must guide interaction to gain accurate information.**
- Note signs of grieving or indicators of severe or prolonged depression **to evaluate need for counseling and/or medications.**
- Determine ethnic background and cultural and religious perceptions or considerations. **May influence how individual deals with what has happened.**
- Identify social aspects of illness or condition (e.g., sexually transmitted diseases, sterility, or chronic conditions).
- Observe interaction of client with SO(s). **Distortions in body image may be unconsciously reinforced by family members, and/or secondary gain issues may interfere with progress.**

Nursing Priority No. 2.

To determine coping abilities and skills:

- Assess the client's current level of adaptation and progress.
- Listen to the client's comments and responses to the situation. **Different situations are upsetting to different people, depending on individual coping skills and past experiences.**

Information that appears in brackets has been added by the authors to clarify and enhance the use of nursing diagnoses.

- Note withdrawn behavior and the use of denial. **This may be a normal response to a situation or may be indicative of mental illness (e.g., schizophrenia).** (Refer to ND ineffective Denial.)
- Note the use of addictive substances, such as alcohol or other drugs, **which may reflect dysfunctional coping.**
- Identify previously used coping strategies and effectiveness.
- Determine individual/family/community resources available to the client.

Nursing Priority No. 3.

To assist client and SO(s) to deal with/accept issues of self-concept related to body image:

- Establish a therapeutic nurse-client relationship, conveying an attitude of caring and developing a sense of trust.
- Visit the client frequently and acknowledge the individual as someone who is worthwhile. **This provides opportunities for listening to concerns and questions.**
- Assist in correcting underlying problems **to promote optimal healing and adaptation.**
- Provide assistance with self-care needs as necessary, while promoting individual abilities and independence.
- Work with the client's self-concept, avoiding moral judgments regarding client's efforts or progress (e.g., "You should be progressing faster"; "You're weak or not trying hard enough"). **Positive reinforcement encourages the client to continue efforts and strive for improvement.**
- Discuss concerns about fear of mutilation, prognosis, or rejection when the client is facing surgery or a potentially poor outcome of procedure/illness, **to address realities and provide emotional support.**
- Acknowledge and accept feelings of dependency, grief, and hostility.
- Encourage verbalization of and role-play anticipated conflicts **to enhance the handling of potential situations.**
- Encourage the client and SO(s) to communicate feelings to each other.
- Assume all individuals are sensitive to changes in appearance, but avoid stereotyping.
- Alert the staff to monitor their own facial expressions and other nonverbal behaviors, **because they need to convey acceptance and not revulsion when the client's appearance is affected.**
- Encourage family members to treat the client normally and not as an invalid.

Information that appears in brackets has been added by the authors to clarify and enhance the use of nursing diagnoses.

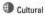

- Encourage the client to look at/touch affected body part **to begin to incorporate changes into body image.**
- Allow the client to use denial without participating (e.g., client may at first refuse to look at a colostomy; the nurse says, "I am going to change your colostomy now" and proceeds with the task). **This provides the individual with time to adapt to the situation.**
- Set limits on maladaptive behavior and assist the client to identify positive behaviors **to aid in recovery.**
- Provide accurate information as desired/requested. Reinforce previously given information.
- Discuss the availability of prosthetics, reconstructive surgery, and physical/occupational therapy or other referrals as dictated by the individual situation.
- Help the client select and use clothing or makeup **to minimize body changes and enhance appearance.**
- Discuss the reasons for infectious isolation and treatment procedures when used and make time to sit down and talk/listen to the client while in the room **to decrease the sense of isolation/loneliness.**

Nursing Priority No. 4.

To promote wellness (Teaching/Discharge Considerations):

- Begin counseling/other therapies (e.g., biofeedback or relaxation) as soon as possible **to provide early/ongoing sources of support.**
- Provide information at the client's level of acceptance and in small segments **to allow easier assimilation.** Clarify misconceptions. Reinforce explanations given by other health team members.
- Include the client in the decision-making process and problem-solving activities.
- Assist the client in incorporating the therapeutic regimen into activities of daily living (e.g., including specific exercises and housework activities). **Promotes continuation of a program.**
- Identify/plan for alterations to home and work environment/activities **to accommodate individual needs and support independence.**
- Assist the client in learning strategies for dealing with feelings and venting emotions.
- Offer positive reinforcement for efforts made (e.g., wearing makeup or using a prosthetic device).
- Refer to appropriate support groups.

Information that appears in brackets has been added by the authors to clarify and enhance the use of nursing diagnoses.

Documentation Focus

Assessment/Reassessment

- Observations, presence of maladaptive behaviors, emotional changes, stage of grieving, level of independence
- Physical wounds, dressings; use of life support–type machine (e.g., ventilator, dialysis machine)
- Meaning of loss or change to client
- Support systems available (e.g., SOs, friends, and groups)

Planning

- Plan of care and who is involved in planning
- Teaching plan

Implementation/Evaluation

- Client's response to interventions, teaching, and actions performed
- Attainment or progress toward desired outcome(s)
- Modifications of plan of care

Discharge Planning

- Long-term needs and who is responsible for actions
- Specific referrals made (e.g., rehabilitation center and community resources)

Sample Nursing Outcomes & Interventions Classifications (NOC/NIC)

NOC—Body Image
NIC—Body Image Enhancement

risk for imbalanced BODY TEMPERATURE

[Diagnostic Division: Safety]

Definition: Vulnerable to failure to maintain body temperature within normal parameters, which may compromise health.

Risk Factors

Acute brain injury; sepsis

Alteration in metabolic rate; condition affecting temperature regulation; increase in oxygen demand; inefficient nonshivering thermogenesis

Information that appears in brackets has been added by the authors to clarify and enhance the use of nursing diagnoses.

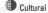

Decreased sweat response; dehydration
Extremes of age or weight; increased body surface area to weight ratio; insufficient supply of subcutaneous fat
Extremes of environmental temperature; improper clothing for environmental temperature;
Inactivity; vigorous activity
Pharmaceutical agent; sedation

NOTE: A risk diagnosis is not evidenced by signs and symptoms as the problem has not occurred; rather, nursing interventions are directed at prevention.

Desired Outcomes/Evaluation Criteria—Client Will:

- Maintain body temperature within normal range.
- Verbalize understanding of individual risk factors and appropriate interventions.
- Demonstrate behaviors for monitoring and maintaining appropriate body temperature.

Actions/Interventions

Nursing Priority No. 1.

To identify causative/risk factors present:

- Determine if present illness/condition results from exposure to environmental factors, surgery, infection, or trauma. **Helps in determining the scope of interventions that may be needed (e.g., simple addition of warm blankets after surgery or hypothermia therapy following brain trauma).**
- Monitor laboratory values (e.g., tests indicative of infection, thyroid or other endocrine tests, or drug screens) **to identify potential internal causes of temperature imbalances.**
- Note the client's age (e.g., premature neonate, young child, or aging individual), **as it can directly impact the ability to maintain/regulate body temperature and respond to changes in the environment.**
- Assess nutritional status **to determine the metabolism effect on body temperature and to identify foods or nutrient deficits that affect metabolism.**
- Refer to NDs Hyperthermia, Hypothermia, risk for Hypothermia, risk for perioperative Hyperthermia, and ineffective Thermoregulation for related assessments and interventions.

Information that appears in brackets has been added by the authors to clarify and enhance the use of nursing diagnoses.

Nursing Priority No. 2.

To prevent occurrence of temperature alteration:

- Monitor temperature regularly, measuring core body temperature whenever needed to observe this vital sign. Exercise care in selecting an appropriate thermometer for the client's age and clinical condition and observe for inconsistencies in readings obtained with various instruments. Observe temperature reading for trends and avoid making therapeutic decisions based solely on thermometer readings. **Traditionally, temperature measurements have been taken orally (good in alert, oriented adult), rectally (accurate but not always easy to obtain), or axillary (readings may be lower than core temperature), with each site offering advantages and disadvantages in terms of accuracy and safety. Newer technologies allow temperatures to be instantly measured. Tympanic temperature measurement is a noninvasive way to measure core temperature, as blood is supplied to the tympanic membrane by the carotid artery.**
- Monitor and maintain comfortable ambient environment (e.g., provide heating/cooling measures such as space heaters/fans) as indicated **to reduce the effect on body temperature alterations.**
- Supervise the use of heating pads, electric blankets, ice bags, and hypothermia blankets, especially in clients who cannot self-protect.
- Dress the client or discuss with the client/caregiver(s) appropriate dressing (e.g., layering clothing, use of hat and gloves in cold weather, light loose clothing in warm weather, or water-resistant outer gear for rainy weather).
- Cover the infant's head with a knit cap, place under adequate blankets, and provide for skin-to-skin contact with the mother. Place the newborn infant under a radiant warmer. **Heat loss in newborns/infants, especially very low weight neonates, is greatest through head and by evaporation and convection.**
- Limit clothing or remove the blanket from a premature infant placed in an incubator **to prevent overheating in a climate-controlled environment.**
- Maintain good nutrition and adequate fluid intake. Offer cool or warm liquids, as appropriate. **Good nutrition and hydration assist in maintaining normal body temperature.**
- Review the client's medications (e.g., diuretics, certain sedatives and antipsychotic agents, some heart and blood pres-

---

Information that appears in brackets has been added by the authors to clarify and enhance the use of nursing diagnoses.

sure medications, or anesthesia) **for possible thermoregulatory side effects.**

- Recommend lifestyle changes, such as cessation of smoking or substance use (such as methamphetamines), normalization of body weight, nutritious meals, and regular exercise **to prevent overheating and loss of regulatory body mechanisms, and to maximize metabolism to meet individual needs.**
- Refer at-risk persons to appropriate community resources (e.g., home care, social services, foster adult care, and housing agencies) **to provide assistance to meet individual needs.**

Nursing Priority No. 3.

To promote wellness (Teaching/Discharge Considerations):

- Discuss potential problems/individual risk factors with client/SO(s).
- Review age and gender issues, as appropriate. **Older or debilitated persons, babies, and young children typically feel more comfortable in higher ambient temperatures. Women notice feeling cooler quicker than men, which may be related to body size, or to differences in metabolism and the rate that blood flows to extremities to regulate body temperature.**
- Instruct in appropriate self-care measures (e.g., adding or removing clothing, adding or removing heat sources, reviewing medication regimen with physician to identify those which can affect thermoregulation, evaluating home/shelter for the ability to manage heat and cold, addressing nutritional and hydration status) **to protect from identified risk factors.**
- Review ways to prevent accidental temperature alterations, such as hypothermia resulting from overzealous cooling to reduce fever or maintaining too warm an environment for a client who has lost the ability to perspire.

Documentation Focus

Assessment/Reassessment

- Identified individual causative and risk factors
- Record of core temperature, initially and prn
- Results of diagnostic studies and laboratory tests

Planning

- Plan of care and who is involved in planning
- Teaching plan, including best ambient temperature, and ways to prevent hypothermia or hyperthermia

Information that appears in brackets has been added by the authors to clarify and enhance the use of nursing diagnoses.

Implementation/Evaluation

- Response to interventions, teaching, and actions performed
- Attainment or progress toward desired outcome(s)
- Modifications to plan of care

Discharge Planning

- Long-term needs and who is responsible for actions
- Specific referrals made

Sample Nursing Outcomes & Interventions Classifications (NOC/NIC)

NOC—Thermoregulation
NIC—Temperature Regulation

ineffective BREASTFEEDING

[Diagnostic Division: Food/Fluid]

Definition: Dissatisfaction or difficulty that a mother, infant, or child experiences with the breastfeeding process.

Related Factors

Insufficient parental knowledge regarding importance of breastfeeding or breastfeeding techniques
Insufficient opportunity for suckling at the breast; inadequate milk supply; delayed lactogenesis II
Prematurity; [late preterm (35 to 37 weeks)]; poor infant sucking reflex
Oropharyngeal defect [e.g., cleft palate/lip, ankyloglossia (tongue tied)]
Supplemental feedings with artificial nipple; pacifier use
Maternal anxiety or ambivalence, fatigue, pain, obesity
Previous history of breastfeeding failure
Interrupted breastfeeding; short maternity leave
Maternal breast anomaly; previous breast surgery

Defining Characteristics

Subjective

Sore nipples persisting beyond the first week of breastfeeding
Insufficient emptying of each breast per feeding
Perceived inadequate milk supply

Information that appears in brackets has been added by the authors to clarify and enhance the use of nursing diagnoses.

 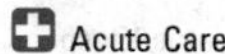 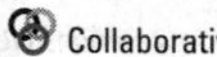 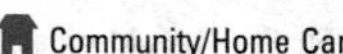  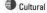

Objective

Insufficient opportunity for suckling at the breast

Infant inability to latch onto maternal breast correctly; unsustained suckling at the breast

Infant arching/crying at the breast; resisting latching on to breast

Infant crying within the first hour after breastfeeding; fussing within one hour of breastfeeding; unresponsive to other comfort measures

Insufficient signs of oxytocin release

Inadequate infant stooling

Insufficient infant weight gain; sustained infant weight loss

Desired Outcomes/Evaluation Criteria—Client Will:

- Verbalize understanding of causative or contributing factors.
- Demonstrate techniques to enhance breastfeeding experience.
- Assume responsibility for effective breastfeeding.
- Achieve mutually satisfactory breastfeeding regimen with infant content after feedings, gaining weight appropriately, and output within normal range.

Actions/Interventions

Nursing Priority No. 1.

To identify maternal causative or contributing factors:

- Assess client knowledge about breastfeeding and extent of instruction that has been given.
- Identify cultural expectations and conflicts about breastfeeding and beliefs or practices regarding lactation, let-down techniques, and maternal food preferences.
- Note incorrect myths/misunderstandings especially in teenage mothers, **who are more likely to have limited knowledge and more concerns about body image issues.**
- Encourage discussion of current and previous breastfeeding experience(s).
- Note previous unsatisfactory experience (including self or others), **because it may lead to negative expectations.**
- Perform physical assessment, noting appearance of breasts and nipples, marked asymmetry of breasts, obvious inverted or flat nipples, or minimal or no breast enlargement during pregnancy.
- Determine whether lactation failure is primary **(i.e., maternal prolactin deficiency/serum prolactin levels, inadequate mammary gland tissue, breast surgery that has damaged**

Information that appears in brackets has been added by the authors to clarify and enhance the use of nursing diagnoses.

the nipple, areola enervation [irremediable], and pituitary disorders) or secondary **(i.e., sore nipples, severe engorgement, plugged milk ducts, mastitis, inhibition of letdown reflex, and maternal/infant separation with disruption of feedings [treatable]).** ***Note:*** **Overweight or obese women are 2.5 and 3.6 times less successful, respectively, in initiating breastfeeding than the general population.**

- Note history of pregnancy, labor, and delivery (vaginal or cesarean section), other recent or current surgery, preexisting medical problems (e.g., diabetes, seizure disorder, cardiac diseases, or presence of disabilities), or adoptive mother.
- Identify maternal support systems or presence and response of SO(s), extended family, and friends. **The infant's father and maternal grandmother (in addition to caring healthcare providers) are important factors that contribute to successful breastfeeding.**
- Ascertain the mother's age, number of children at home, and need to return to work.
- Determine maternal feelings (e.g., fear/anxiety, ambivalence, or depression).

Nursing Priority No. 2.

To assess infant causative/contributing factors:

- Determine suckling problems, as noted in Related Factors/Defining Characteristics.
- Note prematurity and/or infant anomaly (e.g., cleft lip/palate) **to determine special equipment/feeding needs.**
- Review feeding schedule to note increased demand for feeding (at least eight times a day, taking both breasts at each feeding for more than 15 min on each side) or use of supplements with artificial nipple.
- Evaluate observable signs of inadequate infant intake (e.g., baby latches onto mother's nipples with sustained suckling but minimal audible swallowing or gulping noted, infant arching and crying at the breasts with resistance to latching on, decreased urinary output and frequency of stools, or inadequate weight gain).
- Determine whether the baby is content after feeding or exhibits fussiness and crying within the first hour after breastfeeding, **suggesting unsatisfactory breastfeeding process.**
- Note any correlation between maternal ingestion of certain foods and "colicky" response of infant.

Information that appears in brackets has been added by the authors to clarify and enhance the use of nursing diagnoses.

Nursing Priority No. 3.

To assist mother to develop skills of successful breastfeeding:

- Provide emotional support to the mother. Use one-to-one instruction with each feeding during hospital stay and clinic or home visit. Refer adoptive mothers choosing to breastfeed to a lactation consultant **to assist with induced lactation techniques.**
- Discuss early infant feeding cues (e.g., rooting, lip smacking, and sucking fingers/hand) versus late cue of crying. **Early recognition of infant hunger promotes timely/more rewarding feeding experience for infant and mother.**
- Inform the mother how to assess and correct a latch if needed. Demonstrate asymmetric latch aiming infant's lower lip as far from base of the nipple as possible, then bringing infant's chin and lower jaw in contact with breast while mouth is wide open and before upper lip touches breast.
- Recommend avoidance or overuse of supplemental feedings and pacifiers (unless specifically indicated), **which can lessen the infant's desire to breastfeed/increase risk of early weaning. Note: Adoptive mothers may not develop a full breast milk supply, necessitating supplemental feedings.**
- Restrict the use of nipple shields (i.e., only temporarily to help draw the nipple out) and then place the baby directly on the nipple.
- Demonstrate the use of hand expression, hand pump, and piston-type electric breast pump with bilateral collection chamber when necessary **to maintain or increase the milk supply.**
- Discuss/demonstrate breastfeeding aids (e.g., infant sling, nursing pillows, or footstool).
- Suggest using a variety of nursing positions **to find the most comfortable for mother and infant. Positions particularly helpful for plus-sized women or those with large breasts include the "football" hold with the infant's head to the mother's breast and body curved around behind mother or lying down to nurse.**
- Encourage frequent rest periods, sharing household/childcare duties **to limit fatigue and facilitate relaxation at feeding times.**
- Recommend abstinence/restriction of tobacco, caffeine, alcohol, drugs, and excess sugar, as appropriate, **because they may affect milk production and the let-down reflex or be passed on to the infant.**

Information that appears in brackets has been added by the authors to clarify and enhance the use of nursing diagnoses.

- Promote early management of breastfeeding problems. For example:

  Engorgement: Wear a supportive bra, apply heat and/or cool applications to the breasts, and massage from chest wall down to nipple **to enhance let-down reflex;** soothe a "fussy baby" before latching on the breast; properly position the baby on the breast/nipple; alternate the side baby starts nursing on; nurse round the clock and/or pump with piston-type electric breast pump with bilateral collection chambers at least 8 to 12 times a day; and avoid using bottle, pacifier, or supplements.

  Sore nipples: Wear 100% cotton fabrics; do not use soap or alcohol/other drying agents on nipples; avoid the use of nipple shields or nursing pads that contain plastic; cleanse and then pat dry with a clean cloth; apply a thin layer of USP modified lanolin on the nipple, and administer a mild pain reliever as appropriate. **Note:** The infant should latch on to the least sore side or the mother should begin with hand expression **to establish the let-down reflex;** properly position the infant on the breast/nipple and use a variety of nursing positions. Break suction after breastfeeding is complete.

  Clogged ducts: Use a larger bra or extender to avoid pressure on the site; use moist or dry heat; gently massage from above the plug down to the nipple; nurse the infant, hand express, or pump after massage; nurse more often on the affected side.

  Inhibited let-down: Use relaxation techniques before nursing (e.g., maintain quiet atmosphere, massage the breast, apply heat to breasts, have beverage available, assume a position of comfort, place the infant on the mother's chest skin-to-skin). Develop a routine for nursing, and encourage the mother to enjoy her baby.

  Mastitis: Promote bedrest (with infant) for several days; administer antibiotics; provide warm, moist heat before and during nursing; and empty breasts completely. Continue to nurse the baby at least 8 to 12 times a day or pump breasts for 24 hours and then resume breastfeeding as appropriate.

Nursing Priority No. 4.

To condition the infant to breastfeed:

- Scent breast pad with breast milk and leave in bed with infant along with mother's photograph when separated from mother for medical purposes (e.g., prematurity).

Information that appears in brackets has been added by the authors to clarify and enhance the use of nursing diagnoses.

- Increase skin-to-skin contact (kangaroo care).
- Provide practice times at breast for infant to "lick and learn."
- Express small amounts of milk into the baby's mouth.
- Have the mother pump breast after feeding to enhance milk production.
- Use supplemental nutrition system cautiously when necessary.
- Identify special interventions for feeding in the presence of cleft lip/palate. **These measures promote optimal interaction between mother and infant and provide adequate nourishment for the infant, enhancing successful breastfeeding.**

Nursing Priority No. 5.

To promote wellness (Teaching/Discharge Considerations):

- Schedule a follow-up visit with the healthcare provider 48 hr after hospital discharge and 2 weeks after birth **for evaluation of milk intake/breastfeeding process and to answer the mother's questions.**
- Recommend monitoring the number of infant's wet/soiled diapers. **Stools should be yellow in color, and the infant should have at least six wet diapers a day to determine that the infant is receiving sufficient intake.**
- Weigh the infant at least every third day initially as indicated, and record **to verify adequacy of nutritional intake.**
- Educate father/SO about benefits of breastfeeding and how to manage common lactation challenges. **Enlisting the support of the father/SO is associated with a higher ratio of successful breastfeeding at 6 mo.**
- Promote peer and cultural group counseling for teen mothers. **This provides a positive role model that the teen can relate to and feel comfortable with when discussing concerns/feelings.**
- Review the mother's need for rest, relaxation, and time with other children as appropriate.
- Discuss the importance of adequate nutrition and fluid intake, prenatal vitamins, or other vitamin/mineral supplements, such as vitamin C, as indicated.
- Address specific problems (e.g., suckling problems or prematurity facial anomalies).
- Discuss the timing of the introduction of solid foods and the importance of delaying until the infant is at least 4 mo, preferably 6 mo old. If supplementation is necessary, the infant can be finger fed, spoon fed, cup fed, or syringe fed.

Information that appears in brackets has been added by the authors to clarify and enhance the use of nursing diagnoses.

- Inform the mother that return of menses within the first 3 mo after the infant's birth may indicate inadequate prolactin levels.
- Refer to support groups (e.g., La Leche League, parenting support groups, stress reduction, or other community resources, as indicated).
- Provide bibliotherapy/appropriate Web sites for further information.

Documentation Focus

Assessment/Reassessment

- Identified assessment factors, both maternal and infant (e.g., engorgement present, infant demonstrating adequate weight gain without supplementation)

Planning

- Plan of care, specific interventions, and who is involved in planning
- Teaching plan

Implementation/Evaluation

- Mother's/infant's responses to interventions, teaching, and actions performed
- Changes in infant's weight and output
- Attainment or progress toward desired outcome(s)
- Modifications to plan of care

Discharge Planning

- Referrals that have been made and mother's choice of participation

Sample Nursing Outcomes & Interventions Classifications (NOC/NIC)

NOC—Breastfeeding Establishment: Maternal [or] Infant
NIC—Breastfeeding Assistance

interrupted BREASTFEEDING

[Diagnostic Division: Food/Fluid]

Definition: Break in the continuity of providing milk to an infant or young child directly from the breasts, which may compromise breastfeeding success and/or nutritional status of the infant/child.

Information that appears in brackets has been added by the authors to clarify and enhance the use of nursing diagnoses.

  Acute Care 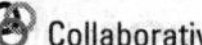 Collaborative 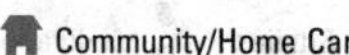 Community/Home Care 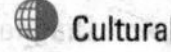 Cultural

Related Factors

Maternal/infant illness
Prematurity
Maternal-infant separation; maternal employment; hospitalization of child
Contraindications to breastfeeding (e.g., pharmaceutical agents)
Need to abruptly wean infant

Defining Characteristics

Subjective

Nonexclusive breastfeeding

Desired Outcomes/Evaluation Criteria—Client Will:

- Identify and demonstrate techniques to sustain lactation until breastfeeding is reinitiated.
- Achieve mutually satisfactory feeding regimen, with infant content after feedings and gaining weight appropriately.
- Achieve weaning and cessation of lactation if desired or necessary.

Actions/Interventions

Nursing Priority No. 1.

To identify causative/contributing factors:

- Assess client knowledge and perceptions about breastfeeding and extent of instruction that has been given.
- Note myths/misunderstandings, especially in some cultures and in teenage mothers, **who are more likely to have limited knowledge and concerns about body image issues.**
- Ascertain cultural expectations/conflicts.
- Encourage the discussion of current/previous breastfeeding experience(s). **This is useful for determining efforts needed to continue breastfeeding, if desired, while circumstances interrupting process are resolved, if possible.**
- Determine maternal responsibilities, routines, and scheduled activities (e.g., caretaking of siblings, employment in/out of home, work/school schedules of family members, ability to visit hospitalized infant).
- Identify factors necessitating interruption, or occasionally cessation, of breastfeeding (e.g., maternal illness, drug use) and desire or need to wean infant. **In general, infants with chronic diseases benefit from breastfeeding. Only a few**

Information that appears in brackets has been added by the authors to clarify and enhance the use of nursing diagnoses.

maternal infections (e.g., HIV, active/untreated tuberculosis for initial 2 weeks of multidrug therapy, active herpes simplex of the breasts, and development of chickenpox within 5 days prior to delivery or 2 days after delivery) are hazardous to breastfeeding infants. Also, the use of antiretroviral medications/chemotherapy agents or maternal substance abuse usually requires weaning of the infant. Exposure to radiation therapy requires interruption of breastfeeding for the length of time radioactivity is known to be present in breast milk and is therefore dependent on the agent used. Note: Mother can "pump and dump" her breast milk to maintain supply and continue to breastfeed after her condition has resolved (e.g., chickenpox).

- Determine support systems available to the mother/family. **The infant's father and maternal grandmother, in addition to caring healthcare providers, are important factors that contribute to successful breastfeeding.**

Nursing Priority No. 2.

To assist the mother to maintain breastfeeding if desired:

- Provide information as needed regarding the need/decision to interrupt breastfeeding.
- Give emotional support to the mother and support her decision regarding cessation or continuation of breastfeeding. **Many women are ambivalent about breastfeeding, and providing information about the pros and cons of both breastfeeding and bottle feeding, along with support for the mother's/couple's decision, will promote a positive experience.**
- Promote peer counseling for teen mothers. **This provides a positive role model that the teen can relate to and feel comfortable with discussing concerns/feelings.**
- Educate the father/SO about the benefits of breastfeeding and how to manage common lactation challenges. **Enlisting the support of the father/SO is associated with a higher ratio of successful breastfeeding at 6 mo.**
- Discuss/demonstrate breastfeeding aids (e.g., infant sling, nursing footstool/pillows, hand expression, manual and/or piston-type electric breast pumps). **This enhances comfort and relaxation for breastfeeding. When circumstances dictate that the mother and infant are separated for a time, whether by illness, prematurity, or returning to work or school, the milk supply can be maintained by use of the**

Information that appears in brackets has been added by the authors to clarify and enhance the use of nursing diagnoses.

pump. Storing the milk for future use enables the infant to continue to receive the value of breast milk. Learning the correct technique is important for successful use of the pump.

- Suggest abstinence/restriction of tobacco, caffeine, excess sugar, alcohol, certain medications, all illicit drugs, as appropriate, when breastfeeding is reinitiated **because they may affect milk production/let-down reflex or be passed on to the infant.**
- Review techniques for expression and storage of breast milk **to provide optimal nutrition and promote continuation of breastfeeding process.**
- Problem-solve return-to-work (or school) issues or periodic infant care requiring bottle/supplemental feeding.
- Provide privacy/calm surroundings when the mother breastfeeds in a hospital/work setting. **Note: Federal Law 2010 requires an employer to provide a place and reasonable break time for an employee to express her breast milk for her baby for 1 yr after birth.**
- Determine if a routine visiting schedule or advance warning can be provided **so that the infant will be hungry/ready to feed.**
- Recommend using expressed breast milk instead of formula or at least partial breastfeeding for as long as mother and child are satisfied. **This prevents permanent interruption in breastfeeding, decreasing the risk of premature weaning.**
- Encourage the mother to obtain adequate rest, maintain fluid and nutritional intake, continue her prenatal vitamins, and schedule breast pumping every 3 hr while awake, as indicated **to sustain adequate milk production and breastfeeding process.**

Nursing Priority No. 3.

To promote successful infant feeding:

- Recommend/provide for infant sucking on a regular basis, especially if gavage feedings are part of the therapeutic regimen. **This reinforces that feeding time is pleasurable and enhances digestion.**
- Discuss the proper use and choice of supplemental nutrition and alternate feeding methods (e.g., bottle/syringe) if desired.
- Review safety precautions (e.g., proper flow of formula from nipple, frequency of burping, holding bottle instead of propping, formula preparation, and sterilization techniques).

Information that appears in brackets has been added by the authors to clarify and enhance the use of nursing diagnoses.

Nursing Priority No. 4.

To promote wellness (Teaching/Discharge Considerations):

- Identify other means (other than breastfeeding) of nurturing and strengthening infant attachment (e.g., comforting, consoling, or play activities).
- Explain anticipated changes in feeding needs/frequency. **Growth spurts require increased intake/more feedings by infant.**
- Refer to support groups (e.g., La Leche League or Lact-Aid), community resources (e.g., a public health nurse; a lactation specialist; Women, Infants, and Children program; and electric pump rental programs).
- Promote the use of bibliotherapy/appropriate Web sites for further information.
- Discuss the timing of the introduction of solid foods and the importance of delaying until the infant is at least 4 mo, preferably 6 mo old, if possible. **The American Academy of Pediatrics and the World Health Organization (WHO) recommend delaying solids until at least 6 mo. If supplementation is necessary, the infant can be finger fed, spoon fed, cup fed, or syringe fed.**

Nursing Priority No. 5.

To assist the mother in the weaning process when desired:

- Provide emotional support to the mother and accept decision regarding cessation of breastfeeding. **Feelings of sadness are common even if weaning is the mother's choice.**
- Discuss reducing the frequency of daily feedings and breast pumping by one session every 2 to 3 days. **This is the preferred method of weaning, if circumstance permits, to reduce problems associated with engorgement.**
- Encourage wearing a snug, well-fitting bra, but refrain from binding breasts **because of increased risk of clogged milk ducts and inflammation.**
- Recommend expressing some milk from breasts regularly each day over a period of 1 to 3 weeks, if necessary, **to reduce discomfort associated with engorgement until milk production decreases.**
- Suggest holding the infant differently during bottle feeding/interactions or having another family member give the infant's bottle feeding **to prevent infant rooting for breast and to prevent stimulation of nipples.**
- Discuss the use of ibuprofen/acetaminophen **for discomfort during the weaning process.**

Information that appears in brackets has been added by the authors to clarify and enhance the use of nursing diagnoses.

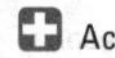 Acute Care  Collaborative 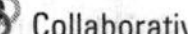 Community/Home Care 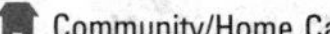 Cultural 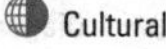

- Suggest the use of ice packs to breast tissue (not nipples) for 15 to 20 min at least four times a day **to help reduce swelling during sudden weaning.**

Documentation Focus

Assessment/Reassessment

- Baseline findings of maternal and infant factors, including mother's milk supply and infant nourishment
- Reason for interruption or cessation of breastfeeding
- Number of wet/soiled diapers daily, log of intake and output, as appropriate; periodic measurement of weight

Planning

- Method of feeding chosen
- Plan of care and who is involved in planning
- Teaching plan

Implementation/Evaluation

- Maternal response to interventions, teaching, and actions performed
- Infant's response to feeding and method
- Whether infant appears satisfied or still seems to be hungry
- Attainment or progress toward desired outcome(s)
- Modifications to plan of care

Discharge Planning

- Plan for follow-up and who is responsible
- Specific referrals made

Sample Nursing Outcomes & Interventions Classifications (NOC/NIC)

NOC—Breastfeeding Maintenance
NIC—Lactation Counseling

readiness for enhanced BREASTFEEDING

[Diagnostic Division: Food/Fluid]

Definition: A pattern of providing milk to an infant or young child directly from the breasts, which may be strengthened.

Information that appears in brackets has been added by the authors to clarify and enhance the use of nursing diagnoses.

Defining Characteristics

Subjective

Mother expresses desire to enhance ability to exclusively breastfeed

Mother expresses desire to provide breast milk for child's nutritional needs

Desired Outcomes/Evaluation Criteria—Client Will:

- Verbalize understanding of breastfeeding techniques; good latch and lactogenesis.
- Demonstrate effective techniques for breastfeeding.
- Demonstrate family involvement and support.
- Attend classes, read appropriate materials, and access resources as necessary.
- Verbalize understanding of the benefits of breast milk.

Actions/Interventions

Nursing Priority No. 1.

To determine individual learning needs:

- Assess the mother's desires/plan for feeding infant. **This provides information for developing a plan of care.**
- Assess the mother's knowledge and previous experience with breastfeeding.
- Identify cultural beliefs/practices regarding lactation, letdown techniques, and maternal food preferences. **In Western cultures, the breast has taken on a sexual connotation, and some mothers may be embarrassed to breastfeed. While breastfeeding may be accepted, in some cultures, certain beliefs may affect specific feeding practices (e.g., in Mexican-American, Navajo, Filipino, and Vietnamese cultures, colostrum is not offered to the newborn; breastfeeding begins only after the milk flow is established).**
- Note myths/misunderstandings, especially in teenage mothers, **who are more likely to have limited knowledge, as well as concerns about body image issues.**
- Evaluate the effectiveness of current breastfeeding efforts.
- Determine the support systems available to the mother/family. **In addition to caring healthcare providers, the infant's father and maternal grandmother are important factors in whether breastfeeding is successful.**

Information that appears in brackets has been added by the authors to clarify and enhance the use of nursing diagnoses.

Nursing Priority No. 2.

To promote effective breastfeeding behaviors:

- Initiate breastfeeding within the first hour after birth. **Throughout the first 2 hr after birth, the infant is usually alert and ready to nurse. Early feedings are of great benefit to the mother and the infant because oxytocin release is stimulated, helping to expel the placenta and prevent excessive maternal blood loss; the infant receives the immunological protection of colostrum, peristalsis is stimulated, lactation is accelerated, and maternal-infant bonding is enhanced.**
- Encourage skin-to-skin contact. Place the infant on the mother's stomach, skin-to-skin, after delivery.
- Demonstrate asymmetric latch aiming infant's lower lip as far from the base of the nipple as possible, then bringing the infant's chin and lower jaw in contact with the breast while the mouth is wide open and before the upper lip touches the breast. **This position allows the infant to use both tongue and jaw more effectively to obtain milk from the breast.**
- Demonstrate how to support and position the infant (e.g., infant sling or nursing footstool or pillows).
- Observe the mother's return demonstration. **This provides practice and the opportunity to correct misunderstandings and add additional information to promote the optimal experience for breastfeeding.**
- Keep the infant with the mother **for unrestricted breastfeeding duration and frequency.**
- Encourage the mother to follow a well-balanced diet containing an extra 500 calories/day, continue her prenatal vitamins, and drink at least 2,000 to 3,000 mL of fluid/day. **There is an increased need for maternal energy, protein, minerals, and vitamins, as well as increased fluid intake during lactation.**
- Provide information as needed about early infant feeding cues (e.g., rooting, lip smacking, sucking on fingers/hand) versus the late cue of crying. **Early recognition of infant hunger promotes a timely/more rewarding feeding experience for the infant and the mother.**
- Promote peer counseling for teen mothers. **This provides a positive role model that the teen can relate to and feel comfortable with discussing concerns/feelings.**

Information that appears in brackets has been added by the authors to clarify and enhance the use of nursing diagnoses.

Nursing Priority No. 3.

To enhance optimum wellness (Teaching/Discharge Considerations):

- Provide for follow-up contact or home visit 48 hr after discharge, as indicated or desired; repeat visits as necessary **to provide support and assist with problem solving.**
- Recommend monitoring the number of infant's wet diapers. **(Some pediatric care providers suggest that six wet diapers in 24 hr indicate adequate hydration.)**
- Encourage the mother/other family members to express feelings/concerns, and active-listen **to determine the nature of concerns.**
- Educate the father/SO about the benefits of breastfeeding and how to manage common lactation challenges. **Enlisting the support of the father/SO is associated with a higher ratio of successful breastfeeding at 6 mo.**
- Review techniques for expression (breast pumping) and storage of breast milk **to help sustain breastfeeding activity.**
- Problem-solve return-to-work issues or periodic infant care requiring bottle/supplemental feeding.
- Recommend using expressed breast milk instead of formula or at least partial breastfeeding for as long as mother and child are satisfied.
- Explain changes in feeding needs/frequency. **Growth spurts require increased intake/more feedings by infant.**
- Review normal nursing behaviors of older breastfeeding infants/toddlers.
- Discuss the importance of delaying the introduction of solid foods until the infant is at least 4 mo, preferably 6 mo old. **(This is recommended by the American Academy of Pediatrics and the World Health Organization.)**
- Recommend avoidance of specific medications or substances (e.g., estrogen-containing contraceptives, bromocriptine, nicotine, and alcohol) **that are known to decrease milk supply. Note: Small amounts of alcohol have not been shown to be detrimental.**
- Emphasize the importance of the client notifying healthcare providers, dentists, and pharmacists of breastfeeding status.
- Problem-solve return-to-work issues or periodic infant care requiring bottle or supplemental feeding. **This enables mothers who need or desire to return to work (for economic or personal reasons) or who simply want to attend activities without the infant to deal with these issues, thus allowing more freedom while maintaining adequate breastfeeding.**

Information that appears in brackets has been added by the authors to clarify and enhance the use of nursing diagnoses.

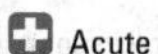

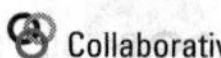

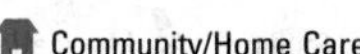

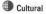

- Refer to support groups, such as the La Leche League, as indicated. Provide the mother with the phone number of a support person or group prior to leaving the hospital.
- Refer to ND ineffective Breastfeeding for more specific information addressing challenges to breastfeeding, as appropriate.

Documentation Focus

Assessment/Reassessment

- Identified assessment factors (maternal and infant)
- Number of wet diapers daily and periodic weight measurement

Planning

- Plan of care, specific interventions, and who is involved in the planning
- Teaching plan

Implementation/Evaluation

- Mother's response to actions, teaching plan, and actions performed
- Effectiveness of infant's efforts to feed
- Attainment or progress toward desired outcome(s)
- Modifications to plan of care

Discharge Planning

- Long-term needs, referrals, and who is responsible for follow-up actions

Sample Nursing Outcomes & Interventions Classifications (NOC/NIC)

NOC—Breastfeeding Maintenance
NIC—Lactation Counseling

insufficient BREAST MILK

[Diagnostic Division: Food/Fluid]

Definition: Low production of maternal breast milk.

Information that appears in brackets has been added by the authors to clarify and enhance the use of nursing diagnoses.

Related Factors

Mother

Insufficient fluid volume [e.g., dehydration, hemorrhage]
Smoking; alcohol consumption
Malnutrition
Treatment regimen [e.g., medication side effects—contraceptives, diuretics]
Pregnancy

Infant

Ineffective latching on to breast, sucking reflex
Insufficient opportunity for suckling at the breast or suckling time at breast
Rejection of breast

Defining Characteristics

Objective

Mother

Expresses breast milk less than prescribed volume
Delay in milk production
Absence of milk production with nipple stimulation

Infant

Frequently seeks to suckle at breast; prolonged breastfeeding time
Suckling time at breast appears unsatisfactory; frequent crying
Refuses to suckle at breast
Voids small amounts of concentrated urine; constipation
Weight gain <500 g in a month

Desired Outcomes/Evaluation Criteria—Client Will:

- Develop plan to correct/change contributing factors.
- Demonstrate techniques to enhance milk production.
- Achieve mutually satisfactory breastfeeding pattern with infant content after feedings and gaining weight appropriately.

Actions/Interventions

Nursing Priority No. 1.

To identify maternal causative or contributing factors:

- Assess the mother's knowledge about breastfeeding and the extent of instruction that has been provided.

Information that appears in brackets has been added by the authors to clarify and enhance the use of nursing diagnoses.

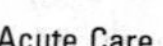
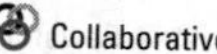
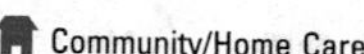
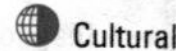

- Identify cultural expectations and conflicts about breastfeeding and beliefs or practices regarding lactation, let-down techniques, and maternal food preferences.
- Note incorrect myths/misunderstandings especially in teenage mothers, **who are more likely to have limited knowledge and more concerns about body image issues.**
- Perform a physical examination, noting the appearance of breasts and nipples, marked asymmetry of breasts, obvious inverted or flat nipples, and minimal or no breast enlargement during pregnancy. **Inadequate mammary gland tissue, breast surgery that has damaged the nipple, and areola enervation result in irremediable primary lactation failure.**
- Assess for other causes of primary lactation failure. **Maternal prolactin deficiency/serum prolactin levels, pituitary or thyroid disorders, and anemia may be corrected with medication.**
- Review lifestyle for common causes of secondary lactation failure. **Smoking, caffeine/alcohol use, birth control pills containing estrogen, medications (e.g., antihistamines, decongestants, or diuretics), stress, and fatigue are known to inhibit milk production.**
- Determine the desire/motivation to breastfeed. **Increasing the milk supply can be intense, requiring commitment to therapeutic regimen and possible lifestyle changes.**

Nursing Priority No. 2.

To identify infant causative or contributing factors:

- Observe the infant at breast to evaluate latching-on skill and the presence of suck/swallow difficulties. **Poor latching on and lack of audible swallowing/gulp are associated with inadequate intake. The infant gets substantial amounts of milk when drinking with an open-pause-close type of suck. Note: Open-pause-close is one suck; the pause is not a pause between sucks.**
- Evaluate the signs of inadequate infant intake. **Infant arching and crying at the breast with resistance to latching on, decreased urinary output/frequency of stools, and inadequate weight gain indicate the need for further evaluation and intervention.**
- Review the feeding schedule—frequency, length of feeding, and taking one or both breasts at each feeding.

Information that appears in brackets has been added by the authors to clarify and enhance the use of nursing diagnoses.

Nursing Priority No. 3.

To increase mother's milk supply:

- Instruct on how to differentiate between perceived and actual insufficient milk supply. **Normal breastfeeding frequencies, suckling times, and amounts not only vary between mothers but are also based on infant's needs/moods. Milk production is likely to be a reflection of the infant's appetite, rather than the mother's ability to produce milk.**
- Provide emotional support to the mother. Use one-to-one instruction with each feeding during the hospital stay and clinic or home visits. Refer adoptive mothers choosing to breastfeed to a lactation consultant **to assist with induced lactation techniques.**
- Inform the mother how to assess and correct a latch if needed. Demonstrate an asymmetric latch aiming the infant's lower lip as far from the base of the nipple as possible, then bringing the infant's chin and lower jaw in contact with the breast while the mouth is wide open and before the upper lip touches the breast. **Correct latching on is the most effective way to stimulate milk supply.**
- Demonstrate the breast massage technique to increase milk supply naturally. **Gently massaging the breast while the infant feeds from it can improve the release of higher-calorie hindmilk from the milk glands.**
- Use the breast pump 8 to 12 times a day. **Expressing with a hospital-grade, double (automatic) pump is ideal for stimulation/reestablishing milk supply.**
- Suggest using a breast pump or hand expression after the infant finishes breastfeeding. **Continued breast stimulation cues the mother's body that more milk is needed, increasing supply.**
- Monitor increased filling of breasts in response to nursing and/or pumping **to help evaluate the effectiveness of interventions.**
- Discuss appropriate/safe use of herbal supplements. **Herbs such as sage, parsley, oregano, peppermint, jasmine, and yarrow may have a negative affect on milk supply if taken in large quantities. A number of herbs have been used for centuries to stimulate milk production, such as fenugreek (*Trigonella foenum-graecum*), the most commonly recommended herbal galactogogue to facilitate lactation.**
- Discuss the possible use of prescribed medications (galactogogues) to increase milk production. **Domperidone (Motilium) is approved by the American Academy of Pediatrics**

Information that appears in brackets has been added by the authors to clarify and enhance the use of nursing diagnoses.

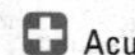

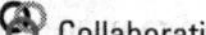
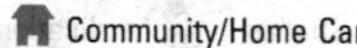
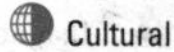

for use in breastfeeding mothers and has fewer side effects. Metoclopramide (Reglan) has been shown to increase milk supply anywhere from 72% to 110%, depending on how many weeks the mother is postpartum.

Nursing Priority No. 4.

To promote optimal success and satisfaction of breastfeeding process for mother and infant:

- Encourage frequent rest periods, sharing household and child-care tasks. **Having assistance can limit fatigue (known to impact milk production) and facilitate relaxation at feeding time.**
- Discuss with the spouse/SO the mother's requirement for rest, relaxation, and time together with family members. **This enhances understanding of mother's needs, and family members feel included and are therefore more willing to support breastfeeding activity/treatment plan.**
- Arrange a dietary consult to review nutritional needs and vitamin/mineral supplements, such as vitamin C, as indicated. **During lactation, there is an increased need for energy requiring supplementation of protein, vitamins, and minerals to provide nourishment for the infant.**
- Stress the importance of adequate fluid intake. **Alternating types of fluids (e.g., water, juice, decaffeinated tea/coffee, and milk) enhances intake, promoting milk production. Note: Beer and wine are not recommended for increasing lactation.**
- Promote peer counseling for teen mothers. **This provides a positive role model that the teen can relate to and feel comfortable with discussing concerns and feelings.**
- Recommend monitoring the number of infant's wet and soiled diapers. **Stools should be yellow in color, and the infant should have at least six wet diapers a day to determine that the infant is receiving sufficient intake.**
- Weigh the infant every 3 days, or as directed by the primary provider/lactation consultant, and record. **This monitors weight gain, verifying the adequacy of intake or the need for additional interventions.**
- Identify products/programs for cessation of smoking. **Smoking can interfere with the release of oxytocin, which stimulates the let-down reflex.**
- Refer to support groups (e.g., La Leche League, parenting support groups, stress reduction, or other community resources), as indicated.

Information that appears in brackets has been added by the authors to clarify and enhance the use of nursing diagnoses.

Documentation Focus

Assessment/Reassessment

- Identified maternal assessment factors—hydration level, medication use, lifestyle choices
- Infant assessment factors—latching-on technique, hydration level/number of wet diapers, weight gain/loss
- Use of supplemental feedings

Planning

- Plan of care, specific interventions, and who is involved in planning
- Individual teaching plan

Implementation/Evaluation

- Mother's/infant's responses to interventions, teaching, and actions performed
- Change in infant's weight
- Attainment or progress toward desired outcomes
- Modification to plan of care

Discharge Planning

- Specific referrals made

Sample Nursing Outcomes & Interventions Classifications (NOC/NIC)

NOC—Breastfeeding Maintenance
NIC—Breastfeeding Assistance

ineffective BREATHING PATTERN

[Diagnostic Division: Respiration]

Definition: Inspiration and/or expiration that does not provide adequate ventilation.

Related Factors

Neuromuscular impairment; spinal cord injury; neurological impairment (e.g., positive EEG, head trauma, seizure disorders) or immaturity
Musculoskeletal impairment; bony/chest wall deformity
Anxiety; [panic attacks]
Pain

Information that appears in brackets has been added by the authors to clarify and enhance the use of nursing diagnoses.

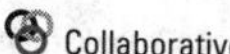

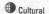

Fatigue; [deconditioning]; respiratory muscle fatigue
Body position that inhibits lung expansion; obesity
Hyperventilation; hypoventilation syndrome [alteration of client's normal O_2:CO_2 ratio (e.g., lung diseases, pulmonary hypertension, airway obstruction, or O_2 therapy in chronic obstructive pulmonary disease (COPD)]

Defining Characteristics

Subjective

Dyspnea; [feeling breathless]
Orthropnea

Objective

Bradypnea; tachypnea
Abnormal breathing pattern (e.g., rate, rhythm, depth)
Prolonged expiration phases; pursed-lip breathing
Decrease in minute ventilation; vital capacity
Decrease in inspiratory/expiratory pressure
Use of accessory muscles to breathe; use of the three-point position
Altered chest excursion; [paradoxical breathing patterns]
Nasal flaring; [grunting]
Increase in anterior-posterior diameter

Desired Outcomes/Evaluation Criteria—Client Will:

- Establish a normal, effective respiratory pattern as evidenced by absence of cyanosis and other signs/symptoms of hypoxia, with arterial blood gasses (ABGs) within client's normal or acceptable range.
- Verbalize awareness of causative factors.
- Initiate needed lifestyle changes.
- Demonstrate appropriate coping behaviors.

Actions/Interventions

Nursing Priority No. 1.

To identify etiology/precipitating factors:

- Determine the presence of factors/physical conditions as noted in Related Factors **that would cause breathing impairments.**
- ∞ 🌐 Identify age and ethnic group of client who may be at increased risk. **Respiratory ailments in general are increased**

Information that appears in brackets has been added by the authors to clarify and enhance the use of nursing diagnoses.

in infants and children with neuromuscular disorders, the frail elderly, and persons living in highly polluted environments. Smoking (and potential for smoking-related disorders) is prevalent among such groups as Appalachians, African Americans, Chinese men, Latinos, and Arabs. Communities of color are especially vulnerable as they tend to live in areas (such as close to freeways or high traffic areas) with high levels of air toxins. People most at risk for infectious pneumonias include the very young and frail elderly.

- Auscultate and percuss chest **to evaluate the presence/characteristics of breath sounds and secretions.**
- Note rate and depth of respirations and type of breathing pattern (e.g., tachypnea, grunting, Cheyne-Stokes, or other irregular patterns).
- Evaluate cough (e.g., tight or moist) and presence of secretions, **indicating possible obstruction.**
- Assist with/review results of necessary testing (e.g., chest x-rays, lung volumes/flow studies, and pulmonary function/sleep studies) **to diagnose the presence/severity of lung diseases.**
- Review laboratory data, such as ABGs **(determines degree of oxygenation and carbon dioxide [CO_2] retention),** drug screens, and pulmonary function studies **(determines vital capacity/tidal volume).**
- Note emotional responses (e.g., gasping, crying, or reports of tingling fingers). **Anxiety may be causing or exacerbating acute or chronic hyperventilation.**
- Assess for concomitant pain/discomfort **that may restrict respiratory effort.**

Nursing Priority No. 2.

To provide for relief of causative factors:

- Administer oxygen at the lowest concentration indicated and prescribed respiratory medications **for management of underlying pulmonary condition, respiratory distress, or cyanosis.**
- Suction airway, as needed, **to clear secretions.**
- Assist with bronchoscopy or chest tube insertion as indicated.
- Elevate the head of the bed and/or have the client sit up in a chair, as appropriate, **to promote physiological and psychological ease of maximal inspiration.**
- Encourage slower/deeper respirations, use of pursed-lip technique, and so on, **to assist the client in "taking control" of the situation.**

Information that appears in brackets has been added by the authors to clarify and enhance the use of nursing diagnoses.

- Monitor pulse oximetry, as indicated, **to verify maintenance/improvement in O_2 saturation.**
- Maintain a calm attitude while dealing with the client and SO(s) **to limit the level of anxiety.**
- Assist the client in the use of relaxation techniques.
- Deal with fear/anxiety that may be present. (Refer to NDs Fear; Anxiety.)
- Encourage a position of comfort. Reposition the client frequently if immobility is a factor.
- Splint the rib cage during deep-breathing exercises/cough, if indicated.
- Medicate with analgesics, as appropriate, **to promote deeper respiration and cough.** (Refer to NDs acute Pain; chronic Pain.)
- Encourage ambulation/exercise, as individually indicated.
- Avoid overeating/gas-forming foods **that may cause abdominal distention and impair breathing efforts.**
- Provide/encourage use of adjuncts, such as incentive spirometer, **to facilitate deeper respiratory effort.**
- Supervise the use of respirator/diaphragmatic stimulator, rocking bed, apnea monitor, and so forth, **when neuromuscular impairment is present.**
- Ascertain that the client possesses and properly operates continuous positive airway pressure (CPAP) machine **when obstructive sleep apnea is causing breathing problems.**
- Maintain emergency equipment in readily accessible location and include age-/size-appropriate endotrachial/trach tubes (e.g., infant, child, adolescent, or adult) **when ventilatory support might be needed.**

Nursing Priority No. 3.

To promote wellness (Teaching/Discharge Considerations):

- Review the etiology of respiratory distress, treatment options, and possible coping behaviors.
- Emphasize the importance of good posture and effective use of accessory muscles **to maximize respiratory effort.**
- Teach conscious control of the respiratory rate, as appropriate.
- Assist the client in breathing retraining (e.g., diaphragmatic, abdominal breathing, inspiratory resistive, and pursed-lip), as indicated.
- Recommend energy conservation techniques and pacing of activities.
- Refer for general exercise program (e.g., upper and lower extremity endurance and strength training), as indicated, **to maximize the client's level of functioning.**

Information that appears in brackets has been added by the authors to clarify and enhance the use of nursing diagnoses.

- Encourage adequate rest periods between activities **to limit fatigue.**
- Discuss the relationship of smoking to respiratory function. Stress the importance of smoking cessation and a smoke-free environment.
- Encourage the client/SO(s) to develop a plan **for smoking cessation.** Provide appropriate referrals.
- Review environmental factors (e.g., exposure to dust, high pollen counts, severe weather, perfumes, animal dander, household chemicals, fumes, secondhand smoke; insufficient home support for safe care) **that may require avoidance of triggers or modification of lifestyle or environment to limit the impact on the client's breathing.**
- Encourage self-assessment and symptom management:

  Use of equipment to identify respiratory decompensation, such as a peak flow meter

  Appropriate use of oxygen (dosage, route, and safety factors)

  Medication regimen, including actions, side effects, and potential interactions of medications, over-the-counter (OTC) drugs, vitamins, and herbal supplements

  Adherence to home treatments such as metered-dose inhalers (MDIs), compressors, nebulizers, and chest physiotherapies

  Dietary patterns and needs; access to foods and nutrients supportive of health and breathing

  Management of personal environment, including stress reduction, rest and sleep, social events, travel, and recreation issues

  Avoidance of known irritants, allergens, and sick persons

  Immunizations against influenza and pneumonia

  Early intervention when respiratory symptoms occur, knowing what symptoms require reporting to medical providers, and seeking emergency care
- Make a referral to pulmonary rehabilitation programs, supply resources, and support groups/contact with individuals who have encountered similar problems.

Documentation Focus

Assessment/Reassessment

- Relevant history of problem
- Respiratory pattern, breath sounds, use of accessory muscles
- Laboratory values
- Use of respiratory aids or supports, ventilator settings, and so forth

---

Information that appears in brackets has been added by the authors to clarify and enhance the use of nursing diagnoses.

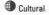

Planning

- Plan of care, specific interventions, and who is involved in the planning
- Teaching plan

Implementation/Evaluation

- Response to interventions, teaching, actions performed, and treatment regimen
- Mastery of skills; level of independence
- Attainment or progress toward desired outcome(s)
- Modifications to plan of care

Discharge Planning

- Long-term needs, including appropriate referrals and action taken, available resources
- Specific referrals provided

Sample Nursing Outcomes & Interventions Classifications (NOC/NIC)

NOC—Respiratory Status: Ventilation
NIC—Ventilation Assistance

decreased CARDIAC OUTPUT and risk for decreased CARDIAC OUTPUT

[Diagnostic Division: Circulation]

Definition: decreased Cardiac Output: Inadequate blood pumped by the heart to meet the metabolic demands of the body. [**Note:** In a hypermetabolic state, although cardiac output may be within normal range, it may still be inadequate to meet the needs of the body's tissues. Cardiac output and tissue perfusion are interrelated, although there are differences. When cardiac output is decreased, tissue perfusion problems will develop; however, tissue perfusion problems can exist without decreased cardiac output.]

Definition: risk for decreased Cardiac Output: Vulnerable to inadequate blood pumped by the heart to meet the metabolic demands of the body, which may compromise health.

Related and Risk Factors

Alteration in heart rate or rhythm
Altered afterload [e.g., systemic vascular resistance]

Information that appears in brackets has been added by the authors to clarify and enhance the use of nursing diagnoses.

Altered contractility [e.g., ventricular-septal rupture, ventricular aneurysm, papillary muscle rupture, valvular disease]
Altered preload [e.g., decreased venous return]
Altered stroke volume

Defining Characteristics (decreased Cardiac Output)

Subjective

Altered heart rate/rhythm: Heart palpitations
Altered preload: Fatigue
Altered afterload: Dyspnea; [feeling breathless]
Altered contractility: Orthopnea; paroxysmal nocturnal dyspnea [PND]
Behavioral/emotional: Anxiety

Objective

Altered heart rate/rhythm: Bradycardia; tachycardia; EKG [ECG] changes (e.g., arrhythmia, conduction abnormality, ischemia)
Altered preload: Jugular vein distention; edema; weight gain; increase or decrease in central venous pressure (CVP); increase or decrease in pulmonary artery wedge pressure (PAWP); heart murmur
Altered afterload: Clammy skin; abnormal skin color (e.g., pale, dusky, cyanosis); prolonged capillary refill; decreased peripheral pulses; alterations in blood pressure readings; increase or decrease in systemic vascular resistance (SVR); increase or decrease in pulmonary vascular resistance (PVR); oliguria
Altered contractility: Adventitious breath sounds; cough; decreased cardiac index; decrease in ejection fraction; decrease in stroke volume index (SVI) or left ventricular stroke work index (LVSWI); S_3 or S_4 sounds [gallop rhythm]
Behavioral/emotional: Restlessness

NOTE: a risk diagnosis is not evidenced by signs and symptoms as the problem has not occurred; rather nursing interventions are directed at prevention.

Desired Outcomes/Evaluation Criteria—Client Will:

- Display hemodynamic stability (e.g., blood pressure, cardiac output, renal perfusion/urinary output, peripheral pulses).

Information that appears in brackets has been added by the authors to clarify and enhance the use of nursing diagnoses.

- Report/demonstrate decreased episodes of dyspnea, angina, and dysrhythmias.
- Demonstrate an increase in activity tolerance.
- Verbalize knowledge of the disease process, individual risk factors, and treatment plan.
- Participate in activities that reduce the workload of the heart (e.g., stress management or therapeutic medication regimen program, weight reduction, balanced activity/rest plan, proper use of supplemental oxygen, cessation of smoking).
- Identify signs of cardiac decompensation, alter activities, and seek help appropriately.

Actions/Interventions

Nursing Priority No. 1.

To identify causative/contributing **or risk** factors:

- Identify clients exhibiting symptoms or at risk as noted in Related/Risk Factors and Defining Characteristics **In addition to an individual who is obviously at risk because of known cardiac problems, there is a potential for cardiac output issues in others (e.g., person with traumatic injuries and hemorrhage; brainstem trauma; spinal cord injury (SCI) at T8 or above; chronic renal failure, alcohol and other drug intoxication, substance withdrawal or overdose; or pregnant woman with hypertensive states).**
- Note age- and ethnic-related cardiovascular considerations. **In infants, failure to thrive with poor ability to suck and feed can be indications of heart problems. When in the supine position, pregnant women incur decreased vascular return during the second and third trimesters, potentially compromising cardiac output. Contractile force is naturally decreased in the elderly with reduced ability to increase cardiac output in response to increased demand. Also, arteries are stiffer, veins are more dilated, and heart valves are less competent, often resulting in systemic hypertension and blood pooling. Generally, higher risk populations for decreased cardiac output due to heart failure include African Americans, Hispanics, Native Americans, and recent immigrants from developing nations, directly related to the higher incidence and prevalence of hypertension and diabetes.**
- Assess the potential for/type of developing shock states: hematogenic, septicemic, cardiogenic, vasogenic, and psychogenic.
- Review laboratory data, including but not limited to complete blood count (CBC), electrolytes, arterial blood gases (ABGs),

Information that appears in brackets has been added by the authors to clarify and enhance the use of nursing diagnoses.

cardiac biomarkers (e.g., creatine kinase and its subclasses, troponins, myoglobin, and LDH); lactate; brain natriuretic peptide (BNP); kidney, thyroid, and liver function studies; cultures (e.g., blood, wound, or secretions); and bleeding and coagulation studies **to identify client at risk, and promote early intervention, if indicated.**

- Review diagnostic studies, including/not limited to: chest radiograph, cardiac stress testing, ECG, echocardiogram, cardiac output and ventricular ejection studies, and heart scan or catheterization. **For example, the ECG may show previous or evolving MI, left ventricular hypertrophy, and valvular stenosis. Doppler flow echocardiogram showing an ejection fraction (EF) less than 40% is indicative of systolic dysfunction.**

Nursing Priority No. 2.

To assess degree of debilitation (decreased Cardiac Outptut):

- Evaluate client reports and evidence of extreme fatigue, intolerance for activity, sudden or progressive weight gain, swelling of extremities, and progressive shortness of breath **to assess for signs of poor ventricular function and/or impending cardiac failure.**
- Determine vital signs/hemodynamic parameters including cognitive status. Note vital sign response to activity or procedures and time required to return to baseline. **This provides a baseline for comparison to follow trends and evaluate response to interventions.**
- Review signs of impending failure/shock, noting decreased cognition and unstable or subnormal blood pressure or hemodynamic parameters; tachypnea; labored respirations; changes in breath sounds (e.g., crackles or wheezing); distant or altered heart sounds (e.g., murmurs or dysrythmias); neck vein and peripheral edema; and reduced urinary output. **Early detection of changes in these parameters promotes timely intervention to limit the degree of cardiac dysfunction.**
- Note the presence of pulsus paradoxus, especially in the presence of distant heart sounds, **suggesting cardiac tamponade.**

Nursing Priority No. 3.

To minimize/correct causative factors, maximize cardiac output (decreased Cardiac Output):

Acute Phase

- Keep client on bed or chair rest in a position of comfort. (In a congestive state, semi-Fowler's position is preferred.) May

Information that appears in brackets has been added by the authors to clarify and enhance the use of nursing diagnoses.

raise legs 20 to 30 degrees in shock situation (if indicated per facility protocol). **This decreases oxygen consumption and the risk of decompensation.**

- Administer oxygen via mask or ventilator, as indicated, **to increase oxygen available for cardiac function/tissue perfusion.**
- Monitor vital signs frequently **to note response to activities and interventions.**
- Perform periodic hemodynamic measurements, as indicated. **Note: If arterial, CVP, pulmonary, and left atrial pressures and cardiac output measures are indicated, the client will be cared for in a critical care unit.**
- Monitor cardiac rhythm continuously **to note the effectiveness of medications and/or assistive devices, such as implanted pacemaker or defibrillator.**
- Administer fluids, diuretics, inotropic drugs, antidysrhythmics, steroids, vasopressors, and/or dilators, as indicated **to support systemic and cardiac circulation.** Evaluate response **to determine therapeutic, adverse, or toxic effects of therapy.**
- Restrict or administer fluids (IV/PO), as indicated **if cardiopulmonary congestion is present.** Provide adequate fluid/free water, depending on client needs.
- Assess urine output hourly or periodically; weigh daily, noting total fluid balance **to allow for timely alterations in therapeutic regimen.**
- Monitor the rate of IV drugs closely, using infusion pumps, as appropriate, **to prevent bolus or overdose.**
- Provide a quiet environment **to promote adequate rest.**
- Schedule activities and assessments **to maximize rest periods.**
- Assist with or perform self-care activities for client.
- Avoid the use of restraints whenever possible if the client is confused. **May increase agitation and increase the cardiac workload.**
- Use sedation and analgesics, as indicated, with caution **to achieve the desired effect without compromising hemodynamic readings.**
- Alter environment/bed linens and administer antipyretics or cooling measures, as indicated, **to maintain body temperature in near-normal range.**
- Encourage the client to breathe in/out during activities that increase risk for the Valsalva effect; limit suctioning/stimulation of coughing reflex in intubated client; administer stool softeners when indicated.

Information that appears in brackets has been added by the authors to clarify and enhance the use of nursing diagnoses.

- Instruct the client to avoid/limit activities that may stimulate a Valsalva response (e.g., bearing down during bowel movement), **which can cause changes in cardiac pressures and/or impede blood flow.**
- Provide psychological support. Maintain a calm attitude, but admit concerns if questioned by the client. **Honesty can be reassuring when so much activity and "worry" are apparent to the client.**
- Provide information about testing procedures and client participation.
- Assist with preparations for and monitor response to support procedures or devices as indicated (e.g., cardioversion, pacemaker, angioplasty and stent placement, coronary artery bypass graft [CABG] or valve replacement, intra-aortic balloon pump [IABP], left ventricular assist device [LVAD]). **Any number of interventions may be required to correct a condition causing heart failure or to support a failing heart during recovery from myocardial infarction, while awaiting transplantation, or for long-term management of chronic heart failure.**
- Explain dietary or fluid restrictions, as indicated.

Nursing Priority No. 4.

To maximize cardiac output or minimize risk factors:

Postacute/Chronic Phase

- Provide for adequate rest.
- Increase activity levels gradually as permitted by individual condition, noting vital sign response to activity.
- Administer medications, as appropriate, and monitor cardiac responses.
- Encourage relaxation techniques **to reduce anxiety, muscle tension.**
- Elevate legs when in sitting position (if heart failure present or extremities are edematous). Apply antiembolic hose or sequential compression devices when indicated, being sure they are individually fitted and appropriately applied. **This limits venous stasis, improves venous return and systemic circulation, and reduces the risk of thrombophlebitis.**
- Avoid a prolonged sitting position for all clients, and supine position for sleep or exercise for gravid clients (second and third trimesters) **to maximize vascular return.**
- Encourage relaxation techniques **to reduce anxiety and conserve energy.**

Information that appears in brackets has been added by the authors to clarify and enhance the use of nursing diagnoses.

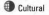

- Provide skin protective measures (e.g., frequent position changes, early ambulation, monitoring of bony prominences, sheepskin or special flotation mattress) **to avoid the development of pressure sores in the setting of impaired circulation and generalized weakness or debilitation.** Refer to ND risk for Pressure Ulcer, as indicated.

Nursing Priority No. 5.

To maintain nutrition and fluid balance:

- Provide for diet restrictions (e.g., low-sodium, bland, soft, low-calorie/low fat diet, with frequent small feedings), as indicated.
- Note reports of anorexia or nausea and withhold oral intake, as indicated.
- Provide fluids and electrolytes, as indicated, **to minimize dehydration and dysrhythmias.**
- Monitor intake/output and calculate 24-hour fluid balance.

Nursing Priority No. 6.

To promote wellness (Teaching/Discharge Considerations):

For client with decreased Cardiac Output:

- Review specifics of drug regimen, diet, exercise/activity plan. Emphasize necessity for long-term management of cardiac conditions.
- Discuss significant signs/symptoms that require prompt reporting to healthcare provider (e.g., muscle cramps, headaches, dizziness, or skin rashes), **which may be signs of drug toxicity and/or electrolyte loss, especially potassium.**
- Emphasize importance of regular medical follow-up care. Review "danger" signs requiring immediate physician notification (e.g., unrelieved or increased chest pain, functional decline, dyspnea, or edema), **which may indicate deteriorating cardiac function, heart failure.**
- Encourage changing positions slowly and dangling legs before standing **to reduce risk for orthostatic hypotension, especially if heart failure present.**
- Give information about positive signs of improvement, such as decreased edema and improved vital signs/circulation, **to provide encouragement.**
- Teach home monitoring of weight, pulse, and/or blood pressure, as appropriate, **to detect change and allow for timely intervention.**
- Arrange time with dietitian **to determine/adjust individually appropriate diet plan.**

Information that appears in brackets has been added by the authors to clarify and enhance the use of nursing diagnoses.

- Promote visits from family/SO(s) who provide positive social interaction.
- Encourage relaxing environment, using relaxation techniques, massage therapy, soothing music, and quiet activities.
- Refer to cardiac rehabilitation program, as indicated.
- Direct client and/or caregivers to resources for emergency assistance, financial help, durable medical supplies, and psychosocial support and respite, especially when client has impaired functional capabilities or requires supporting equipment (e.g., pacemaker, LVAD, or 24-hour oxygen).
- Identify resources for weight reduction, cessation of smoking, and so forth, **to provide support for change.**
- Refer to NDs Activity Intolerance; deficient Diversional Activity; ineffective Coping; ineffective Breathing Pattern; compromised family Coping; deficient/excess Fluid Volume; imbalanced Nutrition: less than body requirements; Overweight; acute/chronic Pain; risk for decreased cardiac Tissue Perfusion; risk for ineffective peripheral Tissue Perfusion; Sexual Dysfunction, as indicated.

For at-risk client

Discuss the individual's particular risk factors (e.g., smoking, stress, obesity, or recent MI) and specific resources for assistance (e.g., written information sheets, direction to helpful Web sites, formalized rehabilitation programs, and home interventions) for management of identified risk factors.

Provide information to clients/caregivers on individual condition, therapies, and expected outcomes.

Educate client/caregivers about drug regimen, including indications, dose and dosing schedules, potential adverse side effects, or drug/drug interactions.

Provide instruction for home monitoring of weight, pulse, and blood pressure, as appropriate.

Discuss significant signs/symptoms that need to be reported to healthcare provider, such as unrelieved or increased chest pain, dyspnea, fever, swelling of ankles, and sudden unexplained cough.

Emphasize the importance of regular medical follow-up care **to monitor the client's condition and provide early intervention when indicated to prevent complications.**

Documentation Focus

Assessment/Reassessment

- Baseline and subsequent findings and individual hemodynamic parameters, heart and breath sounds, ECG pattern,

Information that appears in brackets has been added by the authors to clarify and enhance the use of nursing diagnoses.

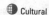

presence/strength of peripheral pulses, skin/tissue status, renal output, and mentation

Planning

- Plan of care and who is involved in planning
- Teaching plan

Implementation/Evaluation

- Client's responses to interventions, teaching, and actions performed
- Status and disposition at discharge
- Attainment or progress toward desired outcome(s)
- Modifications to plan of care

Discharge Planning

- Discharge considerations and who will be responsible for carrying out individual actions
- Long-term needs and available resources
- Specific referrals made

Sample Nursing Outcomes & Interventions Classifications (NOC/NIC)

NOC—Cardiac Pump Effectiveness
NIC—Hemodynamic Regulations
NIC—Cardiac Risk Management

risk for impaired CARDIOVASCULAR FUNCTION

[Diagnostic Division: Circulation]

Definition: Vulnerable to internal or external causes which damage one or more vital organs and the circulatory system itself.

Risk Factors

Age ≥65
Family history of cardiovascular disease; history of cardiovascular disease
Hypertension; dyslipidemia; diabetes mellitus
Insufficient knowledge of modifiable risk factors; obesity; sedentary lifestyle; smoking
Pharmaceutical agent

Information that appears in brackets has been added by the authors to clarify and enhance the use of nursing diagnoses.

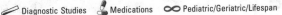

NOTE: A risk diagnosis is not evidenced by signs and symptoms, as the problem has not occurred; rather, nursing interventions are directed at prevention.

Desired Outcomes/Evaluation Criteria—Client Will:

- Be free of cardiovascular symptoms, such as hypertension, chest pain, activity intolerance, altered mental status, changes in heart rate or rhythm, syncope, decreased skin temperature, or diminished peripheral pulses.
- Verbalize knowledge of the disease process, individual risk factors, and treatment plan.
- Participate in activities that promote cardiovascular health (e.g., stress management, therapeutic medication regimen program, weight reduction, balanced activity/rest plan, and cessation of smoking).

Actions/Interventions

Nursing Priority No. 1.

To identify client at risk:

- Note the client's age and gender and family history when assessing risk for cardiovascular disease (CVD). **Risks that cannot be controlled include increasing age, gender, and heredity. The American Heart Association states that "risk for heart disorders increases with age, and men are still considered at higher risk for myocardial infarction and experience them earlier in life."**
- Review with the client his or her past history of conditions associated with cardiovascular impairment, such as heart attack, stroke, diabetes, and peripheral vascular conditions **to help assess current risk for recurrence.**
- Determine if the client has condition known as "metabolic syndrome" (i.e., large waistline, high triglyceride level, low HDL cholesterol level [or is on medications to lower triglycerides or cholesterol]; is hypertensive, and has high fasting blood glucose or A_1C. **Metabolic risk factors are strongly associated with increased risk for heart disease and stroke, especially when combined with other risk factors such as smoking, sedentary lifestyle, and obesity.**
- Inquire about the client's current and past history of smoking. **Smoking is associated with vasoconstriction which causes decreased blood flow and reduced oxygenation of organs, which can impair cardiovascular function.**

Information that appears in brackets has been added by the authors to clarify and enhance the use of nursing diagnoses.

- Note the client's weight and dietary habits **to determine if obesity or poor nutrition are risk factors. Note: Studies have shown that overweight and obesity predispose to or are associated with coronary heart disease, heart failure, and sudden death because of their impact on the cardiovascular system.**

Nursing Priority No. 2.

To determine changes in cardiovascular status:

- Investigate reports of chest pain, headache, or pain in the extremities **to identify potential problem with cardiovascular perfusion.**
- Measure the client's blood pressure at each medical provider visit **to identify the client with high blood pressure (risk factor) or unknown or uncontrolled hypertension.**
- Investigate reports of difficulty breathing; note respiratory rate outside of acceptable parameters, **which can be indicative of oxygen exchange problems with potential for cardiac and/or systemic vascular dysfunction.**
- Review diagnostic studies, including/not limited to electrocardiogram (ECG), echocardiogram, body mass scan or other nutrition screen, or screening heart scan **to determine if cardiovascular concerns are developing.**
- Review laboratory data, including but not limited to lipid studies (e.g., cholesterol, triglycerides), electrolytes, fasting blood glucose, glucose tolerance, insulin resistance, and A_1C; cardiac biomarkers; kidney, thyroid, and liver function studies **to identify imbalances or disease processes, and to take preventive measures when needed. Note: Familial hypercholesterolemia (FH) is an inherited disorder that is thought to lead to aggressive and premature onset cardiovascular disease. Also, it has long been known that an assoiation exits between diabetes mellitus and increased cardiovasular risk.**
- Assess for restlessness, fatigue, changes in level of consciousness, increased capillary refill time, diminished peripheral pulses, and pale, cool skin. **These are signs and symptoms of inadequate systemic perfusion, which can cause or affect cardiovascular function.**
- Assess heart sounds and pulses. **This helps identify conditions associated with inadequate myocardial or systemic tissue perfusion, dehydration, immobility, electrolyte, or acid-base imbalances.**
- Investigate reports of difficulty breathing; note respiratory rate outside of acceptable parameters, **which can be indicative of**

Information that appears in brackets has been added by the authors to clarify and enhance the use of nursing diagnoses.

oxygen exchange problems with potential for cardiopulmonary dysfunction.

- Assess for extremity discoloration, changes in pulses, temperature, or color, and client report of discomfort/pain. **These signs and symptoms are associated with systemic or peripheral vascular conditions.**

Nursing Priority No. 3.

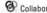

To promote cardiovascular health (Teaching/Discharge Considerations):

- Discuss the risk factors (e.g., family history, obesity, age, smoking, hypertension, diabetes, and clotting disorders) and potential outcomes of atherosclerosis (e.g., systemic and cardiac disease conditions). **This is information necessary for the client to make informed decisions concerning risk factors, and to commit to lifestyle changes necessary to prevent onset of complications or manage symptoms when condition present.**
- Review difference between modifiable and nonmodifiable risk factors **to assist client/SO in understanding those areas in which he/she can take action or make healthy choices.**
- Recommend maintenance of normal weight or weight loss if client is obese **to decrease risk associated with overweight and obesity.**
- Encourage smoking cessation, when indicated, offering information about stop-smoking aids and programs. **Smoking cessation is important in the medical management of many contributors to heart attack and stroke. These include atherosclerosis (fatty buildups in arteries), thrombosis (blood clots), artery spasm (e.g., coronary, carotid, or cerebral), and cardiac dysrhythmias.**
- Encourage the client to engage in regular exercise **to enhance circulation and promote healthy blood pressure and general well-being.**
- Review medications on a regular basis **to manage those that affect cardiac function or those given to prevent blood pressure or thromboembolic problems.**
- Discuss drug use where indicated (including cocaine, methamphetamines, or alcohol) **to educate client regarding effect of drug on cardiovascular system.**
- Encourage the client in high-risk categories (e.g., strong family history, diabetic, or prior history of cardiac event) to

---

Information that appears in brackets has been added by the authors to clarify and enhance the use of nursing diagnoses.

have regular medical examinations **to provide timely intervention, when needed.**

- Refer to educational or community resources, as indicated. **The client/SO may benefit from instruction and support provided by agencies to engage in healthier heart activities (e.g., weight loss, smoking cessation, or exercise).**
- Instruct in blood pressure monitoring at home if indicated; advise purchase of home monitoring equipment; refer to community resources as indicated. **This facilitates management of hypertension which is a major risk factor for damage to blood vessels or organ function.**

Documentation Focus

Assessment/Reassessment

- Individual findings, noting specific risk factors including diet, exercise, smoking
- Vital signs, pulse oximetry, cardiac rhythm, presence of dysrhythmias, capillary refill
- Status of organ function (e.g., mentation, breath sounds, or renal output)

Planning

- Plan of care and who is involved in planning
- Teaching plan

Implementation/Evaluation

- Response to interventions, teaching, and actions performed
- Attainment or progress toward desired outcome(s)
- Modifications to plan of care

Discharge Planning

- Long-term needs and who is responsible for actions to be taken
- Available resources, specific referrals made

Sample Nursing Outcomes & Interventions Classifications (NOC/NIC)

NOC—Circulation Status
NIC—Cardiac Risk Management

Information that appears in brackets has been added by the authors to clarify and enhance the use of nursing diagnoses.

ineffective CHILDBEARING PROCESS and risk for ineffective CHILDBEARING PROCESS

[Diagnostic Division: Sexuality]

Definition: ineffective Childbearing Process: Pregnancy and childbirth process and care of the newborn that does not match the environmental context, norms, and expectations.*

Definition: risk for ineffective Childbearing Process: Vulnerable to not matching the environmental context, norms, and expectations of pregnancy, childbirth process, and care of the newborn.

Related and Risk Factors

Insufficient knowledge of childbearing process; unrealistic birth plan
Unplanned/unwanted pregnancy
Inconsistent prenatal health visits; insufficient prenatal care
Inadequate maternal nutrition
Substance abuse
Insufficient parental role model or cognitive readiness for parenting,
Low maternal confidence
Maternal powerlessness, psychological distress; insufficient support systems
Unsafe environment; domestic violence

Defining Characteristics (ineffective Childbearing Process)

Subjective

During Pregnancy

Inadequate prenatal lifestyle (e.g., nutrition, elimination, sleep, exercise, personal hygiene)
Ineffective management of unpleasant symptoms in pregnancy
Unrealistic birth plan

*The original Japanese term for "childbearing" (*shussan ikujikoudou*), which encompasses both childbirth and rearing of the neonate. It is one of the main concepts of Japanese midwifery.

Information that appears in brackets has been added by the authors to clarify and enhance the use of nursing diagnoses.

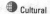

During Labor and Delivery

Inadequate lifestyle for stage of labor (e.g., nutrition, elimination, sleep, exercise, personal hygiene)

After Birth

Inadequate postpartum lifestyle (e.g., nutrition, elimination, sleep, exercise, personal hygiene)

Objective

During Pregnancy

Inadequate prenatal care

Insufficient access of support system

Inadequate preparation of the home environment

Inadequate preparation of newborn care items; insufficient respect for unborn baby

During Labor and Delivery

Inappropriate responce to onset of labor; decrease in proactivity during labor and delivery

Insufficient attachment behavior

Insufficient access of support system

After Birth

Insufficient attachment behavior

Inappropriate baby feeding techniques; inadequate baby care techniques

Unsafe environment for an infant

Inappropriate breast care

Insufficient access of support system

NOTE: A risk diagnosis is not evidenced by signs and symptoms, as the problem has not occurred; rather, nursing interventions are directed at prevention.

Desired Outcomes/Evaluation Criteria—Client Will:

- Acknowledge and address individual risk factors.
- Demonstrate healthy pregnancy free of preventable complications.
- Engage in activities to prepare for birth process and care of newborn.
- Experience complication-free labor and childbirth.
- Verbalize understanding of care requirements to promote health of self and infant.

Information that appears in brackets has been added by the authors to clarify and enhance the use of nursing diagnoses.

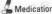

Actions/Interventions

Nursing Priority No. 1.

To determine causative **or risk** factors and individual needs:

Prenatal Concerns

- Determine maternal health/nutritional status, usual pregravid weight, and dietary pattern. **Research studies have found a positive correlation between pregravid maternal obesity and increased perinatal morbidity rates (e.g., hypertension and gestational diabetes) associated with preterm births and macrosomia.**
- Note use of alcohol/other drugs and nicotine. **Maternal pregnancy complications and negative effects on the developing fetus are increased with the use of tobacco, alcohol, and illicit drugs. Note: Prescription medications may also be dangerous to the fetus, requiring a risk/benefit analysis for therapeutic choices and appropriate dosage.**
- Evaluate current knowledge regarding physiological and psychological changes associated with pregnancy. **This provides information to assist in identifying needs and creating an individual plan of care.**
- Identify involvement/response of child's father to pregnancy. **This helps clarify whether or not the father is likely to be supportive or has the potential of posing a threat to the safety and well-being of mother/fetus.**
- Determine individual family stressors, economic situation/ financial needs, and availability/use of resources **to identify necessary referrals.**
- Verify environmental well-being and safety of client/family. **Women experiencing intimate partner violence both prior to and/or during pregnancy are at higher risk for multiple poor maternal and infant health outcomes.**
- Determine cultural expectations/beliefs about child bearing, self-care, and so on. Identify who provides support/instruction within the client's culture (e.g., grandmother/other family member, cuerandero/doula, or other cultural healer). Work with support person(s) as desired by the client, using an interpreter as needed. **This helps ensure quality and continuity of care because support person(s) can reinforce information provided.**
- Ascertain the client's commitments to work, family, and self; roles/responsibilities within family unit; and use of supportive resources. **This helps in setting realistic priorities to assist the client in making adjustments, such as changing work**

Information that appears in brackets has been added by the authors to clarify and enhance the use of nursing diagnoses.

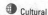

hours, shifting household chores, curtailing some outside commitments.

- Determine the client's/couple's perception of the fetus as a separate entity and extent of preparations being made for this infant. **The absence of activities such as choosing a name or nicknaming the baby in utero and home preparations indicate lack of completion of psychological tasks of pregnancy. Note: Cultural or familial beliefs may limit visible preparations out of concern that a bad outcome might result.**

Labor and Delivery Concerns

- Ascertain the client's understanding and expectations of the labor process and who will participate/provide support. **The client's/couple's coping skills are more challenged during the active and transitional phases as contractions become increasingly intense. Lack of knowledge, misconceptions, or unrealistic expectations can have a negative impact on coping abilities.**
- Determine the presence/appropriateness of the birth plan developed by the client/couple and any associated cultural expectations/preferences. **This identifies areas to address to ensure that choices made are amenable to the specific care setting, reflect reality of client/fetal status, and accommodate individual wishes.**

Postpartum/Newborn Care Concerns

- Determine the plan for discharge after delivery and home care support/needs. **This is important to facilitate discharge and ensure client/infant needs will be met.**
- Appraise the level of the parent's understanding of physiological needs and adaptation to extrauterine life associated with maintenance of body temperature, nutrition, respiratory needs, and bowel and bladder functioning. **This identifies areas of concern/need requiring development of a teaching plan and/or demonstration of care activities.**
- Assess the mother's strengths and needs, noting age, relationship status, and reactions of family members. **This identifies potential risk factors that may influence the client's/couple's ability to assume the role of parenthood. For example, an adolescent still formulating goals and identity may have difficulty accepting the infant as a person. The single parent who lacks support systems may have difficulty assuming sole responsibility for parenting.**

Information that appears in brackets has been added by the authors to clarify and enhance the use of nursing diagnoses.

- Ascertain the nature of emotional and physical parenting that the client/couple received during their childhood. **The parenting role is learned, and individuals use their own parents as role models. Those who experienced a negative upbringing or poor parenting may require additional support to meet the challenges of effective parenting.**

Nursing Priority No. 2.

To promote optimal maternal well-being:

Prenatal

- Emphasize the importance of maternal well-being including discussion of nutrition, regular moderate exercise, comfort measures, rest, breast care, and sexual activity. **Fetal well-being is directly related to maternal health, especially during the first trimester, when developing organ systems are most vulnerable to injury from environmental or hereditary factors:**

  Review nutrition requirements and optimal prenatal weight gain to support maternal-fetal needs. **Inadequate prenatal weight gain and/or below normal prepregnancy weight increases the risk of intrauterine growth retardation (IUGR) in the fetus and delivery of a low-birth-weight (LBW) infant.**

  Encourage moderate exercise such as walking or non-weight-bearing activities (e.g., swimming, bicycling) in accordance with the client's physical condition and cultural beliefs. **Exercise tends to shorten labor, increases likelihood of a spontaneous vaginal delivery, and decreases need for oxytocin augmentation.**

  Recommend a consistent sleep and rest schedule (e.g., 1- to 2-hour daytime nap and 8 hours of sleep each night) in a dark, comfortable room. **This provides rest to meet metabolic needs associated with growth of maternal and fetal tissues.**

- Provide necessary referrals (e.g., dietitian, social services, supplemental nutrition assistance programs) as indicated. **Federal/state food programs promote optimal maternal, fetal, and infant nutrition.**
- Encourage participation in smoking cessation program, alcohol/drug abstinence as appropriate. **This reduces the risk of premature birth, stillbirth, low birth weight, congenital defects, drug withdrawal of newborn, and fetal alcohol syndrome.**

Information that appears in brackets has been added by the authors to clarify and enhance the use of nursing diagnoses.

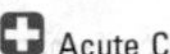

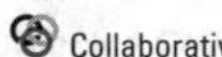

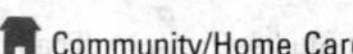

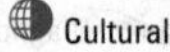

- Explain psychological reactions including ambivalence, introspection, stress reactions, and emotional lability as characteristic of pregnancy. **Helps client/couple understand mood swings and may provide opportunity for partner to offer support and affection at these times. Note: However, the stressors associated with pregnancy may lead to abuse/exacerbate existing abusive behavior.**
- Discuss personal situation and options, providing information about resources available to client. **The partner may be upset about an unplanned pregnancy, have financial concerns regarding supporting the child, or may even be jealous that attention is shifting to the unborn child, creating safety issues for client/family.**
- Identify reportable potential danger signals of pregnancy, such as bleeding, cramping, acute abdominal pain, backache, edema, visual disturbances, headaches, and pelvic pressure. **This helps the client distinguish normal from abnormal findings, thus assisting her in seeking timely, appropriate healthcare.** (Refer to ND risk for disturbed Maternal-Fetal Dyad for additional interventions.)

Labor and Delivery

- Monitor labor progress and maternal and fetal well-being per protocol. Provide continuous intrapartal professional support/doula. **Fear of abandonment can intensify as labor progresses, and client may experience increased anxiety and or loss of control when left unattended.**
- Identify the client's support person/coach and ascertain that the individual is providing support the client requires. **The coach may be the client's husband/SO or doula and needs to provide physical and emotional support for the mother and aid in initiation of bonding with the neonate.**

Postpartum

- Promote sleep and rest. **This reduces the metabolic rate and allows energy and oxygen to be used for the healing process.**
- Ascertain the client's perception of labor and delivery, length of labor, and fatigue level. **There is a correlation between length of labor and the ability of some clients to assume responsibility for self-care/infant-care tasks and activities.**
- Assess the client's readiness for learning. Assist the client in identifying needs. **The postpartum period provides an opportunity to foster maternal growth, maturation, and competence.**

Information that appears in brackets has been added by the authors to clarify and enhance the use of nursing diagnoses.

- Provide information about self-care, including perineal care and hygiene; physiological changes, including normal progression of lochial flow; needs for sleep and rest; importance of progressive postpartum exercise program; and role changes. **This helps prevent infection, fosters healing and recuperation, and contributes to positive adaptation to physical and emotional changes enhancing feelings of general well-being.**
- Review nipple and breast care, special dietary needs for lactating mother, factors that facilitate or interfere with successful breastfeeding, use of breast pump and appropriate suppliers, proper storage of expressed milk or preparation/storage of formula, as indicated. **This prevents nipple cracking and soreness enhancing comfort, facilitates role of breastfeeding mother, and helps ensure an adequate milk supply.**
- Discuss normal psychological changes and needs associated with the postpartal period. **The client's emotional state may be somewhat labile at this time and often is influenced by physical well-being. Anticipating such changes may reduce the stress associated with this transition period that necessitates learning new roles and taking on new responsibilities**
- Discuss sexuality needs and plans for contraception. Provide information about available methods, including advantages/disadvantages. **Client/couple may need clarification regarding available contraception methods and the fact that pregnancy could occur even prior to the 4- to 6-week postpartum visit.**
- Reinforce the importance of postpartum examination by a healthcare provider and interim follow-up as appropriate. **A follow-up visit is necessary to evaluate recovery of reproductive organs, healing of episiotomy/laceration repair, general well-being, and adaptation to life changes.**

Nursing Priority No. 3.

To promote appropriate participation in childbearing process:

Prenatal

- Develop nurse-client relationship and maintain an open attitude toward beliefs of the client/couple. **Acceptance is important to developing and maintaining a relationship and supporting independence.**
- Explain office visit routine and rationale for ongoing screening and close monitoring (e.g., urine testing, blood pressure monitoring, weight, fetal growth). Emphasize the importance

Information that appears in brackets has been added by the authors to clarify and enhance the use of nursing diagnoses.

of keeping regular appointments. **This reinforces the relationship between health assessment and positive outcomes for mother and baby.**

- Suggest father/siblings attend office visits and listen to fetal heart tones (FHTs) as appropriate. **This promotes a sense of involvement and helps make baby a reality for family members.**
- Provide anticipatory guidance regarding health habits/lifestyle and employment concerns:

  Review physical changes to be expected during each trimester. **Prepares client/couple for managing common discomforts associated with pregnancy.**

  Discuss signs/symptoms requiring evaluation by primary provider during prenatal period (e.g., excessive vomiting, fever, unresolved illness of any kind, and decreased fetal movement). **This allows for timely intervention.**

  Identify anticipatory adaptations for SO/family necessitated by pregnancy. **Family members will need to be flexible in adjusting own roles and responsibilities in order to assist client to meet her needs related to the demands of pregnancy.**

  Provide information about potential teratogens, such as alcohol, nicotine, illicit drugs, the STORCH group of viruses (syphilis, toxoplasmosis, other, rubella, cytomegalovirus [CMV], herpes simplex), and HIV. **This helps the client make informed decisions/choices about behaviors/environment that can promote healthy offspring. Note: Research supports the attribution of a wide range of negative effects in the neonate to alcohol, recreational drug use, and smoking.**
- Provide information about the need for additional laboratory studies, diagnostic tests, or procedure(s). Review risks and potential side effects **to facilitate the decision-making process.**
- Discuss signs of labor onset, how to distinguish between false and true labor, when to notify healthcare provider, and when to leave for birth center/hospital as appropriate; and stages of labor and delivery. **This helps ensure timely arrival and enhances coping with the labor/delivery process.**
- Determine anticipated infant feeding plan. Discuss physiology and benefits of breastfeeding. **Breastfeeding provides a protective effect against respiratory illnesses, ear infections, gastrointestinal diseases, and allergies including asthma, eczema, and atopic dermatitis.**

Information that appears in brackets has been added by the authors to clarify and enhance the use of nursing diagnoses.

- Encourage attendance at prenatal and childbirth classes. Provide information about father/sibling or grandparent participation in classes and delivery if client desires. **Knowledge gained helps reduce fear of the unknown and increases confidence that client/couple can manage the preparation for the birth of their child. This helps family members to realize they are an integral part of the pregnancy and delivery.**

Labor and Delivery

- Support use of positive coping mechanisms. **This enhances feelings of competence and fosters self-esteem.**
- Demonstrate behaviors and techniques (e.g., breathing, focused imagery, music, other distractions; aromatherapy; abdominal effleurage, back or leg rubs, sacral pressure, repositioning, back rest; oral care, linen changes, shower/tub use) that a partner can use **to assist with pain control and relaxation.**

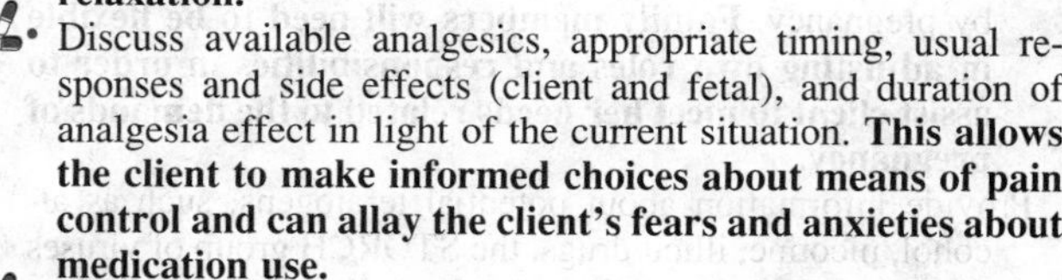

- Discuss available analgesics, appropriate timing, usual responses and side effects (client and fetal), and duration of analgesia effect in light of the current situation. **This allows the client to make informed choices about means of pain control and can allay the client's fears and anxieties about medication use.**
- Honor the client's decision about the use or nonuse of medication in a nonjudgmental manner. Continue encouragement for efforts and use of relaxation techniques. **This enhances the client's sense of control and may prevent or reduce the need for medication.**

After Birth

- Monitor and document the client's/couple's interactions with the infant. **The presence of bonding acquaintance behaviors (e.g., making eye contact, using a high-pitched voice and en face [face-to-face] position as culturally appropriate, calling infant by name, and holding infant closely) are indicators of beginning attachment process.**
- Initiate early breastfeeding or oral feeding according to facility protocol and client preference. **Initiating feeding for breastfed infants usually occurs in the delivery room. Otherwise, 5 to 15 mL of sterile water may be offered in the nursery to assess effectiveness of sucking, swallowing, gag reflexes, and patency of esophagus.**
- Provide for unlimited participation of father and siblings. Ascertain whether siblings attended orientation program. **This**

Information that appears in brackets has been added by the authors to clarify and enhance the use of nursing diagnoses.

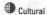

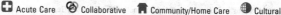

facilitates family development and ongoing process of acquaintance.

Nursing Priority No. 4.

To promote optimal well-being of newborn (Teaching/Discharge Considerations):

- Provide information about newborn interactional capabilities, states of consciousness, and means of stimulating cognitive development. **This helps parents recognize and respond to infant cues during interactional process and fosters optimal interaction, attachment behaviors, and cognitive development in the infant.**
- Note the father's/partner's response to birth and to the parenting role. **The client's ability to adapt positively to parenting may be strongly influenced by the partner's reaction.**
- Discuss normal variations and characteristics of the infant, such as caput succedaneum, cephalohematoma, pseudomenstruation, breast enlargement, physiological jaundice, and milia. **This helps parents recognize normal variations and may reduce anxiety.**
- Demonstrate/supervise infant care activities related to feeding and holding; bathing, diapering, and clothing; care of umbilical cord stump; and care of circumcised male infant. **This promotes an understanding of the principles and techniques of newborn care, fosters parents' skills as caregivers, and enhances self-confidence.**
- Note the frequency, amount, and length of feedings. Encourage demand feedings instead of scheduled feedings. Note frequency, amount, and appearance of regurgitation. **Hunger and length of time between feedings vary from feeding to feeding, and excessive regurgitation increases replacement needs.**
- Evaluate neonate and maternal satisfaction following feedings. **This provides an opportunity to answer client questions, offer encouragement for efforts, identify needs, and problem-solve situations.**
- Appraise the level of parent's understanding of physiological needs and adaptation to extrauterine life associated with maintenance of body temperature, nutrition, respiratory needs, and bowel and bladder functioning.
- Emphasize the newborn's need for follow-up laboratory tests, regular evaluations by the healthcare provider, and timely immunizations.

Information that appears in brackets has been added by the authors to clarify and enhance the use of nursing diagnoses.

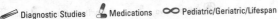

- Identify manifestations of illness and infection and when to contact healthcare provider. Demonstrate proper technique for taking temperature, administering oral medication, or providing other care activities for the infant as required. **Early recognition of illness and prompt use of healthcare facilitate timely treatment and positive outcomes.**
- Provide oral and written/pictorial information and reliable Web sites about infant care and development, feeding, and safety issues. Offer appropriate resources in client's dominant language and reflecting cultural beliefs. **This maximizes learning, providing the opportunity to review information as needed.**
- Refer the breastfeeding client to a lactation consultant/support group (e.g., La Leche League, Lact-Aid) **to promote a successful breastfeeding outcome.**
- Discuss available community support groups/parenting class as indicated. **This increases the parents' knowledge of child rearing and child development and provides a supportive atmosphere while parents incorporate new roles.**

Documentation Focus

Assessment/Reassessment

- Assessment findings, general health, previous pregnancy experience, any risks or safety concerns
- Knowledge of pre-/postpartum needs and newborn care
- Cultural beliefs and expectations
- Specific birth plan and individuals to be involved in delivery
- Arrangement for postpartum period and preparation for newborn

Planning

- Plan of care and who is involved in planning
- Individual teaching plans for pregnancy, labor/delivery, postpartum self-care, and infant care

Implementation/Evaluation

- Response to interventions, teaching, and actions performed
- Attainment or progress toward desired outcomes
- Modifications to plan of care

Discharge Planning

- Long-term needs and who is responsible for actions to be taken
- Available resources, specific referrals made

Information that appears in brackets has been added by the authors to clarify and enhance the use of nursing diagnoses.

Sample Nursing Outcomes & Interventions Classifications (NOC/NIC)

NOC—Childbirth Preparation
NIC—Knowledge: Pregnancy

readiness for enhanced CHILDBEARING PROCESS

[Diagnostic Division: Sexuality]

Definition: A pattern of preparing for and maintaining a healthy pregnancy, childbirth process, and care of the newborn for ensuring well-being, which can be strengthened.

Defining Characteristics

During Pregnancy

Subjective

Expresses desire to enhance prenatal lifestyle (e.g., nutrition, elimination, sleep, exercise, and personal hygiene)
Expresses desire to enhance knowledge of childbearing process
Expresses desire to enhance management of unpleasant pregnancy symptoms
Expresses desire to enhance preparation for newborn

During Labor and Delivery

Subjective

Expresses desire to enhance lifestyle appropriate for stage of labor (e.g., nutrition, elimination, sleep, exercise, personal hygiene) that is appropriate for the stage of labor
Expresses desire to enhance proactivity during labor and delivery

After Birth

Subjective

Expresses desire to enhance attachment behavior, baby care/feeding techniques, environmental safety for the baby
Expresses desire to enhance postpartum lifestyle (e.g., nutrition, elimination, sleep, exercise, personal hygiene), breast care
Expresses desire to enhance use of support system

Information that appears in brackets has been added by the authors to clarify and enhance the use of nursing diagnoses.

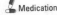

Desired Outcomes/Evaluation Criteria—Client Will

- Demonstrate healthy pregnancy free of preventable complications.
- Engage in activities to prepare for birth process and care of newborn.
- Experience complication-free labor and childbirth.
- Verbalize understanding of care requirements to promote health of self and infant.

Actions/Interventions

Nursing Priority No. 1.

To determine individual needs:

Prenatal

- Evaluate current knowledge and cultural beliefs regarding normal physiological and psychological changes of pregnancy, as well as beliefs about activities, self-care, and so on.
- Determine the degree of motivation for learning. **The client may have difficulty learning unless the need for it is clear.**
- Identify who provides support/instruction within the client's culture (e.g., grandmother/other family member, cuerandero/doula, or other cultural healer). Work with the support person(s) when possible, using an interpreter as needed. **This helps ensure quality and continuity of care because the support person(s) may be more successful than the healthcare provider in communicating information.**
- Determine the client's commitments to work, family, community, and self; roles/responsibilities within family unit; and use of supportive resources. **This helps in setting realistic priorities to assist the client in making adjustments, such as changing work hours, shifting household chores, and curtailing some outside commitments.**
- Evaluate the client's/couple's response to pregnancy, individual and family stressors, and cultural implications of pregnancy/childbirth. **The ability to adapt positively depends on support systems, cultural beliefs, resources, and effective coping mechanisms developed in dealing with past stressors.**
- Determine the client's/couple's perception of the fetus as a separate entity and the extent of preparations being made for

Information that appears in brackets has been added by the authors to clarify and enhance the use of nursing diagnoses.

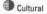

this infant. **Activities such as choosing a name or nicknaming the baby in utero and home preparations indicate completion of psychological tasks of pregnancy. Note: Cultural or familial beliefs may limit visible preparations out of concern that a bad outcome might result.**

- Assess the client's economic situation and financial needs in order to make necessary referrals.
- Determine usual pregravid weight and dietary patterns. **Research studies have found a positive correlation between pregravid maternal obesity and increased perinatal morbidity rates (e.g., hypertension and gestational diabetes) associated with preterm births and macrosomia.**

Labor and Delivery

- Ascertain the client's understanding and expectations of the labor process.
- Review the birth plan developed by the client/partner. Note cultural expectations and preferences. **This verifies that choices made are amenable to the specific care setting, accommodate individual wishes, and reflect client/fetal status.**

Postpartum/Newborn Care

- Determine the plan for discharge after delivery and home care support/needs. **Early planning can facilitate discharge and help ensure that client/infant needs will be met.**
- Ascertain the client's perception of labor and delivery, length of labor, and client's fatigue level. **There is a correlation between length of labor and the ability of some clients to assume responsibility for self-care/infant care tasks and activities.**
- Assess the mother's strengths and needs, noting age, marital status/relationship, presence and reaction of siblings and other family members, available sources of support, and cultural background. **This identifies potential risk factors and sources of support, which influence the client's/couple's ability to assume the role of parenthood. For example, an adolescent still formulating goals and an identity may have difficulty accepting the infant as a person. The single parent who lacks support systems may have difficulty assuming sole responsibility for parenting.**
- Appraise the level of parent's understanding of infant's physiological needs and adaptation to extrauterine life associated with maintenance of body temperature, nutrition, respiratory needs, and bowel and bladder functioning.
- Evaluate the nature of emotional and physical parenting that client/couple received during their childhood. **The parenting**

Information that appears in brackets has been added by the authors to clarify and enhance the use of nursing diagnoses.

role is learned, and individuals use their own parents as role models. Those who experienced a negative upbringing or poor parenting may require additional support to meet the challenges of effective parenting.

- Note the father's/partner's response to birth and to the parenting role. **The client's ability to adapt positively to parenting may be strongly influenced by the father's/partner's reaction.**
- Assess the client's readiness and motivation for learning. Assist the client/couple in identifying needs. **The postpartal period provides an opportunity to foster maternal growth, maturation, and competence.**

Nursing Priority No. 2.

To promote maximum participation in the childbearing process:

Prenatal

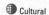

- Maintain an open attitude toward the beliefs of the client/couple. **Acceptance is important to developing and maintaining relationships and supporting independence.**
- Explain the office visit routine, and the rationale for ongoing screening and close monitoring (e.g., urine testing, blood pressure monitoring, weight, and fetal growth). Emphasize the importance of keeping regular appointments. **This reinforces the relationship between health assessment and positive outcome for mother and baby.**
- Suggest that father and siblings attend prenatal office visits and listen to fetal heart tones (FHTs) as appropriate. **This promotes a sense of involvement and helps make the baby a reality for family members.**
- Provide information about need for additional laboratory studies, diagnostic tests, or procedure(s). Review risks and potential side effects.
- Discuss any medications that may be needed to control or treat medical conditions. **Helpful in choosing treatment options because need must be weighed against possible harmful effects on the fetus.**
- Provide anticipatory guidance, including discussion of nutrition, regular moderate exercise, comfort measures, rest, employment, breast care, sexual activity, and health habits/lifestyle. **Information encourages acceptance of responsibility and promotes self-care:**

Review nutrition requirements and optimal prenatal weight gain to support maternal-fetal needs. **Inadequate prenatal weight gain and/or below normal prepregnancy weight increases the risk of intrauterine growth restriction**

Information that appears in brackets has been added by the authors to clarify and enhance the use of nursing diagnoses.

(IUGR) in the fetus and delivery of a low-birth-weight (LBW) infant.

Encourage moderate exercise such as walking, or non-weight-bearing activities (e.g., swimming or bicycling) in accordance with the client's physical condition and cultural beliefs. **This tends to shorten labor, increases the likelihood of a spontaneous vaginal delivery, and decreases the need for oxytocin augmentation.**

Recommend a consistent sleep and rest schedule (e.g., 1- to 2-hr daytime nap and 8 hr of sleep each night) in a dark, comfortable room.

Identify anticipatory adaptations for SO/family necessitated by pregnancy. **Family members will need to be flexible in adjusting their own roles and responsibilities in order to assist the client to meet her needs related to the demands of pregnancy.**

Provide/reinforce information about potential teratogens, such as alcohol, nicotine, illicit drugs, the STORCH group of viruses (syphilis, toxoplasmosis, other, rubella, cytomegalovirus, herpes simplex), and HIV. **This helps the client make informed decisions/choices about behaviors/environment that can promote healthy offspring. Note: Research supports the attribution of a wide range of negative effects in the neonate to alcohol, recreational drug use, and smoking.**

- Use various methods for learning, including pictures, to discuss fetal development. **Visualization enhances the reality of the child and strengthens the learning process.**
- Discuss the signs of labor onset, how to distinguish between false and true labor, when to notify the healthcare provider and to leave for the hospital/birth center, and stages of labor/delivery. **Helps ensure timely arrival and enhances coping with the labor/delivery process.**
- Review signs/symptoms requiring evaluation by the primary provider during the prenatal period (e.g., excessive vomiting, fever, unresolved illness of any kind, and decreased fetal movement). **This allows for timely intervention.**

Labor and Delivery

- Identify the client's support person/coach and ascertain that the individual is providing support that the client requires. **The coach may be the client's husband/SO or doula, and support can take the form of physical and emotional support for the mother and aid in initiation of bonding with the neonate.**

Information that appears in brackets has been added by the authors to clarify and enhance the use of nursing diagnoses.

- Demonstrate or review behaviors and techniques (e.g., breathing, focused imagery, music, other distractions; aromatherapy; abdominal effleurage, back or leg rubs, sacral pressure, repositioning, and back rest; oral and perineal care and linen changes; and shower/hot tub use) that the partner can use **to assist with pain control and relaxation.**
- Discuss available analgesics, usual responses and side effects (client and fetal), and duration of analgesic effect in light of current situation. **This allows the client to make an informed choice about the means of pain control; this can allay the client's fears and anxieties about medication use.**
- Support the client's decision about the use or nonuse of medication in a nonjudgmental manner. Continue encouragement for efforts and use of relaxation techniques. **Enhances the client's sense of control and may prevent or decrease the need for medication.**

Postpartum/Newborn Care

- Initiate early breastfeeding or oral feeding according to hospital protocol. **Initial feeding for breastfed infants usually occurs in the delivery room. Otherwise, 5 to 15 mL of sterile water may be offered in the nursery to assess the effectiveness of sucking, swallowing, gag reflexes, and patency of esophagus.**
- Note frequency, amount, and length of feedings. Encourage demand feedings instead of scheduled feedings. Note frequency, amount, and appearance of regurgitation. **Hunger and length of time between feedings vary from feeding to feeding, and excessive regurgitation increases replacement needs.**
- Evaluate neonate and maternal satisfaction following feedings. **This provides the opportunity to answer client questions, offer encouragement for efforts, identify needs, and problem-solve situations.**
- Demonstrate and supervise infant care activities related to feeding and holding; bathing, diapering, and clothing; care of circumcised male infant; and care of umbilical cord stump. Provide written/pictorial information for parents to refer to after discharge.
- Provide information about newborn interactional capabilities, states of consciousness, and means of stimulating cognitive development. **This helps parents recognize and respond to infant cues during an interactional process, and fosters optimal interaction, attachment behaviors, and cognitive development in infant.**

Information that appears in brackets has been added by the authors to clarify and enhance the use of nursing diagnoses.

- Promote sleep and rest. **This reduces the metabolic rate and allows nutrition and oxygen to be used for the healing process rather than for energy needs.**
- Provide for unlimited participation for father and siblings. Ascertain whether siblings attended an orientation program. **This facilitates family development and the ongoing process of acquaintance and attachment.**
- Monitor and document the client's/couple's interactions with the infant. Note the presence of bonding or acquaintance behaviors (e.g., making eye contact, using high-pitched voice and en face [face-to-face] position as culturally appropriate, calling the infant by name, and holding the infant closely).

Nursing Priority No. 3.

To enhance optimal well-being:

Prenatal

- Emphasize the importance of maternal well-being. **Fetal well-being is directly related to maternal well-being, especially during the first trimester, when developing organ systems are most vulnerable to injury from environmental or hereditary factors.**
- Review physical changes to be expected during each trimester. **This prepares the client/couple for managing common discomforts associated with pregnancy.**
- Explain psychological reactions including ambivalence, introspection, stress reactions, and emotional lability as characteristic of pregnancy. **This helps the client/couple understand mood swings and may provide opportunities for the partner to offer support and affection at these times.**
- Provide necessary referrals (e.g., dietitian, social services, food stamps, or Women, Infants, and Children [WIC] food programs) as indicated. **A supplemental federally funded food program helps promote optimal maternal, fetal, and infant nutrition.**
- Review reportable danger signals of pregnancy, such as bleeding, cramping, acute abdominal pain, backache, edema, visual disturbance, headaches, and pelvic pressure. **This help the client distinguish normal from abnormal findings, thus assisting her in seeking timely, appropriate healthcare.**
- Encourage attendance at prenatal and childbirth classes. Provide information about father/sibling or grandparent participation in classes and delivery if the client desires.
- Provide a list of appropriate reading materials for client, couple, and siblings regarding adjusting to a newborn. **Infor-**

Information that appears in brackets has been added by the authors to clarify and enhance the use of nursing diagnoses.

mation helps the individual realistically analyze changes in family structure, roles, and behaviors.

Labor and Delivery

- Monitor labor progress and maternal and fetal well-being per protocol. Provide continuous intrapartal professional support/doula. **Fear of abandonment can intensify as labor progresses, and the client may experience increased anxiety and/or loss of control when left unattended.**
- Reinforce the use of positive coping mechanisms. **This enhances feelings of competence and fosters self-esteem.**

Postpartum/Newborn Care

- Provide information about self-care, including perineal care and hygiene; physiological changes, including normal progression of lochial discharge; needs for sleep and rest; importance of progressive postpartal exercise program; and role changes.
- Review normal psychological changes and needs associated with the postpartal period. **The client's emotional state may be somewhat labile at this time and often is influenced by physical well-being.**
- Discuss sexuality needs and plans for contraception. Provide information about available methods, including advantages and disadvantages.
- Reinforce the importance of postpartal examination by healthcare provider and interim follow-up as appropriate. **Follow-up visit is necessary to evaluate the recovery of reproductive organs, healing of episiotomy/laceration repair, general well-being, and adaptation to life changes.**
- Provide oral and written information about infant care and development, feeding, and safety issues.
- Offer appropriate references reflecting cultural beliefs.
- Discuss the physiology and benefits of breastfeeding, nipple and breast care, special dietary needs, factors that facilitate or interfere with successful breastfeeding, use of breast pump, and appropriate suppliers. **This helps ensure an adequate milk supply, prevents nipple cracking and soreness, facilitates comfort, and establishes the role of the breastfeeding mother.**
- Refer the client to support groups (e.g., La Leche League or Lact-Aid) or lactation consultant **to promote a successful breastfeeding outcome.**
- Identify available community resources as indicated (e.g., WIC program). **WIC and other federal programs support**

Information that appears in brackets has been added by the authors to clarify and enhance the use of nursing diagnoses.

well-being through client education and enhanced nutritional intake for the infant.

- Discuss normal variations and characteristics of the infant, such as caput succedaneum, cephalohematoma, pseudomenstruation, breast enlargement, physiological jaundice, and milia. **This helps parents recognize normal variations and may reduce anxiety.**
- Emphasize the newborn's need for follow-up evaluation by the healthcare provider and timely immunizations.
- Identify manifestations of illness and infection and the times at which a healthcare provider should be contacted. Demonstrate the proper technique for taking temperature, administering oral medications, or providing other care activities for infant as required. **Early recognition of illness and prompt use of healthcare facilitate treatment and positive outcome.**
- Refer the client/couple to community postpartal parent groups. **This increases the parent's knowledge of child rearing and child development and provides a supportive atmosphere while parents incorporate new roles.**

Documentation Focus

Assessment/Reassessment

- Assessment findings, general health, previous pregnancy experience
- Cultural beliefs and expectations
- Specific birth plan and individuals to be involved in delivery
- Arrangements for postpartal recovery period

Planning

- Plan of care and who is involved in planning
- Teaching plan

Implementation/Evaluation

- Response to interventions, teaching, and actions performed
- Attainment or progress toward desired outcome(s)
- Modifications to plan of care

Discharge Planning

- Long-term needs and who is responsible for actions to be taken
- Available resources, specific referrals made

Information that appears in brackets has been added by the authors to clarify and enhance the use of nursing diagnoses.

Sample Nursing Outcomes & Interventions Classifications (NOC/NIC)

NOC—Knowledge: Pregnancy
NIC—Childbirth Preparation

impaired COMFORT

[Diagnostic Division: Pain/Discomfort]

Definition: Perceived lack of ease, relief, and transcendence in physical, psychospiritual, environmental, cultural, and social dimensions.

Related Factors

Illness-related symptoms; treatment regimen
Insufficient environmental/situational control
Insufficient privacy
Noxious environmental stimuli
Insufficient resources (e.g., financial, social, knowledge)

Defining Characteristics

Subjective
Distressing symptoms; feeling of hunger, discomfort; itching; Feeling cold or hot
Alteration in sleep pattern; inability to relax
Anxiety; fear; uneasy in situation

Objective
Restlessness; irritability; sighing, moaning, crying

Desired Outcomes/Evaluation Criteria—Client Will:

- Engage in behaviors or lifestyle changes to increase level of ease.
- Verbalize sense of comfort or contentment.
- Participate in desirable and realistic health-seeking behaviors.

Actions/Interventions

Nursing Priority No. 1.
To assess etiology/precipitating contributory factors:

- Determine the type of discomfort the client is experiencing, such as physical pain, feeling of discontent, lack of ease with

Information that appears in brackets has been added by the authors to clarify and enhance the use of nursing diagnoses.

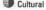

self, environment, or sociocultural settings, or inability to rise above one's problems or pain (lack of transcendence). Have the client rate total comfort, using a scale of 0 to 10, with 10 being as comfortable as possible, or a "general comfort" questionnaire using a Likert-type scale. **A comfort scale is similar to a pain rating scale and can help the client identify the focus of discomfort (e.g., physical, emotional, or social).**

- Note cultural/religious beliefs and values that impact perceptions and expectations of comfort.
- Ascertain locus of control. **The presence of an external locus of control may hamper efforts to achieve a sense of peace or contentment.**
- Discuss concerns with the client and active-listen to identify underlying issues (e.g., physical and emotional stressors or external factors such as environmental surroundings; social interactions) that could impact the client's ability to control own well-being. **This helps to determine the client's specific needs and ability to change own situation.**
- Establish context(s) in which lack of comfort is realized: physical (pertaining to bodily sensations); psychospiritual (pertaining to internal awareness of self and meaning in one's life, relationship to a higher order or being), environmental (pertaining to external surroundings, conditions, and influences), or sociocultural (pertaining to interpersonal, family, and societal relationships).

Physical

- Determine how the client is managing pain and pain components. **Lack of control may be related to other issues or emotions such as fear, loneliness, anxiety, noxious stimuli, or anger.**
- Ascertain what has been tried or is required for comfort or rest (e.g., head of bed up/down, music on/off, white noise, rocking motion, or a certain person or thing).

Psychospiritual

- Determine how psychological and spiritual indicators overlap (e.g., meaningfulness, faith, identity, and self-esteem) for the client.
- Ascertain if the client/SO desires support regarding spiritual enrichment, including prayer, meditation, or access to a spiritual counselor of choice.

Environmental

- Determine that the client's environment both respects privacy and provides natural lighting with readily accessible view to outdoors—**an aspect that can be manipulated to enhance comfort.**

Information that appears in brackets has been added by the authors to clarify and enhance the use of nursing diagnoses.

Sociocultural

- Ascertain the meaning of comfort in the context of interpersonal, family, cultural values, and societal relationships.
- Validate client/SO understanding of client's situation and ongoing methods of managing condition, as appropriate and/or desired by client. **This considers client/family needs in this area and/or shows appreciation for their desires.**

Nursing Priority No. 2.

To assist client to alleviate discomfort:

- Review knowledge base and note coping skills that have been used previously to change behavior/promote well-being. **This brings these to client's awareness and promotes use in the current situation.**
- Acknowledge the client's strengths in the present situation and build on these in planning for the future.

Physical

- Collaborate in treating or managing medical conditions involving oxygenation, elimination, mobility, cognitive abilities, electrolyte balance, thermoregulation, and hydration **to promote physical stability.**
- Work with the client to prevent pain, nausea, itching, and thirst/other physical discomforts.
- Review medications or treatment regimen **to determine possible changes or options to reduce side effects.**
- Suggest that the parent be present during procedures **to comfort child.**
- Provide age-appropriate comfort measures (e.g., back rub, change of position, cuddling, and use of heat/cold) **to provide nonpharmacological pain management.**
- Discuss interventions/activities such as Therapeutic Touch (TT), massage, healing touch, biofeedback, self-hypnosis, guided imagery, and breathing exercises; play therapy; and humor **to promote ease and relaxation and to refocus attention.**
- Assist the client to use and modify medication regimen **to make the best use of pharmacological pain or symptom management.**
- Assist the client/SO(s) to develop a plan for activity and exercise within individual ability, emphasizing the necessity of allowing sufficient time to finish activities.
- Maintain open and flexible visitation with client's desired persons.

Information that appears in brackets has been added by the authors to clarify and enhance the use of nursing diagnoses.

- Encourage/plan care to allow individually adequate rest periods **to prevent fatigue.** Schedule activities for periods when the client has the most energy **to maximize participation.**
- Discuss routines to promote restful sleep.

Psychospiritual

- Interact with the client in a therapeutic manner. **The nurse could be the most important comfort intervention for meeting client's needs. For example, assuring the client that nausea can be treated successfully with both pharmacological and nonpharmacological methods may be more effective than simply administering an antiemetic without reassurance and a comforting presence.**
- Encourage verbalization of feelings and make time for listening/interacting.
- Identify ways (e.g., meditation, sharing oneself with others, being out in nature/garden, other spiritual activities) to achieve connectedness or harmony with self, others, nature, or a higher power.
- Establish realistic activity goals with the client. **This enhances commitment to promoting optimal outcomes.**
- Involve the client/SO(s) in schedule planning and decisions about timing and spacing of treatments **to promote relaxation/reduce sense of boredom.**
- Encourage the client to do whatever possible (e.g., self-care, sit up in chair, or walk). **This enhances self-esteem and independence.**
- ∞ Use age-appropriate distraction with music, reading, chatting, or texting with family and friends, watching TV or movies, or playing video or computer games **to limit dwelling on and transcend unpleasant sensations and situations.**
- Encourage the client to develop assertiveness skills, prioritizing goals/activities, and to make use of beneficial coping behaviors. **This promotes a sense of control and improves self-esteem.**
- Identify opportunities for the client to participate in experiences that enhance control and independence.

Environmental

- Provide a quiet environment, calm activities.
- Provide for periodic changes in the personal surroundings when the client is confined. Use the individual's input in creating the changes (e.g., seasonal bulletin boards, color changes, rearranging furniture, or pictures). **This promotes a client's sense of self-control and environmental comfort.**

Information that appears in brackets has been added by the authors to clarify and enhance the use of nursing diagnoses.

- Suggest activities, such as bird feeders or baths for bird-watching, a garden in a window box/terrarium, or a fish bowl/aquarium, **to stimulate observation as well as involvement and participation in activity.**

Sociocultural

- Encourage age-appropriate diversional activities (e.g., TV/radio, computer games, play time, or socialization/outings with others).
- Avoid overstimulation/understimulation (cognitive and sensory).
- Make appropriate referrals to available support groups, hobby clubs, and service organizations.

Nursing Priority No. 3.

To promote wellness (Teaching/Discharge Considerations):

- Provide information about conditions/health risk factors or concerns in desired format (e.g., pictures, TV programs, articles, handouts, or audio/visual materials; classes, group discussions, Internet Web sites, and other databases) as appropriate. **The use of multiple modalities enhances acquisition/retention of information and gives the client choices for accessing and applying information.**

Physical

- Promote overall health measures (e.g., nutrition, adequate fluid intake, elimination, and appropriate vitamin and iron supplementation).
- Discuss potential complications and the possible need for medical follow-up or alternative therapies. **Timely recognition and intervention can promote wellness.**
- Assist the client/SO(s) to identify and acquire necessary equipment (e.g., lifts, commode chair, safety grab bars, or personal hygiene supplies) to meet individual needs. Refer to appropriate suppliers.

Psychospiritual

- Collaborate with others when the client expresses interest in lessons, counseling, coaching, and/or mentoring **to meet/enhance emotional and/or spiritual comfort.**
- Promote and encourage the client's contributions toward meeting realistic goals.
- Encourage the client to take time to be introspective in the search for contentment/transcendence.

Environmental

- Create a compassionate, supportive, and therapeutic environment incorporating client's cultural and age or developmental factors.

Information that appears in brackets has been added by the authors to clarify and enhance the use of nursing diagnoses.

- Correct environmental hazards that could influence safety or negatively affect comfort.
- Arrange for home visit or evaluation as needed.
- Discuss long-term plan for taking care of environmental needs.

Sociocultural

- Advocate for a growth-promoting environment in conflict situations and consider issues from client/family and cultural perspective.
- Identify resources or referrals (e.g., knowledge and skills, financial resources or assistance, personal or psychological support group, social activities).

Documentation Focus

Assessment/Reassessment

- Individual findings including client's description of current status/situation and factors impacting sense of comfort
- Pertinent cultural and religious beliefs and values
- Medication use and nonpharmacological measures

Planning

- Plan of care, specific interventions, and who is involved in planning
- Teaching plan

Implementation/Evaluation

- Responses to interventions, teaching, and actions performed
- Attainment or progress toward desired outcome(s)
- Modifications to plan of care

Discharge Planning

- Long-term needs and who is responsible for actions to be taken
- Specific referrals made

Sample Nursing Outcomes & Interventions Classifications (NOC/NIC)

NOC—Comfort Status
NIC—Environmental Management: Comfort

Information that appears in brackets has been added by the authors to clarify and enhance the use of nursing diagnoses.

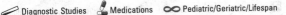

readiness for enhanced COMFORT

[Diagnostic Division: Pain/Discomfort]

Definition: A pattern of ease, relief, and transcendence in physical, psychospiritual, environmental, and/or social dimensions, which be strengthened.

Defining Characteristics

Subjective

- Expresses desire to enhance comfort, feeling of contentment
- Expresses desire to enhance relaxation
- Expresses desire to enhance resolution of complaints

Desired Outcomes/Evaluation Criteria—Client Will:

- Verbalize sense of comfort or contentment.
- Demonstrate behaviors of optimal level of ease.
- Participate in desirable and realistic health-seeking behaviors.

Actions/Interventions

Nursing Priority No. 1.

To determine current level of comfort and motivation for change:

- Determine the type of comfort client is experiencing: (1) relief (as from pain), (2) ease (a state of calm or contentment), or (3) transcendence (a state in which one rises above one's problems or pain).
- Ascertain motivation or expectations for improvement.
- Establish context(s) in which comfort is realized: (1) physical (pertaining to bodily sensations), (2) psychospiritual (pertaining to internal awareness of self and meaning in one's life, relationship to a higher order or being), (3) environmental (pertaining to external surroundings, conditions, and influences), and (4) sociocultural (pertaining to interpersonal, family, and societal relationships).

Physical

- Verify that the client is managing pain and pain components effectively. **Success in this area usually addresses other issues and emotions (e.g., fear, loneliness, anxiety, noxious stimuli, or anger).**

Information that appears in brackets has been added by the authors to clarify and enhance the use of nursing diagnoses.

- Ascertain what is used or required for comfort or rest (e.g., head of bed up or down, music on or off, white noise, rocking motion, certain person or thing, or ability to express and/or manage conflicts).

Psychospiritual

- Determine how psychological and spiritual indicators overlap (e.g., meaningfulness, faith, identity, or self-esteem) for a client in enhancing comfort.
- Determine the influence of cultural beliefs and values.
- Ascertain that the client/SO has received desired support regarding spiritual enrichment, including prayer, meditation, and access to a spiritual counselor of choice.

Environmental

- Determine that the client's environment respects privacy and provides natural lighting and a readily accessible view to the outdoors **(an aspect that can be manipulated to enhance comfort).**

Sociocultural

- Ascertain the meaning of comfort in the context of interpersonal, family, cultural values, spatial, and societal relationships.
- Validate client/SO understanding of client's diagnosis and prognosis and ongoing methods of managing condition, as appropriate and/or desired by client. **This considers client/family needs in this area and/or shows appreciation for their desires.**

Nursing Priority No. 2.

To assist client in developing plan to improve comfort:

- Review knowledge base and note coping skills that have been used previously to change behavior and promote well-being. **This brings these to the client's awareness and promotes use in the current situation.**
- Acknowledge the client's strengths in the present situation that can be used to build on in planning for the future.

Physical

- Collaborate in treating and managing medical conditions involving oxygenation, elimination, mobility, cognitive abilities, electrolyte balance, thermoregulation, and hydration **to promote physical stability.**
- Work with the client to prevent pain, nausea, itching, thirst, or other physical discomforts.

Information that appears in brackets has been added by the authors to clarify and enhance the use of nursing diagnoses.

- Suggest that the parent be present during procedures **to comfort the child.**
- Suggest age-appropriate comfort measures (e.g., back rub, change of position, cuddling, or the use of heat/cold) **to provide nonpharmacological pain management.**
- Review interventions and activities such as therapeutic touch, biofeedback, self-hypnosis, guided imagery, breathing exercises, play therapy, and humor **that promote ease and relaxation, and can refocus attention.**
- Assist the client to use or modify the medication regimen **to make the best use of pharmacological pain management.**
- Assist the client/SO(s) to develop or modify the plan for activity and exercise within individual ability, emphasizing the necessity of allowing sufficient time to finish activities.
- Maintain open and flexible visitation with client's desired persons.
- Encourage adequate rest periods **to prevent fatigue.**
- Plan care to allow individually adequate rest periods. Schedule activities for periods when the client has the most energy **to maximize participation.**
- Discuss routines to promote restful sleep.

Psychospiritual

- Interact with the client in a therapeutic manner. **The nurse could be the most important comfort intervention for meeting the client's needs. For example, assuring the client that nausea can be treated successfully with both pharmacological and nonpharmacological methods may be more effective than simply administering an antiemetic without reassurance and comforting presence.**
- Encourage verbalization of feelings and make time for listening and interacting.
- Identify ways (e.g., meditation, sharing oneself with others, being out in nature/garden, or other spiritual activities) **to achieve connectedness or harmony with self, others, nature, or a higher power.**
- Establish realistic activity goals with client. **This enhances a commitment to promoting optimal outcomes.**
- Involve the client/SO(s) in schedule planning and decisions about timing and spacing of treatments **to promote relaxation and involvement in plan.**
- Encourage the client to do whatever possible (e.g., self-care, sit up in chair, walk, etc.). **This enhances self-esteem and independence.**
- Use age-appropriate distraction with music, chatting, or texting with family and friends, watching TV, or playing video

Information that appears in brackets has been added by the authors to clarify and enhance the use of nursing diagnoses.

or computer games **to limit dwelling on, or transcend unpleasant sensations and situations.**
- Encourage the client to make use of beneficial coping behaviors and assertiveness skills, prioritizing goals and activities. **This promotes a sense of control and improves self-esteem.**
- Offer or identify opportunities for the client to participate in experiences that enhance control and independence.

Environmental

- Provide a quiet environment and calm activities.
- Provide for periodic changes in the personal surroundings when the client is confined. Use the individual's input in creating the changes (e.g., seasonal bulletin boards, color changes, rearranging furniture, or pictures). **This enhances a sense of comfort and control over the environment.**
- Suggest activities, such as bird feeders or baths for bird-watching, a garden in a window box/terrarium, or a fish bowl/aquarium **to stimulate observation as well as involvement and participation in activity.**

Sociocultural

- Encourage age-appropriate diversional activities (e.g., TV/radio, play time/games, or socialization/outings with others).
- Avoid cognitive or sensory overstimulation and understimulation.
- Make appropriate referrals to available support groups, hobby clubs, or service organizations.

Nursing Priority No. 3.

To promote optimum wellness (Teaching/Discharge Considerations):

Physical

- Promote overall health measures (e.g., nutrition, adequate fluid intake, elimination, appropriate vitamin/iron supplementation).
- Discuss potential complications and possible need for medical follow-up care or alternative therapies. **Timely recognition and intervention can promote wellness.**
- Assist client/SO(s) in identifying and acquiring necessary equipment (e.g., lifts, commode chair, safety grab bars, and personal hygiene supplies) **to meet individual needs.**

Psychospiritual

- Collaborate with others when the client expresses interest in lessons, counseling, coaching, and/or mentoring **to meet/enhance emotional and/or spiritual comfort.**

Information that appears in brackets has been added by the authors to clarify and enhance the use of nursing diagnoses.

- Encourage the client's contributions toward meeting realistic goals.
- Encourage the client to take time to be introspective in the search for contentment/transcendence.

Environmental

- Promote a compassionate, supportive, and therapeutic environment incorporating client's cultural, age, and developmental factors.
- Correct environmental hazards **that could influence safety or negatively affect comfort.**
- Arrange for home visit/evaluation, as needed.
- Discuss long-term plan for taking care of environmental needs.

Sociocultural

- Advocate for growth-promoting environment in conflict situations and consider issues from client/family and cultural perspective.
- Support client/SO access to resources (e.g., knowledge and skills, financial resources/assistance, personal/psychological support, social systems).

Documentation Focus

Assessment/Reassessment
- Individual findings, including client's description of current status/situation
- Motivation and expectations for change
- Medication use/nonpharmacological measures

Planning
- Plan of care, specific interventions, and who is involved in planning
- Teaching plan

Implementation/Evaluation
- Responses to interventions, teaching, and actions performed
- Attainment or progress toward desired outcome(s)
- Modifications to plan of care

Discharge Planning
- Long-term needs and who is responsible for actions to be taken
- Specific referrals made

Information that appears in brackets has been added by the authors to clarify and enhance the use of nursing diagnoses.

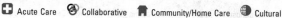

  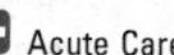 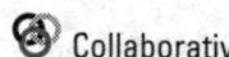 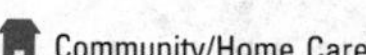  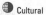
Acute Care Collaborative Community/Home Care Cultural

Sample Nursing Outcomes & Interventions Classifications (NOC/NIC)

NOC—Comfort Status
NIC—Self-Modification Assistance

impaired verbal COMMUNICATION

[Diagnostic Division: Social Interaction]

Definition: Decreased, delayed, or absent ability to receive, process, transmit, and or use a system of symbols.

Related Factors

Alteration in development
Physical barrier (e.g., tracheostomy, intubation); oropharyngeal defect
Physiological condition (e.g., decreased circulation to brain, weakened musculoskeletal system); central nervous system impairment
Vulnerability; emotional disturbance; psychotic disorder
Environmental barrier
Cultural incongruence
Insufficient information
Treatment regimen
Alteration in self-concept; low self-esteem
Alteration in perception
Absence of significant other

Defining Characteristics

Objective

Inability to speak language of caregiver
Difficulty speaking/verbalizing; stuttering; slurred speech
Does not speak; refusal to speak; inability to speak
Difficulty forming sentences or words (e.g., aphonia, dyslalia, dysarthria)
Difficulty expressing thoughts verbally (e.g., aphasia, dysphasia, apraxia, dyslexia)
Inappropriate verbalization [e.g., incessant, loose association of ideas; flight of ideas]
Difficulty comprehending or maintaining communication
Absence of eye contact; difficulty in selective attending; partial/total visual deficit

---

Information that appears in brackets has been added by the authors to clarify and enhance the use of nursing diagnoses.

Inability/difficulty in use of facial or body expressions
Dyspnea
Disoriented to person, space, time
[Inability to modulate speech; message inappropriate to content]
[Use of nonverbal cues (e.g., pleading eyes, gestures, or turning away)]

Desired Outcomes/Evaluation Criteria—Client Will:

- Verbalize or indicate an understanding of the communication difficulty and plans for ways of handling.
- Establish method of communication in which needs can be expressed.
- Participate in therapeutic communication (e.g., using silence, acceptance, restating, reflecting, active-listening, and I-messages).
- Demonstrate congruent verbal and nonverbal communication.
- Use resources appropriately.

Actions/Interventions

Nursing Priority No. 1.

To assess causative/contributing factors:

- Identify physiological or neurological conditions impacting speech such as severe shortness of breath, cleft palate, facial trauma, neuromuscular weakness, stroke, brain tumors or infections, dementia, brain trauma, deafness, or hard of hearing.
- ∞ Determine age and developmental considerations: (1) child too young for language or has developmental delays affecting speech and language skills or comprehension; (2) autism or other mental impairments; (3) older client doesn't or isn't able to speak, verbalizes with difficulty, or has difficulty hearing or comprehending language or concepts.
- Review history for neurological conditions that could affect speech, such as stroke, tumor, multiple sclerosis (MS), or hearing or vision impairment.
- Note results of neurological tests (e.g., electroencephalogram [EEG]; or computed tomography/magnetic resonance imaging scans; language/speech tests [e.g., Boston Diagnostic Aphasia Examination, the Action Naming Test]) **to assess and delineate underlying conditions affecting verbal communication.**
- Note whether aphasia is motor **(expressive: loss of images for articulated speech)**, sensory **(receptive: unable to un-**

Information that appears in brackets has been added by the authors to clarify and enhance the use of nursing diagnoses.

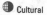

derstand words and does not recognize the defect), conduction (**slow comprehension: uses words inappropriately but knows the error)**, and/or global (**total loss of ability to comprehend and speak)**. Evaluate the degree of impairment.

- Evaluate mental status and note the presence of psychiatric conditions (e.g., bipolar, schizoid/affective behavior). Assess psychological response to communication impairment and willingness to find an alternate means of communication.
- Note the presence of endotracheal tube/tracheostomy or other physical blocks to speech (e.g., cleft palate or jaws wired).
- Assess the environmental factors that may affect the ability to communicate (e.g., room noise level).
- Identify environmental barriers: recent or chronic exposure to hazardous noise in home, job, recreation, and healthcare setting (e.g., rock music, jackhammer, snowmobile, lawn mower, truck traffic or busy highway, heavy equipment, or medical equipment). **Noise not only affects hearing, but it also increases blood pressure and breathing rate, can have negative cardiovascular effects, disturbs digestion, increases fatigue, causes irritability, and reduces attention to tasks.**
- Determine the primary language spoken. **Knowing the client's primary language and fluency in other languages is important to communication. For example, while some individuals may seem to be fluent in conversational English, they may still have limited understanding, especially the language of health professionals, and have difficulty answering questions, describing symptoms, or following directions.**
- Ascertain whether the client is a recent immigrant, noting country of origin, and what cultural/ethnic group the client identifies with (**e.g., recent immigrant may identify with home country and its people, beliefs, and healthcare practices)**.
- Determine cultural factors affecting communication such as beliefs concerning touch and eye contact. **Certain cultures may prohibit client from speaking directly to healthcare provider; some Native Americans, Appalachians, or young African Americans may interpret direct eye contact as disrespectful, impolite, an invasion of privacy, or aggressive; Latinos, Arabs, and Asians may shout and gesture when excited.**
- Assess the style of speech (as outlined in Defining Characteristics).
- Determine the presence of psychological or emotional barriers, history or presence of psychiatric conditions (e.g.,

Information that appears in brackets has been added by the authors to clarify and enhance the use of nursing diagnoses.

bipolar disorder, schizoid or affective behavior); high level of anxiety, frustration, or fear; presence of angry, hostile behavior. Note the effects on speech and communication.
- Interview the parent to determine the child's developmental level of speech and language comprehension.
- Note parental speech patterns and the manner of communicating with the child, including gestures.

Nursing Priority No. 2.

To assist client to establish a means of communication to express needs, wants, ideas, and questions:

- Ascertain that you have the client's attention before communicating.
- Establish rapport with client, initiate eye contact, shake hands, address by preferred name, and meet the family members present; ask simple questions, smile, and engage in brief social conversation if appropriate. **This helps establish a trusting relationship with client/family, demonstrating caring about the client as a person.**
- Determine the ability to read and write. Evaluate musculoskeletal states, including manual dexterity (e.g., ability to hold a pen and write).
- Advise other healthcare providers of client's communication deficits (e.g., deafness, aphasia, intubation/presence of mechanical ventilation) and needed means of communication (e.g., writing pad, signing, yes/no responses, gestures, or picture board) **to minimize the client's frustration and promote understanding.**
- Obtain a translator or provide written translation or picture chart **when writing is not possible or the client speaks a different language than that spoken by the healthcare provider.**
- Facilitate hearing and vision examinations **to obtain necessary aids.**
- Ascertain that hearing aid(s) are in place and batteries are charged and/or glasses are worn when needed **to facilitate and improve communication.** Assist the client to learn to use and adjust to aids.
- Reduce environmental noise that can interfere with comprehension. Provide adequate lighting, especially if the client is reading lips or attempting to write.
- Establish a relationship with the client, listening carefully and attending to the client's verbal/nonverbal expressions. **This conveys interest and concern.**

Information that appears in brackets has been added by the authors to clarify and enhance the use of nursing diagnoses.

 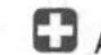 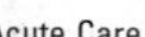 Acute Care 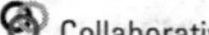 Collaborative 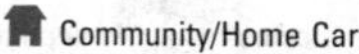 Community/Home Care 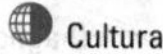 Cultural

- Maintain eye contact, preferably at the client's level. Be aware of cultural factors that may preclude eye contact (e.g., found in some American Indians, Indo-Chinese, Arabs, and natives of Appalachia).
- Keep communication simple, speaking in short sentences, using appropriate words, and using all modes for accessing information: visual, auditory, and kinesthetic.
- Refrain from shouting when directing speech to confused, deaf, or hearing-impaired client. Speak slowly and clearly, pitching voice low **to increase the likelihood of being understood.**
- Maintain a calm, unhurried manner. Provide sufficient time for the client to respond. Downplay errors and avoid frequent corrections. **Individuals with expressive aphasia may talk more easily when they are rested and relaxed and when they are talking to one person at a time.**
- Determine the meaning of words used by the client and congruency of communication and nonverbal messages.
- Validate the meaning of nonverbal communication; do not make assumptions **because they may be wrong.** Be honest; if you do not understand, seek assistance from others.
- Individualize techniques using breathing for relaxation of the vocal cords, rote tasks (such as counting), and singing or melodic intonation **to assist aphasic clients in relearning speech.**
- Anticipate needs and stay with the client until effective communication is reestablished, and/or client feels safe/comfortable.
- Plan for and provide alternative methods of communication, incorporating information about type of disability present:

  Provide pad and pencil or slate board **when the client is able to write but cannot speak.**

  Use letter or picture board **when the client can't write and picture concepts are understandable to both parties.**

  Establish hand or eye signals **when the client can understand language but cannot speak or has physical barrier to writing.**

  Remove isolation mask **when the client is deaf and reads lips.**

  Obtain or provide access to tablet or computer **if communication impairment is long-standing or the client is used to this method.**
- Identify and use previous successful communication solutions used if the situation is chronic or recurrent.

Information that appears in brackets has been added by the authors to clarify and enhance the use of nursing diagnoses.

- Provide reality orientation by responding with simple, straightforward, honest statements.
- Provide environmental stimuli, as needed, **to maintain contact with reality,** or reduce stimuli **to lessen anxiety that may worsen problem.**
- Use confrontation skills, when appropriate, within an established nurse-client relationship **to clarify discrepancies between verbal and nonverbal cues.**
- Refer for appropriate therapies and support services. **Client and family may have multiple needs (e.g., sources for further examinations and rehabilitation services, local community or national support groups and services for disabled, or financial assistance with obtaining necessary aids for improving communication).**

Nursing Priority No. 3.

To promote wellness (Teaching/Discharge Considerations):

- Review information about condition, prognosis, and treatment with client/SO(s).
- Teach client and family the needed techniques for communication, whether it be speech or language techniques, or alternate modes of communicating. Encourage the family to involve the client in family activities using enhanced communication techniques. **This reduces stress of difficult situation and promotes earlier return to more normal life patterns.**
- Reinforce that loss of speech does not imply loss of intelligence.
- Discuss individual methods of dealing with impairment, capitalizing on client's and caregiver's strengths.
- Discuss ways to provide environmental stimuli as appropriate **to maintain contact with reality or reduce environmental stimuli or noise. Unwanted sound affects physical health, increases fatigue, reduces attention to tasks, and makes speech communication more difficult.**
- Recommend placing a tape recorder with a prerecorded emergency message near the telephone. Include the client's name, address, telephone number, and critical information (e.g., type of airway, person cannot speak) and a request for immediate emergency assistance.
- Use and assist client/SO(s) to learn therapeutic communication skills of acknowledgment, active-listening, and I-messages. **This improves general communication skills.**

Information that appears in brackets has been added by the authors to clarify and enhance the use of nursing diagnoses.

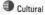

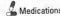

- Involve family/SO(s) in plan of care as much as possible. **This enhances participation and commitment to communication with a loved one.**
- Refer to appropriate resources (e.g., speech/language therapist, support groups such as stroke club, individual/family, and/or psychiatric counseling).
- Refer to NDs ineffective Coping; disabled family Coping; Anxiety; Fear.

Documentation Focus

Assessment/Reassessment

- Assessment findings, pertinent history information (i.e., physical, psychological, cultural concerns)
- Meaning of nonverbal cues, level of anxiety client exhibits

Planning

- Plan of care and interventions (e.g., type of alternative communication/translator)
- Teaching plan

Implementation/Evaluation

- Response to interventions, teaching, and actions performed
- Attainment or progress toward desired outcome(s)
- Modifications to plan of care

Discharge Planning

- Discharge needs, referrals made; additional resources available

Sample Nursing Outcomes & Interventions Classifications (NOC/NIC)

NOC—Communication
NIC—Communication Enhancement: Speech Deficit

readiness for enhanced COMMUNICATION

[Diagnostic Division: Teaching/Learning]

Definition: A pattern of exchanging information and ideas with others, which can be strengthened.

Information that appears in brackets has been added by the authors to clarify and enhance the use of nursing diagnoses.

Defining Characteristics

Subjective

Expresses desire to enhance communication

Desired Outcomes/Evaluation Criteria—Client/SO/Caregiver Will:

- Verbalize or indicate an understanding of the communication process.
- Identify ways to improve communication.

Actions/Interventions

Nursing Priority No. 1.

To assess how client is managing communication/challenges:

- Ascertain circumstances that result in a client's desire to improve communication. **Many factors are involved in communication, and identifying specific needs/expectations helps in developing realistic goals and determining likelihood of success.**
- Evaluate mental status. **Disorientation, acute or chronic confusion, or psychotic conditions may be affecting speech and the communication of thoughts, needs, and desires.**
- Determine the client's developmental level of speech and language comprehension. **This provides baseline information for developing a plan for improvement.**
- Determine the ability to read and write preferred language. **Evaluating grasp of language as well as musculoskeletal states, including manual dexterity (e.g., ability to hold a pen and write), provides information about the nature of client's situation. The educational plan can address language skills. Neuromuscular deficits will require an individual program in order to improve.**
- Determine country of origin, dominant language, whether client is recent immigrant, and what cultural/ethnic group the client identifies with. **A recent immigrant may identify with home country and its people, language, beliefs, and healthcare practices, thus affecting language skills and the ability to improve interactions in a new country.**
- Ascertain if an interpreter is needed/desired. **The law mandates that interpretation services be made available. A trained, professional interpreter who translates precisely and possesses a basic understanding of medical terminology and healthcare ethics is preferred to enhance client and provider satisfaction.**

Information that appears in brackets has been added by the authors to clarify and enhance the use of nursing diagnoses.

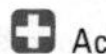

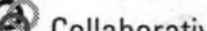
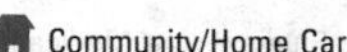
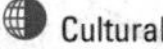

- Determine comfort level in expression of feelings and concepts in nonproficient language. **Concern about language skills can impact their perception of their own ability to communicate.**
- Note any physical barriers to effective communication (e.g., talking tracheostomy or wired jaws) or physiological or neurological conditions (e.g., severe shortness of breath, neuromuscular weakness, stroke, brain trauma, hearing impairment, cleft palate, and facial trauma). **The client may be dealing with speech/language comprehension difficulties or have voice production problems (pitch, loudness, or quality) that call attention to voice rather than what the speaker is saying. These barriers may need to be addressed to enable the client to improve communication skills.**
- Clarify the meaning of words used by the client to describe important aspects of life and health/well-being (e.g., pain, sorrow, or anxiety). **Words can easily be misinterpreted when the sender and receiver have different ideas about their meanings. Restating what one has heard can clarify whether an expressed statement has been correctly understood or misinterpreted.**
- Determine the presence of emotional lability (e.g., anger outbursts) and the frequency of unstable behaviors. **Emotional and psychiatric issues can affect communication and interfere with understanding.**
- Evaluate congruency of verbal and nonverbal messages. **Communication is enhanced when verbal and nonverbal messages are congruent.**
- Evaluate need or desire for pictures or written communications and instructions as part of the treatment plan. **Alternative methods of communication can help the client feel understood and promote feelings of satisfaction with interaction.**

Nursing Priority No. 2.

To improve the client's ability to communicate thoughts, needs, and ideas:

- Maintain a calm, unhurried manner. Provide sufficient time for the client to respond. **An atmosphere in which the client is free to speak without fear of criticism provides the opportunity to explore all the issues involved in making decisions to improve communication skills.**
- Pay attention to the speaker. Be an active listener. **The use of active-listening communicates acceptance and respect for the client, establishing trust and promoting openness and**

Information that appears in brackets has been added by the authors to clarify and enhance the use of nursing diagnoses.

honest expression. It communicates a belief that the client is a capable and competent person.

- Sit down, maintain eye contact as culturally appropriate, preferably at client's level, and spend time with the client. **This conveys a message that the nurse has time and interest in communicating.**
- Observe body language, eye movements, and behavioral cues. **This may reveal unspoken concerns; for example, when pain is present, the client may react with tears, grimacing, stiff posture, turning away, or angry outbursts.**
- Help the client identify and learn to avoid the use of nontherapeutic communication. **These barriers are recognized as detriments to open communication, and learning to avoid them maximizes the effectiveness of communication between client and others.**
- Obtain an interpreter with language or signing abilities, as needed. **This may be needed to enhance understanding of words and language concepts or to ascertain that interpretation of communication is accurate.**
- Suggest the use of pad and pencil, slate board, or letter/picture board when interacting or attempting to interface in new situations. **When the client has physical impairments that challenge verbal communication, an alternate means can provide clear concepts that are understandable to both parties.**
- Obtain or provide access to a voice-enabled computer, when indicated. **Use of these devices may be more helpful when communication challenges are long-standing and/or when client is used to working with them.**
- Respect the client's cultural communication needs. **Culture can dictate beliefs of what is normal or abnormal (i.e., in some cultures, eye-to-eye contact is considered disrespectful, impolite, or an invasion of privacy; silence and tone of voice have various meanings, and slang words can cause confusion).**
- Encourage the use of glasses, hearing aids, dentures, or electronic speech devices, as needed. **These devices maximize sensory perception or speech formation and can improve understanding and enhance speech patterns.**
- Reduce distractions and background noises (e.g., close the door and turn down the radio or TV). **A distracting environment can interfere with communication, limiting attention to tasks and making speech and communication more difficult. Reducing noise can help both parties hear clearly, thus improving understanding.**

Information that appears in brackets has been added by the authors to clarify and enhance the use of nursing diagnoses.

- Associate words with objects—using repetition and redundancy—and point to objects or demonstrate desired actions if communication requires visual aids. **The speaker's own body language can be used to enhance the client's understanding.**
- Use confrontation skills carefully, when appropriate, within an established nurse-client relationship. **This can be used to clarify discrepancies between verbal and nonverbal cues, enabling the client to look at areas that may require change.**

Nursing Priority No. 3.

To promote optimum communication:

- Discuss with family/SO and other caregivers effective ways in which the client communicates. **Identifying positive aspects of current communication skills enables family members and other caregivers to learn and move forward in desire to enhance ways of interacting.**
- Encourage client/SO(s) to familiarize themselves with and use new communication technologies. **This enhances family relationships and promotes self-esteem for all members as they are able to communicate regardless of the problems (e.g., progressive disorder) that could interfere with the ability to interact.**
- Reinforce client/SO(s) learning and using therapeutic communication skills of acknowledgment, active-listening, and I-messages. **This improves general communication skills, emphasizes acceptance, and conveys respect, enabling family relationships to improve.**
- Refer to appropriate resources (e.g., speech therapist, language classes, individual/family and/or psychiatric counseling). **This may be needed to help overcome challenges as the family reaches toward a desired goal of enhanced communication.**

Documentation Focus

Assessment/Reassessment

- Assessment findings, pertinent history information (i.e., physical, psychological, cultural concerns)
- Meaning of nonverbal cues, level of anxiety client exhibits

Planning

- Plan of care and interventions (e.g., type of alternative communication, use of translator)
- Teaching plan

Information that appears in brackets has been added by the authors to clarify and enhance the use of nursing diagnoses.

Implementation/Evaluation
- Progress toward desired outcome(s)
- Modifications to plan of care

Discharge Planning
- Discharge needs, referrals made, additional resources available

Sample Nursing Outcomes & Interventions Classifications (NOC/NIC)

NOC—Communication
NIC—Communication Enhancement [specify]

acute CONFUSION and risk for acute CONFUSION

[Diagnostic Division: Neurosensory]

Definition: acute Confusion: Abrupt onset of reversible disturbances of consciousness, attention, cognition, and perception that develop over a short period of time.

Definition: risk for acute Confusion: Vulnerable to reversible disturbances of consciousness, attention, cognition, and perception that develop over a short period of time, which may compromise health.

Related Factors (acute Confusion)

Age ≥60 years
Alteration in sleep-wake cycle
Delirium [including mania/other psychiatric disorder]; dementia
Substance abuse
[Endocrine or metabolic crisis, liver or renal failure; hypoxemia, hypercarbia; shock]

Defining Characteristics (acute Confusion)

Subjective
Hallucinations [visual or auditory]
[Exaggerated emotional responses]

Objective
Agitation; restlessness
Alteration in cognitive functioning, or level of consciousness

Information that appears in brackets has been added by the authors to clarify and enhance the use of nursing diagnoses.

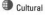

Alteration in psychomotor functioning
Misperception
Inability to initiate goal-directed or purposeful behavior
Inability to follow-through with goal-directed or purposeful behavior

Risk Factors (risk for acute Confusion)

Age ≥60 years; male gender
Alteration in cognitive functioning; dementia
Alteration in sleep-wake cycle; sensory deprivation
Dehydration; malnutrition
History of cerebral vascular accident
History of metabolic functioning (e.g., azotemia, decreased hemoglobin, electrolyte imbalance, increase in blood urea nitrogen/creatinine)
Impaired mobility; inappropriate use of restraints; pain
Pharmaceutical agent
Substance abuse
Infection; urinary retention

> **NOTE:** A risk diagnosis is not evidenced by signs and symptoms, as the problem has not occurred; rather, nursing interventions are directed at prevention.

Desired Outcomes/Evaluation Criteria—Client Will:

- Regain and maintain usual reality orientation and level of consciousness.
- Verbalize understanding of causative or risk factors when known.
- Initiate lifestyle or behavior changes to prevent or reduce risk of problem.

Actions/Interventions

Nursing Priority No. 1.

To assess causative/contributing **or risk** factors:

- Identify factors present such as recent surgery or trauma; use of large numbers of medications (polypharmacy); intoxication with/withdrawal from a substance (e.g., prescription and over-the-counter [OTC] drugs; alcohol or illicit drugs); history or current seizure activity; episodes of fever or pain, or presence of acute infection (especially occult urinary tract infection [UTI] in elderly

Information that appears in brackets has been added by the authors to clarify and enhance the use of nursing diagnoses.

clients); traumatic events; or person with dementia experiencing sudden change in environment, unfamiliar surroundings, or people. **Acute confusion is a symptom associated with numerous causes (e.g., hypoxia; metabolic/endocrine/ neurological conditions, toxins; electrolyte abnormalities; systemic or central nervous system [CNS] infections; nutritional deficiencies; or acute psychiatric disorders).**

- Assess mental status. **Typical symptoms of delirium include anxiety, disorientation, tremors, hallucinations, delusions, and incoherence. Onset is usually sudden, developing over a few hours or days, and resolving over varying periods of time.**
- Evaluate vital signs **for indicators of poor tissue perfusion (i.e., hypotension, tachycardia, or tachypnea) or stress response (tachycardia, tachypnea).**
- Determine the client's functional level, including the ability to provide self-care and move about at will. **Conditions and situations that limit a client's mobility and independence (e.g., acute or chronic physical or psychiatric illnesses and their therapies; trauma or extensive immobility, confinement in unfamiliar surroundings, and sensory deprivation) potentiate the prospect of acute confusional state.**
- Determine current medications/drug use—especially antianxiety agents, barbiturates, certain antipsychotic agents, methyldopa, disulfiram, cocaine, alcohol, amphetamines, hallucinogens, or opiates **associated with a high risk of confusion and delirium**—and schedule of use, such as cimetidine + antacid or digoxin + diuretics **(combinations can increase the risk of adverse reactions and interactions).**
- Evaluate for exacerbation of psychiatric conditions (e.g., mood or dissociative disorders or dementia). **Identification of the presence of mental illness provides opportunity for correct treatment and medication.**
- Investigate the possibility of alcohol or other drug intoxication or withdrawal.
- Ascertain life events (e.g., death of spouse/other family member, absence of known care provider, move from lifelong home, catastrophic natural disaster) **that can affect client's perceptions, attention, and concentration.**
- Assess diet and nutritional status **to identify possible deficiencies of essential nutrients and vitamins (e.g., thiamine) that could affect mental status.**
- Evaluate sleep and rest status, noting insomnia, sleep deprivation, or oversleeping. (Refer to NDs Insomnia; Sleep Deprivation, as appropriate.)

Information that appears in brackets has been added by the authors to clarify and enhance the use of nursing diagnoses.

- Monitor laboratory values (e.g., CBC, blood cultures; oxygen saturation and, in some cases, ABGs with carbon monoxide; BUN and Cr levels; electrolytes; thyroid function studies; liver function studies, ammonia levels; serum glucose; urinalysis for infection and drug analysis; specific drug toxicologies and drug levels [including peak and trough, as appropriate]) **to identify imbalances that have potential for causing confusion.**

Nursing Priority No. 2.

To determine degree of impairment **(acute Confusion):**

- Talk with SO(s) to determine historic baseline, observed changes, and onset or recurrence of changes **to understand and clarify current situation.**
- Collaborate with medical and psychiatric providers. Review results of diagnostic studies (e.g., delirium assessment tools, such as the Confusion Assessment Method [CAM], delirium index [DI], Mini-Mental State Examination [MMSE]; brain scans or imaging studies; electroencephalogram [EEG]; or lumbar puncture and cerebrospinal fluid [CSF] studies) **to evaluate the extent of impairment in orientation, attention span, ability to follow directions, send and receive communication, and appropriateness of response.**
- Note occurrence and timing of agitation, hallucinations, and violent behaviors. **("Sundown syndrome" may occur, with client oriented during daylight hours but confused during nighttime.)**
- Determine threat to safety of client/others. **Delirium can cause the client to become verbally and physically aggressive, resulting in behavior threatening to safety of self and others.**

Nursing Priority No. 3.

To maximize level of function, prevent further deterioration, correct existing risk factors:

- Assist with treatment of the underlying problem (e.g., drug intoxication/substance abuse, infectious process, hypoxemia, biochemical imbalances, nutritional deficits, or pain management).
- Monitor/adjust medication regimen and note response. Determine medications that can be changed or eliminated **when polypharmacy, side effects, or adverse reactions are determined to be associated with current condition.**

Information that appears in brackets has been added by the authors to clarify and enhance the use of nursing diagnoses.

- Orient client to surroundings, staff, necessary activities, as needed. Present reality concisely and briefly. Avoid challenging illogical thinking—**defensive reactions may result.**
- Encourage family/SO(s) to participate in reorientation as well as providing ongoing input (e.g., current news and family happenings). **The client may respond positively to a well-known person and familiar items.**
- Maintain a calm environment and eliminate extraneous noise or other stimuli **to prevent overstimulation.** Provide normal levels of essential sensory and tactile stimulation—include personal items, pictures, and so forth.
- Mobilize an elderly client (especially after orthopedic injury) as soon as possible. **An older person with low level of activity prior to crisis is at particular risk for acute confusion and may fare better when out of bed.**
- Encourage the client to use vision or hearing aids when needed **to assist the client in interpretation of environment and communication.**
- Give simple directions. Allow sufficient time for the client to respond, communicate, and make decisions.
- Provide for safety needs (e.g., supervision, seizure precautions, placing call bell within reach, positioning needed items within reach/clearing traffic paths, and ambulating with devices).
- Establish and maintain elimination patterns. **Disruption of elimination may be a cause for confusion, or changes in elimination may also be a symptom of acute confusion.**
- Note behavior that may be indicative of a potential for violence and take appropriate actions. (Refer to ND risk for other-directed/self-directed Violence.)
- Assist with treatment of alcohol or drug intoxication and/or withdrawal, as indicated.
- Administer psychotropics cautiously **to control restlessness, agitation, and hallucinations.**
- Avoid or limit the use of restraints—**they may worsen the situation and increase the likelihood of untoward complications.**
- Provide undisturbed rest periods.
- Refer to NDs impaired Memory; impaired verbal Communication, for additional interventions.

Nursing Priority No. 4.

To promote wellness (Teaching/Discharge Considerations):

- Assist with treatment of underlying medical conditions and/or management of risk factors **to reduce or limit conditions associated with confusion.**

Information that appears in brackets has been added by the authors to clarify and enhance the use of nursing diagnoses.

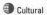

- Explain reason(s) for confusion, if known. **Although acute confusion usually subsides over time as the client recovers from the underlying cause and/or adjusts to a situation, it can initially be frightening to a client/SO. Therefore, information about the cause and appropriate treatment to improve the condition may be helpful in managing a sense of fear and powerlessness.**
- Discuss the need for ongoing medical review of the client's medications **to limit the possibility of misuse or potential for adverse actions or reactions.**
- Assist in identifying ongoing treatment needs and emphasize the necessity of periodic evaluation **to support early intervention.**
- Educate SO/caregivers to monitor client at home for sudden change in cognition and behavior. **An acute change is a classic presentation of delirium and should be considered a medical emergency. Early intervention can often prevent long-term complications.**
- Emphasize the importance of keeping vision/hearing aids in good repair **to improve the client's interpretation of environmental stimuli and communication.**
- Review ways to maximize the sleep environment (e.g., preferred bedtime rituals, comfortable room temperature, bedding and pillows, and elimination or reduction of extraneous noise or stimuli and interruptions.)
- Provide appropriate referrals (e.g., cognitive retraining, substance abuse treatment and support groups, medication monitoring program, Meals on Wheels, home health, or adult day care).

Documentation Focus

Assessment/Reassessment

- Existing conditions, risk factors for individual
- Nature, duration, frequency of problem
- Current and previous level of function and effect on independence and lifestyle (including safety concerns)

Planning

- Plan of care and who is involved in planning
- Teaching plan

Implementation/Evaluation

- Response to interventions and actions performed
- Attainment or progress toward desired outcomes
- Modifications to plan of care

Information that appears in brackets has been added by the authors to clarify and enhance the use of nursing diagnoses.

Discharge Planning

- Long-term needs and who is responsible for actions to be taken
- Available resources and specific referrals

Sample Nursing Outcomes & Interventions Classifications (NOC/NIC)

NOC—Acute Confusion Level
NOC—Cognition
NIC—Delirium Management
NIC—Reality Oreintation

chronic CONFUSION

[Diagnostic Division: Neurosensory]

Definition: Irreversible, long-standing, and/or progressive deterioration of intellect and personality characterized by a decreased ability to interpret environmental stimuli and decreased capacity for intellectual thought processes and manifested by disturbances of memory, orientation, and behavior.

Related Factors

Alzheimer's disease
Korsakoff's psychosis
Multi-infarct dementia
Cerebral vascular attack
Brain injury (e.g., cerebrovascular impairment, neurological illness, trauma, tumor)

Defining Characteristics

Objective

Alteration in interpretation or response to stimuli
Progressive alteration in cognitive function; chronic cognitive impairment; organic brain disorder
Normal level of consciousness
Impaired social functioning
Alteration in short-term/long-term memory
Alteration in personality

Information that appears in brackets has been added by the authors to clarify and enhance the use of nursing diagnoses.

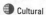

Desired Outcome/Evaluation Criteria—Client Will:

- Remain safe and free from harm.
- Maintain usual level of orientation.

Family/Significant Other Will:

- Verbalize an understanding of the disease process, prognosis, and client's needs.
- Identify and participate in interventions to deal effectively with the situation.
- Provide for maximal independence while meeting the safety needs of the client.

Actions/Interventions

Nursing Priority No. 1.

To assess degree of impairment:

- Evaluate responses on diagnostic examinations (e.g., memory impairments, reality orientation, attention span, calculations, and quality of life). **A combination of tests (e.g., Confusion Assessment Method [CAM], the Mini-Mental State Examination [MMSE], the Alzheimer's Disease Assessment Scale [ADAS-cog], the Brief Dementia Severity Rating Scale [BDSRS], or the Neuropsychiatric Inventory [NPI]) is often needed to complete an evaluation of the client's overall condition relating to a chronic/irreversible condition.**
- Test the client's ability to receive and send effective communication. **The client may be nonverbal or require assistance with/interpretation of verbalizations.**
- Talk with significant others (SO[s]) regarding baseline behaviors, length of time since onset, and progression of problem, their perception of prognosis, and other pertinent information and concerns for client. **If the history reveals an insidious decline over months to years, and if abnormal perceptions, inattention, and memory problems are concurrent with confusion, a diagnosis of dementia is likely.**
- Ascertain interventions previously used or tried.
- Evaluate response to care providers and receptiveness to interventions **to determine areas of concern to be addressed.**
- Determine anxiety level in relation to situation and problem behaviors **that may be indicative of potential for violence.**

Information that appears in brackets has been added by the authors to clarify and enhance the use of nursing diagnoses.

Nursing Priority No. 2.

To limit effects of deterioration/maximize level of function:

- Assist in treating conditions (e.g., infections, malnutrition, electrolyte imbalances, and adverse medication reactions) **that may contribute to/exacerbate confusion, discomfort, and agitation.**
- Provide a calm environment, minimize relocations, and eliminate extraneous noise/stimuli **that may increase the client's level of agitation/confusion.**
- Be open and honest in discussing the client's disease, abilities, and prognosis.
- Use touch judiciously. Tell the client what is being done before initiating contact **to reduce sense of surprise and negative reaction.**
- Avoid challenging illogical thinking **because defensive reactions may result.**
- Use positive statements; offer guided choices between two options. Simplify the client's tasks and routines **to accommodate fluctuating abilities and to reduce agitation associated with multiple options or demands.**
- Be supportive when the client is attempting to communicate and be sensitive to increasing frustration, fears, and misperceived threats.
- Encourage family/SO(s) to provide ongoing orientation and input to include current news and family happenings.
- Maintain reality-oriented relationship and environment (e.g., clocks, calendars, personal items, and seasonal decorations). Encourage participation in resocialization groups.
- Allow the client to reminisce or exist in own reality, if not detrimental to well-being.
- Provide safety measures (e.g., close supervision, identification bracelet, alarm on unlocked exits; medication lockup, removal of car or car keys; and lower temperature on hot water tank).
- Set limits on unsafe and/or inappropriate behavior, being alert to potential for violence.
- Avoid use of restraints as much as possible. Use vest (instead of wrist) restraints, or investigate the use of alternatives (such as bed nets, electronic bed pads, laptop trays) when required. **Although restraints may prevent falls, they can increase client's agitation and distress and are a safety risk.**
- Administer medications, as ordered (e.g., antidepressants or antipsychotics). Monitor for therapeutic action, as well as adverse reactions, side effects, and interactions. **Medications**

Information that appears in brackets has been added by the authors to clarify and enhance the use of nursing diagnoses.

 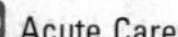 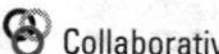 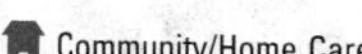  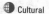

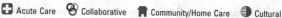

may be used judiciously to manage symptoms of psychosis, depression, or aggressive behavior.

- Refer to NDs acute Confusion; impaired Memory; impaired verbal Communication, for additional interventions.

Nursing Priority No. 3.

To assist SO(s) to develop coping strategies:

- Determine family resources, availability, and willingness to participate in meeting client's needs.
- Involve family/SO(s) in planning and care activities as needed/desired. Maintain frequent interactions with SO(s) **in order to relay information, change care strategies, obtain SO feedback, and offer support.**
- Discuss caregiver burden and signs of burnout, when appropriate. (Refer to NDs caregiver Role Strain; risk for caregiver Role Strain.)
- Provide educational materials, bibliographies, list of available local resources, help lines, Web sites, and so on, as desired, **to assist SO(s) in dealing and coping with long-term care issues.**
- Identify appropriate community resources (e.g., Alzheimer's Association [AA], stroke or brain injury support groups, senior support groups, specialist day services, home care, and respite care; adult placement and short-term residential care; clergy, social services, occupational and physical therapists; assistive technology and tele-care; attorney services for advance directives, and durable power of attorney) **to provide client/SO with support and assist with problem-solving.**

Nursing Priority No. 4.

To promote wellness (Teaching/Discharge Considerations):

- Discuss the nature of the client's condition (e.g., chronic stable, progressive, or degenerative), treatment concerns, and follow-up needed **to promote maintaining client at highest possible level of functioning.**
- Determine age-appropriate ongoing treatment and socialization needs and appropriate resources.
- Review medications with SO/caregiver(s), including dosage, route, action, expected and reportable side effects, and potential drug interactions **to prevent or limit complications associated with multiple psychiatric and central nervous system medications.**

Information that appears in brackets has been added by the authors to clarify and enhance the use of nursing diagnoses.

- Develop plan of care with family **to meet client's and SO's individual needs.**
- Provide appropriate referrals (e.g., Meals on Wheels, adult day care, home care agency, or respite care).

Documentation Focus

Assessment/Reassessment

- Individual findings, including current level of function and rate of anticipated changes
- Safety issues

Planning

- Plan of care and who is involved in planning

Implementation/Evaluation

- Response to interventions and actions performed
- Attainment or progress toward desired outcomes
- Modifications to plan of care

Discharge Planning

- Long-term needs, referrals made and who is responsible for actions to be taken
- Available resources, specific referrals made

Sample Nursing Outcomes & Interventions Classifications (NOC/NIC)

NOC—Cognitive Orientation
NIC—Dementia Management

CONSTIPATION and risk for CONSTIPATION

[Diagnostic Division: Elimination]

Definition: Constipation: Decrease in normal frequency of defecation accompanied by difficult or incomplete passage of stool and/or passage of excessively hard, dry stool.

Definition: at risk for Constipation: Vulnerable to a decrease in frequency of defecation, accompanied by difficulty passing stool, which may compromise health.

Information that appears in brackets has been added by the authors to clarify and enhance the use of nursing diagnoses.

Author note: After reviewing current research and all NDs involving constipation it appears that chronic functional Constipation is actually the more commonly occurring form. To this end the assessment and interventions here reflect only what is presented in the Related Factors and Defining Characteristics. More in depth assessment and interventions will be found in chronic functional Constipation.

Related Factors and Risk Factors

Functional

Abdominal muscle weakness
Average daily physical activity is less than recommended for gender and age
Habitually ignores urge to defecate; irregular defecation habits; inadequate toileting habits
Recent environmental change

Mechanical

Electrolyte imbalance
Hemorrhoids; pregnancy; obesity
Neurological impairment (e.g., positive EEG, head trauma, seizure disorders); Hirschsprung's disease; tumor
Prostate enlargement; postsurgical bowel obstruction; [colostomy]
Rectal abscess, ulcer; rectal prolapse; rectal anal fissure or stricture; rectocele

Pharmacological

Pharmaceutical agent; laxative abuse; iron salts (risk for constipation)

Physiological

Eating habit change (e.g., foods, eating times); insufficient dietary habits; insufficient fiber or fluid intake; dehydration
Inadequate dentition or oral hygiene
Decrease in gastrointestinal motility

Psychological

Emotional disturbance; depression; confusion

Information that appears in brackets has been added by the authors to clarify and enhance the use of nursing diagnoses.

Defining Characteristics (Constipation)

Subjective

Abdominal pain; pain with defecation;
Change in bowel pattern; decrease in frequency or volume of stool; hard, formed stool; inability to defecate;
Increase in abdominal pressure; feeling of rectal fullness or pressure; straining with defecation
Indigestion; vomiting; headache; fatigue

Objective

Hard, formed stool
Straining with defecation
Hypoactive or hyperactive bowel sounds; borborygmi
Distended abdomen; abdominal tenderness with/without palpable muscle resistance; palpable abdominal or rectal mass
Percussed abdominal dullness
Presence of soft paste-like stool in rectum; liquid stool; bright red blood with stool
Severe flatus; anorexia
Atypical presentations in older adults (e.g., changes in mental status, urinary incontinence, unexplained falls, or elevated body temperature)

NOTE: A risk diagnosis is not evidenced by signs and symptoms, as the problem has not occurred; rather, nursing interventions are directed at prevention.

Desired Outcomes/Evaluation Criteria—Client Will:

- Establish or regain normal pattern of bowel functioning.
- Verbalize understanding of etiology and appropriate interventions or solutions for individual situation.
- Demonstrate behaviors or lifestyle changes to prevent recurrence of problem.
- Participate in bowel program as indicated.

Actions/Interventions

Nursing Priority No. 1.

To identify causative/contributing or individual risk factors:

- Review medical, surgical, and social history **to identify conditions commonly associated with constipation, including (1) problems with colon or rectum (e.g., obstruction, scar tissue**

Information that appears in brackets has been added by the authors to clarify and enhance the use of nursing diagnoses.

or stricture; presence of diversion [e.g., descending/sigmoid colostomy]; diverticulitis, irritable bowel syndrome, tumors, anal fissure); (2) metabolic or endocrine disorders (e.g., diabetes mellitus, hypothyroidism, or uremia); (3) limited physical activity (e.g., bedrest, poor mobility, chronic disability); (4) chronic pain problems (especially when client is on pain medications); (5) pregnancy and childbirth, recent abdominal or perianal surgery; and (6) neurological disorders (e.g., stroke, traumatic brain injury, Parkinson's disease, MS, and spinal cord abnormalities).

- Note the client's age. **Constipation is more likely to occur in individuals older than 65 but can occur in any age from infant to elderly. A bottle-fed infant is more prone to constipation than a breastfed infant, especially when formula contains iron. Toddlers are at risk because of developmental factors (e.g., too young, too interested in other things, rigid schedule during potty training), and children and adolescents are at risk because of unwillingness to take break from play, poor eating and fluid intake habits, and withholding because of perceived lack of privacy. Many older adults experience constipation as a result of diminished nerve sensations, immobility, dehydration, and electrolyte imbalances; incomplete emptying of the bowel, or failing to attend to signals to defecate.**
- Review daily dietary regimen, noting if diet is deficient in fiber. **Inadequate dietary fiber (vegetable, fruits, and whole grains) and highly processed foods contribute to poor intestinal function. Note: Clients with descending or sigmoid colostomy must avoid constipation. Some may find it helpful to create their own dietary bulk laxative by combining unprocessed millers bran, applesauce, and prune juice.** Refer to ND: chronic functional Constipation for further assessments and interventions regarding dietary issues in constipation.
- Note general oral/dental health issues. **Dental problems can impact dietary intake (e.g., loss of teeth or other oral conditions can force individuals to eat soft foods or liquids, mostly lacking in fiber).**
- Determine fluid intake **to note deficits.** Refer to ND: chronic functional Constipation for further assessments and interventions regarding fluid issues in constipation.
- Evaluate the client's medications or drug usage **that could cause/exacerbate constipation.** Refer to ND: chronic functional Constipation for further assessments and interventions regarding medication issues in constipation.

Information that appears in brackets has been added by the authors to clarify and enhance the use of nursing diagnoses.

- Note energy and activity levels and exercise pattern. **Lack of physical activity or regular exercise is often a factor in constipation.** Refer to ND: chronic functional Constipation for assessments and interventions regarding activity issues in constipation.
- Identify areas of life changes or stressors (e.g., personal relationships, occupational factors, or financial problems). **Individuals may fail to allow time for good bowel habits and/or suffer gastrointestinal effects from stress.**
- Determine access to bathroom, privacy, and ability to perform self-care activities.
- Investigate reports of pain with defecation. **Hemorrhoids, rectal fissures or prolapse, skin breakdown, or other abnormal findings may be hindering passage of stool or causing client to hold stool.**
- Determine laxative/enema use. Note signs and reports of overuse of stimulant laxatives. **This is most common among older adults preoccupied with having daily bowel movements.**
- Auscultate abdomen for presence, location, and characteristics of bowel sounds **reflecting bowel activity.**
- Palpate abdomen **for presence of distention or masses.**
- Check digital rectum for presence of fecal impaction, as indicated, **to evaluate rectal tone and detect tenderness, blood, or detect fecal impaction.**
- Assist with medical work-up (e.g., x-rays, abdominal imaging, proctosigmoidoscopy, anorectal function tests, colonic transit studies, and stool sample tests) **for identification of other possible causative factors.**

Nursing Priority No. 2.

To determine usual pattern of elimination:

- Discuss usual elimination habits (e.g., normal urge time) and problems (e.g., client unable to eliminate unless in own home, passing hard stool after prolonged effort, or anal pain).
- Note color, odor, consistency, amount, and frequency of stool. **This provides a baseline for comparison, and promotes recognition of changes.**
- Identify elements that usually stimulate bowel activity (e.g., caffeine, walking, and laxative use) and any interfering factors (e.g., taking opioid pain medications, being unable to ambulate to the bathroom, or pelvic surgery).
- Ascertain client's degree of concern (e.g., long-standing condition that client has "lived with" may not cause undue concern, whereas an acute postsurgical occurrence of constipation

---

Information that appears in brackets has been added by the authors to clarify and enhance the use of nursing diagnoses.

can cause great distress). **The client's response may or may not reflect the severity of the condition.**

- Note the pharmacological agents the client has used (e.g., fiber pills, laxatives, suppositories, or enemas) **to determine the effectiveness of the current regimen, and whether laxative use is appropriate and helpful.**
- Encourage the client to maintain an elimination diary, if appropriate, **to facilitate monitoring of long-term problem.**

Nursing Priority No. 3.

To facilitate an acceptable pattern of elimination:

- Promote lifestyle changes:

  Limit foods with little or no fiber, or diet high in fats (e.g., ice cream, cheese, meats, fast foods, and processed foods).

  Promote adequate fluid intake, including water, high-fiber fruit, and vegetable juices, fruit/vegetable smoothies, popsicles. Suggest drinking warm, stimulating fluids (e.g., decaffeinated coffee, hot water, or tea).

  Encourage daily activity and exercise within limits of individual ability.

  Encourage the client to not ignore urge. Provide privacy and routinely scheduled time for colostomy irrigation or defecation (bathroom or commode preferable to bedpan).

  Refer to ND: chronic functional Constipation for related interventions.

- Encourage sitz bath after stools **for soothing effect to rectal area.**
- Administer or recommend medications (e.g., stool softeners, mild stimulants, or bulk-forming agents), as ordered or routinely, when appropriate **to prevent constipation (e.g., client taking pain medications, especially opiates, or who is inactive, or immobile).**
- Apply lubricant/anesthetic ointment to anus, if needed.
- Review the client's current medication regime with the physician **to determine if drugs contributing to constipation can be discontinued or changed.**
- Establish bowel program to include predictable interval timing for colostomy irrigation or toileting; use of particular position for defecation; abdominal massage; biofeedback for pelvic floor dysfunction; and medications, as appropriate, **when long-term or permanent bowel dysfunction is present.**
- Refer to primary care provider for medical therapies (e.g., added emolient, saline, or hyperosmolar laxatives, enemas, or suppositories) **to best treat acute situation.**

Information that appears in brackets has been added by the authors to clarify and enhance the use of nursing diagnoses.

Nursing Priority No. 5.

To promote wellness (Teaching/Discharge Considerations):

- Discuss client's particular physiology and acceptable variations in elimination.
- Provide information about relationship of diet, exercise, fluid, and healthy elimination, as indicated.
- Provide social and emotional support **to help the client manage actual or potential disabilities associated with long-term bowel management.**
- Discuss rationale for and encourage continuation of successful interventions.
- Work to implement bowel management program that is easily replicated in home and community setting.
- Identify specific actions to be taken if problem does not resolve **to promote timely intervention, thereby enhancing client's independence.**

Documentation Focus

Assessment/Reassessment

- Usual and current bowel pattern, duration of the problem, and individual contributing factors, including diet and exercise/activity level
- Characteristics of stool
- Individual contributing or risk factors

Planning

- Plan of care, specific interventions, and changes in lifestyle that are necessary to correct individual situation, and who is involved in planning
- Teaching plan

Implementation/Evaluation

- Responses to interventions, teaching, and actions performed
- Change in bowel pattern, character of stool
- Attainment or progress toward desired outcomes
- Modifications to plan of care

Discharge Planning

- Individual long-term needs, noting who is responsible for actions to be taken
- Recommendations for follow-up care
- Specific referrals made

Information that appears in brackets has been added by the authors to clarify and enhance the use of nursing diagnoses.

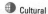

Sample Nursing Outcomes & Interventions Classifications (NOC/NIC)

NOC—Bowel Elimination
NIC—Constipation/Impaction Management

chronic functional CONSTIPATION and risk for functional CONSTIPATION

[Diagnostic Division: Elimination]

Definition: chronic functional Constipation: Infrequent or difficult evacuation of feces, which has been present for at least 3 of the prior 12 months.

Definition: risk for functional Constipation: Vulnerable to infrequent or difficult evacuation of feces, which has been present for nearly 3 of the prior 12 months, which may compromise health.

Related Factors (chronic functional Constipation)

Anal fissure/stricture; hemorrhoids; proctitis
Insufficient dietary/fluid intake; dehydration; low fiber diet; low calorie intake; diet disproportionately high in protein and fat; failure to thrive
Inflammatory bowel disease; chronic intestinal pseudoobstruction; ischemic stenosis; postinflammatory stenosis; surgical stenosis; colorectal cancer; extra intestinal mass; Hirschprung's disease
Sedentary lifestyle; impaired mobility; Parkinson's disease; slow colon transit time
Spinal cord injury; paraplegia; multiple sclerosis; autonomic neuropathy; myotonic dystrophy; cerebral vascular accident
Pharmaceutical agent; polypharmacy
Pregnancy; perineal damage; pelvic floor dysfunction
Hypercalcemia; hypothyroidism; panhypopituitarism
Diabetes mellitus; chronic renal insufficiency; scleroderma; dermatomyositis
Depression; dementia; habitually ignores urge to defecate

Risk Factors (risk for chronic functional Constipation)

Aluminum-containing antacids; antieleptics; anthihypertensives; anti-Parkinsonian agents (anticholinergic or dopamin-

Information that appears in brackets has been added by the authors to clarify and enhance the use of nursing diagnoses.

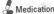

ergic); calcium-channel antagonists; diuretics; iron preparations; non-steroidal anti-inflammatories (NSAIDs); opoids; tricyclic antidepressants; polypharmacy
Chronic intestinal pseudo-obstruction; slow colon transit times
Decreased food intake; dehydration; insufficient fluid intake
Depression; failure to thrive
Diet proportionally high in protein and fat; low-fiber diet; low caloric intake
Habitual ignoring of urge to defecate
Impaired immobility; inactive lifestyle

Defining Characteristics (chronic functional Constipation)

Subjective

Pain with defecation
Prolonged straining
[Feeling as though stool is still in rectum after bowel movement]
[Feeling as though something is blocking stool from passing]
[Using fingers to help with stool passage]

Objective

Type 1 or 2 Bristol Stool Chart

- CHILD: ≤4 years: Presence of ≥2 criteria on roman III Pediatric classification system for ≥1 month; or child ≥4 years ≥2 criteria for ≥2 months:

  ≤2 defecations per week
  ≥1 episode of fecal incontinence per week
  Stool retentive posturing
  Painful or hard bowel movements
  Presence of a large fecal mass in the rectum
  Large diameter stools that may obstruct the toilet

- ADULT: Presence of ≥2 of the following symptoms on Rome III classification system:

  Lumpy or hard stool in ≥25% defecations
  Straining during ≥25% of defecations
  Sensation of anorectal obstruction/blockage for ≥25% of defecations

Information that appears in brackets has been added by the authors to clarify and enhance the use of nursing diagnoses.

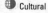

Manual maneuvers to facilitate ≥25% of defecations (digital manipulation, pelvic floor support)
≥3 defecations per week

Abdominal distention
Palpable abdominal mass
Fecal impaction
Fecal incontinence (in children)
Leakage of stool with digital stimulation
Positive fecal occult blood testing

Desired Outcomes/Evaluation Criteria—Client Will:

- Establish or regain a normal pattern of bowel functioning.
- Document that bowel function has improved through the use of a bowel function diary noting an increase in the frequency of stools, and/or decrease in straining at stool.
- Verbalize an understanding of etiology and appropriate interventions or solutions for the individual situation.

Actions/Interventions

Nursing Priority No. 1.

To identify causative/contributing or risk factors:

- Review medical/surgical history **to identify conditions commonly associated with functional constipation. Primary causes are related to problems inherent to the intestine; subdivided into normal-transit constipation, slow-transit constipation, and anorectal dysfunction. Secondary causes include (1) gastrointestinal disorders (e.g., intestinal tumors; idiopathic megacolon; rectal prolapse, anal fissure; and irritable bowel syndrome); (2) metabolic and endocrine disorders (e.g., diabetes, chronic renal insufficiency); (3) neurological conditions (e.g., stroke, dementia syndromes, multiple sclerosis, spinal cord injuries); (4) psychogenic disorders (e.g., anxiety, depression); (5) dehydration; and (6) the use of a variety of medications.**
- ∞ Note the client's age, gender, and general health status. **Constipation is more likely to occur in individuals older than**

Information that appears in brackets has been added by the authors to clarify and enhance the use of nursing diagnoses.

65 years of age but may occur in a client of any age with chronic, debilitating conditions. Approximately 95% of childhood constipation is functional in nature without any obvious cause. Note: Prevalence estimates by gender support a female-to-male ratio of 3.1:1.

- Evaluate current medications or drug usage **for agents that could slow the passage of stool and cause or exacerbate constipation (e.g., opioids, anti-inflammatories, calcium channel blockers, calcium and iron supplements, anticholinergics, antidepressants, antipsychotics, antihistamines, anticonvulsants, diuretics, chemotherapy, contrast media, and steroids).**
- Note interventions the client has tried **to relieve the current situation (e.g., fiber pills, laxatives, suppositories, or enemas),** and document success or lack of effectiveness.
- Assist with medical workup (e.g., lower GI series x-rays, abdominal imaging [e.g., defecography], colonoscopy, or sigmoidoscopy; anorectal function tests [e.g., anal manometry, blood expulsion tests]; and colonic transit studies) **for identification of possible causative factors and to show how well food moves through the colon.**

Nursing Priority No. 2.

To assess current pattern of elimination:

- Note color, odor, consistency, amount, and frequency of stool following each bowel movement during assessment phase. **Provides a baseline for comparison, promoting recognition of changes.**
- Auscultate abdomen for presence, location, and characteristics of bowel sounds **reflecting bowel activity.**
- Palpate abdomen for hardness, distention, and masses, **indicating possible obstruction or retention of stool.**
- Perform digital rectal examination, as indicated, **to evaluate rectal tone and detect tenderness, blood, or fecal impaction.**
- Remove impacted stool digitally, when necessary, after applying lubricant and anesthetic ointment to anus **to soften impaction and decrease rectal pain.**

Nursing Priority No. 3.

To reduce actual **or risk** of unacceptable pattern of elimination:

- Collaborate in the treatment of underlying medical cause where appropriate (e.g., surgery to repair rectal prolapse, biofeedback

---

Information that appears in brackets has been added by the authors to clarify and enhance the use of nursing diagnoses.

to retrain anorectal or pelvic floor dysfunction, medications, and combinations of therapies as indicated) **to improve body and bowel function. Note: Treatment is highly individual. For example, clients with slow-transit constipation tend to benefit from fiber, osmotic laxatives, and stimulant laxatives (e.g., bisacodyl), whereas those with evacuation disorders usually do not need medication other than fiber supplementation following pelvic floor retraining.**

- Review the client's current medication regime with the physician **to determine if drugs contributing to constipation can be discontinued or changed.**
- Administer medications as indicated by the client's particular bowel dysfunction, such as stool softeners (e.g., docusate sodium [Colase, Surfak]), mild stimulants (e.g., bisacodyl [Dulcolax, Bisco-Lax], osmotic agents (e.g., polyethylene glycol [PEG, Miralax] opioid antagonist (e.g., methylanaltrexone [Relistor]
- Administer enemas (e.g., hyperosmolar agents [e.g., Fleet enema] or suppositories), as indicated.
- Promote lifestyle changes:

  Instruct in and encourage a personalized dietary program that involves adjustment of dietary fiber and bulk in diet (e.g., fruits, vegetables, and whole grains) and fiber supplements (e.g., wheat bran, psyllium) **to improve consistency of stool and increase transit time through colon, if slow transit through colon is causing symptoms.**

  Promote adequate fluid intake, including water, high-fiber fruit, and vegetable juices, fruit/vegetable smoothies, popsicles. Suggest drinking warm, stimulating fluids (e.g., decaffeinated coffee, hot water, or tea) **to avoid dehydration, promote moist, soft feces, and facilitate passage of stool.**
- Instruct in/assist with other means of triggering defecation (e.g., abdominal massage, digital stimulation, placement of rectal stimulant suppositories) **to provide predictable and effective elimination and reduce evacuation problems when long-term or permanent bowel dysfunction is present.**
- Refer to physical therapy or other medical/surgical practitioners for additional interventions as indicated. **Physical therapy may be useful in improving mobility, pelvic floor retraining, and activity levels. Biofeedback treatment can result in a cure for constipation associated with certain evacuation disorders. Surgical interventions may be used in some instances to treat long-term, intractable constipation due to neurogenic bowel.**

Information that appears in brackets has been added by the authors to clarify and enhance the use of nursing diagnoses.

Nursing Priority No. 4.

To promote wellness (Teaching/Discharge Considerations):

- Discuss the client's particular anatomy and physiology of bowel and acceptable variations in elimination.
- Provide information and resources to client/SO about relationship of diet, exercise, fluid, and appropriate use of laxatives, as indicated.
- Provide social and emotional support **to help client manage actual or potential disabilities associated with long-term bowel management.** Discuss rationale for and encourage continuation of successful interventions.
- Encourage the client to maintain an elimination diary, if appropriate, **to facilitate management of long-term condition, and reveal the most helpful interventions.**
- Collaborate with medical providers and client/caregiver in designing bowel management program to be easily replicated in home and community setting.
- Identify specific actions to be taken if the problem does not resolve (e.g., return to physician for additional testing and interventions) **to promote timely intervention, thereby enhancing the client's independence.**

Documentation Focus

Assessment/Reassessment

- Usual and current bowel pattern, duration of the problem, and interventions used
- Characteristics of stool
- Individual contributing factors

Planning

- Plan of care, specific interventions or changes in lifestyle necessary to correct individual situation, and who is involved in planning
- Teaching plan

Implementation/Evaluation

- Responses to interventions, teaching, and actions performed
- Change in bowel pattern, character of stool
- Attainment or progress toward desired outcomes
- Modifications to plan of care

Discharge Planning

- Individual long-term needs, noting who is responsible for actions to be taken

---

Information that appears in brackets has been added by the authors to clarify and enhance the use of nursing diagnoses.

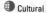

- Recommendations for follow-up care
- Specific referrals made

Sample Nursing Outcomes & Interventions Classifications (NOC/NIC)

NOC—Bowel Elimination
NIC—Bowel Management

perceived CONSTIPATION

[Diagnostic Division: Elimination]

Definition: Self-diagnosis of constipation combined with abuse of laxatives, enemas, and/or suppositories to ensure a daily bowel movement.

Related Factors

Cultural or family health beliefs
Impaired thought process

Defining Characteristics

Subjective

Expects daily bowel movement
Expects daily bowel movement at same time every day
Laxative, enema, or suppository abuse

Desired Outcomes/Evaluation Criteria—Client Will:

- Verbalize understanding of physiology of bowel function.
- Identify acceptable interventions to promote adequate bowel function.
- Decrease reliance on laxatives or enemas.
- Establish individually appropriate pattern of elimination.

Actions/Interventions

Nursing Priority No. 1.

To identify factors affecting individual beliefs:

- Determine the client's understanding of a "normal" bowel pattern and cultural expectations. **This helps to identify areas for discussion or intervention. For example, what is con-**

Information that appears in brackets has been added by the authors to clarify and enhance the use of nursing diagnoses.

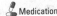

sidered "normal" varies with the individual, cultural, and familial factors with differences in expectations and dietary habits. In addition, individuals can think they are constipated when, in fact, their bowel movements are regular and soft, possibly revealing a problem with thought processes or perception. Some people believe they are constipated, or irregular, if they do not have a bowel movement every day, because of ideas instilled from childhood. The elderly client may believe that laxatives or purgatives are necessary for elimination, when in fact the problem may be long-standing habits (e.g., insufficient fluids, lack of exercise and/or fiber in the diet).

- Discuss the client's use of laxatives. **Perceived constipation typically results in self-medicating with various laxatives. Although laxatives may correct the acute problem, chronic use leads to habituation, requiring ever-increasing doses that result in drug dependency and, ultimately, a hypotonic colon.**
- Identify interventions used by the client to correct the perceived problem **to identify strengths and areas of concern to be addressed.**

Nursing Priority No. 2.

To promote wellness (Teaching/Discharge Considerations):

- Discuss the following with the client/SO/caregiver **to clarify issues regarding actual and perceived bowel functioning, and to provide support during behavior modification/ bowel retraining:**

  Review anatomy and physiology of bowel function and acceptable variations in elimination.

  Identify detrimental effects of habitual laxative or enema use, and discuss alternatives.

  Provide information about the relationship of diet, hydration, and exercise to improved elimination.

  Encourage the client to maintain an elimination calendar or diary, if appropriate.

  Provide support by active-listening and discussing the client's concerns or fears.

  Provide social and emotional support.

  Encourage the use of stress-reduction activities and refocusing of attention while the client works to establish an individually appropriate pattern.
- Offer educational materials and resources for client/SO to peruse at home **to assist the client in making informed con-**

Information that appears in brackets has been added by the authors to clarify and enhance the use of nursing diagnoses.

clusions about symptoms, as well as constipation management options.

- Refer to medical/psychiatric providers, as indicated. **A client with a fixed perception of constipation where none actually exists may require further assessment and intervention.**
- Refer to ND Constipation for additional interventions, as appropriate.

Documentation Focus

Assessment/Reassessment

- Assessment findings, client's perceptions of the problem
- Current bowel pattern, stool characteristics

Planning

- Plan of care, specific interventions, and who is involved in the planning
- Teaching plan

Implementation/Evaluation

- Client's responses to interventions, teaching, and actions performed
- Changes in bowel pattern, character of stool
- Attainment or progress toward desired outcome(s)
- Modifications to plan of care

Discharge Planning

- Referral for follow-up care

Sample Nursing Outcomes & Interventions Classifications (NOC/NIC)

NOC—Health Beliefs
NIC—Bowel Management

CONTAMINATION and risk for CONTAMINATION

[Diagnostic Division: Safety]

Definition: Contamination: Exposure to environmental contaminants in doses sufficient to cause adverse health effects.

Definition: risk for Contamination: Vulnerable to exposure to environmental contaminants which may compromise health.

Information that appears in brackets has been added by the authors to clarify and enhance the use of nursing diagnoses.

Related and Risk Factors

External

Carpeted flooring; flaking, peeling surface in presence of young children (e.g., paint, plaster); playing where environmental contaminants are used

Chemical contamination of food or water; ingestion of contaminated material (e.g., radioactive, food, water)

Economically disadvantaged

Exposure to areas with high contaminant level or atmospheric pollutants; inadequate breakdown of contaminant;

Exposure to bioterrorism, or disaster (natural or man-made), or radiation; unprotected exposure to chemical (e.g., arsenic)

Inadequate household or personal hygiene practices.

Inadequate municipal services (e.g., trash removal, sewage treatment facilities)

Use of environmental contaminants in the home; use of noxious material (e,g, lacquer, paint) in an insufficiently ventilated area or without effective protection

Internal

Age (children less than 5 years, older adults); gestational age during exposure

Female gender; pregnancy

Inadequate nutrition

Preexisting disease states; smoking

Concomitant exposure or previous exposures to contaminants

> **NOTE:** A risk diagnosis is not evidenced by signs and symptoms, as the problem has not occurred; rather, nursing interventions are directed at prevention.

Defining Characteristics (Contamination)

> **Author note:** Defining characteristics are dependent on the causative agent. Agents cause a variety of individual organ responses as well as systemic responses.

Subjective/Objective

Pesticides: [Major categories of pesticides: insecticides, herbicides, fungicides, antimicrobials, rodenticides; major pesticides: organophosphates, carbamates, organochlorines,

---

Information that appears in brackets has been added by the authors to clarify and enhance the use of nursing diagnoses.

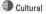

pyrethrum, arsenic, glycophosphates, bipyridyis, chlorophenoxy compounds]

Dermatological, gastrointestinal, neurological, pulmonary, or renal effects of pesticide

Chemicals: [Major chemical agents: petroleum-based agents, anticholinesterases; type I agents act on proximal tracheobronchial portion of the respiratory tract, type II agents act on alveoli, type III agents produce systemic effects]

Dermatological, gastrointestinal, immunological, neurological, pulmonary, or renal effects of chemical exposure

Biologicals: [Toxins from living organisms—bacteria, viruses, fungi]

Dermatological, gastrointestinal, neurological, pulmonary, or renal effects of exposure to biologicals

Pollution: [Major locations: air, water, soil; major agents: asbestos, radon, tobacco [smoke], heavy metal, lead, noise, exhaust fumes]

Neurological or pulmonary effects of pollution exposure

Waste: [Major categories of waste: trash, raw sewage, industrial waste]

Dermatological, gastrointestinal, hepatic, or pulmonary effects of waste exposure

Radiation: [External exposure through direct contact with radioactive material]

Immunological, genetic, neurological, or oncological effects of radiation exposure

Desired Outcomes/Evaluation Criteria—Client Will:

- Be free of injury.
- Verbalize an understanding of individual factors that contributed to injury and take steps to correct situation(s).
- Demonstrate behaviors or lifestyle changes to reduce risk factors and protect self from injury.
- Modify environment, as indicated, to enhance safety.

Client/Community Will:

- Identify hazards that lead to exposure or contamination.
- Correct environmental hazards, as identified.
- Demonstrate necessary actions to promote community safety.
- Support community activities for disaster preparedness.

Information that appears in brackets has been added by the authors to clarify and enhance the use of nursing diagnoses.

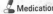

Actions/Interventions

In reviewing this ND, it is apparent there is overlap with other diagnoses. We have chosen to present generalized interventions. Although there are commonalities to contamination situations, we suggest that the reader refer to other primary diagnoses as indicated, such as ineffective Airway Clearance; ineffective Breathing Pattern; impaired Gas Exchange; impaired Home Maintenance; risk for Infection; risk for Injury; risk for Poisoning; impaired/risk for impaired Skin Integrity; risk for Suffocation; ineffective Tissue Perfusion [specify]; risk for Trauma.

Nursing Priority No. 1.

To evaluate degree/source of exposure **or source of risk:**

- Ascertain the type of contaminant(s) (e.g., chemical, biological, or air pollutant) **which has exposed (or is posing a potential hazard to) client and/or community.**
- Determine manner of exposure when contamination has occurred (e.g., inhalation, ingestion, or topical), whether exposure was accidental or intentional, and immediate/delayed reactions. **This determines the course of action to be taken by all emergency/other care providers. Note: Intentional exposure to hazardous materials requires notification of law enforcement for further investigation and possible prosecution.**
- ∞ Note age and gender: **Children less than 5 years are at greater risk for adverse effects from exposure to contaminants because (1) smaller body size causes them to receive a more concentrated "dose" than adults; (2) they spend more time outside than most adults, increasing exposure to air and soil pollutants; (3) they spend more time on the floor, increasing exposure to toxins in carpets and low cupboards; (4) they consume more water and food per pound than adults, increasing their body-weight-to-toxin ratio; and (5) fetus's/infant's and young children's developing organ systems can be disrupted. Older adults have a normal decline in function of immune, integumentary, cardiac, renal, hepatic, and pulmonary systems; an increase in adipose tissue mass; and a decline in lean body mass. Females, in general, have a greater proportion of body fat, increasing the chance of accumulating more lipid-soluble toxins than males.**
- Ascertain geographical location (e.g., home, work) where exposure occurred. **Individual and/or community intervention may be needed to correct problem.**

Information that appears in brackets has been added by the authors to clarify and enhance the use of nursing diagnoses.

- Note socioeconomic status and availability and use of resources. **Living in poverty increases potential for multiple exposures, delayed/lack of access to healthcare, and poor general health, potentially increasing the severity of adverse effects of exposure.**
- Determine factors associated with particular contaminant:

  Pesticides: Determine if client has ingested contaminated foods (e.g., fruits, vegetables, or commercially raised meats), or inhaled agent (e.g., aerosol bug sprays, in vicinity of crop spraying).

  Chemicals: Ascertain if client uses environmental contaminants in the home or at work (e.g., pesticides, chemicals, chlorine household cleaners) and fails to use/inappropriately uses protective clothing.

  Biologicals: Determine if client may have been exposed to biological agents (bacteria, viruses, fungi) or bacterial toxins (e.g., botulinum, ricin). **Exposure occurring as a result of an act of terrorism would be rare; however, individuals may be exposed to bacterial agents or toxins through contaminated or poorly prepared foods.**

  Pollution air/water: Determine if client has been exposed/is sensitive to atmospheric pollutants (e.g., radon, benzene [from gasoline], carbon monoxide, automobile emissions [numerous chemicals], chlorofluorocarbons [refrigerants, solvents], ozone or smog particles [acids, organic chemicals; particles in smoke; commercial plants, such as pulp and paper mills]).

  Investigate possibility of home-based exposure to air pollution. **Toxins may include carbon monoxide (e.g., poor ventilation, especially in the winter months [poor heating systems, use of charcoal grill indoors, car left running in garage]; cigarette or cigar smoke indoors; ozone [spending a lot of time outdoors, such as playing children, adults participating in moderate to strenuous work or recreational activities]).**

  Waste: Determine if the client lives in an area where trash or garbage accumulates or is exposed to raw sewage or industrial wastes that **can contaminate soil and water.**

  Radiation: Ascertain if the client/household member experienced accidental exposure (e.g., occupation in radiography; living near, or working in, nuclear industries or electrical generation plants).
- Observe for signs and symptoms of infective agent and sepsis such as fatigue, malaise, headache, fever, chills, diaphoresis, skin rash, and altered level of consciousness. **Initial symp-**

Information that appears in brackets has been added by the authors to clarify and enhance the use of nursing diagnoses.

toms of some diseases that mimic influenza may be misdiagnosed if healthcare providers do not maintain an index of suspicion.

- Note the presence and degree of chemical burns and initial treatment provided.
- Obtain/assist with diagnostic studies, as indicated. **This provides information about the type and degree of exposure/organ involvement or damage.**
- Identify psychological response (e.g., anger, shock, acute anxiety, confusion, or denial) to accidental or mass exposure incident. **Although these are normal responses, they may recycle repeatedly and result in post-trauma syndrome if not dealt with adequately.**
- Alert the proper authorities to the presence of or exposure to contamination, as appropriate. **Depending on the agent involved, there may be reporting requirements to local, state, or national agencies, such as the local health department, the Environmental Protection Agency (EPA), and Centers for Disease Control and Prevention (CDC).**

Nursing Priority No. 2.

To assist in treating effects of exposure **(Contamination):**

- Implement a coordinated decontamination plan (e.g., removal of clothing, showering with soap and water), when indicated, following consultation with medical toxicologist, hazardous materials team, and industrial hygiene and safety officer **to prevent further harm to client and to protect healthcare providers.**
- Ensure availability and use of personal protective equipment (PPE) (e.g., high-efficiency particulate air [HEPA] filter masks, special garments, and barrier materials including gloves/face shield) **to protect from exposure to biological, chemical, and radioactive hazards.**
- Provide for isolation or group/cohort individuals with same diagnosis or exposure, as resources require. **Limited resources may dictate open ward-like environment; however, the need to control the spread of infection still exists. Only plague, smallpox, and viral hemorrhagic fevers require more than standard infection-control precautions.**
- Provide/assist with therapeutic interventions, as individually appropriate. **Specific needs of the client and the level of care available at a given time/location determine response.**
- Refer pregnant client for individually appropriate diagnostic procedures or screenings. **This helps to determine effects of**

Information that appears in brackets has been added by the authors to clarify and enhance the use of nursing diagnoses.

teratogenic exposure on fetus, allowing for informed choices/preparations.

- Screen breast milk in lactating client following radiation exposure. **Depending on type and amount of exposure, breastfeeding may need to be briefly interrupted or, occasionally, terminated.**
- Cooperate with and refer to appropriate agencies (e.g., CDC; U.S. Army Medical Research Institute of Infectious Diseases [USAMRIID]; Federal Emergency Management Agency [FEMA]; U.S. Department of Health and Human Services [DHHS]; Office of Emergency Preparedness [OEP]; EPA) **to prepare for/manage mass casualty incidents.**

Nursing Priority No. 3. (risk for Contamination)

To assist client to reduce or correct individual risk factors:

- Assist the client to develop a plan to address individual safety needs and injury/illness prevention in home, community, and work settings.
- Repair or replace unsafe household items and situations (e.g., flaking/peeling paint or plaster; filter for unsafe tap water).
- Review effects of secondhand smoke and importance of refraining from smoking in home/car **where others are likely to be exposed.**
- Encourage the removal or proper cleaning of carpeted floors, especially for small children and persons with respiratory conditions. **Carpets hold up to 100 times as much fine-particle material as a bare floor and can contain metals and pesticides.**
- Encourage timely cleaning and replacement of air filters on furnace and/or air-conditioning unit. **Good ventilation cuts down on indoor air pollution from carpets, machines, paints, solvents, cleaning materials, and pesticides.**
- Recommend periodic inspection of well water or tap water **to identify possible contaminants.**
- Encourage the client to install carbon monoxide monitors and other air pollutant detectors in the home, as appropriate.
- Recommend placing a dehumidifier in damp areas **to retard growth of molds.**
- Review proper handling of household chemicals:

  Read chemical labels. Know primary hazards (especially in commonly used household cleaning and gardening products).

  Follow directions printed on product label (e.g., avoid use of certain chemicals on food preparation surfaces, refrain from spraying garden chemicals on windy days).

Information that appears in brackets has been added by the authors to clarify and enhance the use of nursing diagnoses.

Use products labeled "nontoxic" wherever possible. Choose the least hazardous products for the job, preferably multiuse products **to reduce number of different chemicals used and stored.**

Use a form of chemical that most reduces risk of exposure (e.g., cream instead of liquid or aerosol).

Wear protective clothing, gloves, and safety glasses when using chemicals. Avoid mixing chemicals at all times, and use in well-ventilated areas.

Store chemicals in locked cabinets. Keep chemicals in original labeled containers and do not pour into other containers.

∞ Place safety stickers on chemicals **to warn children of harmful contents.**

- Review proper food handling, storage, and cooking techniques.
- ∞ Stress the importance of pregnant or lactating women following fish and wildlife consumption guidelines provided by state and U.S. territorial or Native American tribes. **Ingestion of noncommercial fish or wildlife can be a significant source of pollutants.**

Nursing Priority No. 4.

To promote wellness (Teaching/Discharge Considerations):

Client/Caregiver

- Identify individual safety needs and injury/illness prevention in home, community, and work settings.
- Review individual nutritional needs, appropriate exercise program, and need for rest. **These are essentials for well-being and recovery.**
- ∞ Emphasize the importance of supervising infant/child or individuals with cognitive limitations.
- Discuss protective actions for specific "bad air days" (e.g., limiting or avoiding outdoor activities).
- Refer to smoking-cessation program, as needed.
- Stress the importance of posting emergency and poison control numbers in a visible location.
- Encourage learning CPR and first aid.
- Encourage the client/caregiver to develop a personal/family disaster plan, to gather needed supplies to provide for self and family during a community emergency, and to learn how specific public health threats might affect client and actions **to reduce the risk to health and safety.**
- Review pertinent job-related safety regulations. Emphasize the necessity of wearing appropriate protective equipment.

Information that appears in brackets has been added by the authors to clarify and enhance the use of nursing diagnoses.

- Instruct the client to always refer to local authorities and health experts for specific up-to-date information for the community and to follow their advice.
- Refer to counselor/support groups **for ongoing assistance in dealing with traumatic incident/aftereffects of exposure.**
- Provide bibliotherapy including written resources and appropriate Web sites **for review and self-paced learning.**

Home

- Discuss general safety concerns with client/SO **to ensure that people are educated about potential risks and ways to manage risks.**
- Review effects of secondhand smoke and importance of refraining from smoking in home/car where others are likely to be exposed.
- Install carbon monoxide monitors and other indoor air pollutant detectors in the home, as appropriate.
- Install a dehumidifier in damp areas **to retard the growth of molds.**
- Encourage timely replacement of air filters on furnace and/or air-conditioning unit. **Good ventilation cuts down on indoor air pollution from carpets, machines, paints, solvents, cleaning materials, and pesticides.**
- Discuss protective actions for specific "bad air" days (e.g., limiting or avoiding outdoor activities). **Measures may include limiting or avoiding outdoor activities, especially in sensitive groups (e.g., children who are active outdoors, adults involved in moderate or strenuous outdoor activities, and persons with respiratory diseases).**
- Repair, replace, or correct unsafe household items or situations (e.g., storage of solvents in soda bottles, flaking or peeling paint or plaster, and filtering unsafe tap water).
- Encourage the removal of or cleaning of carpeted floors, especially for small children and persons with respiratory conditions. **Carpets hold up to 100 times as much fine-particle material as a bare floor and can contain metals and pesticides.**
- Identify commercial cleaning resources, if appropriate, **for safe cleaning of contaminated articles/surfaces.**
- Recommend periodic inspection of well water and tap water **to identify possible contaminants.**

Community

- Encourage community members/groups to engage in problem-solving activities.
- Promote community education programs in different modalities, languages, cultures, and educational levels geared **to in-**

Information that appears in brackets has been added by the authors to clarify and enhance the use of nursing diagnoses.

creasing awareness of safety measures and resources available to individuals/community.

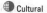

- Review pertinent job-related health department and Occupational Safety and Health Administration (OSHA) regulations.
- Ascertain that there is a comprehensive disaster plan for the community that includes a chain of command, equipment, communication, training, decontamination area(s), and safety and security plans **to ensure an effective response to any emergency (e.g., flood, toxic spill, infectious disease outbreak, radiation release).**
- Refer to appropriate agencies (e.g., CDC; U.S. Army Medical Research Institute of Infectious Diseases; FEMA; U.S. DHHS; OEP; EPA) **to prepare for and manage mass casualty incidents.**

Documentation Focus

Assessment/Reassessment

- Details of specific exposure including location and circumstances.
- Client's/caregiver's understanding of individual risks and safety concerns.

Planning

- Plan of care and who is involved in planning
- Teaching plan

Implementation/Evaluation

- Individual responses to interventions, teaching, and actions performed
- Specific actions and changes that are made
- Attainment or progress toward desired outcome(s)
- Modifications to plan of care

Discharge Planning

- Long-range plans for discharge needs, lifestyle and community changes, and who is responsible for actions to be taken
- Specific referrals made

Sample Nursing Outcomes & Interventions Classifications (NOC/NIC)

NOC—Symptom Severity
NOC—Risk Control
NIC—Environmental Risk Protection

Information that appears in brackets has been added by the authors to clarify and enhance the use of nursing diagnoses.

compromised family COPING

[Diagnostic Division: Social Interaction]

Definition: A usually supportive primary person (family member, significant other, or close friend) provides insufficient, ineffective, or compromised support, comfort, assistance, or encouragement that may be needed by the client to manage or master adaptive tasks related to his or her health challenge.

Related Factors

Coexisting situations affecting the significant person; preoccupation by support person with concern outside of family
Developmental crisis; situational crisis faced by support person
Prolonged disease that exhausts the capacity of support person
Exhaustion of support person's capacity
Insufficient understanding/misunderstanding of information by support person
Insufficient information available to support person; misinformation obtained by support person
Insufficient reciprocal support; insufficient support given by client to support person
Family disorganization, role change

Defining Characteristics

Subjective

Client complaint/concern about support person's response to health problem
Support person reports inadequate knowledge or understanding that interferes with effective behaviors
Support person reports preoccupation with own personal reaction to client's need

Objective

Assistive behaviors by support person produce unsatisfactory results
Protective behavior by support person incongruent with client's abilities
Limitation in communication between support person and client
Support person withdraws from client

Information that appears in brackets has been added by the authors to clarify and enhance the use of nursing diagnoses.

Desired Outcomes/Evaluation Criteria—Family Will:

- Identify and verbalize resources within themselves to deal with the situation.
- Interact appropriately with the client, providing support and assistance as indicated.
- Provide opportunity for client to deal with situation in own way.
- Verbalize knowledge and understanding of illness, disability, or disease.
- Express feelings honestly.
- Identify need for outside support and seek such.

Actions/Interventions

Nursing Priority No. 1.

To assess causative/contributing factors:

- Identify underlying situation(s) that may contribute to the inability of the family to provide needed assistance to the client. **Circumstances may have preceded the illness and now have a significant effect (e.g., client had a heart attack during sexual activity; mate is afraid any activity may cause repeat).**
- Note cultural factors related to family relationships that may be involved in problems of caring for member who is ill.
- Note the length of illness, such as cancer, multiple sclerosis (MS), and/or other long-term situations that may exist.
- Assess information available to and understood by the family/SO(s).
- Discuss family perceptions of situation. **Expectations of client and family members may differ and/or be unrealistic.**
- Identify role of the client in family and how illness has changed the family organization.
- Note other factors besides the client's illness that are affecting the abilities of family members **to provide needed support.**

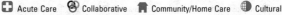

Nursing Priority No. 2.

To assist family to reactivate/develop skills to deal with current situation:

- Listen to client's/SO(s)' comments, remarks, and expression of concern(s). Note nonverbal behaviors and/or responses and congruency.

Information that appears in brackets has been added by the authors to clarify and enhance the use of nursing diagnoses.

 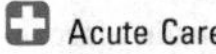 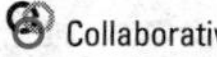 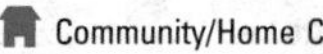 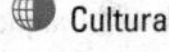

- Encourage family members to verbalize feelings openly and clearly.
- Discuss underlying reasons for behaviors with family **to help them understand and accept and deal with client behaviors.**
- Assist the family and client to understand "who owns the problem" and who is responsible for resolution. Avoid placing blame or guilt.
- Encourage the client and family to develop problem-solving skills **to deal with the situation.**

Nursing Priority No. 3.

To promote wellness (Teaching/Discharge Considerations):

- Provide information for family/SO(s) about specific illness or condition.
- Involve client and family in planning care as often as possible. **This enhances commitment to a plan.**
- Promote the assistance of family in providing client care, as appropriate. **This identifies ways of demonstrating support while maintaining a client's independence (e.g., providing favorite foods and engaging in diversional activities).**
- Refer to appropriate resources for assistance, as indicated (e.g., counseling, psychotherapy, financial, and spiritual).
- Refer to NDs Fear; Anxiety; Death Anxiety; ineffective Coping; readiness for enhanced family Coping; disabled family Coping; Grieving, as appropriate.

Documentation Focus

Assessment/Reassessment

- Assessment findings, including current and past coping behaviors, emotional response to situation and stressors, and support systems available

Planning

- Plan of care, who is involved in planning, and areas of responsibility
- Teaching plan

Implementation/Evaluation

- Responses of family members/client to interventions, teaching, and actions performed

---

Information that appears in brackets has been added by the authors to clarify and enhance the use of nursing diagnoses.

- Attainment or progress toward desired outcome(s)
- Modifications to plan of care

Discharge Planning

- Long-term plan and who is responsible for actions
- Specific referrals made

Sample Nursing Outcomes & Interventions Classifications (NOC/NIC)

NOC—Family Coping
NIC—Family Involvement Promotion

defensive COPING

[Diagnostic Division: Ego Integrity]

Definition: Repeated projection of falsely positive self-evaluation based on a self-protective pattern that defends against underlying perceived threats to positive self-regard.

Related Factors

Conflict between self-perception and value system; uncertainty
Fear of failure, humiliation, or repercussions; insufficient self-confidence
Unrealistic self-expectations
Insufficient resilience
Insufficient confidence in others; insufficient support

Defining Characteristics

Subjective

Denial of obvious problems/weaknesses
Projection of blame/responsibility
Hypersensitive to a discourtesy/criticism
Grandiosity
Rationalization of failures

Objective

Superior attitude toward others; ridicule of others; hostile laughter
Difficulty establishing/maintaining relationships

Information that appears in brackets has been added by the authors to clarify and enhance the use of nursing diagnoses.

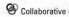

Alteration in reality testing; reality distortion
Insufficient participation in or follow-through with treatment

Desired Outcomes/Evaluation Criteria—Client Will:

- Verbalize understanding of own problems and stressors.
- Identify areas of concern or problems.
- Demonstrate acceptance of responsibility for own actions, successes, and failures.
- Participate in treatment program or therapy.
- Maintain involvement in relationships.

Actions/Interventions

- Refer to ND ineffective Coping for additional interventions.

Nursing Priority No. 1.

To determine degree of impairment:

- Assess the ability to comprehend current situation and/or developmental level of functioning.
- Determine level of anxiety and effectiveness of current coping mechanisms.
- Perform or review results of testing such as Taylor Manifest Anxiety Scale and Marlowe-Crowne Social Desirability Scale, as indicated, to identify coping styles.
- Determine coping mechanisms used (e.g., projection, avoidance, or rationalization) and purpose of coping strategy (e.g., may mask low self-esteem) **to note how these behaviors affect the current situation.**
- Observe interactions with others **to note difficulties and ability to establish satisfactory relationships.**
- Note availability of family/friends' support for client in current situation. **SO(s) may not be supportive when a person is denying problems or exhibiting unacceptable behaviors.**
- Note expressions of grandiosity in the face of contrary evidence (e.g., "I'm going to buy a new car" when the individual has no job or available finances).
- Assess physical condition. **A defensive coping style has been connected with a decline or alteration in physical well-being and illnesses, especially chronic health concerns (e.g., congestive heart failure, diabetes, and chronic fatigue syndrome).**

Information that appears in brackets has been added by the authors to clarify and enhance the use of nursing diagnoses.

Nursing Priority No. 2.

To assist client to deal with current situation:

- Develop a therapeutic relationship to enable client **to test new behaviors in a safe environment.** Use positive, nonjudgmental approach and "I" language **to promote sense of self-esteem.**
- Assist the client to identify and consider the need to address a problem differently.
- Use therapeutic communication skills such as active-listening to assist the client to describe all aspects of the problem.
- Acknowledge individual strengths and incorporate awareness of personal assets and strengths in plan.
- Provide an explanation of the rules of the treatment program, when indicated, and consequences of lack of cooperation.
- Set limits on manipulative behavior; be consistent in enforcing consequences when rules are broken and limits tested.
- Encourage control in all situations possible; include the client in decisions and planning **to preserve autonomy.**
- Convey an attitude of acceptance and respect (unconditional positive regard) **to avoid threatening the client's self-concept and to preserve existing self-esteem.**
- Encourage identification and expression of feelings.
- Provide healthy outlets for the release of hostile feelings (e.g., punching bags and pounding boards). Involve the client in an outdoor recreation program or activities.
- Provide opportunities for the client to interact with others in a positive manner, **promoting self-esteem.**
- Identify and discuss responses to the situation and maladaptive coping skills. Suggest alternative responses to the situation **to help the client select more adaptive strategies for coping.**
- Use confrontation judiciously **to help the client begin to identify defense mechanisms (e.g., denial/projection) that are hindering the development of satisfying relationships.**
- Assist with treatments for physical illnesses, as appropriate.

Nursing Priority No. 3.

To promote wellness (Teaching/Discharge Considerations):

- Use cognitive-behavioral therapy. **This helps change negative thinking patterns when rigidly held beliefs are used by the client to defend against low self-esteem.**
- Encourage the client to learn relaxation techniques, use guided imagery, and give positive affirmation of self **in order to incorporate and practice new behaviors.**

Information that appears in brackets has been added by the authors to clarify and enhance the use of nursing diagnoses.

- Promote involvement in activities or classes where the client can practice new skills and develop new relationships.
- Refer to additional resources (e.g., substance rehabilitation, family/marital therapy), as indicated.

Documentation Focus

Assessment/Reassessment

- Assessment findings, presenting behaviors
- Client perception of the present situation and usual coping methods, degree of impairment
- Health concerns

Planning

- Plan of care and interventions and who is involved in development of the plan
- Teaching plan

Implementation/Evaluation

- Response to interventions, teaching, and actions performed
- Attainment or progress toward desired outcome(s)
- Modifications to plan of care

Discharge Planning

- Referrals and follow-up program

Sample Nursing Outcomes & Interventions Classifications (NOC/NIC)

NOC—Acceptance: Health Status
NIC—Self-Awareness Enhancement

disabled family COPING

[Diagnostic Division: Social Interaction]

Definition: Behavior of primary person (family member, significant other, or close friend) that disables his or her capacities and the client's capacities to effectively address tasks essential to either person's adaptation to the health challenge.

Related Factors

Chronically unexpressed feelings by support person
Differing coping styles between support person and client

Information that appears in brackets has been added by the authors to clarify and enhance the use of nursing diagnoses.

Differing coping styles between support persons
Ambivalent family relationships
Inconsistent management of family's resistance to treatment

Defining Characteristics

Subjective

Expresses despair regarding family reactions or lack of involvement

Objective

Psychosomatic symptoms
Intolerance; rejection; abandonment; desertion; agitation; aggression; hostility; depression
Performing routines without regard for client's needs; disregard for client's needs
Neglect of basic needs of client, or treatment regimen
Neglect of relationship with family member
Family behaviors detrimental to well-being
Distortion of reality about client's health problem
Impaired ability to structure a meaningful life; impaired individualization; prolonged hyperfocus on client
Adopts illness symptoms of client
Client's dependence

Desired Outcomes/Evaluation Criteria—Family Will:

- Verbalize more realistic understanding and expectations of the client.
- Visit or contact client regularly.
- Participate positively in care of client, within limits of family's abilities and client's needs.
- Express feelings and expectations openly and honestly, as appropriate.
- Access available resources/services to assist with required care.

Actions/Interventions

Nursing Priority No. 1.

To assess causative/contributing factors:

- Ascertain pre-illness behaviors and interactions of the family. **This provides a comparative baseline.**

Information that appears in brackets has been added by the authors to clarify and enhance the use of nursing diagnoses.

- Identify current behaviors of the family members (e.g., withdrawal—not visiting, brief visits, and/or ignoring client when visiting; anger and hostility toward client and others; ways of touching between family members, expressions of guilt).
- Discuss family perceptions of the situation. **The expectations of the client and family members may/may not be realistic.**
- Note cultural factors related to family relationships that may be involved in problems of caring for member who is ill.
- Note other factors that may be stressful for the family (e.g., financial difficulties or lack of community support, as when illness occurs when out of town). **This provides an opportunity for appropriate referrals.**
- Determine the readiness of family members to be involved with the care of the client.

Nursing Priority No. 2.

To provide assistance to enable family to deal with the current situation:

- Establish rapport with family members who are available. **This promotes a therapeutic relationship and support for problem-solving solutions.**
- Acknowledge the difficulty of the situation for the family. **This reduces blaming/feelings of guilt.**
- Active-listen concerns; note both overconcern and lack of concern, which may interfere with the ability to resolve the situation.
- Allow free expression of feelings, including frustration, anger, hostility, and hopelessness. Place limits on acting-out/inappropriate behaviors **to minimize the risk of violent behavior.**
- Give accurate information to SO(s) from the beginning.
- Act as liaison between family and healthcare providers **to provide explanations and clarification of treatment plan.**
- Provide brief, simple explanations about use and alarms when equipment (such as a ventilator) is involved. Identify appropriate professional(s) **for continued support/problem solving.**
- Provide time for private interaction between client/family.
- Include SO(s) in the plan of care; provide instruction **to assist them to learn necessary skills to help the client.**
- Accompany the family when they visit **to be available for questions, concerns, and support.**
- Assist SO(s) to initiate therapeutic communication with the client.

Information that appears in brackets has been added by the authors to clarify and enhance the use of nursing diagnoses.

- Refer the client to protective services as necessitated by risk of physical harm. **Removing the client from home enhances individual safety and may reduce stress on the family to allow the opportunity for therapeutic intervention.**

Nursing Priority No. 3.

To promote wellness (Teaching/Discharge Considerations):

- Assist the family to identify coping skills being used and how these skills are/are not helping them deal with the current situation.
- Answer the family's questions patiently and honestly. Reinforce information provided by other healthcare providers.
- Reframe negative expressions into positive, whenever possible. **A positive frame contributes to supportive interactions and can lead to better outcomes.**
- Respect family needs for withdrawal and intervene judiciously. **The situation may be overwhelming, and time away can be beneficial to continued participation.**
- Encourage the family to deal with the situation in small increments rather than the whole picture at one time.
- Assist the family to identify familiar items that would be helpful to the client (e.g., a family picture on the wall), especially when hospitalized for a long period of time, **to reinforce/ maintain orientation.**
- Refer the family to appropriate resources, as needed (e.g., family therapy, financial counseling, or a spiritual advisor).
- Refer to ND Grieving, as appropriate.

Documentation Focus

Assessment/Reassessment

- Assessment findings, current and past behaviors, including family members who are directly involved and support systems available
- Emotional response(s) to situation or stressors
- Specific health or therapy challenges

Planning

- Plan of care, specific interventions, and who is involved in planning
- Teaching plan

Implementation/Evaluation

- Responses of individuals to interventions, teaching, and actions performed

Information that appears in brackets has been added by the authors to clarify and enhance the use of nursing diagnoses.

- Attainment or progress toward desired outcome(s)
- Modifications to plan of care

Discharge Planning

- Ongoing needs, resources, other follow-up recommendations, and who is responsible for actions
- Specific referrals made

Sample Nursing Outcomes & Interventions Classifications (NOC/NIC)

NOC—Family Normalization
NIC—Family Therapy

ineffective community COPING

[Diagnostic Division: Social Interaction]

Definition: A pattern of community activities for adaptation and problem-solving that is unsatisfactory for meeting the demands or needs of the community.

Related Factors

Insufficient community resources (e.g., respite, recreation, social support services)
Inadequate resources for problem-solving
Nonexistent community systems
History of exposure to disaster (e.g., natural/man-made)

Defining Characteristics

Subjective

Community does not meet expectations of its members
Perceived community vulnerability/powerlessness
Excessive stressors

Objective

Deficient community participation
Excessive community conflict
Elevated community illness rate
High incidence of community problems (e.g., homicides, vandalism, robbery, terrorism, abuse, unemployment, poverty, militancy, mental illness)

Information that appears in brackets has been added by the authors to clarify and enhance the use of nursing diagnoses.

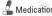

Desired Outcomes/Evaluation Criteria—Community Will:

- Recognize negative and positive factors affecting community's ability to meet its own demands or needs.
- Identify alternatives to inappropriate activities for adaptation/problem-solving.
- Report a measurable increase in necessary/desired activities to improve community functioning.

Actions/Interventions

Nursing Priority No. 1.

To identify causative or precipitating factors:

- Evaluate community activities **as related to meeting collective needs within the community itself and between the community and the larger society.**
- Note community reports of community functioning (e.g., transportation, financial needs, or emergency response), including areas of weakness or conflict.
- Identify effects of Related Factors on community activities.
- Determine the availability and use of resources.
- Identify unmet demands or needs of the community.

Nursing Priority No. 2.

To assist the community to reactivate/develop skills to deal with needs:

- Determine community strengths. **Provides a base upon which to build additional effective coping strategies.**
- Identify and prioritize community goals.
- Encourage community members to join groups and engage in problem-solving activities **to strengthen efforts and broaden the base of support.**
- Develop a plan jointly with the community **to deal with deficits in support to meet identified goals.**

Nursing Priority No. 3.

To promote wellness as related to community health:

- Create plans managing interactions within the community itself and between the community and the larger society **to meet collective needs.**
- Assist the community to form partnerships within the community and between the community and the larger society.

Information that appears in brackets has been added by the authors to clarify and enhance the use of nursing diagnoses.

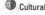

This promotes long-term development of the community to deal with current and future problems.

- Promote community involvement in developing a comprehensive disaster plan **to ensure an effective response to any emergency (e.g., flood, tornado, toxic spill, or infectious disease outbreak).** (Refer to ND Contamination for additional interventions.)
- Provide channels for dissemination of information to the community as a whole (e.g., print media; radio/television reports and community bulletin boards; speakers' bureau; and reports to committees, councils, and advisory boards), keeping material on file and accessible to the public.
- Make information available in different modalities and geared to differing educational levels and cultural and ethnic populations of the community.
- Seek out and evaluate underserved populations, including the homeless.

Documentation Focus

Assessment/Reassessment

- Assessment findings, including perception of community members regarding problems
- Availability and use of resources

Planning

- Plan of care and who is involved in planning
- Teaching plan

Implementation/Evaluation

- Response of community entities to plan, interventions, and actions performed
- Attainment or progress toward desired outcome(s)
- Modifications to plan of care

Discharge Planning

- Long-term plans and who is responsible for actions to be taken

Sample Nursing Outcomes & Interventions Classifications (NOC/NIC)

NOC—Community Competence
NIC—Community Health Development

Information that appears in brackets has been added by the authors to clarify and enhance the use of nursing diagnoses.

ineffective COPING

[Diagnostic Division: Ego Integrity]

Definition: Inability to form a valid appraisal of the stressors, inadequate choices of practiced responses, and/or inability to use available resources.

Related Factors

Situational or maturational crisis; inadequate opportunity to prepare for stressor
High degree of threat; inaccurate threat appraisal
Ineffective tension release strategies
Inadequate confidence in ability to deal with a situation; insufficient sense of control; uncertainty
Inadequate resources; insufficient social support
Ineffective tension release strategies
Inability to conserve adaptive energies
Gender differences in coping strategies
Severe/chronic pain

Defining Characteristics

Subjective

Inability to deal with a situation, ask for help
Alteration in sleep pattern; fatigue
Substance abuse

Objective

Insufficient goal-directed behavior, problem-solving, or problem resolution
Ineffective coping strategies
Inability to meet role expectation/basic needs
Insufficient access of social support
Alteration in concentration; inability to attend to information; difficulty organizing information
Change in communication pattern
Frequent illness
Risk-taking behavior
Destructive behavior toward self/others

Desired Outcomes/Evaluation Criteria—Client Will:

- Assess the current situation accurately.
- Identify ineffective coping behaviors and consequences.

Information that appears in brackets has been added by the authors to clarify and enhance the use of nursing diagnoses.

- Verbalize awareness of own coping abilities.
- Verbalize feelings congruent with behavior.
- Meet psychological needs as evidenced by appropriate expression of feelings, identification of options, and use of resources.

Actions/Interventions

Nursing Priority No. 1.

To determine degree of impairment:

- Determine individual stressors (e.g., family, social, work environment, life changes, or nursing or healthcare management).
- Evaluate the ability to understand events; provide a realistic appraisal of situation.
- Identify developmental level of functioning. **(People tend to regress to a lower developmental stage during illness or crisis.)**
- Assess current functional capacity and note how it is affecting the individual's coping ability.
- Determine alcohol intake, drug use, smoking habits, and sleeping and eating patterns. **These mechanisms are often used when the individual is not coping effectively with stressors.**
- Ascertain the impact of illness on sexual needs and relationship.
- Assess the level of anxiety and coping on an ongoing basis.
- Note speech and communication patterns. Be aware of negative/catastrophizing thinking.
- Observe and describe behavior in objective terms. Validate observations.

Nursing Priority No. 2.

To assess coping abilities and skills:

- Ascertain the client's understanding of the current situation and its impact on life and work.
- Active-listen and identify the client's perceptions of what is happening.
- Evaluate the client's decision-making ability.
- Determine previous methods of dealing with life problems **to identify successful techniques that can be used in the current situation.**

Information that appears in brackets has been added by the authors to clarify and enhance the use of nursing diagnoses.

Nursing Priority No. 3.

To assist client to deal with current situation:

- Call the client by name. Ascertain how the client prefers to be addressed. **Using the client's name enhances sense of self and promotes individuality and self-esteem.**
- Encourage communication with the staff/SO(s).
- Use reality orientation (e.g., clocks, calendars, and bulletin boards) and make frequent references to time and place, as indicated. Place needed and familiar objects within sight for visual cues.
- Provide for continuity of care with the same personnel taking care of the client as often as possible.
- Explain disease process, procedures, and events in a simple, concise manner. Devote time for listening. **This may help the client to express emotions, grasp the situation, and feel more in control.**
- Provide for a quiet environment and position equipment out of view as much as possible **when anxiety is increased by noisy surroundings or the sight of medical equipment.**
- Schedule activities so periods of rest alternate with nursing care. Increase activity slowly.
- Assist the client in the use of diversion, recreation, and relaxation techniques.
- Emphasize positive body responses to medical conditions, but do not negate the seriousness of the situation (e.g., stable blood pressure during gastric bleed or improved body posture in depressed client).
- Encourage the client to try new coping behaviors and gradually master the situation.
- Confront the client when behavior is inappropriate, pointing out the difference between words and actions. **This provides an external locus of control, enhancing safety.**
- Assist in dealing with change in concept of body image, as appropriate. (Refer to ND disturbed Body Image.)

Nursing Priority No. 4.

To provide for meeting psychological needs:

- Treat the client with courtesy and respect. Converse at the client's level, providing meaningful conversation while performing care. **This enhances the therapeutic relationship.**
- Help the client learn how to substitute positive thoughts for negative ones (i.e., "I can do this"; "I am in charge of myself"). Take advantage of teachable moments.
- Allow the client to react in his or her own way without judgment by staff. Provide support and diversion, as indicated.

Information that appears in brackets has been added by the authors to clarify and enhance the use of nursing diagnoses.

- Encourage verbalization of fears and anxieties and expression of feelings of denial, depression, and anger. Let the client know that these are normal reactions.
- Provide opportunity for expression of sexual concerns.
- Help the client to set limits on acting-out behaviors and learn ways to express emotions in an acceptable manner. **This promotes an internal locus of control.**

Nursing Priority No. 5.

To promote wellness (Teaching/Discharge Considerations):

- Give updated or additional information needed about events, cause (if known), and potential course of illness as soon as possible. **Knowledge helps reduce anxiety/fear and allows the client to deal with reality.**
- Provide and encourage an atmosphere of realistic hope.
- Give information about purposes and side effects of medications/treatments.
- Stress the importance of follow-up care.
- Encourage and support the client in evaluating lifestyle, occupation, and leisure activities.
- Discuss ways to deal with identified stressors (e.g., family, social, work environment, or nursing or healthcare management).
- Provide for gradual implementation and continuation of necessary behavior/lifestyle changes. **This enhances commitment to plan.**
- Discuss or review anticipated procedures and client concerns, as well as postoperative expectations when surgery is recommended.
- Refer to outside resources and/or professional therapy, as indicated or ordered.
- Determine need/desire for religious representative/spiritual counselor and arrange for visit.
- Provide information and/or refer for consultation, as indicated, for sexual concerns. Provide privacy when the client is not in his or her own home.
- Refer to other NDs, as indicated (e.g., chronic Pain; Anxiety; impaired verbal Communication; risk for other-/self-directed Violence).

Documentation Focus

Assessment/Reassessment

- Baseline findings, specific stressors, degree of impairment, and client's perceptions of situation

Information that appears in brackets has been added by the authors to clarify and enhance the use of nursing diagnoses.

- Coping abilities and previous ways of dealing with life problems

Planning

- Plan of care, specific interventions, and who is involved in planning
- Teaching plan

Implementation/Evaluation

- Client's responses to interventions, teaching, and actions performed
- Medication dose, time, and client's response
- Attainment or progress toward desired outcome(s)
- Modifications to plan of care

Discharge Planning

- Long-term needs and actions to be taken
- Support systems available, specific referrals made, and who is responsible for actions to be taken

Sample Nursing Outcomes & Interventions Classifications (NOC/NIC)

NOC—Coping
NIC—Coping Enhancement

readiness for enhanced COPING

[Diagnostic Division: Ego Integrity]

Definition: A pattern of cognitive and behavioral efforts to manage demands related to well-being, which can be strengthened.

Defining Characteristics

Subjective

Expresses desire to enhance knowledge of stress management strategies, management of stressors
Expresses desire to enhance use of emotion-oriented/problem-oriented strategies
Expresses desire to enhance social support
Awareness of possible environmental change

Information that appears in brackets has been added by the authors to clarify and enhance the use of nursing diagnoses.

Desired Outcomes/Evaluation Criteria—Client Will:

- Assess current situation accurately.
- Identify effective coping behaviors currently being used.
- Verbalize feelings congruent with behavior.
- Meet psychological needs as evidenced by appropriate expression of feelings, identification of options, and use of resources.

Actions/Interventions

Nursing Priority No. 1.

To determine needs and desire for improvement:

- Evaluate the ability to understand events and provide a realistic appraisal of the situation. **This provides information about client's perception and cognitive ability and whether the client is aware of the facts of the situation. This is essential for facilitating growth.**
- Determine stressors that are currently affecting the client. **Accurate identification of the situation that the client is dealing with provides information for planning interventions to enhance coping abilities.**
- Ascertain motivation/expectations for change.
- Identify social supports available to the client. **Available support systems, such as family and friends, can provide the client with the ability to handle current stressful events, and often "talking it out" with an empathetic listener will help the client move forward to enhance coping skills.**
- Review coping strategies the client is aware of and currently using. **The desire to improve one's coping ability is based on an awareness of the current status of the stressful situation.**
- Determine alcohol intake, other drug use, smoking habits, and sleeping and eating patterns. **Use of these substances impairs the ability to deal with anxiety and affects the ability to cope with life's stressors. Identification of impaired sleeping and eating patterns provides clues needed for change.**
- Assess the level of anxiety and coping on an ongoing basis. **This provides information for baseline to develop a plan of care to improve coping abilities.**
- Note speech and communication patterns. **This assesses the ability to understand and provides information necessary to help the client make progress in a desire to enhance coping abilities.**

Information that appears in brackets has been added by the authors to clarify and enhance the use of nursing diagnoses.

- Evaluate the client's decision-making ability. **Understanding the client's ability provides a starting point for developing a plan and determining what information the client needs to develop more effective coping skills.**

Nursing Priority No. 2.

To assist client to develop enhanced coping skills:

- Active-listen and clarify the client's perceptions of current status. **Reflecting the client's statements and thoughts can provide a forum for understanding perceptions in relation to reality for planning care and determining accuracy of interventions needed.**
- Review previous methods of dealing with life problems. **This enables the client to identify successful techniques used in the past, promoting feelings of confidence in own ability.**
- Discuss the desire to improve the client's ability to manage stressors of life. **Understanding the client's desire to seek new information to enhance life will help the client determine what is needed to learn new skills of coping.**
- Discuss an understanding of the concept of knowing what can and cannot be changed. **Acceptance of reality that some things cannot be changed allows the client to focus energies on dealing with things that can be changed.**
- Help the client develop problem-solving skills. **Learning the process for problem solving will promote successful resolution of potentially stressful situations that arise.**

Nursing Priority No. 3.

To promote optimum wellness:

- Discuss predisposing factors related to any individual's response to stress. **Understanding that genetic influences, past experiences, and existing conditions determine whether a person's response is adaptive or maladaptive will give the client a base on which to continue to learn what is needed to improve life.**
- Encourage the client to create a stress management program. **An individualized program of relaxation, meditation, and involvement with caring for others/pets will enhance coping skills and strengthen the client's ability to manage challenging situations.**
- Recommend involvement in activities of interest, such as exercise/sports, music, and art. **Individuals must decide for themselves what coping strategies are adaptive for them. Most people find enjoyment and relaxation in these kinds of activities.**

Information that appears in brackets has been added by the authors to clarify and enhance the use of nursing diagnoses.

- Discuss the possibility of doing volunteer work in an area of the client's choosing. **Many people report satisfaction in helping others, and the client may find pleasure in such involvement.**
- Refer to classes and/or reading material, as appropriate. **This may be helpful to further learning and pursuing a goal of enhanced coping ability.**

Documentation Focus

Assessment/Reassessment

- Baseline information, client's perception of need to enhance abilities
- Coping abilities and previous ways of dealing with life problems
- Motivation and expectations for change

Planning

- Plan of care, specific interventions, and who is involved in planning
- Teaching plan

Implementation/Evaluation

- Client's responses to interventions, teaching, and actions performed
- Attainment or progress toward desired outcome(s)
- Modifications to plan of care

Discharge Planning

- Long-term needs and actions to be taken
- Support systems available, specific referrals made, and who is responsible for actions to be taken

Sample Nursing Outcomes & Interventions Classifications (NOC/NIC)

NOC—Coping
NIC—Coping Enhancement

readiness for enhanced community COPING

[Diagnostic Division: Social Interaction]

Definition: A pattern of community activities for adaptation and problem solving for meeting the demands or needs of the community, which can be improved.

Information that appears in brackets has been added by the authors to clarify and enhance the use of nursing diagnoses.

Defining Characteristics

Subjective

Expresses desire to enhance problem-solving for identified issue, planning for predictable stressors

Expresses desire to enhance community responsibility for stress management, resources for managing stressors

Expresses desire to enhance communication among community members, between aggregates and larger community

Expresses desire to enhance availability of community recreation/relaxation programs

Desired Outcomes/Evaluation Criteria—Community Will:

- Identify positive and negative factors affecting management of current and future problems and stressors.
- Have an established plan in place to deal with identified problems and stressors.
- Describe management of challenges in characteristics that indicate effective coping.
- Report a measurable increase in ability to deal with problems and stressors.

Actions/Interventions

Nursing Priority No. 1.

To determine existence of and deficits or weaknesses in the management of current and future problems/stressors:

- Review the community plan for dealing with problems and stressors.
- Determine the community's strengths and weaknesses.
- Identify limitations in the current pattern of community activities (such as transportation, water needs, and roads) **that can be improved through adaptation and problem-solving.**
- Evaluate community activities as related to the management of problems and stressors within the community itself and between the community and the larger society.

Nursing Priority No. 2.

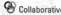

To assist the community in adaptation and problem solving for management of current and future needs/stressors:

- Define and discuss current needs and anticipated or projected concerns. **Agreement on scope/parameters of needs is essential for effective planning.**

Information that appears in brackets has been added by the authors to clarify and enhance the use of nursing diagnoses.

- Prioritize goals **to facilitate accomplishment.**
- Identify available resources (e.g., persons, groups, financial, and governmental, as well as other communities).
- Make a joint plan with the community to deal with adaptation and problem solving **for management of problems and stressors.**
- Seek out and involve underserved and at-risk groups within the community. **This supports communication and commitment of community as a whole.**

Nursing Priority No. 3.

To promote well-being of community:

- Assist the community to form partnerships within the community and between the community and the larger society **to promote long-term developmental growth of the community.**
- Support the development of plans for maintaining these interactions.
- Establish a mechanism for self-monitoring of community needs and evaluation of efforts. **This facilitates proactive rather than reactive responses by the community.**
- Use multiple formats, such as TV, radio, print media, billboards and computer bulletin boards, speakers' bureaus, and reports to community leaders/groups on file and accessible to the public **to keep the community informed regarding plans, needs, and outcomes.**

Documentation Focus

Assessment/Reassessment

- Assessment findings and community's perception of situation
- Identified areas of concern, community strengths and challenges

Planning

- Plan of care and who is involved and responsible for each action
- Teaching plan

Implementation/Evaluation

- Response of community entities to the actions performed
- Attainment or progress toward desired outcomes
- Modifications to plan of care

Information that appears in brackets has been added by the authors to clarify and enhance the use of nursing diagnoses.

Discharge Planning

- Short- and long-term plans to deal with current, anticipated, and potential needs and who is responsible for follow-through
- Specific referrals made, coalitions formed

Sample Nursing Outcomes & Interventions Classifications (NOC/NIC)

NOC—Community Competence
NIC—Program Development

readiness for enhanced family COPING

[Diagnostic Division: Social Interaction]

Definition: A pattern of management of adaptive tasks by primary person (family member, SO, or close friend) involved with the client's health change, which can be strengthened.

Defining Characteristics

Subjective

Expresses desire to acknowledge growth impact of crisis
Expresses desire to enhance connection with others who have experienced a similar situation
Expresses desire to choose experiences that optimize wellness
Expresses desire to enhance health promotion, enrichment of lifestyle

Desired Outcomes/Evaluation Criteria—Family Member Will:

- Express willingness to look at own role in the family's growth.
- Verbalize desire to undertake tasks leading to change.
- Report feelings of self-confidence and satisfaction with progress being made.

Actions/Interventions

Nursing Priority No. 1.

To assess situation and adaptive skills being used by the family members:

- Determine individual situation and stage of growth family is experiencing or demonstrating. **The changes that are occur-**

Information that appears in brackets has been added by the authors to clarify and enhance the use of nursing diagnoses.

ring may help the family adapt, grow, and thrive when faced with these transitional events.

- Ascertain motivation and expectations for change.
- Note expressions such as "Life has more meaning for me since this has occurred," **to identify changes in values.**
- Observe communication patterns of the family. Listen to the family's expressions of hope and planning and their effects on relationships and life.
- Identify cultural/religious health beliefs and expectations. **For example, Navajo parents may define family as nuclear, extended, or a clan, and it is important to identify who are the primary child-rearing persons.**

Nursing Priority No. 2.

To assist family member to develop/strengthen potential for growth:

- Provide time to talk with the family **to discuss their view of the situation.**
- Establish a relationship with the family/client **to foster trust and growth.**
- Provide a role model with which the family member may identify.
- Discuss the importance of open communication and of not having secrets.
- Demonstrate techniques, such as active-listening, I-messages, and problem solving, **to facilitate effective communication.**
- Establish social goals of achieving and maintaining harmony with oneself, family, and community.

Nursing Priority No. 3.

To promote wellness (Teaching/Discharge Considerations):

- Assist the family member to support the client in meeting his or her own needs within ability and/or constraints of the illness or situation.
- Provide experiences for the family **to help them learn ways of assisting or supporting the client.**
- Identify other individuals or groups with similar conditions (e.g., Reach for Recovery, CanSurmount, Al-Anon, MS Society) and assist the client/family member to make contact. **This provides ongoing support for sharing common experiences, problem solving, and learning new behaviors.**

Information that appears in brackets has been added by the authors to clarify and enhance the use of nursing diagnoses.

- Assist the family member to learn new, effective ways of dealing with feelings and reactions.
- Encourage the family member to pursue personal interests, hobbies, and leisure activities **to promote individual well-being and strengthen coping abilities.**

Documentation Focus

Assessment/Reassessment

- Adaptive skills being used, stage of growth
- Family communication patterns
- Motivation and expectations for change

Planning

- Plan of care, specific interventions, and who is involved in planning
- Teaching plan

Implementation/Evaluation

- Client's/family's responses to interventions, teaching, and actions performed
- Attainment or progress toward desired outcome(s)
- Modifications to plan of care

Discharge Planning

- Identified needs/referrals for follow-up care and/or support systems
- Specific referrals made

Sample Nursing Outcomes & Interventions Classifications (NOC/NIC)

NOC—Family Normalization
NIC—Normalization Promotion

Information that appears in brackets has been added by the authors to clarify and enhance the use of nursing diagnoses.

DEATH ANXIETY

[Diagnostic Division: Ego Integrity]

Definition: Vague uneasy feeling of discomfort or dread generated by perceptions of a real or imagined threat to one's existence.

Related Factors

Anticipation of pain, suffering, adverse consequences of anesthesia, impact of death on others

Confronting the reality of terminal disease; experiencing dying process; perceived imminence of death

Discussions on the topic of death; observations related to death; near-death experience

Uncertainty of prognosis; nonacceptance of own mortality

Uncertainty about the existence of a higher power, life after death, an encounter with a higher power

Defining Characteristics

Subjective

Fear of developing a terminal illness, the dying process, pain/suffering related to dying, loss of mental/[physical] abilities when dying, premature death, or prolonged dying process

Negative thoughts related to death and dying

Deep sadness; powerlessness

Concerns about strain on the caregiver; worried about the impact of one's own death on significant other

Desired Outcomes/Evaluation Criteria—Client Will:

- Identify and express feelings (e.g., sadness, guilt, fear) freely/effectively.
- Look toward/plan for the future one day at a time.
- Formulate a plan dealing with individual concerns and eventualities of dying as appropriate.

Actions/Interventions

Nursing Priority No. 1.

To assess causative/contributing factors:

- Determine how client sees self in usual lifestyle role functioning and perception and meaning of anticipated loss to him or her and SO(s).

Information that appears in brackets has been added by the authors to clarify and enhance the use of nursing diagnoses.

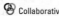

- Ascertain current knowledge of situation **to identify misconceptions, lack of information, and other pertinent issues.**
- Determine the client's role in the family constellation. Observe patterns of communication in family and response of family/SO to client's situation and concerns. **In addition to identifying areas of need/concern, this also reveals strengths useful in addressing the concerns.**
- Assess the impact of client reports of subjective experiences and past experience with death (or exposure to death), for example, witnessed violent death, viewed body in casket as a child, and so on.
- Identify cultural factors/expectations and impact on current situation and feelings.
- Note physical and mental condition and complexity of therapeutic regimen.
- Determine the ability to manage own self-care, end-of-life and other affairs, and awareness/use of available resources.
- Observe behavior indicative of the level of anxiety present (mild to panic) **as it affects the client's/SO(s)' ability to process information and participate in activities.**
- Identify coping skills currently used and how effective they are. Be aware of defense mechanisms being used by the client.
- Note the use of alcohol or other drugs of abuse, reports of insomnia, excessive sleeping, and avoidance of interactions with others, **which may be behavioral indicators of use of withdrawal to deal with problems.**
- Note the client's religious and spiritual orientation and involvement in religious activities; note also the presence of conflicts regarding spiritual beliefs.
- Listen to client/SO reports/expressions of anger and concern, alienation from God, or belief that impending death is a punishment for wrongdoing.
- Determine sense of futility; feelings of hopelessness or helplessness; lack of motivation to help self. **These may indicate the presence of depression and need for intervention.**
- Active-listen comments regarding sense of isolation.
- Listen for expressions of inability to find meaning in life or suicidal ideation.

Nursing Priority No. 2.

To assist client to deal with situation:

- Provide an open and trusting relationship.
- Use therapeutic communication skills of active-listening, silence, and acknowledgment. Respect the client's desire or re-

---

Information that appears in brackets has been added by the authors to clarify and enhance the use of nursing diagnoses.

quest not to talk. Provide hope within parameters of the individual situation.

- Encourage expressions of feelings (anger, fear, sadness, etc.). Acknowledge anxiety/fear. Do not deny or reassure client that everything will be all right. Be honest when answering questions/providing information. **This enhances trust and therapeutic relationship.**
- Provide information about the normalcy of feelings and individual grief reaction.
- Make time for nonjudgmental discussion of philosophical issues and questions about the spiritual impact of the illness/situation.
- Review life experiences of loss and previous use of coping skills, noting the client's strengths and successes.
- Provide a calm, peaceful setting and privacy as appropriate. **This promotes relaxation and the ability to deal with a situation.**
- Assist the client to engage in spiritual growth activities, if desired, and experience prayer/meditation and forgiveness to heal past hurts. Provide information that anger with God is a normal part of the grieving process. **This reduces feelings of guilt/conflict, allowing the client to move forward toward resolution.**
- Refer to therapists, spiritual advisors, and counselors **to facilitate grief work.**
- Refer to community agencies/resources **to assist client/SO(s) for planning for eventualities (legal issues, funeral plans, etc.).**

Nursing Priority No. 3.

To promote independence:

- Support the client's efforts to develop realistic steps to put plans into action.
- Direct the client's thoughts beyond the present state to enjoyment of each day and the future when appropriate.
- Provide opportunities for the client to make simple decisions. **This enhances sense of control.**
- Develop an individual plan using the client's locus of control **to assist the client/family through the process.**
- Treat expressed decisions and desires with respect and convey to others as appropriate.
- Assist with completion of Advance Directives, CPR instructions, and durable medical power of attorney.

Information that appears in brackets has been added by the authors to clarify and enhance the use of nursing diagnoses.

Documentation Focus

Assessment/Reassessment
- Assessment findings, including client's fears and signs/symptoms being exhibited
- Responses and actions of family/SO(s)
- Availability and use of resources

Planning
- Plan of care and who is involved in planning

Implementation/Evaluation
- Client's response to interventions, teaching, and actions performed
- Attainment or progress toward desired outcome(s)
- Modifications to plan of care

Discharge Planning
- Identified needs and who is responsible for actions to be taken
- Specific referrals made

Sample Nursing Outcomes & Interventions Classifications (NOC/NIC)

NOC—Dignified Life Closure
NIC—Dying Care

DECISIONAL CONFLICT

[Diagnostic Division: Ego Integrity]

Definition: Uncertainty about course of action to be taken when choice among competing actions involves risk, loss, or challenge to values and beliefs.

Related Factors

Unclear personal values/beliefs; perceived threat to value system
Inexperience with or interference in decision-making
Insufficient information; conflicting information sources
Conflict with moral obligation
Moral principle, rule, value support mutually inconsistent actions
Insufficient support system deficit
Age; developmental stage/level of functioning

Information that appears in brackets has been added by the authors to clarify and enhance the use of nursing diagnoses.

Defining Characteristics

Subjective

Uncertainty about choices; recognizes undesired consequences of actions being considered
Distress while attempting a decision
Questioning of moral principle, rule, value, or personal beliefs/values while attempting a decision

Objective

Vacillating among choices; delay in decision making
Self-focused
Physical signs of tension or distress (e.g., increase in heart rate, restlessness)

Desired Outcomes/Evaluation Criteria—Client Will:

- Verbalize awareness of positive and negative aspects of choices and alternative actions.
- Acknowledge and ventilate feelings of anxiety and distress associated with making a difficult decision.
- Identify personal values and beliefs concerning issues.
- Make decision(s) and express satisfaction with choices.
- Meet psychological needs as evidenced by appropriate expression of feelings, identification of options, and use of resources.
- Display relaxed manner or calm demeanor free of physical signs of distress.

Actions/Interventions

Nursing Priority No. 1.

To assess causative/contributing factors:

- ∞ Determine usual ability to manage own affairs. Clarify who has legal right to intervene on behalf of a child, elder, or impaired individual (e.g., parent/spouse, other relative, designee for durable medical power of attorney, or court appointed guardian/advocate). **Family disruption and conflicts can complicate decision process.**
- Note expressions of indecision, dependence on others, availability/involvement of support persons (e.g., client may have lack of/conflicting advice). Ascertain dependency of other(s) on client and/or issues of codependency.

Information that appears in brackets has been added by the authors to clarify and enhance the use of nursing diagnoses.

- Active-listen/identify reason for indecisiveness. **This helps the client to clarify the problem and work toward a solution.**
- Determine the effectiveness of the current problem-solving techniques.
- Note the presence/intensity of physical signs of anxiety (e.g., increased heart rate and muscle tension).
- Listen for expressions of the client's inability to find meaning in life/reason for living, feelings of futility, or alienation from God and others around the client. (Refer to ND Spiritual Distress, as indicated.)
- Review information the client has about the healthcare decision. **Accurate and clearly understood information about the situation will help the client make the best decision for self.**

Nursing Priority No. 2.

To assist client to develop/effectively use problem-solving skills:

- Promote a safe and hopeful environment, as needed, while the client regains inner control.
- Encourage verbalization of conflicts or concerns.
- Accept verbal expressions of anger or guilt, setting limits on maladaptive behavior **to promote client safety.**
- Clarify and prioritize individual goals, noting where the subject of the "conflict" falls on this scale. **Choices may have risky, uncertain outcomes; may reflect a need to make value judgments; or may generate regret over having to reject positive choice and accept negative consequences.**
- Identify strengths and presence of positive coping skills (e.g., use of relaxation technique or willingness to express feelings).
- Identify positive aspects of this experience and assist the client to view it as a learning opportunity **to develop new and creative solutions.**
- Correct misperceptions the client may have and provide factual information. **This provides for better decision making.**
- Provide opportunities for the client to make simple decisions regarding self-care and other daily activities. Accept the choice not to do so. Advance complexity of choices, as tolerated.
- ∞ Encourage the child to make developmentally appropriate decisions concerning own care. **This fosters the child's sense of self-worth, and enhances the child's ability to learn and exercise coping skills.**

Information that appears in brackets has been added by the authors to clarify and enhance the use of nursing diagnoses.

- Discuss time considerations, setting a time line for small steps and considering consequences related to not making/postponing specific decisions **to facilitate resolution of conflict.**
- Have the client list some alternatives to the present situation or decisions, using a brainstorming process. Include the family in this activity as indicated (e.g., placement of parent in a long-term care facility, use of intervention process with addicted member). (Refer to NDs interrupted Family Processes; dysfunctional Family Processes; compromised family Coping; Moral Distress.)
- Practice the use of the problem-solving process with the current situation/decision.
- Discuss or clarify cultural or spiritual concerns, accepting the client's values in a nonjudgmental manner.

Nursing Priority No. 3.

To promote wellness (Teaching/Discharge Considerations):

- Promote opportunities for using conflict-resolution skills, identifying steps as the client does each one.
- Provide positive feedback for efforts and progress noted. **This promotes a continuation of efforts.**
- Encourage involvement of family/SO(s), as desired/available, **to provide support for the client.**
- Support the client for decisions made, especially if consequences are unexpected and/or difficult to cope with.
- Encourage attendance at stress reduction or assertiveness classes.
- Refer to other resources, as necessary (e.g., clergy, psychiatric clinical nurse specialist/psychiatrist, family/marital therapist, or addiction support groups).

Documentation Focus

Assessment/Reassessment

- Assessment findings, behavioral responses, degree of impairment in lifestyle functioning
- Individuals involved in the conflict
- Personal values and beliefs

Planning

- Plan of care, specific interventions, and who is involved in the planning process
- Teaching plan

Information that appears in brackets has been added by the authors to clarify and enhance the use of nursing diagnoses.

Implementation/Evaluation
- Client's and involved individual's responses to interventions, teaching, and actions performed
- Ability to express feelings, identify options; use of resources
- Attainment or progress toward desired outcome(s)
- Modifications to plan of care

Discharge Planning
- Long-term needs, referrals made, actions to be taken, and who is responsible for doing
- Specific referrals made

Sample Nursing Outcomes & Interventions Classifications (NOC/NIC)

NOC—Decision-Making
NIC—Decision-Making Support

readiness for enhanced DECISION-MAKING

[Diagnostic Division: Ego Integrity]

Definition: A pattern of choosing a course of action for meeting short- and long-term health-related goals, which can be strengthened.

Defining Characteristics

Subjective
Expresses desire to enhance decision-making, use of reliable evidence for decisions, risk-benefit analysis of decisions

Expresses desire to enhance understanding of choices for decision-making, meaning of choices

Expresses desire to enhance congruency of decisions with values/goal, or sociocultural values/goal

Desired Outcomes/Evaluation Criteria—Client Will:
- Explain possible choices for decision-making.
- Identify risks and benefit of decisions.
- Express beliefs about the meaning of choices.
- Make decisions that are congruent with personal and sociocultural values or goals.
- Use reliable evidence in making decisions.

Information that appears in brackets has been added by the authors to clarify and enhance the use of nursing diagnoses.

 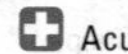  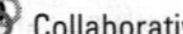 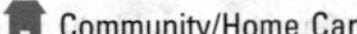 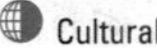

Actions/Interventions

Nursing Priority No. 1.

To assess causative/contributing factors:

- Determine the client's usual ability to manage own affairs. **This provides the baseline for understanding the client's decision-making process and measures growth.**
- Note expressions of decision, dependability, and availability of support persons.
- Active-listen and identify reason(s) the client would like to improve decision-making abilities and expectations of change. **As the client articulates/clarifies reasons for improvement, direction is provided for change.**
- Note the presence of physical signs of excitement. **This enhances energy for quest for improvement and personal growth.**
- Discuss the meaning of life and reasons for living, belief in God or higher power, and how these relate to current desire for improvement.

Nursing Priority No. 2.

To assist client to improve/effectively use problem-solving skills:

- Promote a safe and hopeful environment. **This provides an opportunity for the client to discuss concerns/thoughts freely.**
- Provide opportunities for the client to recognize his or her own inner control in the decision-making process. **Individuals with an internal locus of control believe they have some degree of control in outcomes and that their own actions/choices help determine what happens in their lives.**
- Encourage verbalization of ideas, concerns, and particular decisions that need to be made.
- Clarify and prioritize the individual's goals, noting possible conflicts or challenges that may be encountered.
- Identify positive aspects of this experience, encouraging the client to view it as a learning opportunity.
- Assist the client in learning how to find factual information (e.g., use of the library or reliable Internet Web sites).
- Review the process of problem-solving and how to do a risk-benefit analysis of decisions.
- ∞ Encourage children to make age-appropriate decisions. **Learning problem-solving at an early age will enhance sense of self-worth and ability to exercise coping skills.**
- Discuss and clarify spiritual beliefs, accepting the client's values in a nonjudgmental manner.

Information that appears in brackets has been added by the authors to clarify and enhance the use of nursing diagnoses.

Nursing Priority No. 3.

To promote optimum wellness:

- Identify opportunities for using conflict-resolution skills, emphasizing each step as it is used.
- Provide positive feedback for efforts. **This enhances the use of skills and learning efforts.**
- Encourage involvement of family/SO(s), as desired or appropriate, in the decision-making process **to help all family members improve conflict-resolution skills.**
- Suggest participation in stress management or assertiveness classes, as appropriate.
- Refer to other resources, as necessary (e.g., clergy, psychiatric clinical nurse specialist or psychiatrist, or family or marital therapist).

Documentation Focus

Assessment/Reassessment

- Assessment findings, behavioral responses
- Motivation and expectations for change
- Individuals involved in improving conflict skills
- Personal values and beliefs

Planning

- Plan of care, intervention, and who is involved in the planning
- Teaching plan

Implementation/Evaluation

- Clients and involved individual's responses to interventions, teaching, and actions performed
- Ability to express feelings, identify options, and use resources
- Attainment or progress toward desired outcome(s)
- Modifications to plan of care

Discharge Planning

- Long-term needs, noting who is responsible for actions to be taken
- Specific referrals made

Sample Nursing Outcomes & Interventions Classifications (NOC/NIC)

NOC—Decision-Making
NIC—Decision-Making Support

Information that appears in brackets has been added by the authors to clarify and enhance the use of nursing diagnoses.

 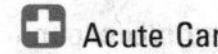

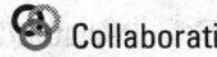

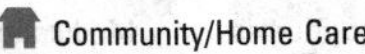

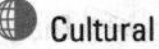

ineffective DENIAL

[Diagnostic Division: Ego Integrity]

Definition: Conscious or unconscious attempt to disavow the knowledge or meaning of an event to reduce anxiety and/or fear, leading to the detriment of health.

Related Factors

Anxiety; perceived inadequacy in dealing with strong emotions
Insufficient sense of control; fear of losing autonomy
Excessive stress; ineffective coping strategies
Threat of unpleasant reality
Fear of separation/death
Insufficient emotional support

Defining Characteristics

Subjective

Minimizes symptoms; displaces source of symptoms
Does not admit impact of disease on life
Displaces fear of impact of the condition
Denies fear of death/invalidism

Objective

Delay in seeking or refusal of healthcare
Does not perceive relevance of symptoms/danger
Use of dismissive gestures or comments when speaking of distressing event
Inappropriate affect
Use of treatment not advised by healthcare professional

Desired Outcomes/Evaluation Criteria—Client Will:

- Acknowledge reality of situation or illness.
- Express realistic concern or feelings about symptoms/illness.
- Seek appropriate assistance for presenting problem.
- Display appropriate affect.

Actions/Interventions

Nursing Priority No. 1.

To assess causative/contributing factors:

- Identify situational crisis or problem and client's perception of the situation.

Information that appears in brackets has been added by the authors to clarify and enhance the use of nursing diagnoses.

- Determine the stage and degree of denial.
- Compare the client's description of symptoms or conditions to the reality of the clinical picture.
- Note the client's comments about the impact of illness or problem on lifestyle.

Nursing Priority No. 2.

To assist client to deal appropriately with situation:

- Use therapeutic communication skills of active-listening and I-messages **to develop a trusting nurse-client relationship.**
- Provide a safe, nonthreatening environment. **This encourages the client to talk freely without fear of judgment.**
- Encourage expressions of feelings, accepting the client's view of the situation without confrontation. Set limits on maladaptive behavior **to promote safety.**
- Present accurate information, as appropriate, without insisting that the client accept what has been presented. **This avoids confrontation, which may further entrench the client in denial.**
- Discuss the client's behaviors in relation to illness (e.g., diabetes, hypertension, or alcoholism) and point out the results of these behaviors.
- Encourage the client to talk with SO(s)/friends. **This may clarify concerns and reduce isolation and withdrawal.**
- Involve the client in group sessions **so the client can hear other views of reality and test his or her own perceptions.**
- Avoid agreeing with inaccurate statements/perceptions **to prevent perpetuating false reality.**
- Provide positive feedback for constructive moves toward independence **to promote repetition of behavior.**

Nursing Priority No. 3.

To promote wellness (Teaching/Discharge Considerations):

- Provide written information about illness or situation **for client and family to refer to as they consider options.**
- Involve family members/SO(s) in long-range planning for meeting individual needs.
- Refer to appropriate community resources (e.g., Diabetes Association, MS Society, or Alcoholics Anonymous) **to help the client with long-term adjustment.**
- Refer to ND ineffective Coping.

Information that appears in brackets has been added by the authors to clarify and enhance the use of nursing diagnoses.

Documentation Focus

Assessment/Reassessment

- Assessment findings, degree of personal vulnerability and denial
- Impact of illness or problem on lifestyle

Planning

- Plan of care and who is involved in the planning
- Teaching plan

Implementation/Evaluation

- Client's response to interventions, teaching, and actions performed
- Use of resources
- Attainment or progress toward desired outcome(s)
- Modifications to plan of care

Discharge Planning

- Long-term needs and who is responsible for actions taken
- Specific referrals made

Sample Nursing Outcomes & Interventions Classifications (NOC/NIC)

NOC—Acceptance: Health Status
NIC—Anxiety Reduction

impaired DENTITION

[Diagnostic Division: Food/Fluid]

Definition: Disruption in tooth development/eruption patterns or structural integrity of individual teeth.

Related Factors

Insufficient dietary habits; malnutrition
Pharmaceutical agent; habitual use of staining substances (e.g., tobacco, coffee, tea, red wine)
Insufficient oral hygiene; oral temperature sensitivity
Insufficient knowledge of dental health; excessive intake of fluoride or use of abrasive oral cleaning agents
Barrier to self-care; difficulty accessing dental care

Information that appears in brackets has been added by the authors to clarify and enhance the use of nursing diagnoses.

Economically disadvantaged
Genetic predisposition; bruxism
[Traumatic injury to face/jaw; surgical intervention]

Defining Characteristics

Subjective

Toothache

Objective

Halitosis
Enamel discoloration; erosion of enamel; excessive oral plaque/calculus
Abraded teeth; dental or root caries; tooth fracture; loose tooth; absence of teeth
Premature loss of primary teeth; incomplete tooth eruption for age
Malocclusion; tooth misalignment; facial asymmetry

Desired Outcomes/Evaluation Criteria—Client Will:

- Display healthy gums, mucous membranes, and teeth in good repair.
- Report adequate nutritional and fluid intake.
- Verbalize and demonstrate effective dental hygiene skills.
- Follow through on referrals for appropriate dental care.

Action/Interventions

Nursing Priority No. 1.

To assess causative/contributing factors:

- Inspect the oral cavity. Note the presence or absence of teeth and/or dentures and ascertain the significance of finding in terms of nutritional needs and aesthetics.
- Evaluate the current status of dental hygiene and oral health **to determine the need for instruction or coaching, assistive devices, and/or referral to dental care providers.**
- ∞ Document age, developmental and cognitive status, and manual dexterity. Evaluate nutritional and health state, noting the presence of conditions such as bulimia or chronic vomiting, musculoskeletal impairments, or problems with mouth (e.g., bleeding disorders, cancer lesions, abscesses, and facial trauma), **which are factors affecting a client's dental health and the ability to provide effective oral care.**

Information that appears in brackets has been added by the authors to clarify and enhance the use of nursing diagnoses.

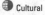

- Document the presence of factors affecting dentition (e.g., chronic use of tobacco, coffee, or tea; bulimia/chronic vomiting; abscesses; tumors; braces; bruxism [chronic grinding of teeth]) **to determine possible interventions and/or treatment needs.**
- Note the current situation that could impact dental health (e.g., presence of endotrachial [ET] intubation, facial fractures, or chemotherapy) **and that require special mouth care procedures.**
- Document (photograph) facial injuries before treatment **to provide a "pictorial baseline" for future comparison and evaluation.**

Nursing Priority No. 2.

To treat/manage dental care needs:

- Ascertain the client's usual method of oral care **to provide continuity of care or to build on the client's existing knowledge base and current practices in developing a plan of care.**
- Assist with or provide oral care, as indicated:

  Offer tap water or saline rinses and diluted alcohol-free mouthwashes.

  Provide gentle gum massage and tongue brushing with a soft toothbrush, using fluoride toothpaste to manage tartar buildup, if appropriate.

  Use foam sticks **to swab gums and oral cavity when brushing is not possible or is inadvisable.**

  Assist with brushing and flossing **when the client is unable to do self-care.**

  Demonstrate and assist with electric or battery-powered mouth care devices (e.g., toothbrush, plaque remover, or Waterpik®), as indicated.

  Remind the client to brush teeth as indicated. **Cues, modeling, or pantomime may be helpful if the client is young, elderly, or cognitively or emotionally impaired.**

  Assist with or provide denture care, when indicated (e.g., remove and clean after meals and at bedtime).
- Provide an appropriate diet for optimal nutrition, considering the client's special needs, such as pregnancy, age and developmental concerns, and ability to chew (e.g., liquids or soft foods), and offer low-sugar, low-starch foods and snacks; limit between-meal eating, sugary foods, and bedtime snacks **to minimize tooth decay and to improve overall health.**
- Increase fluids, as needed, **to enhance hydration and general well-being of oral mucous membranes.**

Information that appears in brackets has been added by the authors to clarify and enhance the use of nursing diagnoses.

- Reposition ET tubes and airway adjuncts routinely, carefully padding and protecting teeth or prosthetics. Suction with care, when indicated.
- Avoid thermal stimuli when teeth are sensitive. Recommend the use of specific toothpastes **designed to reduce sensitivity of teeth.**
- Maintain good jaw and facial alignment when fractures are present.
- Administer antibiotics, as needed, **to treat dental and gum infections.**
- Recommend the use of analgesics and topical analgesics, as needed, **when dental pain is present.**
- Administer antibiotic therapy prior to dental procedures in susceptible individuals (e.g., prosthetic heart valve clients) and/or ascertain that bleeding disorders or coagulation deficits are not present **to prevent excess bleeding.**
- Refer to appropriate care providers (e.g., dental hygienists, dentists, periodontists, and oral surgeons).

Nursing Priority No. 3.

To promote wellness (Teaching/Discharge Considerations):

- Instruct the client/caregiver in home-care interventions **to treat the condition and/or prevent further complications.**
- Review resources that are needed for the client to perform adequate dental hygiene care (e.g., toothbrush/paste, clean water, dental floss, and/or personal care assistant).
- Recommend that the client (of any age) limit sugary and high-carbohydrate foods in diet and snacks **to reduce the buildup of plaque and the risk of cavities caused by acids associated with the breakdown of sugar and starch.**
- Instruct older client and caregiver(s) concerning special needs and importance of daily mouth care and regular dental follow-up.
- Advise the mother regarding age-appropriate concerns (e.g., refrain from letting baby fall asleep with milk or juice in bottle; use water and pacifier during the night; avoid sharing eating utensils and toothbrushes among family members; teach children to brush teeth while young; provide the child with safety devices such as helmet, face mask, or mouth guard to prevent facial injuries).
- Discuss with pregnant women special needs and regular dental care **to maintain maternal dental health and promote strong teeth and bones in fetal development.**
- Encourage cessation of tobacco, especially smokeless, and enrollment in smoking-cessation classes **to reduce the inci-**

Information that appears in brackets has been added by the authors to clarify and enhance the use of nursing diagnoses.

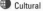

dence of gum disorders, oral cancer, and other health problems.

- Discuss advisability of dental checkup and care prior to initiating chemotherapy or radiation treatments **to minimize oral and dental tissue damage.**
- Refer to resources to maintain dental hygiene (e.g., dental care providers, oral health care supplies, and/or financial assistance programs).

Documentation Focus

Assessment/Reassessment

- Individual findings, including individual factors influencing dentition problems
- Baseline photos; description of oral cavity and structures

Planning

- Plan of care and who is involved in planning
- Teaching plan

Implementation/Evaluation

- Responses to interventions, teaching, and actions performed
- Attainment or progress toward desired outcome(s)
- Modifications to plan of care

Discharge Planning

- Individual long-term needs, noting who is responsible for actions to be taken
- Specific referrals made

Sample Nursing Outcomes & Interventions Classifications (NOC/NIC)

NOC—Oral Hygiene
NIC—Oral Health Restoration

risk for delayed DEVELOPMENT

[Diagnostic Division: Teaching/Learning]

Definition: Vulnerable to delay of 25% or more in one or more of the areas of social or self-regulatory behavior or in cognitive, language, or gross or fine motor skills, which may compromise health.

Information that appears in brackets has been added by the authors to clarify and enhance the use of nursing diagnoses.

Risk Factors

Prenatal

Maternal age ≤ 15 or ≥ 35 years
Unplanned or unwanted pregnancy; insufficient or late-term prenatal care
Inadequate nutrition; economically disadvantaged
Functional illiteracy
Genetic or endocrine disorder; infection; substance abuse

Individual

Prematurity; congenital or genetic disorder
Visual or hearing impairment; recurrent otitis media
Inadequate nutrition; failure to thrive
Chronic illness; treatment regimen
Brain injury (e.g., hemorrhage, shaken baby syndrome, abuse, or accident); seizures
Positive drug screening; substance abuse; lead poisoning
Involvement with the foster care system; history of adoption
Behavior disorder (e.g., attention deficit, oppositional defiant)
Technology dependence (e.g., ventilator, augmentative communication)
Natural disaster

Environmental

Economically disadvantaged
Exposure to violence

Caregiver

Learning disability
Presence of abuse (e.g., physical, psychological, or sexual)
Mental health issue (e.g., depression, psychosis, personality disorder, or substance abuse)

NOTE: A risk diagnosis is not evidenced by signs and symptoms, as the problem has not occurred; rather, nursing interventions are directed at prevention.

Desired Outcomes/Evaluation Criteria—Client Will:

- Perform self-regulatory behavior and motor, social, cognitive, and language skills appropriate for age within scope of present capabilities.

Information that appears in brackets has been added by the authors to clarify and enhance the use of nursing diagnoses.

Caregiver Will:

- Verbalize an understanding of age-appropriate development and expectations.
- Identify individual risk factors for developmental delay or deviation.
- Formulate plan(s) for prevention of developmental deviation.
- Initiate interventions and lifestyle changes promoting appropriate development.

Actions/Interventions

Nursing Priority No. 1.

To assess causative/contributing risk factors:

- Identify condition(s) that could contribute to developmental deviations. **This list is extensive and widely variable (see Risk Factors). The potential for developmental issues might be apparent at birth. However, risks are not confined to the child's birth events, but also encompass parent/family issues and environment (e.g., family history of developmental disorders; mother with mental illness or retardation, child with acute or chronic severe illness and lengthy hospitalizations; family poverty with inadequate living quarters, nutrition, nurturing, or supervision; family instability or violence; shaken baby syndrome and other maltreatment or child abuse; or institutional home or foster system during early life or prior to adoption).**
- Participate in screening the child's development level by means of observation and history related by concerned parents/other significant others. **Developmental delay occurs when a child fails to achieve one or more developmental milestones within an expected time period, may be in one or more areas (e.g., cognitive, social and emotional, speech and language, fine motor skills or gross motor skills) and may be the result of one or multiple factors.**
- Obtain information from a variety of sources. **Parents are often the first to think that there is a problem with their baby's development and should be encouraged to have routine well-baby checkups and screening for developmental delays. Teachers, family members, day care or foster care providers, and others interacting with a client (older than infant) may have valuable input regarding behaviors that may indicate problems or developmental issues.**
- Identify cultural beliefs, norms, and values. **Culture shapes parenting practices, understanding of health and illness,**

Information that appears in brackets has been added by the authors to clarify and enhance the use of nursing diagnoses.

perceptions related to development, and beliefs about individuals affected by developmental disorders.

- Note the severity and pervasiveness of the situation (e.g., potential for long-term stress leading to abuse or neglect, versus situational disruption during period of crisis or transition). **Situations require different interventions in terms of the intensity and length of time that assistance and support may be critical to the parent/caregiver.**
- Evaluate the environment in which long-standing care will be provided. **The physical, emotional, financial, and social needs of a family are impacted and intertwined with the needs of the client.**
- Refer for and assist with in-depth evaluation, if indicated, using an authoritative text (e.g., Gesell, Mussen-Conger) or assessment tools (e.g., Ages and Stages Questionnaire [ASQ-3], Parents Evaluation of Developmental Status [PEDS], Temperament and Atypical Behavior Scale [TABS], Denver II Developmental Screening Test, or Bender's Visual Motor Gestalt Test). **This provides a guide for comparative measurement as the child/individual progresses. There are tools to evaluate the child's skills in certain areas, such as motor development, speech, language, math, and so on. However, a diagnosis is often determined over months or years. Also, a child who is delayed in an area at a certain age may "catch up" in later years.**

Nursing Priority No. 2.

To assist in preventing and/or limiting developmental delays:

- At clinic visits, note chronological age and review with parents the expectations for "normal development" in infancy and early childhood **to help determine developmental expectations and how the expectations may be altered by the child's condition. For high-risk individuals, including children affected by biological (e.g., low birth weight) and psychosocial (e.g., foster care or homelessness) risk factors, earlier and more frequent developmental screening may be warranted.**
- Describe realistic, age-appropriate patterns of development to parent/caregiver and promote activities and interactions that support developmental tasks where client is at this time. **This is important in planning interventions in keeping with the individual's current status and potential. Each child will have his or her own unique strengths and challenges.**
- Collaborate with related professional resources, as indicated (e.g., physical, occupational, rehabilitation, speech therapists;

Information that appears in brackets has been added by the authors to clarify and enhance the use of nursing diagnoses.

home health agencies; social services, nutritionist; special-education teacher, family therapists; technological and adaptive equipment specialists; vocational counselor). **Multidisciplinary team care increases the likelihood of developing a well-rounded plan of care that meets the client/family's specialized and varied needs, minimizing identified risks.**

- Encourage setting of short-term realistic goals for achieving developmental potential. **Small incremental steps are often easier to deal with.**

Nursing Priority No. 3.

To promote wellness (Teaching/Discharge Considerations):

- Engage in and encourage prevention strategies (e.g., abstinence from drugs, alcohol, tobacco for pregnant women/child, referral for treatment programs, referral for violence prevention counseling, anticipatory guidance for potential challenges [vision, hearing, or failure to thrive]). **Promoting wellness starts with preventing complications and/or limiting the severity of anticipated problems. Such strategies can often be initiated by nurses where the potential is first identified, in the community setting.**
- Evaluate the client's progress on a continual basis. Identify target symptoms requiring intervention **to make referrals in a timely manner and/or to make adjustments in the plan of care, as indicated.**
- Provide information regarding development, as appropriate, including pertinent reference materials.
- Emphasize the importance of follow-up screening appointments as indicated **to promote ongoing evaluation, support, or management of situation.**
- Discuss proactive wellness actions to take (e.g., periodic laboratory studies to monitor nutritional status or getting immunizations on schedule to prevent serious infections) **to avoid preventable complications.**
- Maintain positive, hopeful attitude. Encourage the setting of short-term realistic goals for achieving developmental potential. **Small, incremental steps are often easier to deal with, and successes enhance hopefulness and well-being.**
- Provide information as appropriate, including pertinent reference materials and reliable Web sites. **Bibliotherapy provides an opportunity to review data at own pace, enhancing the likelihood of retention.**
- Identify available community resources, as appropriate (e.g., early intervention programs, seniors' activity/support groups, gifted and talented programs, sheltered workshop, children's

Information that appears in brackets has been added by the authors to clarify and enhance the use of nursing diagnoses.

services, and medical equipment/supplier). **This can provide assistance to support the family and help identify community responsibilities (e.g., services required to be provided to school-age child if developmental disabilities are diagnosed).**

Documentation Focus

Assessment/Reassessment

- Assessment findings, individual needs including developmental level and potential for improvement
- Caregiver's understanding of situation and individual role

Planning

- Plan of care and who is involved in the planning
- Teaching plan

Implementation/Evaluation

- Client's response to interventions, teaching, and actions performed
- Caregiver response to teaching
- Attainment or progress toward desired outcome(s)
- Modifications to plan of care

Discharge Planning

- Identified long-range needs and who is responsible for actions to be taken
- Specific referrals made, sources for assistive devices, educational tools

Sample Nursing Outcomes & Interventions Classifications (NOC/NIC)

NOC—Child Development [specify age]
NIC—Developmental Enhancement: Child [or] Adolescent

DIARRHEA

[Diagnostic Division: Elimination]

Definition: Passage of loose, unformed stools.

Information that appears in brackets has been added by the authors to clarify and enhance the use of nursing diagnoses.

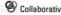

Related Factors

Psychological
Increase in stress level; anxiety

Situational
Laxative or substance abuse; exposure to toxin, contaminant
Treatment regimen
Enteral feedings
Travel

Physiological
Gastrointestinal inflammation, irritation
Infection; parasite
Malabsorption

Defining Characteristics

Subjective
Abdominal pain
Bowel urgency; cramping

Objective
Hyperactive bowel sounds
Loose liquid stools >3 in 24 hours

Desired Outcomes/Evaluation Criteria—Client Will:

- Reestablish and maintain normal pattern of bowel functioning.
- Verbalize understanding of causative factors and rationale for treatment regimen.
- Demonstrate appropriate behavior to assist with resolution of causative factors (e.g., proper food preparation or avoidance of irritating foods).

Actions/Interventions

Nursing Priority No. 1.
To assess causative factors/etiology:

- Ascertain onset and pattern of diarrhea, noting whether acute or chronic. **Acute diarrhea (caused by viral, bacterial, or parasitic infections [e.g., *Norwalk, Rotavirus; Salmonella,***

Information that appears in brackets has been added by the authors to clarify and enhance the use of nursing diagnoses.

***Shigella, Giardia;* amebiasis, respectively]; bacterial food-borne toxins [e.g., *Staphylococcus aureus, Escherichia coli*]; medications [e.g., antibiotics, chemotherapy agents, cholchicine, laxatives]; and enteral tube feedings) lasts from a few days up to a week. Chronic diarrhea (caused by irritable bowel syndrome, infectious diseases affecting the colon [e.g., inflammatory bowel disease], colon cancer and treatments, severe constipation, malabsorption disorders, laxative abuse, certain endocrine disorders [e.g., hyperthyroidism, Addison's disease]) almost always lasts more than 3 weeks.**

- Obtain history and observe stools for volume, frequency (e.g., more than normal number of stools per day), characteristics (e.g., slightly soft to watery stools), and precipitating factors (e.g., travel, recent antibiotic use, day care center attendance) related to occurrence of diarrhea.
- Note the client's age. **Diarrhea in an infant or young child and older or debilitated client can cause complications of dehydration and electrolyte imbalances.**
- Determine if incontinence is present. (Refer to ND bowel Incontinence.)
- Note reports of abdominal or rectal pain associated with episodes. **Pain is often present with inflammatory bowel disease, irritable bowel syndrome, and mesenteric ischemia.**
- Auscultate abdomen **for presence, location, and characteristics of bowel sounds.**
- Observe for the presence of associated factors, such as fever or chills, abdominal pain and cramping, bloody stools, emotional upset, physical exertion, and so forth.
- Evaluate diet history, noting food allergies or intolerances and food and water safety issues, and note general nutritional intake and fluid and electrolyte status.
- Review medications, noting side effects and possible interactions. **Many drugs (e.g., antibiotics [e.g., cephalosporins, erythromycin, penicillins, quinolones, tetracyclines], digitalis, angiotensin-converting enzyme [ACE] inhibitors, nonsteroidal anti-inflammatory drugs [NSAIDs], hypoglycemia agents, and cholesterol-lowering drugs) can cause or exacerbate diarrhea, particularly in the elderly and in those who have had surgery on the intestinal tract.**
- Determine recent exposure to different or foreign environments, change in drinking water or food intake, and similar illness of others **that may help identify causative environmental factors.**

Information that appears in brackets has been added by the authors to clarify and enhance the use of nursing diagnoses.

- Note history of recent gastrointestinal surgery, concurrent or chronic illnesses and treatment, food or drug allergies, and lactose intolerance.
- Review results of laboratory testing **(e.g., parasites, cultures for bacteria, toxins, fat, blood) for acute diarrhea. Chronic diarrhea testing may include upper and lower gastrointestinal studies, stool examination for parasites, colonoscopy with biopsies, and so forth.**

Nursing Priority No. 2.

To eliminate causative factors:

- Restrict solid food intake, as indicated, **to allow for bowel rest and reduced intestinal workload.**
- Provide for changes in dietary intake **to avoid foods or substances that precipitate diarrhea.**
- Limit caffeine and high-fiber foods; avoid milk and fruits, as appropriate.
- Adjust strength or rate of enteral tube feedings; change formula, as indicated, **when diarrhea is associated with tube feedings.**
- Assess for and remove fecal impaction, especially in an elderly client **where impaction may be accompanied by diarrhea.** (Refer to NDs Constipation; bowel Incontinence.)
- Recommend change in drug therapy, as appropriate (e.g., choice of antibiotic).
- Assist in treatment of underlying conditions (e.g., infections, malabsorption syndrome, cancer) and complications of diarrhea. **Therapies can include treatment of fever, pain, and infectious or toxic agents; rehydration; oral refeeding; and so forth.**
- Promote use of relaxation techniques (e.g., progressive relaxation exercise, visualization techniques) **to decrease stress and anxiety.**

Nursing Priority No. 3.

To maintain hydration/electrolyte balance:

- Note reports of thirst, less frequent or absent urination, dry mouth and skin, weakness, light-headedness, and headaches. **These are signs/symptoms of dehydration and need for rehydration.**
- Observe for or question parents about young child crying with no tears, fever, decreased urination, or no wet diapers for 6 to 8 hr; listlessness or irritability; sunken eyes; dry mouth and tongue; and suspected or documented weight loss. **The child**

Information that appears in brackets has been added by the authors to clarify and enhance the use of nursing diagnoses.

needs urgent or emergency treatment for dehydration if these signs are present and the child is not taking fluids.

- Assess for the presence of postural hypotension, tachycardia, skin hydration/turgor, and condition of mucous membranes **indicating dehydration.**
- Weigh the infant's diapers **to determine the amount of output and fluid replacement needs.**
- Review laboratory studies for abnormalities. **Chronic diarrhea may require more invasive testing, including upper and/or lower gastrointestinal radiographs, ultrasound, endoscopic evaluations, biopsy, and so on.**
- Administer antidiarrheal medications, as indicated, **to decrease gastrointestinal motility and minimize fluid losses.**
- Encourage oral intake of fluids containing electrolytes, such as juices, bouillon, or commercial preparations, as appropriate.
- Administer enteral and parenteral fluids, as indicated.

Nursing Priority No. 4.

To maintain skin integrity:

- Assist, as needed, with pericare after each bowel movement.
- Provide prompt diaper/incontinence brief change and gentle cleansing, **because skin breakdown can occur quickly when diarrhea is present.**
- Apply lotion or ointment as skin barrier, as needed.
- Provide dry linen, as necessary.
- Expose perineum and buttocks to air; use heat lamp with caution, if needed to keep area dry.
- Refer to ND impaired Skin Integrity.

Nursing Priority No. 5.

To promote return to normal bowel functioning:

- Increase oral fluid intake and return to normal diet, as tolerated.
- Encourage intake of nonirritating liquids.
- Discuss possible change in infant formula. **Diarrhea may be a result of or be aggravated by intolerance to a specific formula.**
- Recommend products such as natural fiber, plain natural yogurt, and Lactinex **to restore normal bowel flora.**
- Administer medications, as ordered, **to treat infectious process, decrease motility, and/or absorb water.**
- Provide privacy during defecation and psychological support, as necessary.

Information that appears in brackets has been added by the authors to clarify and enhance the use of nursing diagnoses.

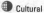

Nursing Priority No. 6.

To promote wellness (Teaching/Discharge Considerations):

- Review causative factors and appropriate interventions **to prevent recurrence.**
- Discuss individual stress factors and coping behaviors.
- Review food preparation, emphasizing adequate cooking time and proper refrigeration or storage **to prevent bacterial growth and contamination.**
- Emphasize importance of hand hygiene **to prevent spread of infectious causes of diarrhea such as *Clostridium difficile* or *S. aureus*.**
- Discuss the possibility of dehydration and the importance of proper fluid replacement.
- Suggest the use of incontinence pads (depending on the severity of the problem) **to protect bedding or furniture.**

Documentation Focus

Assessment/Reassessment

- Assessment findings, including characteristics and pattern of elimination
- Causative and aggravating factors
- Methods used to treat problem

Planning

- Plan of care and who is involved in planning
- Teaching plan

Implementation/Evaluation

- Client's response to treatment, teaching, and actions performed
- Attainment or progress toward desired outcome(s)
- Modifications to plan of care

Discharge Planning

- Recommendations for follow-up care

Sample Nursing Outcomes & Interventions Classifications (NOC/NIC)

NOC—Bowel Elimination
NIC—Diarrhea Management

Information that appears in brackets has been added by the authors to clarify and enhance the use of nursing diagnoses.

risk for DISUSE SYNDROME

[Diagnostic Division: Activity/Rest]

Definition: Vulnerable to deterioration of body systems as the result of prescribed or unavoidable musculoskeletal inactivity, which may compromise health.

NOTE: Complications from immobility can include decreased strength or endurance, activity intolerance, impaired sitting or standing or walking; pressure ulcer, impaired urinary or bowel function; respiratory complications such as pneumonia; systemic infections; blood clots; orthostatic hypotension; disorientation, body image disturbance, ineffective coping, and powerlessness.

Risk Factors

Alteration in level of consciousness
Mechanical or prescribed immobility; paralysis
Pain

NOTE: A risk diagnosis is not evidenced by signs and symptoms, as the problem has not occurred; rather, nursing interventions are directed at prevention.

Desired Outcomes/Evaluation Criteria—Client Will:

- Display intact skin and tissues or achieve timely wound healing.
- Maintain or reestablish effective elimination patterns.
- Be free of signs/symptoms of infectious processes.
- Demonstrate absence of pulmonary congestion with breath sounds clear.
- Demonstrate adequate peripheral perfusion with stable vital signs, skin warm and dry, palpable peripheral pulses.
- Maintain usual reality orientation.
- Maintain or regain optimal level of cognitive, neurosensory, and musculoskeletal functioning.
- Express sense of control over the present situation and potential outcome.

Information that appears in brackets has been added by the authors to clarify and enhance the use of nursing diagnoses.

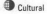

- Recognize and incorporate change into self-concept in accurate manner without negative self-esteem.

Actions/Interventions

Nursing Priority No. 1.

To evaluate probability of developing complications:

- Identify underlying conditions/pathology (e.g., cancer, trauma, fractures with casting, immobilization devices, surgery, chronic disease conditions, malnutrition, neurological conditions [e.g., stroke/other brain injury, postpolio syndrome, multiple sclerosis (MS), or spinal cord injury], chronic pain conditions, or use of predisposing medications [e.g., steroids]) **that cause or exacerbate problems associated with inactivity and immobility. Note: "Disuse syndrome" is a classic pattern of muscular deconditioning and atrophy resulting from inactivity or immobilization. Once muscle is lost, it is difficult to gain it back.**
- Identify potential concerns, including cognition, mobility, and exercise status. **Disuse syndrome can include muscle and bone atrophy, stiffening of joints, brittle bones, reduction of cardiopulmonary function, loss of red blood cells (RBCs), decreased sex hormones, decreased resistance to infections, increased proportion of body fat in relation to muscle mass, and chemical changes in the brain, which adversely impact the client's activities of daily living (ADLs), social life, and quality of life.**
- ∞ Note specific and potential concerns including client's age, cognition, mobility and exercise status. **Age-related physiological changes along with limitations imposed by illness or confinement predispose older adults to deconditioning and functional decline.**
- Determine if the client's condition is acute/short term or whether it may be a long-term/permanent condition. **Relatively short-term conditions (e.g., simple fracture treated with cast) may respond quickly to rehabilitative efforts. Long-term conditions (e.g., stroke, aged person with dementia, cancers, demyelinating or degenerative diseases, spinal cord injury (SCI), and psychological problems such as depression or learned helplessness) have a higher risk of complications for the client and caregiver.**
- Assess and document (ongoing) the client's ongoing functional status, including cognition, vision, and hearing; social support; psychological well-being; abilities in performance of

---

Information that appears in brackets has been added by the authors to clarify and enhance the use of nursing diagnoses.

activities of daily living **for comparative baseline to use to evaluate response to treatment and identify preventive interventions or necessary services.**

- Evaluate the client's risk for injury. **Risk is greater in a client with cognitive difficulties, lack of safe or stimulating environment, inadequate or unsafe use of mobility aids, and/or sensory-perception problems.**
- Ascertain attitudes of individual/SO about condition (e.g., cultural values, stigma). Note misconceptions. **The client may be influenced (positively or negatively) by peer group, cultural, and family role expectations.**
- Evaluate the client's/family's understanding and ability to manage care for a prolonged period. Ascertain availability and use of support systems. **Caregivers may be influenced by their own physical or emotional limitations, degree of commitment to assisting the client toward optimal independence, or available time.**
- Review psychological assessment of client's emotional status. **Potential problems that may arise from presence of condition need to be identified and dealt with to avoid further debilitation. Common associated psychological changes include depression, anxiety, and avoidance behaviors.**

Nursing Priority No. 2.

To provide individually appropriate preventive/corrective interventions:

Skin

- Inspect skin on a frequent basis, noting changes. Monitor skin over bony prominences.
- Reposition frequently as individually indicated **to relieve pressure.**
- Provide skin care daily and prn, drying well and using gentle massage and lotion **to stimulate circulation.**
- Use pressure-reducing devices (e.g., egg crate, gel, water, or air mattress or cushions).
- Review nutritional status and promote diet with adequate protein, calorie, and vitamin and mineral intake **to aid in healing and promote general good health of skin and tissues.**
- Provide or reinforce teaching regarding dietary needs, position changes, and cleanliness.
- Refer to NDs impaired Skin Integrity, impaired Tissue Integrity, and risk for Pressure Ulcer for additional interventions.

Information that appears in brackets has been added by the authors to clarify and enhance the use of nursing diagnoses.

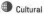

Elimination

- Observe elimination pattern, noting changes and potential problems.
- Encourage a balanced diet, including fruits and vegetables high in fiber and with adequate fluids **for optimal stool consistency and to facilitate passage through colon.**
- Encourage intake of adequate fluids, including water and cranberry juice **to reduce risk of urinary infections.**
- Maximize mobility at earliest opportunity.
- Evaluate need for stool softeners or bulk-forming laxatives.
- Implement consistent bowel management or bladder training programs, as indicated.
- Monitor urinary output and characteristics **to identify changes associated with infection.**
- Refer to NDs Constipation; Diarrhea; bowel Incontinence; impaired Urinary Elimination; Urinary Retention for additional interventions.

Respiration

- Monitor breath sounds and characteristics of secretions **for early detection of complications (e.g., atelectasis, pneumonia).**
- Encourage ambulation and an upright position. Reposition, cough, and deep breathe on a regular schedule **to facilitate clearing of secretions and to improve lung function.**
- Encourage use of incentive spirometry. Suction, as indicated, **to clear airways.**
- Demonstrate techniques for, and assist with, postural drainage.
- Assist with, and instruct family and caregivers in, quad coughing techniques and diaphragmatic weight training **to maximize ventilation in the presence of a spinal cord injury.**
- Discourage smoking. Encourage the client to join a smoking-cessation program, as indicated.
- Refer to NDs ineffective Airway Clearance, ineffective Breathing Pattern, impaired Gas Exchange, impaired spontaneous Ventilation for additional interventions.

Vascular (Tissue Perfusion)

- Assess cognition and mental status (ongoing). **Changes can reflect state of cardiac health or cerebral oxygenation impairment or can be indicative of mental or emotional state that could adversely affect safety and self-care.**

Information that appears in brackets has been added by the authors to clarify and enhance the use of nursing diagnoses.

- Determine core and skin temperature. Investigate development of cyanosis or changes in mentation **to identify changes in oxygenation status.**
- Evaluate circulation and nerve function of affected body parts on a routine, ongoing basis. **Changes in temperature, color, sensation, and movement can be the effect of immobility, disease, aging, or injury.**
- Encourage adequate fluid intake **to prevent dehydration and circulatory stasis.**
- Monitor blood pressure before, during, and after activity—sitting, standing, and lying—if possible, **to ascertain response to and tolerance of activity.**
- Assist with position changes as needed. Raise head gradually. Institute use of tilt table where appropriate. **Injury may occur as a result of orthostatic hypotension.**
- Institute peripheral vascular support measures (e.g., elastic hose, Ace wraps, sequential compression devices [SCDs]) **to enhance venous return and reduce risk for deep vein thrombosis.**
- Have client perform bed or chair exercises if not contraindicated **to help prevent loss of, or maintain muscle strength and tone.**
- Mobilize quickly and as often as possible, using mobility aids and frequent rest stops to assist the client in continuing activity. **Upright position and weight bearing help maintain bone strength, improve circulation, and prevent postural hypotension.**
- Evaluate the role of physiological and psychological pain in the mobility problem. Implement pain management program as individually indicated.
- Refer to NDs risk for Activity Intolerance; decreased Cardiac Output; risk for Peripheral Neurovascular Dysfunction; ineffective peripheral Tissue Perfusion for additional interventions.

Musculoskeletal (Mobility/Range of Motion, Strength/Endurance)

- Perform range of motion (ROM) exercises and involve client in active exercises with physical or occupational therapy (e.g., muscle strengthening) **to promote bone health, muscle strengthening, flexibility, optimal conditioning, and functional ability.**
- Maximize involvement in self-care **to restore or maintain strength, functional abilities, and early independence in self-care activities.**

Information that appears in brackets has been added by the authors to clarify and enhance the use of nursing diagnoses.

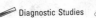

- Intersperse activity with rest periods. Pace activities as possible **to increase strength and endurance in a gradual manner and reduce failure of planned exercise because of exhaustion or overuse of weak muscles or injured area.**
- Identify need and use of supportive devices (e.g., cane, walker, or functional positioning splints) as appropriate **to assist with safe mobility and functional independence.**
- Evaluate the role of physiological and psychological pain in the mobility problem. Implement pain management program as individually indicated.
- Refer to NDs risk for Falls; impaired physical Mobility; impaired Sitting, Standing, and Walking; acute Pain; chronic Pain, chronic Pain Syndrome for additional interventions.

Sensory-Perception

- Orient client as necessary to situation, time, place, and person. Provide cues for orientation (e.g., clock and calendar). **Disturbances of sensory stimulation, interpretation, and thought processes are associated with immobility as well as aging, being ill, disease processes/treatments, and medication effects.**
- Provide appropriate level of environmental stimulation (e.g., music, TV/radio, personal possessions, and visitors) **to decrease the sensory deprivation associated with immobility and isolation.**
- Avoid or monitor closely the use of restraints, and immobilize the client as little as possible **to reduce the possibility of agitation and injury.**
- Promote regular sleep hours, use of sleep aids, and usual presleep rituals **to promote normal sleep and rest cycle.**
- Refer to NDs chronic Confusion, deficient Diversional Activity, Insomnia, [disturbed Sensory Perception] for additional interventions.

Self-Esteem, Powerlessness, Hopelessness, Social Isolation

- Determine factors that may contribute to impairment of client's self-esteem and social interactions. **Many factors can be involved, including the client's age, relationship status, usual health state; presence of disabilities, including pain; financial, environmental, and physical problems; or current situation causing immobility and client's state of mind concerning the importance of the current situation in regard to the rest of client's life and desired lifestyle.**

Information that appears in brackets has been added by the authors to clarify and enhance the use of nursing diagnoses.

- Ascertain if changes in client's situation are likely to be short term and temporary, or long term, or permanent. **This can affect both the client and care provider's coping abilities and willingness to engage in activities that prevent or limit effects of immobility.**
- Explain or review all care procedures. **This involves the client in his or her own care, enhances sense of control, and promotes independence.**
- Provide for, and assist with, mutual goal setting involving SO(s). **This promotes a sense of control and enhances commitment to goals.**
- Provide consistency in caregivers whenever possible.
- Ascertain that client can communicate needs adequately (e.g., call light, writing tablet, picture/letter board, or interpreter).
- Encourage verbalization of feelings and questions. **This aids in reducing anxiety and promotes learning about condition and specific needs.**
- Refer for mental, psychological, or spiritual services as indicated **to provide counseling, support, and medications.**
- Refer to NDs Powerlessness; impaired verbal Communication; ineffective Role Performance; Self-Esteem [specify]; impaired Social Interaction and Social Isolation for additional interventions.

Body Image

- Evaluate for presence or potential for physical, emotional, and behavioral conditions that may contribute to isolation and degeneration. **Disuse syndrome often affects those individuals who are already isolated for one reason or another (e.g., serious illness or injury with disfigurement, frail elderly living alone, individual with severe depression, or a person with unacceptable behavior or without a support system).**
- Orient to body changes through verbal description, written information; encourage looking at and discussing changes **to promote acceptance and understanding of needs.**
- Promote interactions with peers and normalization of activities within individual abilities. **Physical activity and social interactions stimulate the body to produce chemical substances that produce increased feelings of well-being, vitality, and alertness.**
- Refer to NDs disturbed Body Image; situational low Self-Esteem; Social Isolation; disturbed Personal Identity.

Nursing Priority No. 3.

To promote wellness (Teaching/Discharge Considerations):

Information that appears in brackets has been added by the authors to clarify and enhance the use of nursing diagnoses.

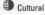

- Promote self-care and SO-supported activities **to gain or maintain independence.**
- Provide or review information about individual needs and areas of concerns (e.g., client's mental status, living environment, and nutritional needs) **to enhance safety and prevent or limit effects of disuse.**
- Encourage involvement in regular exercise program, including flexibility, resistance, and strengthening activities and active or assistive ROM, **to limit consequences of disuse and maximize level of function.**
- Review signs/symptoms requiring medical evaluation/follow-up **to promote timely interventions and limit adverse effects of the situation.**
- Review therapeutic regimen. **Treatment may be required for underlying condition(s), stress management, medications, therapies, and needed lifestyle changes.**
- Refer to appropriate rehabilitation/home-care resources **to provide assistance (e.g., help with care activities, exercise, meal preparation, financial help, transportation, or respite care; nutritionist).**
- Inform client/SO about supply sources for assistive devices and necessary equipment.

Documentation Focus

Assessment/Reassessment

- Assessment findings, noting individual areas of concern, functional level, degree of independence, support systems, and available resources

Planning

- Plan of care and who is involved in planning
- Teaching plan

Implementation/Evaluation

- Client's response to interventions, teaching, and actions performed
- Changes in level of functioning
- Attainment or progress toward desired outcome(s)
- Modifications to plan of care

Discharge Planning

- Long-term needs and who is responsible for actions to be taken
- Specific referrals made, resources for specific equipment needs

---

Information that appears in brackets has been added by the authors to clarify and enhance the use of nursing diagnoses.

Sample Nursing Outcomes & Interventions Classifications (NOC/NIC)

NOC—Immobility Consequences: Physiological
NIC—Exercise Promotion

deficient DIVERSIONAL ACTIVITY

[Diagnostic Division: Activity/Rest]

Definition: Decreased stimulation from (or interest or engagement in) recreational or leisure activities. [**Note:** Internal/external factors may be beyond the individual's control.]

Related Factors

Insufficient diversional activity [e.g., lack of resources]
Prolonged hospitalization/institutionalization; [frequent, lengthy treatments; homebound/bedridden]
Extremes of age
[Physical limitations; fatigue; chronic pain]

Defining Characteristics

Subjective

Boredom [e.g., wishes there were something to do, to read]

Objective

Current setting does not allow engagement in activities

Desired Outcomes/Evaluation Criteria—Client Will:

- Recognize own psychological response (e.g., hopelessness and helplessness, anger, depression) and initiate appropriate coping actions.
- Engage in satisfying activities within personal limitations.

Actions/Interventions

Nursing Priority No. 1.

To assess precipitating/etiological factors:

- Assess client's physical, cognitive, emotional, and environmental status. **Validates the reality of environmental dep-**

Information that appears in brackets has been added by the authors to clarify and enhance the use of nursing diagnoses.

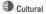

rivation when it exists or considers potential for loss of desired diversional activities in order to plan for prevention or early interventions. Note: Studies show that key problems faced by clients who are hospitalized (or immobilized) for extended periods of time include boredom, stress, and depression. These negative states can impede recovery and lead clients to report symptoms more frequently.

- Note impact of disability or illness on lifestyle (e.g., young child with leukemia, elderly person with fractured hip, individual with severe depression). **This provides a comparative baseline for assessments and interventions.**
- Note age and developmental level, gender, cultural factors, and the importance of a given activity in the client's life. **Cultural issues include gender roles, communication styles, privacy and personal space, expectations and views regarding time and activities, control of the immediate environment family traditions, and social patterns. When illness interferes with an individual's ability to engage in usual activities, the person may have difficulty engaging in meaningful substitute activities.**
- Determine the client's actual ability to participate and interest in available activities, noting attention span, physical limitations and tolerance, level of interest or desire, and safety needs. **The presence of acute illness, depression, problems of mobility, protective isolation, or sensory deprivation may interfere with desired activity.**

Nursing Priority No. 2.

To motivate and stimulate client involvement in solutions:

- Institute and continue appropriate actions to deal with concomitant conditions such as anxiety, depression, grief, dementia, physical injury, isolation and immobility, malnutrition, or acute or chronic pain. **These interfere with the individual's ability to engage in meaningful diversional activities.**
- Acknowledge the reality of the situation and feelings of the client **to establish therapeutic relationship and support hopeful emotions.**
- Review history of lifelong activities and hobbies client has enjoyed. Discuss reasons the client is not doing these activities now and determine whether the client can and would like to resume these activities.
- Encourage a mix of desired activities and stimuli (e.g., music, news, educational presentations—TV/tapes, movies, com-

Information that appears in brackets has been added by the authors to clarify and enhance the use of nursing diagnoses.

puter or Internet access, books and other reading materials, visitors, games, arts and crafts, sensory enrichment [e.g., massage, aromatherapy], grooming and beauty care, cooking, social outings, gardening, or discussion groups, as appropriate). **Activities need to be personally meaningful and not physically or emotionally overwhelming for the client to derive the most benefit.**

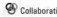

- Participate in decisions about timing and spacing of visitors, leisure, and care activities **to promote relaxation and reduce sense of boredom, as well as to prevent overstimulation and exhaustion.**
- Encourage the client to assist in scheduling required and optional activity choices (e.g., if client's favorite TV show occurs at bath time, reschedule the bath for a later time), **enhancing client's sense of control.**
- Refrain from making changes in the schedule without discussing with the client. **It is important for staff to be responsible in making and following through on commitments to client.**
- Provide a change of scenery (indoors and outdoors where possible) to **provide positive sensory stimulation, reduce sense of boredom, and improve sense of normalcy and control.**
- Identify requirements for mobility (wheelchair, walker, van, volunteers, etc.) **to make it possible for the individual to participate safely in desired activities.**
- Provide for periodic changes in the personal environment when the client is confined. Use the individual's input in creating the changes (e.g., seasonal bulletin boards, color changes, rearranging furniture, or pictures).
- Suggest activities, such as bird feeders or baths for bird watching, a garden in a window box or terrarium, or a fish bowl or aquarium **to stimulate observation as well as involvement and participation in activity, such as identification of birds, choice of seeds, and so forth.**
- Accept hostile expressions while limiting aggressive acting-out behavior. **Permission to express feelings of anger and hopelessness allows for beginning resolution. However, destructive behavior is counterproductive to self-esteem and problem-solving.**
- Involve recreational, occupational, play, music, and/or movement therapist as appropriate **to help identify enjoyable activities for client; procure assistive devices and/or modify activities for individual situation.**

Nursing Priority No. 3.

To promote wellness (Teaching/Discharge Considerations):

Information that appears in brackets has been added by the authors to clarify and enhance the use of nursing diagnoses.

- Explore options for useful activities using the person's strengths and abilities.
- Make appropriate referrals to available support groups, hobby clubs, or service organizations.
- Refer to NDs ineffective Coping; Hopelessness; Powerlessness; Social Isolation.

Documentation Focus

Assessment/Reassessment

- Specific assessment findings, including blocks to desired activities
- Individual choices for activities

Planning

- Plan of care, specific interventions, and who is involved in planning

Implementation/Evaluation

- Client's responses to interventions, teaching, and actions performed
- Attainment or progress toward desired outcome(s)
- Modifications to plan of care

Discharge Planning

- Long-term needs and who is responsible for actions to be taken
- Referrals and community resources

Sample Nursing Outcomes & Interventions Classifications (NOC/NIC)

NOC—Leisure Participation
NIC—Recreation Therapy

risk for DRY EYE

[Diagnostic Division: Safety]

Definition: Vulnerable to eye discomfort or damage to the cornea and conjunctiva due to reduced quantity or quality of tears to moisten the eye, which may compromise health.

Information that appears in brackets has been added by the authors to clarify and enhance the use of nursing diagnoses.

Risk Factors

Aging; female gender; hormonal change; vitamin A deficiency
Autoimmune disease (e.g., rheumatoid arthritis, diabetes mellitus); history of allergy
Contact lens wearer; ocular surface damage
Environmental factor (e.g., air conditioning, excessive wind, sunlight exposure, air pollution, low humidity)
Lifestyle choice (e.g., smoking, caffeine use, prolonged reading/[computer use])
Neurological lesion with sensory or motor reflex loss (e.g., lagophthalmos, lack of spontaneous blink reflex)
Treatment regimen; mechanical ventilation

> **NOTE:** A risk diagnosis is not evidenced by signs and symptoms, as the problem has not occurred; rather, nursing interventions are directed at prevention.

Desired Outcomes/Evaluation Criteria–Client Will:

- Be free of discomfort or damage to eye related to dryness.
- Verbalize understanding of risk factors and ways to prevent dry eye.

Actions/Interventions

Nursing Priority No. 1.

To identify causative/precipitating factors related to risk:

- Obtain a history of eye conditions when assessing client concerns overall. Note reports of dry sensation, burning, itching, pain, foreign body sensation, light sensitivity (photophobia), and blurred vision. **These symptoms can be associated with dry eye syndrome and, if present, require further evaluation and possible treatment.**
- Note the presence of conditions listed in risk factors above **to identify client with possible dry eye syndrome. Dry eye is most commonly caused by insufficient aqueous tear production. This can occur because of damage to the eye surface (e.g., chemical burn) or may be associated with disease conditions, neurological disorders, or environmental factors.**
- ∞ Note the client's gender and age. **Studies show a higher prevalence of dry eye syndrome in females than in males, especially aged over 50.**

Information that appears in brackets has been added by the authors to clarify and enhance the use of nursing diagnoses.

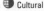

- Determine the client's current situation (e.g., admitted to facility for procedures/surgery, recent neurological event, mechanical ventilation, facial or eye trauma; eye infections, lower eyelid malposition) **that places the client at high risk for dry eye associated with low or absent blink reflex and/or decreased tear production.**
- Determine the client's history/presence of seasonal or environmental allergies, **which may cause or exacerbate conjunctivitis.**
- Review living and work environments to identify factors (e.g., exposure to smoke, wind, or chemicals; poor lighting; long periods of computer use or eye-straining work).
- Assess the client's medications, noting the use of certain drugs (e.g., antihistamines, beta blockers, antidepressants, and oral contraceptives) **known to decrease tear production.**
- Refer for diagnostic evaluation and interventions as indicated.

Nursing Priority No. 2.

To promote eye health/comfort:

- Assist in/refer for treatment of underlying cause of dry eyes. **Interventions could range from changing a medication that's causing decreased tear production to surgery to correct an anatomic abnormality of the eyelid that interferes with blinking. Or referral may be needed (e.g., to rheumatologist or endocrinologist for treatment of autoimmune condition or diabetes).**
- Administer artificial tears, lubricating eyedrops, or ointments as indicated, **when the client is unable to blink or otherwise protect eyes while in healthcare facility.**

Nursing Priority No. 3.

To promote wellness (Teaching/Discharge Criteria):

- Instruct high-risk client in self-management interventions **to prevent or limit symptoms of dry eye:**

  Avoid air blowing in eyes **such as might occur with hair dryers, car heaters, air conditioners, or fans directed toward eyes.**

  Wear eyeglasses or safety shield glasses on windy days **to reduce effects of the wind** and goggles while swimming **to protect eyes from chemicals in the water.**

  Take proper care of contact lenses and adhere to prescribed wearing time.

  Add moisture to indoor air, especially in winter.

  Take eye breaks during long reading and computer tasks or when watching TV for long periods of time.

Information that appears in brackets has been added by the authors to clarify and enhance the use of nursing diagnoses.

Blink repeatedly for a few seconds **to help spread tears evenly over eye.**
Position computer screen below eye level. **This may help slow the evaporation of tears between eye blinks.**
Stop smoking and avoid smoking environments. **Smoke can worsen dry eye symptoms.**

Documentation Focus

Assessment/Reassessment

- Individual risk factors identified
- Client concerns or difficulty making and following through with plan

Planning

- Plan of care and who is involved in planning
- Teaching plan

Implementation/Evaluation

- Response to interventions, teaching, and actions performed
- Attainment or progress toward outcomes

Discharge Planning

- Referrals to other resources
- Long-term need and who is responsible for actions

Sample Nursing Outcomes & Interventions Classifications (NOC/NIC)

NOC—Risk Control
NIC—Eye Care

risk for peripheral neurovascular DYSFUNCTION

[Diagnostic Division: Neurosensory]

Definition: Vulnerable to disruption in the circulation, sensation, and motion of an extremity, which may compromise health.

Risk Factors

Burns; trauma; vascular obstruction
Fracture; immobilization; orthopedic surgery
Mechanical compression (e.g., tourniquet, cane, cast, brace, dressing, restraint)

Information that appears in brackets has been added by the authors to clarify and enhance the use of nursing diagnoses.

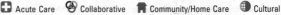

 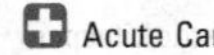 Acute Care 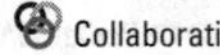 Collaborative 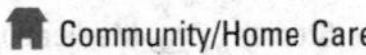 Community/Home Care 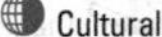 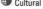 Cultural

NOTE: A risk diagnosis is not evidenced by signs and symptoms, as the problem has not occurred; rather, nursing interventions are directed at prevention.

Desired Outcomes/Evaluation Criteria—Client Will:

- Maintain function as evidenced by sensation and movement within normal range for the individual.
- Develop plan to address individual risk factors.
- Demonstrate and participate in behaviors and activities to prevent complications.
- Relate signs/symptoms that require medical reevaluation.

Actions/Interventions

Nursing Priority No. 1.

To determine significance/degree of potential for compromise:

- Assess for individual risk factors: (1) trauma to extremity(ies) that causes internal tissue damage (e.g., high-velocity and penetrating trauma); fractures (especially long-bone fractures) with hemorrhage, or external pressures from burn eschar; (2) immobility (e.g., long-term bedrest, tight dressings, splints, or casting); (3) presence of conditions affecting peripheral circulation, such as atherosclerosis, Raynaud's disease, or diabetes; (4) smoking, obesity, and sedentary lifestyle; and (5) presence of conditions affecting peripheral circulation, such as atherosclerosis, cardiovascular or cerebrovascular disease; diabetes, sickle cell disease, deep vein thrombosis (DVT), coagulation disorders, or use of anticoagulants, **which potentiate risk of circulation insufficiency and occlusion.**
- Monitor for tissue bleeding and spread of hematoma formation, **which can compress blood vessels and raise compartment pressures.**
- Note position and location of casts, braces, and traction apparatus **to ascertain potential for pressure on tissues.**
- Review recent and current drug regimen, noting the use of anticoagulants and vasoactive agents.

Nursing Priority No. 2.

To prevent deterioration/maximize circulation of affected limb(s):

- Conduct a comprehensive upper or lower extremity assessment in at-risk client, including color, sensation, and func-

Information that appears in brackets has been added by the authors to clarify and enhance the use of nursing diagnoses.

tional ability. **Early detection of circulatory issues may prevent the onset or severity of functional impairments associated with arterial or venous disorders of the extremities.**

- Perform neurovascular assessment in a person immobilized for any reason (e.g., surgery, diabetic neuropathy, or fractures) or individuals with suspected neurovascular problems. **This provides a baseline for future comparisons.**
- Evaluate for differences between affected extremity and unaffected extremity, noting pain, pulses, pallor, paresthesia, paralysis, and changes in motor and sensory function.
- Ask the client to localize pain or discomfort and to report numbness and tingling or presence of pain with exercise or rest (atherosclerotic changes). (Refer to ND ineffective peripheral Tissue Perfusion, as appropriate.)
- Monitor the presence and quality of peripheral pulse distal to injury or impairment via palpation or Doppler. **An intact pulse usually indicates adequate circulation. Occasionally, a pulse may be palpated even though circulation is blocked by a soft clot through which pulsations may be felt; or perfusion through larger arteries may continue after increased compartment pressure has collapsed the arteriole/venule circulation in the muscle.**
- Assess capillary return, skin color, and warmth in the limb(s) at risk and compare with unaffected extremities. **Pallor with cool, shiny, taut skin and slow venous refill is indicative of circulatory impairment. Cold, pale, bluish color with purpura indicates arterial insufficiency.**
- Test sensation of peroneal nerve by pinch or pinprick in the dorsal web between first and second toe, and assess the ability to dorsiflex toes if indicated (e.g., presence of leg fracture). **Changes in sensation cover a wide continuum and may include feeling of tingling, numbness, "pins and needles," burning, or diminished or absent sensation. Changes that might not be apparent to the client could include loss of protective sensation in feet as determined by screening with tuning fork or percussion hammer.**
- Evaluate extremity range of motion. **Movement may be limited or absent because of tissue edema and nerve compression or because of nerve impingement such as would occur with spinal nerve compression.**
- Monitor for tissue edema and/or tightness. **Swelling or tightness may indicate obstruction, such as might occur with DVT, or compartment syndrome.**

Information that appears in brackets has been added by the authors to clarify and enhance the use of nursing diagnoses.

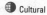

- Collaborate in interventions to minimize edema formation and elevated tissue pressure:

  Maintain elevation of injured extremity(ies).

  Apply cold packs around injury/fracture site as indicated.

  Remove jewelry from affected limb.

  Avoid or limit use of restraints. Pad limb and evaluate status frequently if restraints are required.

  Observe position and location of supporting ring of orthopedic splints or sling. Readjust, as indicated.

- Maximize circulation:

  Use techniques such as repositioning and padding **to relieve pressure.**

  Encourage client to routinely exercise digits or joints distal to injury.

  Encourage ambulation as soon as possible.

  Apply antiembolic hose or sequential pressure device, as indicated.

  Administer intravenous fluids, blood products, as needed, **to maintain circulating volume and tissue perfusion.**

  Administer anticoagulants or antithrombic agents, as indicated, **to prevent DVT or treat thrombotic vascular obstructions.**

  Split or bivalve cast, or reposition traction or restraints, as appropriate, **to quickly release pressure.**

  Prepare for surgical intervention (e.g., fibulectomy or fasciotomy), as indicated, **to relieve pressure and restore circulation.**

- Monitor for development of complications:

  Inspect tissues around cast edges for rough places, and pressure points. Investigate reports of "burning sensation" under cast.

  Evaluate for tenderness, swelling, and pain on dorsiflexion of foot (positive Homans' sign).

  Monitor hemoglobin/hematocrit, coagulation studies (e.g., prothrombin time).

  Investigate sudden signs of limb ischemia (e.g., decreased skin temperature, pallor, or increased pain), reports of pain that are extreme for type of injury, increased pain on passive movement of extremity, development of paresthesia, muscle tension or tenderness with erythema, or change in pulse quality distal to injury. Place the limb in a neutral position, avoiding elevation. Report symptoms to physician at once **to provide for timely intervention/limit severity of problem.**

Information that appears in brackets has been added by the authors to clarify and enhance the use of nursing diagnoses.

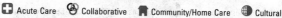

- Assist with measurements of intracompartmental pressures, as indicated. **This provides for early intervention and evaluates the effectiveness of therapy.**

Nursing Priority No. 3.

To promote wellness (Teaching/Discharge Considerations):

- Review proper body alignment, elevation of limbs, as appropriate.
- Keep linens off affected extremity with bed cradle or cut-out box, as indicated.
- Discuss necessity of avoiding constrictive clothing, sharp angulation of legs or crossing legs.
- Demonstrate proper application of antiembolic hose.
- Review safe use of heat or cold therapy, as indicated.
- Instruct client/SO(s) to check shoes and socks for proper fit and/or wrinkles.
- Demonstrate and recommend continuation of exercises **to maintain function and circulation of limbs.**

Documentation Focus

Assessment/Reassessment

- Specific risk factors, nature of injury to limb
- Assessment findings, including comparison of affected and unaffected limb, characteristics of pain in involved area

Planning

- Plan of care and who is involved in the planning
- Teaching plan

Implementation/Evaluation

- Response to interventions, teaching, and actions performed
- Attainment or progress toward desired outcome(s)
- Modification of plan of care

Discharge Planning

- Long-term needs, referrals made, and who is responsible for actions to be taken
- Specific referrals made

Sample Nursing Outcomes & Interventions Classifications (NOC/NIC)

NOC—Neurological Status: Peripheral
NIC—Peripheral Sensation Management

Information that appears in brackets has been added by the authors to clarify and enhance the use of nursing diagnoses.

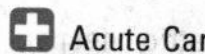

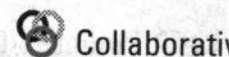

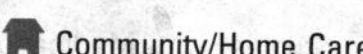

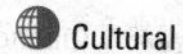

risk for ELECTROLYTE IMBALANCE

[Diagnostic Division: Food/Fluid]

Definition: Vulnerable to changes in serum electrolyte levels that may compromise health.

Risk Factors

Insufficient fluid volume; diarrhea; vomiting
Excessive fluid volume
Endocrine regulatory dysfunction (e.g., glucose intolerance, increase in IGF-1, androgen, DHEA, and cortisol); renal dysfunction
Compromised regulatory mechanisms [e.g., diabetes insipidus, syndrome of inappropriate secretion of antidiuretic hormone]
Treatment regimen

NOTE: A risk diagnosis is not evidenced by signs and symptoms, as the problem has not occurred; rather, nursing interventions are directed at prevention.

Desired Outcomes/Evaluation Criteria—Client Will:

- Display laboratory results within normal range for individual.
- Be free of complications resulting from electrolyte imbalance.
- Identify individual risks and engage in appropriate behaviors or lifestyle changes to prevent or reduce frequency of electrolyte imbalances.

Actions/Interventions

Nursing Priority No. 1.

To assess causative/contributing factors:

- Identify the client with current or newly diagnosed condition commonly associated with electrolyte imbalances, such as inability to eat or drink, febrile illness, active bleeding or other fluid loss, including vomiting, diarrhea, gastrointestinal drainage, or burns.
- Assess specific client risk, noting chronic disease processes that may lead to electrolyte imbalances, including kidney dis-

Information that appears in brackets has been added by the authors to clarify and enhance the use of nursing diagnoses.

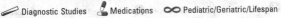

ease, metabolic or endocrine disorders, chronic alcoholism, cancer or cancer treatments, conditions causing hemolysis such as massive trauma, multiple blood transfusions, and sickle cell disease.

- Note the client's age and developmental level, which may increase the risk for electrolyte imbalance. **This risk group can include the very young or premature infant, the elderly, or individuals unable to meet their own needs or monitor their health status, including clients who are unconscious for an unknown cause or period of time, a trauma victim, and so on.**
- Review the client's medications **for those associated with electrolyte imbalance. Note: There are many, including (and not limited to) diuretics, laxatives, corticosteroids, barbiturates, certain antidepressants (e.g., SSRIs), antihypertensive agents, antiepileptics, some hormones/birth control pills, some antibiotics, and antifungal agents.**

Nursing Priority No. 2.

To identify potential electrolyte deficit:

- Assess mental status, noting client/caregiver report of change—altered attention span, recall of recent events, and other cognitive functions. **This can be associated with electrolyte imbalance; for example, it is the most common sign associated with sodium imbalances.**
- Monitor heart rate and rhythm by palpation and auscultation. **Tachycardia, bradycardia, and other dysrhythmias are associated with potassium, calcium, and magnesium imbalances.**
- Auscultate breath sounds, assess rate and depth of respirations and ease of respiratory effort, observe color of nailbeds and mucous membranes, and note pulse oximetry or blood gas measurement, as indicated. **Certain electrolyte imbalances, such as hypokalemia, can cause or exacerbate respiratory insufficiency.**
- Review the electrocardiogram (ECG). **Because the ECG reflects electrophysiological, anatomical, metabolic, and hemodynamic alterations, it is routinely used for the diagnosis of electrolyte and metabolic disturbances, as well as myocardial ischemia, cardiac dysrhythmias, structural changes of the myocardium, and drug effects.**
- Assess gastrointestinal symptoms, noting presence, absence, and character of bowel sounds; presence of acute or chronic diarrhea; and persistent vomiting, high nasogastric tube out-

---

Information that appears in brackets has been added by the authors to clarify and enhance the use of nursing diagnoses.

put. **Any disturbance of the gastrointestinal functioning carries with it the potential for electrolyte imbalances.**

- Review the client's food intake. Note the presence of anorexia, vomiting, or recent fad or unusual diet; look for signs of chronic malnutrition. **These conditions can point to potential electrolyte imbalances, either deficiencies or excesses, such as high sodium content.**
- Evaluate motor strength and function, noting steadiness of gait, hand grip strength, and reactivity of reflexes. **These neuromuscular functions can provide clues to electrolyte imbalances, including calcium, magnesium, phosphorus, sodium, and potassium.**
- Assess fluid intake and output. **Many factors, such as inability to drink, diuresis or chronic kidney failure, trauma, and surgery, affect an individual's fluid balance, disrupting electrolyte transport, function, and excretion.**
- Review laboratory results for abnormal findings. **Electrolytes include sodium, potassium, calcium, chloride, bicarbonate (carbon dioxide), and magnesium. These chemicals are essential in many bodily functions including fluid balance, movement of fluid within and between body compartments, nerve conduction, muscle contraction—including the heart, blood clotting, and pH balance. Excitable cells, such as nerve and muscle, are particularly sensitive to electrolyte imbalances.**
- Assess for specific imbalances:

Sodium (Na^+) **This is a dominant extracellular cation and cannot freely cross the cell membrane.**

Review laboratory results—normal range in adults is 135 to 145 mEq/L. **Elevated sodium (hypernatremia) can occur if the client has an overall deficit of total body water owing to inadequate fluid intake or water loss and can be associated with low potassium, metabolic acidosis, and hypoglycemia.**

Monitor for physical or mental disorders impacting fluid intake. **Impaired thirst sensation or an inability to express thirst or obtain needed fluids may lead to hypernatremia.**

Note the presence of medical conditions that may impact sodium level. **Hyponatremia may be associated with disorders such as congestive heart failure, liver and kidney failure, pneumonia, metabolic acidosis, and intestinal conditions resulting in prolonged gastrointestinal suction. Hypernatremia can result from simple conditions**

Information that appears in brackets has been added by the authors to clarify and enhance the use of nursing diagnoses.

such as febrile illness, causing fluid loss and/or restricted fluid intake, or complicated conditions such as kidney and endocrine diseases, affecting sodium intake or excretion.

Note the presence of cognitive dysfunction such as confusion, restlessness, and abnormal speech **which may be a cause or effect of sodium imbalance.**

Assess for orthostatic blood pressure changes, tachycardia, or low urine output, or other clinical findings, such as generalized weakness, swollen tongue, weight loss, and seizures. **These signs suggest hypernatremia.**

Assess for nausea, abdominal cramping, lethargy, and orthostatic blood pressure changes—if fluid volume is also depleted; confusion, decreased level of consciousness, or headache. **These are signs and symptoms suggestive of hyponatremia, which can lead to seizures and a coma if untreated.**

Review drug regimen. **Drugs such as anabolic steroids, angiotensin, cisplatin, and mannitol may increase sodium level. Diuretics, laxatives, theophylline, and triamterine can decrease sodium level.**

Potassium (K^+) **Most abundant intracellular cation, obtained through diet, is excreted via the kidneys.**

Review laboratory results—the normal range in adults is 3.5 to 5 mEq/L.

Note current medical conditions that may impact potassium level. **Metabolic acidosis, burn or crush injuries, massive hemolysis, diabetes, kidney disease/renal failure, cancer, and sickle cell trait are associated with hyperkalemia, fasting, diarrhea or nasogastric suctioning, alkalosis, administration of IV potassium boluses, or transfusions of whole blood or packed red blood cells increases the risk of hypokalemia.**

Identify conditions or situations **that potentiate risk for hyperkalemia, including ingestion of an unusual diet with high-potassium, low-sodium foods or use of potassium supplements, including over-the-counter (OTC) herbals or salt substitutes.**

Monitor ECG, as indicated. **Abnormal potassium levels, both low and high, are associated with changes in the ECG.**

Evaluate reports of abdominal cramping, fatigue, hyperactive bowel motility, muscle twitching, and cramps, followed by muscle weakness. Note the presence of depressed reflexes,

Information that appears in brackets has been added by the authors to clarify and enhance the use of nursing diagnoses.

ascending flaccid paralysis of legs and arms. **These signs/symptoms suggest hyperkalemia.**

Note the presence of weakness and fatigue (most common), anorexia, abdominal distention, diminished bowel sounds, palpitations, postural hypotension, muscle cramps, and pain (severe hypokalemia); also note flaccid paralysis. **These may be manifestations of hypokalemia.**

Review the drug regimen. **Use of potassium-sparing diuretics, other medications, such as nonsteroidal anti-inflammatory agents (NSAIDs), angiotensin-converting enzyme (ACE) inhibitors, angiotensin-receptor blockers (ARBs), heparin, and certain antibiotics such as pentamidine may increase potassium level. Medications such as some COPD medications (e.g., albuterol, terbutaline), steroids, certain antimicrobials (e.g., penicillins, aminoglycosides), laxatives, and some diuretics may cause hypokalemia.**

Calcium (Ca^{2+}) **Most abundant cation in the body, participates in almost all vital processes, working with sodium to regulate depolarization and the generation of action potentials**

Review laboratory results—the normal range for adults is 8.5 to 10.5 mg/dL.

Note the presence of medical conditions impacting calcium level. **Acidosis, Addison's disease, cancers (e.g., bone, lymphoma, and leukemias), hyperparathyroidism, lung disease (e.g., TB, histoplasmosis), thyrotoxicosis, and polycythemia may lead to an increased calcium level. Chronic diarrhea, intestinal disorders such as Crohn's disease; pancreatitis, alcoholism, renal failure, or renal tubular disease; recent orthopedic surgery or bone healing, history of thyroid surgery or irradiation of upper middle chest and neck; and psychosis may result in decreased calcium levels.**

Monitor for excessive urination (polyuria), constipation, lethargy, muscle weakness, anorexia, headache, and coma, **which can be associated with hypercalcemia.**

Monitor for cardiac dysrhythmias, hypotension, and heart failure; muscle cramps, facial spasms—positive Chvostek's sign; numbness and tingling sensations, muscle twitching—positive Trousseau's sign; seizures, or tetany, **which suggest hypocalcemia.**

Review the drug regimen. **Drugs such as anabolic steroids, some antacids, lithium, oral contraceptives, vitamins A**

Information that appears in brackets has been added by the authors to clarify and enhance the use of nursing diagnoses.

and D, and amoxapine, can increase calcium levels. Drugs such as albuterol, glucocorticoids, insulin, phosphates, trazodone, laxative overuse, or long-term anticonvulsant therapy can decrease calcium levels.

Magnesium (Mg^{2+}) **The second most abundant intracellular cation after potassium, magnesium controls absorption or function of sodium, potassium, calcium, and phosphorus.**

Review laboratory results—normal range in adults is 1.5 to 2 mEq/L.

Note the presence of medical conditions impacting magnesium level. **Diabetic acidosis, multiple myeloma, renal insufficiency, eclampsia, asthma, GI hypomotility; adrenal insufficiency, extensive soft tissue injury, severe burns, shock, sepsis, and cardiac arrest are associated with hypermagnesemia. Conditions resulting in decreased intake (starvation, alcoholism, and parenteral feeding), excess gastrointestinal losses (diarrhea, vomiting, nasogastric suction, and malabsorption), renal losses (inherited renal tubular defects among others), or miscellaneous causes (including calcium abnormalities, chronic metabolic acidosis, and diabetic ketoacidosis) can lead to hypomagnesemia.**

Note GI and renal function. **The main controlling factors of magnesium are GI absorption and renal excretion. Low levels of magnesium, potassium, calcium, and phosphorus may be manifest at the same time if absorption is impaired. High levels of magnesium, calcium, phosphate, and potassium often occur together in the setting of kidney disease.**

Monitor for nausea, vomiting, weakness, and vasodilation, **which suggest a mild to moderate elevation of magnesium level (from 3.5 to 5 mEq/L).**

Monitor ECG, as indicated. **The presence of heart blocks, especially if accompanied by ventilatory failure and stupor, suggests severe hypermagnesemia (more than 10 mEq/L). Hypomagnesemia can lead to potentially fatal ventricular dysrhythmias, coronary artery vasospasm, and sudden death.**

Review the drug regimen. **Drugs such as aspirin and progesterone may increase magnesium level; albuterol, digoxin, diuretics, oral contraceptives, aminoglycosides, proton-pump inhibitors, immunosuppressants, cisplatin, and cyclosporines are some of the medications that may decrease magnesium levels.**

Information that appears in brackets has been added by the authors to clarify and enhance the use of nursing diagnoses.

Nursing Priority No. 3.

To prevent imbalances:

- Collaborate in the treatment of underlying conditions **to prevent or limit effects of electrolyte imbalances caused by disease or organ dysfunction.**
- Observe and intervene with elderly hospitalized person on admission and during facility stay. **Elderly are more prone to electrolyte imbalances related to fluid imbalances, use of multiple medications including diuretics, heart and blood pressure medications, lack of appetite or interest in eating or drinking; or lack of appropriate dietary and/or medication supervision.**
- Provide or recommend balanced nutrition, using the best route for feeding. Monitor intake, weight, and bowel function. **Obtaining and utilizing electrolytes and other minerals depends on the client regularly receiving them in a readily available form, including food and supplements via ingestion, enteral, or parenteral routes.**
- Measure and report all fluid losses, including emesis, diarrhea, wound, or fistula drainage. **Loss of fluids rich in electrolytes can lead to imbalances.**
- Maintain fluid balance **to prevent dehydration and shifts of electrolytes.**
- Use pump or controller device when administering IV electrolyte solutions **to provide medication at desired rate and prevent untoward effects of excessive or too rapid delivery.**

Nursing Priority No. 4.

To promote wellness (Teaching/Discharge Considerations):

- Discuss ongoing concerns for the client with chronic health problems, such as kidney disease, diabetes, or cancer; individuals taking multiple medications; and/or client deciding to take medications or drugs differently than prescribed. **Early intervention can help prevent serious complications.**
- Consult with dietitian or nutritionist for specific teaching needs. **Learning how to incorporate foods that increase electrolyte intake or identifying food or condiment alternatives increases client's self-sufficiency and likelihood of success.**
- Review the client's medications at each visit **for possible change in dosage or drug choice based on the client's response, change in condition, or development of side effects.**
- Discuss medications with primary care provider **to determine if different pharmaceutical intervention is appropriate.**

Information that appears in brackets has been added by the authors to clarify and enhance the use of nursing diagnoses.

For example, changing to potassium-sparing diuretic or withholding a diuretic may correct imbalance.

- Teach the client/caregiver to take or administer drugs as prescribed—especially diuretics, antihypertensives, and cardiac drugs **to reduce the potential of complications associated with medication-induced electrolyte imbalances.**
- Instruct the client/caregiver in reportable symptoms. **For example, a sudden change in mentation or behavior 2 days after starting a new diuretic could indicate hyponatremia, or an elderly person taking digitalis (for atrial fibrillation) and a diuretic may be hypokalemic.**
- Provide information regarding calcium supplements, as indicated. **It is popular wisdom to instruct people, women in particular, to take calcium for prevention of osteoporosis. However, calcium absorption cannot take place without vitamins D and K and magnesium. A client taking calcium may need additional information or resources.**

Documentation Focus

Assessment/Reassessment

- Identified or potential risk factors for individual
- Assessment findings, including vital signs, mentation, muscle strength and reflexes, presence of fatigue, respiratory distress
- Results of laboratory tests and diagnostic studies

Planning

- Plan of care, specific interventions, and who is involved in the planning
- Teaching plan

Implementation/Evaluation

- Client's responses to treatment, teaching, and actions performed
- Attainment or progress toward desired outcome(s)
- Modifications to plan of care

Discharge Planning

- Long-term needs, identifying who is responsible for actions to be taken
- Specific referrals made

Sample Nursing Outcomes & Interventions Classifications (NOC/NIC)

NOC—Electrolyte and Acid/Base Balance
NIC—Electrolyte Monitoring

Information that appears in brackets has been added by the authors to clarify and enhance the use of nursing diagnoses.

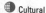

impaired urinary ELIMINATION

[Diagnostic Division: Elimination]

Definition: Dysfunction in urine elimination.

Related Factors

Multiple causality; sensory motor impairment; anatomic obstruction; urinary tract infection; [fluid/volume states; psychogenetic factors; surgical diversion]

Defining Characteristics

Subjective

Frequent voiding; urinary urgency
Hesitancy
Dysuria
Nocturia; [enuresis]

Objective

Urinary incontinence
Urinary retention

Desired Outcomes/Evaluation Criteria—Client Will:

- Verbalize understanding of condition.
- Identify specific causative factors.
- Achieve normal elimination pattern or participate in measures to correct or compensate for defects.
- Demonstrate behaviors and techniques to prevent urinary infection.
- Manage care of urinary catheter, or stoma, and appliance following urinary diversion.

Actions/Interventions

Nursing Priority No. 1.

To assess causative/contributing factors:

- Identify conditions that may be present, such as urinary tract infection, interstitial cystitis or painful bladder syndrome; dehydration; surgery (including urinary diversion); neurological involvement (e.g., multiple sclerosis [MS], stroke, Parkinson's disease, paraplegia/tetraplegia); mental or emotional

Information that appears in brackets has been added by the authors to clarify and enhance the use of nursing diagnoses.

dysfunction (e.g., impaired cognition, delirium or confusion, depression, Alzheimer's disease); prostate disorders; recent or multiple pregnancies; and pelvic trauma.

- Determine pathology of bladder dysfunction relative to medical diagnosis identified. **This identifies direction for further evaluation and treatment options to discover specifics of individual situation. For example, in neurological or demyelinating diseases such as MS, the problem may be related to the inability to store urine, empty the bladder, or both.**
- Assist with physical examination (e.g., cough test for incontinence, palpation for bladder retention or masses, prostate size, and observation for urethral stricture).
- Note age and gender of client. **Incontinence and urinary tract infections are more prevalent in women and older adults; painful bladder syndrome (PBS) or interstitial cystitis (IC) is more common in women.**
- Investigate pain, noting location, duration, intensity; presence of bladder spasms; or back or flank pain **to assist in differentiating between bladder and kidney as cause of dysfunction.**
- Have the client complete the Pelvic Pain and Urgency/Frequency (PUF) patient symptom survey, as indicated. **This helps in evaluating the presence and severity of PBS/IC symptoms.**
- Note reports of exacerbations and spontaneous remissions of symptoms of urgency and frequency, which may or may not be accompanied by pain, pressure, or spasm.
- Determine the client's usual daily fluid intake (both amount and beverage choices, use of caffeine). Note the condition of skin and mucous membranes and the color of urine **to help determine level of hydration.**
- Review medication regimen **for drugs that can alter bladder or kidney function (e.g., antihypertensive agents such as angiotensin-converting enzyme [ACE] inhibitors, beta-adrenergic blockers; anticholinergics, antihistamines; antiparkinsonian drugs; antidepressants or antipsychotics; sedatives, hypnotics, opioids; caffeine and alcohol).**
- Send urine specimen (midstream clean-voided or catheterized) for culture and sensitivities in the presence of signs of urinary tract infection—cloudy, foul odor; bloody urine.
- Rule out gonorrhea in men when urethritis with a penile discharge is present and there are no bacteria in the urine.
- Obtain specimen for antibody-coated bacteria assay **to diagnose bacterial infection of the kidney or prostate.**

Information that appears in brackets has been added by the authors to clarify and enhance the use of nursing diagnoses.

- Assist with potassium sensitivity test (instillation of potassium solution into bladder), as appropriate. **Eighty percent of patients with PBS/IC will react positively with painful symptoms.**
- Review laboratory tests for hyperglycemia, hyperparathyroidism, or other metabolic conditions; changes in renal function; culture for presence of infection or sexually transmitted infections (STIs); urine cytology for cancer.
- Review results of diagnostic studies (e.g., uroflowmetry; cystometrogram; postvoid residual ultrasound (bladder scan); pressure flow and leak point pressure measurement; videourodynamics; electromyography; kidney, ureter, and bladder [KUB] imaging) **to identify presence and type of elimination problem.**

Nursing Priority No. 2.

To assess degree of interference/disability:

- Ascertain the client's previous pattern of elimination **for comparison with current situation.** Note reports of problems (e.g., frequency, urgency, painful urination; leaking or incontinence; changes in size and force of urinary stream; problems emptying bladder completely; nocturia or enuresis).
- Ascertain the client's/SO's perception of problem and degree of disability (e.g., client is restricting social, employment, or travel activities; having sexual or relationship difficulties; incurring sleep deprivation; experiencing depression).
- Note influence of culture/ethnicity or gender on client's view of problems of incontinence. **Limited evidence exists to understand and help people cope with the physical and psychosocial consequences of this chronic, socially isolating, and potentially devastating disorder.**
- Have the client keep a voiding diary for a prescribed number of days to record fluid intake, voiding times, precise urine output, and dietary intake. **This helps determine baseline symptoms, severity of frequency or urgency, and whether diet is a factor (if symptoms worsen).**

Nursing Priority No. 3.

To assist in treating/preventing urinary alteration:

- Refer to specific NDs urinary Incontinence [specify]; Urinary Retention, for additional related interventions.
- Encourage fluid intake up to 1,500–2,000 mL/day (within cardiac tolerance), including cranberry juice, **to help maintain renal function, prevent infection and formation of uri-**

Information that appears in brackets has been added by the authors to clarify and enhance the use of nursing diagnoses.

nary stones, avoid encrustation around catheter, or flush urinary diversion appliance.

- Discuss possible dietary restrictions (e.g., especially coffee, alcohol, carbonated drinks, citrus, tomatoes, and chocolate) based on individual symptoms.
- Assist with developing toileting routines (e.g., timed voiding, bladder training, prompted voiding, habit retraining), as appropriate. **For adults who are cognitively intact and physically capable of self-toileting, bladder training, timed voiding, and habit retraining may be beneficial.**
- Encourage the client to verbalize fears and concerns (e.g., disruption in sexual activity or inability to work). **Open expression allows the client to deal with feelings and begin problem-solving.**
- Implement and monitor interventions for specific elimination problem (e.g., pelvic floor exercises or other bladder retraining modalities; medication regimen, including antimicrobials [single dose is frequently being used for UTI], sulfonamides, antispasmodics); and evaluate client's response **to modify treatment, as needed.**
- Discuss possible surgical procedures and medical regimen, as indicated (e.g., client with benign prostatic hypertrophy bladder or prostatic cancer, PBS/IC). **For example, cystoscopy with bladder hydrodistention may be used for PBS/IC, or an electrical stimulator may be implanted to treat chronic urinary urge incontinence, nonobstructive urinary retention, and symptoms of urgency and frequency.**

Nursing Priority No. 4.

To assist in management of long-term urinary alterations:

- Keep bladder deflated by use of an indwelling catheter connected to closed drainage. Investigate alternatives when possible. **Measures such as intermittent catheterization, surgical interventions, urinary drugs, voiding maneuvers, condom catheter may be preferable to the indwelling catheter to provide more effective control and prevent the possibility of recurrent infections.**
- Provide latex-free catheter and care supplies. **This reduces the risk of developing sensitivity to latex, which can develop in individuals requiring frequent catheterization or who have long-term indwelling catheters.**
- Check frequently for bladder distention and observe for overflow **to reduce the risk of infection and/or autonomic hyperreflexia.**

Information that appears in brackets has been added by the authors to clarify and enhance the use of nursing diagnoses.

- Adhere to a regular bladder or diversion appliance emptying schedule **to avoid accidents.**
- Provide for routine diversion appliance care and assist the client to recognize and deal with problems, such as alkaline salt encrustation, ill-fitting appliance, malodorous urine, and infection.

Nursing Priority No. 5.

To promote wellness (Teaching/Discharge Considerations):

- Emphasize the importance of keeping the area clean and dry **to reduce the risk of infection and/or skin breakdown.**
- Instruct female clients with UTI to drink large amounts of fluid, void immediately after intercourse, wipe from front to back, promptly treat vaginal infections, and take showers rather than tub baths **to limit risk or avoid reinfection.**
- Recommend smoking cessation program, as appropriate. **Cigarette smoking can be a source of bladder irritation.**
- Encourage SO(s) who participate in routine care to recognize complications (including latex allergy) necessitating medical evaluation or intervention.
- Instruct in proper application and care of appliance for urinary diversion. Encourage liberal fluid intake, avoidance of foods or medications that produce strong odor, use of white vinegar or deodorizer in pouch **to promote odor control.**
- Identify sources for supplies and programs or agencies providing financial assistance. **Lack of access to necessities can be a barrier to management of incontinence, and having help to obtain needed equipment can assist with daily care.**
- Recommend avoidance of gas-forming foods in the presence of ureterosigmoidostomy **as flatus can cause urinary incontinence.**
- Recommend use of silicone catheter. **Although these catheters are more expensive than rubber catheters, they are more comfortable and generally cause fewer problems with infection when permanent or long-term catheterization is required.**
- Demonstrate proper positioning of catheter drainage tubing and bag **to facilitate drainage and prevent reflux.**
- Refer client/SO(s) to appropriate community resources, such as ostomy specialist, support group, sex therapist, or psychiatric clinical nurse specialist, **to deal with changes in body image and function, when indicated.**

Information that appears in brackets has been added by the authors to clarify and enhance the use of nursing diagnoses.

Documentation Focus

Assessment/Reassessment

- Individual findings, including previous and current pattern of voiding, nature of problem, and effect on desired lifestyle
- Cultural factors or concerns

Planning

- Plan of care and who is involved in planning
- Teaching plan

Implementation/Evaluation

- Response to interventions, teaching, and actions performed
- Attainment or progress toward desired outcome(s)
- Modifications to plan of care

Discharge Planning

- Long-term needs and who is responsible for actions to be taken
- Available resources and specific referrals made
- Individual equipment needs and sources

Sample Nursing Outcomes & Interventions Classifications (NOC/NIC)

NOC—Urinary Elimination
NIC—Urinary Elimination Management

readiness for enhanced urinary ELIMINATION

[Diagnostic Division: Elimination]

Definition: A pattern of urinary functions for meeting eliminatory needs, which can be strengthened.

Defining Characteristics

Subjective

Expresses desire to enhance urinary elimination

Desired Outcomes/Evaluation Criteria—Client Will:

- Verbalize understanding of condition that has potential for altering elimination.

Information that appears in brackets has been added by the authors to clarify and enhance the use of nursing diagnoses.

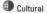

- Maintain normal or acceptable elimination pattern emptying bladder, voiding in appropriate amounts.
- Alter lifestyle or environment to accommodate individual needs.

Actions/Interventions

Nursing Priority No. 1.

To assess status and adaptive skills being used by client:

- Identify physical conditions (e.g., surgery, childbirth, recent or multiple pregnancies, pelvic trauma, neurogenic bladder from central nervous system disorders or neuropathies [such as stroke, spinal cord injury, diabetes], prostate disease or surgery, mental or emotional dysfunction) **that can impact the client's elimination patterns.**
- Determine the client's usual pattern of elimination and compare with the current situation **to determine the client's readiness for improving elimination patterns and/or how pattern can be improved.** Review voiding diary, if indicated. **This provides the baseline for future comparison.**
- Observe voiding patterns, time, color, and amount voided, if indicated (e.g., postsurgical or postpartum client) **to document normalization of elimination.**
- Ascertain methods of self-management (e.g., limiting or increasing liquid intake, acting on urge in timely manner, established voiding schedule, regularly spaced catheterization) **to identify strengths and areas of concern in elimination management.**
- Determine client's usual daily fluid intake. **Amount and timing of fluid intake, as well as beverage choices, are important in managing elimination.**

Nursing Priority No. 2.

To assist client to improve management of urinary elimination:

- Encourage fluid intake, including water and cranberry juice, **to help maintain renal function and prevent infection.**
- Regulate liquid intake at prescheduled times **to promote a predictable voiding pattern.**
- Restrict fluid intake 2 to 3 hours before bedtime, if indicated, **to reduce voiding during the night.**
- Assist with modifying current routines, as appropriate. **The client may benefit from additional information in enhancing success, such as responding to cues or urge to void, adjusting schedule of voiding or catheterization (shorter or longer), relaxation and/or distraction techniques,**

Information that appears in brackets has been added by the authors to clarify and enhance the use of nursing diagnoses.

standing or sitting upright during voiding to ensure that bladder is completely empty, and/or practicing pelvic muscle strengthening exercises.

- Provide assistance or devices, as indicated (e.g., providing means of summoning assistance; placing bedside commode, urinal, or bedpan within client's reach; using elevated toilet seats; mobility devices) **when client is frail or mobility is impaired.**
- Modify or recommend diet changes, if indicated, **such as limiting caffeine intake because of its bladder irritant effect or weight loss to reduce overactive bladder symptoms and incontinence by decreasing pressure on the bladder.**
- Modify medication regimens, as appropriate (e.g., administer prescribed diuretics in the morning **to lessen nighttime voiding**). Reduce or eliminate use of hypnotics, if possible, **as client may be too sedated to recognize and respond to urge to void.**
- Refer to appropriate resources (e.g., medical supply company, ostomy nurse, or rehabilitation team) **for assistance, as desired/needed to promote self-care.**

Nursing Priority No. 3.

To promote optimum wellness:

- Encourage continuation of successful toileting program and identify possible alterations to meet individual needs (e.g., use of adult briefs for extended outing or travel with limited access to toilet). **This promotes proactive problem-solving and supports self-esteem and normalization of social interactions and desired lifestyle activities.**
- Instruct client/SO(s)/caregivers in cues that client needs, such as voiding on routine schedule, showing client location of the bathroom, providing adequate room lighting, signs, color coding of door **to assist client in continued continence, especially when in unfamiliar surroundings.**
- Review with client/SO(s) the signs and symptoms of urinary complications and need for expedient medical follow-up care. **This promotes timely intervention to limit or prevent adverse events.**

Documentation Focus

Assessment/Reassessment

- Individual findings including adaptive skills being used

Information that appears in brackets has been added by the authors to clarify and enhance the use of nursing diagnoses.

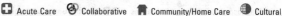

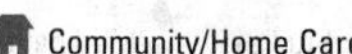
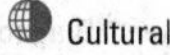

Planning

- Plan of care and who is involved in planning
- Teaching plan

Implementation/Evaluation

- Responses to treatment plan, interventions, and actions performed
- Attainment or progress toward desired outcome(s)
- Modifications to plan of care

Discharge Planning

- Available resources, equipment needs and sources

Sample Nursing Outcomes & Interventions Classifications (NOC/NIC)

NOC—Urinary Elimination
NIC—Urinary Elimination Management

impaired EMANCIPATED DECISION-MAKING and risk for impaired EMANCIPATED DECISION-MAKING

[Diagnostic Division: Ego Integrity]

Definition: impaired Emancipated Decision-Making: A process of choosing a healthcare decision that does not include personal knowledge and/or consideration of social norms, or does not occur in a flexible environment, resulting in decisional dissatisfaction.

Definition: risk for impaired Emancipated Decision-Making: Vulnerable to a process of choosing a healthcare decision that does not include personal knowledge and/or consideration of social norms, or does not occur in a flexible environment resulting in decisional dissatisfaction.

Related Factors: (impaired Emancipated Decision-Making)

Traditional hierarchical family or healthcare systems
Limited decision-making experience
Decrease in understanding of all available healthcare options
Inability to adequately verbalize perceptions about healthcare options

Information that appears in brackets has been added by the authors to clarify and enhance the use of nursing diagnoses.

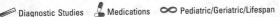

Inadequate time to discuss healthcare options; insufficient privacy to openly discuss healthcare options

Risk Factors: (risk for impaired Emancipated Decision-Making)

Traditional hierarchical family or healthcare systems
Limited decision-making experience; insufficient self-confidence in decision-making
Insufficient information regarding healthcare options
Inadequate time to discuss healthcare options
Insufficient confidence or privacy to openly discuss healthcare options

NOTE: A risk diagnosis is not evidenced by signs and symptoms, as the problem has not occurred; rather, nursing interventions are directed at prevention.

Defining Characteristics (impaired Emancipated Decision-Making)

Subjective

Feeling constrained in describing own option
Inability to choose a healthcare option that best fits current lifestyle
Inability to describe how option will fit into current lifestyle
Excessive concern about what others think is the best decision
Excessive fear of what others think about decision

Objective

Delay in enacting chosen healthcare option
Distress when listening to other's opinion
Limited verbalization about healthcare option in other's presence

Desired Outcomes/Evaluation Criteria—Client Will: (impaired Emancipated Decision-Making)

- Verbalize concern about healthcare decision making.
- Express understanding of available healthcare options.
- Discuss healthcare options openly and with confidence.
- Participate in decision making freely and openly.

Information that appears in brackets has been added by the authors to clarify and enhance the use of nursing diagnoses.

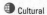

Desired Outcomes/Evaluation Criteria—Client Will: (risk for impaired Emancipated Decision-Making)

- Acknowledge awareness of difficulty in healthcare decision making.
- Seek information for making healthcare decisions.
- Discuss options openly with family/others as appropriate.
- Develop confidence as decisions are make.

Actions/Interventions

Nursing Priority No. 1.

To assess causative/contributing **or risk** factors:

- Determine usual ability to make decisions and factors that are currently interfering with making a personal choice. **The individual may not have sufficient knowledge, or may be influenced by family pressures which may prevent making an independent decision.**
- Note expressions of indecision, dependence on others, availability and involvement of support persons. **Caregivers need to be sensitive to the physical, emotional, cognitive effects of the situation on decision-making capabilities.**
- Discuss the issue of whether the individual wants to be involved in decision making. **External influences may pressure the person to give up his or her own responsibility for the decision.**
- Identify previous decisions the individual has made and the environment in which those and current decisions were/are made. **This provides information about the client's ability and circumstances surrounding decision making.**
- Active-listen, identify reasons for indecisiveness. **This helps the client to clarify the problem and begin to look at alternatives for the situation.**
- Identify cultural values, beliefs, moral obligations, or ethical concerns that may be creating conflict in the current situation. **These issues need to be resolved before the client will be comfortable with the decision.**
- Review information the client has to support the decision to be made. **This provides an opportunity to clarify and correct misinformation or inaccurate perceptions which can affect the outcome.**

Nursing Priority No. 2.

To assist client to become empowered and able to make effective decisions:

Information that appears in brackets has been added by the authors to clarify and enhance the use of nursing diagnoses.

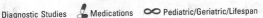

- Promote safe and hopeful environment as needed, including therapeutic nurse-client relationship. **The client needs to feel safe and supported to be comfortable in his or her own ability to make satisfactory decisions.**
- Encourage verbalization of conflicts and concerns. **This helps to identify and clarify these issues so the individual can reach a satisfying solution.**
- Clarify and prioritize individual goals. **This enables the client to look at the importance of the issues of the conflict and reach realistic problem-solving.**
- Identify strengths and use of positive coping skills, relaxation techniques, and willingness to express feelings. **This encourages the individual to view him- or herself as a capable person who can make a desired decision.**
- Discuss time constraints related to the decision to be made. **Healthcare decisions (i.e., breastfeeding) may need to be made quickly depending on the circumstances.**
- Help the client to learn the problem-solving process. **This provides a structure for the individual to look at alternatives for making a decision in the current situation and for other decisions that need to be made in the future.**
- Discuss and clarify spiritual concerns, accepting the client's values in a nonjudgmental manner. **The client will be willing to consider his or her own situation when accepted as an individual of worth.**

Nursing Priority No. 3.

To promote wellness (Teaching/Discharge Considerations):

- Provide opportunities for practicing problem-solving skills. **This helps the client to become more confident and solve current and future situations.**
- Encourage the family to become involved as desired/available. **This facilitates an understanding of the individual's needs and abilities, promoting support and acceptance of the ability of the family member.**
- Discuss attendance at assertiveness and stress-reduction classes. **Learning these skills helps the client to become able to make decisions in a more decisive manner.**
- Refer to other resources as indicated (e.g., public health, healthcare providers, support group, clergy, psychiatrist/clinical specialist psychiatric nurse). **The client may need additional help to manage difficult decision-making and/or support for long-term needs.**

Information that appears in brackets has been added by the authors to clarify and enhance the use of nursing diagnoses.

Documentation Focus

Assessment/Reassessment

- Assessment findings, behavioral responses and degree of impairment in lifestyle functioning
- Individual involved in the conflict
- Personal values and beliefs, moral or ethical concerns

Planning

- Plan of care, specific interventions, and who is involved in the planning process
- Teaching plan

Implementation/Evaluation

- Client's and individual's involved responses to interventions, teaching, and actions performed
- Ability to express feelings and identify options
- Use of resources
- Attainment or progress toward desired outcome(s)
- Modifications to plan of care

Discharge Planning

- Long-term needs, actions to be taken, and who is responsible for doing
- Specific referrals made

Sample Nursing Outcomes & Interventions Classifications (NOC/NIC)

NOC—Decision-Making
NIC—Decision-Making Support

readiness for enhanced EMANCIPATED DECISION-MAKING

[Diagnostic Division: Ego Integrity]

Definition: A process of choosing a healthcare decision that includes personal knowledge and/or consideration of social norms, which can be strengthened.

Defining Characteristics

Subjective

Expresses desire to enhance:

Decision-making; confidence in decision-making

Information that appears in brackets has been added by the authors to clarify and enhance the use of nursing diagnoses.

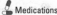

Ability to understand all available healthcare options
Privacy to discuss healthcare options; confidence to discuss healthcare options openly
Ability to verbalize own options without constraint; comfort to verbalize healthcare options in the presence of others
Ability to choose healthcare options that best fit current lifestyle; ability to enact chosen healthcare options

Desired Outcomes/Evaluation Criteria—Client Will:

- Gather information including opinions of others while making own decision.
- Express comfort with taking adequate time to make decision.
- Make decision that is congruent with lifestyle, personal and sociocultural values and goals.
- Acknowledge comfort with own decision.

Actions/Interventions

Nursing Priority No. 1.

To determine current decision-making abilities and needs:

- Determine usual ability to manage own affairs and make own decisions. **Provides baseline for understanding client's usual manner of making decisions.**
- Identify status of client, married, unmarried, and position in the household. **Although there does not seem to be a significant difference between married and unmarried women in decision-making, women often depend on the masculine members of the household to make the decisions. This suggests a lack of empowerment in women.**
- Note availability of support person. **May provide individual with positive feedback regarding the validity of the choice.**
- Active-listen and identify reason(s) client is ready to improve decision-making ability. **Provides opportunity for individual to clarify and understand how decisions are made and how the individual can help to achieve desired goals.**
- (Cultural) Identify cultural values, beliefs, moral obligations and ethical principles that guide or affect decision-making process. **Although individuals believe they are able to look at the issues with an unbiased eye, it has been shown that one's unconscious biases may interfere with making a decision that is desired.**
- Discuss meaning of life and reasons for living and how these relate to desire for improvement. **Cutting-edge research**

Information that appears in brackets has been added by the authors to clarify and enhance the use of nursing diagnoses.

demonstrates that the mind within the brain affects how these issues impact the individual's decision-making process.

Nursing Priority No. 2.

To assist client to improve/effectively use problem-solving skills:

- Promote safe and hopeful environment and help client identify own inner control. **The individual can take into consideration the context, pertinent facts when he or she feels safe and believes the decision-making is in his or her control and make a rational and well-thought-out decision.**
- Encourage verbalization of ideas, concerns, particular decisions that need to be made. **Identifying these issues can help client make desired choices.**
- Correct misconceptions and biases client may have. **People often have unconscious biases that can interfere with decision-making. Helping to clarify these ideas will make for efficient decisions.**
- Identify positive aspects of this learning opportunity. **Every day individuals make decisions, often without giving thought to what is needed to make a good decision. Decision-making can be developed by using rational and lateral thinking.**
- Discuss the process of practicing making decisions. **Decision-making is a skill that we use every day at home, work, school, and in every aspect of our lives, so the more one knows about an effective process, the better one's decisions can be.**
- ∞ Encourage children to make age-appropriate decisions. **The earlier they learn the problem-solving process, self-esteem and coping skills will be enhanced.**
- Discuss client's spiritual beliefs and values. **Accepting these in a nonjudgmental manner can help the individual look at what he or she believes in relation to these issues and decision-making.**

Nursing Priority No. 3.

To promote optimum well-being (Teaching/Discharge Considerations):

- Identify opportunities for using problem-solving skills. **Emphasizing each step as it is used will facilitate the learning process.**

Information that appears in brackets has been added by the authors to clarify and enhance the use of nursing diagnoses.

- Involve family and significant others as desired by client. **Helps all those involved to improve their decision-making skills, enhance relationships, and client can live a fuller life.**
- Recommend client attend assertiveness and/or stress reduction classes as desired. **Provides opportunity to learn new ways of dealing with problems, enhancing decision-making abilities and life in general.**
- Refer to other resources as necessary (e.g., public health, healthcare providers, clergy, support group, clergy, psychiatrist/clinical specialist psychiatric nurse). **May need additional assistance for specific problems and/or support long-term needs.**

Documentation Focus

Assessment/Reassessment

- Assessment findings, behavioral responses
- Motivation for change
- Personal values, beliefs

Planning

- Plan of care, specific interventions and actions to be performed
- Teaching plan

Implementation/Evaluation

- Response to interventions, teaching, and actions performed
- Ability to express feelings and confidence in decision-making process
- Attainment or progress toward desired outcomes
- Modifications to plan of care

Discharge Planning

- Long-term needs and who is responsible for actions to be taken
- Specific referrals made

Sample Nursing Outcomes & Interventions Classifications (NOC/NIC)

NOC—Decision-Making
NIC—Decision-Making Support

Information that appears in brackets has been added by the authors to clarify and enhance the use of nursing diagnoses.

labile EMOTIONAL CONTROL

[Diagnostic Division: Ego Integrity]

Definition: Uncontrollable outbursts of exaggerated and involuntary emotional expression.

Related Factors

Fatigue; insufficient muscles strength; musculoskeletal impairment
Functional impairment; physical disability
Stressors; social distress; alteration in self-esteem
Brain injury
Emotional disturbance; mood disorder; psychiatric disorder
Insufficient knowledge of disease or about symptom control
Pharmaceutical agent; substance abuse

Defining Characteristics

Subjective

Embarrassment regarding emotional expression
Excessive laughing/crying without feeling happiness
Expression of emotion incongruent with triggering factor

Objective

Uncontrollable/involuntary crying, laughing
Tearfulness
Absence of eye contact
Difficulty in use of facial expressions
Withdrawal from social or occupational situations

Desired Outcomes/Evaluation Criteria—Client Will:

- Acknowledge problem with emotional control.
- Identify feelings that occur with episodes of uncontrollable emotions.
- Follow medication regimen.
- Participate in recommended activities/rehabilitation.

Actions/Interventions

Nursing Priority No. 1.

To assess causative/contributing factors:

- Determine individual factors related to client situation. **Many different physiological/psychological factors may be in-**

Information that appears in brackets has been added by the authors to clarify and enhance the use of nursing diagnoses.

volved in the loss of emotional control for a given person. Identifying these factors will help to develop a plan of care that is specific to this individual.

- Assess demographic, clinical, psychiatric, and stroke lesion characteristics. **Assessment of these characteristics helps to identify individual areas that are affected, possibly related to injury to anterior regions of the cerebral hemispheres.**
- Note when episodes of loss of control occur. **This helps in determining the frequency of incidents and factors associated with the condition.**
- Identify client's perception of incidents. **Most people are embarrassed by these outbursts, believing they could control them. Individuals with certain neurological conditions or brain injuries are prone to these episodes.**
- Evaluate for depression. **Depression may be a factor for these individuals, but pseudobulbar affect needs to be recognized as treatments are different for these conditions.**

Nursing Priority No. 2.

To determine effective control of labile episodes:

- Develop plan of care to meet needs of individual situation. **This assists in providing effective care for specific problems the person is experiencing.**
- Establish a therapeutic nurse/client relationship. **This promotes trust and willingness to share concerns about problems that arise.**
- Note feelings of emotional exhaustion and social isolation. **The individual may not recognize this is a medical condition and may tend to remove himself or herself from situations that trigger the episodes.**
- Assure the client that the symptoms are real and need to be treated. **Healthcare providers may not know about this condition and the person may not recognize that these are symptoms and do not report them for intervention.**
- Correct misperceptions and provide accurate information. **This promotes understanding and helps the client to be proactive in care.**

Nursing Priority No. 3.

To promote wellness (Teaching/Discharge Considerations):

- Involve the family in the treatment plan. **This provides support for the client and promotes understanding of the uncontrollable episodes.**

Information that appears in brackets has been added by the authors to clarify and enhance the use of nursing diagnoses.

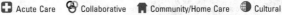

 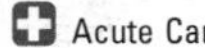 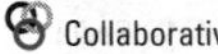 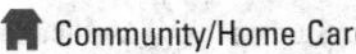 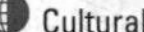

- Discuss the use of medication. **Until recently, there was no treatment until Nuedexta was approved to treat pseudobulbar affect (PBA). Its active ingredient is dextromethorphan; however, the formulation is different from any over-the-counter medications.**
- Encourage involvement in social activities. **This enhances the ability to participate with others.**
- Refer for physical therapy and rehabilitation. **The client may exhibit emotional lability following stroke and can benefit from these activities.**
- Refer to other resources as necessary: group therapy, psychiatric therapy, assertiveness training. **This additional help will enable the client to develop a more positive lifestyle.**

Documentation Focus

Assessment/Reassessment

- Assessment findings, characteristics/frequency of episodes, other pertinent information

Planning

- Plan of care, specific interventions, and who is involved in the planning process
- Teaching plan

Implementation/Evaluation

- Response to intervention, teaching, and actions performed
- Ability to express feelings, control emotions
- Use of resources
- Attainment or progress toward desired outcomes
- Modifications to plan of care

Discharge Planning

- Long-term needs, who is responsible for, actions to be taken
- Specific referrals made

Sample Nursing Outcomes & Interventions Classifications (NOC/NIC)

NOC—Mood Equilibrium
NIC—Mood Management

Information that appears in brackets has been added by the authors to clarify and enhance the use of nursing diagnoses.

risk for FALLS

[Diagnostic Division: Safety]

Definition: Vulnerable to increased susceptibility to falling, which may cause physical harm and compromise health.

Risk Factors

Adults

Age 65 or over; living alone
History of falls
Use of assistive device (e.g., walker, cane, wheelchair)
Lower-limb prosthesis

Physiological

Acute illness; postoperative recovery period
Alteration in blood glucose level; anemia
Arthritis; condition affecting the foot; decrease in lower extremity strength; difficulty with gait
Diarrhea; incontinence; urinary urgency
Faintness when extending or turning neck; orthostatic hypotension
Hearing or visual impairment
Impaired balance or mobility; proprioceptive deficit; neuropathy
Sleeplessness

Cognitive

Alteration in cognitive functioning

Pharmaceutical Agents

Alcohol consumption
Pharmaceutical agent

Environment

Use of restraints
Exposure to unsafe weather-related condition (e.g., wet floors, ice)
Cluttered environment; use of throw rugs; insufficient antislip material in bathroom
Unfamiliar setting; insufficient lighting

Information that appears in brackets has been added by the authors to clarify and enhance the use of nursing diagnoses.

Children

Age ≤2 ; male gender when <1 year of age [Note: Centers for Disease Control and Prevention (CDC) statistics suggest male gender is a factor for children age 1 to 19 but gender not significant during first year of life]

Absence of stairway gate or window guard: insufficient automobile restraints

Inadequate supervision

> **NOTE:** A risk diagnosis is not evidenced by signs and symptoms, as the problem has not occurred; rather, nursing interventions are directed at prevention.

Desired Outcomes/Evaluation Criteria—Client/Caregivers Will:

- Verbalize understanding of individual risk factors that contribute to the possibility of falls.
- Demonstrate behaviors and lifestyle changes to reduce risk factors and protect self from injury.
- Modify environment as indicated to enhance safety.
- Be free of injury.

Actions/Interventions

Nursing Priority No. 1.

To evaluate source/degree of risk:

- Observe the individual's general health status, **noting multiple factors that might affect safety, such as chronic or debilitating conditions, use of multiple medications, recent trauma (especially a fall within the past year), prolonged bedrest/immobility, unstable balance on standing. or a sedentary lifestyle.**
- Evaluate the client's current disorders/conditions that could enhance risk potential for falls. **Acute, even short-term, situations can affect any client, such as sudden dizziness, positional blood pressure changes, new medication, change in glasses prescription, recent use of alcohol/other drugs, and so on.**
- ∞ Note factors associated with age, gender, and developmental level. **Infants, young children (e.g., climbing on objects, falling against objects), young adults (e.g., sports activities), and elderly are at greatest risk because of**

Information that appears in brackets has been added by the authors to clarify and enhance the use of nursing diagnoses.

developmental issues and impaired or lack of ability to self-protect.

- Evaluate the client's general and hip muscle strength, postural stability, gait and standing balance, and gross and fine motor coordination. Review history of past or current physical injuries (e.g., musculoskeletal injuries; orthopedic surgery) **altering coordination, gait, and balance.**
- Review the client's medication regimen ongoing, noting number and type of drugs that could impact fall potential. **Studies have confirmed that use of four or more medications (polypharmacy) increases the risk of falls.**
- Evaluate use, misuse, or failure to use assistive aids, when indicated. **The client may have an assistive device but is at high risk for falls while adjusting to altered body state and use of unfamiliar device; or the client might refuse to use devices for various reasons (e.g., waiting for help or perception of weakness).**
- Evaluate the client's cognitive status (e.g., brain injury, neurological disorders; depression). **This affects the client's ability to perceive his or her own limitations or recognize danger.**
- Assess mood, coping abilities, and personality styles. **An individual's temperament, typical behavior, stressors, and level of self-esteem can affect attitude toward safety issues, resulting in carelessness or increased risk taking without consideration of consequences.**
- Ascertain the client's/SO's level of knowledge about and attendance to safety needs. **This may reveal a lack of understanding, insufficient resources, or simple disregard for personal safety (e.g., "I can't watch him every minute," "We can't hire a home assistant," "It's not manly...," etc.).**
- Consider hazards in the care setting and/or home/other environment. **Identifying needs or deficits provides opportunities for intervention and/or instruction (e.g., concerning clearing of hazards, intensifying client supervision, obtaining safety equipment, or referring for vision evaluation).**
- Review results of various fall risk assessment tools (e.g., Morse Fall Scale [MFS], Functional Ambulation Profile (FAP); the Johns Hopkins Hospital Fall Risk Assessment Tool; the Tinetti Balance and Gait Instrument [not a comprehensive listing]). **Fall-risk scales are widely used in acute care and long-term settings and include numbered rating**

Information that appears in brackets has been added by the authors to clarify and enhance the use of nursing diagnoses.

scales that place the client in risk categories (from low to high). By way of example, An MFS score of >51 indicates the client is at high risk for falls and requires high fall-prevention interventions.**

- Note socioeconomic status and availability and use of resources in other circumstances. **This can affect current coping abilities.**

Nursing Priority No. 2.

To assist client/caregiver to reduce or correct individual risk factors:

- Assist in treatments and provide information regarding the client's disease/condition(s) **that may result in increased risk of falls.**
- Review consequences of previously determined risk factors (e.g., falls caused by failure to make provisions for previously identified impairments or safety needs) **for follow-up instruction or interventions.**
- Review medication regimen and how it affects client. Instruct in the monitoring of effects and side effects. **The use of certain medications (e.g., narcotics/opiates, psychotropics, antihypertensives, and diuretics) can contribute to weakness, confusion, and balance and gait disturbances.** Review medications with client and primary care provider **to determine if changes (e.g., different medication or dosage) could reduce the client's fall risk.**
- Practice client safety. **This demonstrates behaviors for client/caregiver(s) to emulate.**
- Recommend or implement needed interventions and safety devices **to manage conditions that could contribute to falling and to promote safe environment for individual and others:**

  Evaluate vision and encourage use of prescription eyewear, as needed. **Note: The client with bifocals, trifocals, or implanted lenses may have difficulty perceiving steps or uneven surfaces, increasing risk for falls even when wearing glasses.**

  Situate the bed to enable the client to exit toward his or her stronger side whenever possible.

  Place the bed in the lowest possible position, use a raised-edge mattress, pad floor at side of bed, or place mattress on floor as appropriate.

  Use half side rail instead of full side rails or upright pole **to assist individual in arising from bed.**

Information that appears in brackets has been added by the authors to clarify and enhance the use of nursing diagnoses.

- Provide chairs with firm, high seats and lifting mechanisms when indicated.
- Provide appropriate day or night lighting.
- Assist with transfers and ambulation; show client/SO ways to move safely.
- Provide and instruct in use of mobility devices and safety devices, like grab bars and call light or personal assistance systems.
- Clear the environment of hazards (e.g., obstructing furniture, small items on the floor, electrical cords, and throw rugs).
- Lock wheels on movable equipment (e.g., wheelchairs and beds).
- Encourage the use of treaded slippers, socks, and shoes, and maintain nonskid floors and floor mats.
- Provide foot and nail care.
- Provide or encourage the use of analgesics before activity if pain is interfering with desired activities. **Balance and movement can be impaired by pain associated with multiple conditions such as trauma or arthritis.**
- Determine the caregiver's expectations of children, cognitive impairment, and/or elderly family members and compare with actual abilities. **The reality of the client's abilities and needs may be different from perception or desires of caregivers.**
- Discuss need for and sources of supervision (e.g., babysitters, before- and after-school programs, elderly day care, and personal companions).
- Perform home visit when appropriate. Determine that home safety issues are addressed, including supervision, access to emergency assistance, and client's ability to manage self-care in the home. **This may be needed to adequately determine client's needs and available resources.**
- Refer to rehabilitation team, physical or occupational therapist, as appropriate, **to improve the client's balance, strength, or mobility; to improve or relearn ambulation; and to identify and obtain appropriate assistive devices for mobility, environmental safety, or home modification.**

Nursing Priority No. 3.

To promote wellness (Teaching/Discharge Considerations):

- Refer to other resources as indicated. **Client/caregivers may need financial assistance, home modifications, referrals for counseling, home care, sources for safety equipment, or placement in extended-care facility.**

Information that appears in brackets has been added by the authors to clarify and enhance the use of nursing diagnoses.

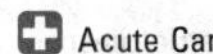

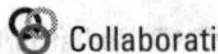

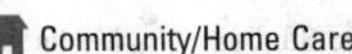

Cultural

- Provide educational resources (e.g., home safety checklist, equipment directions for proper use, appropriate Web sites) **for later review and reinforcement of learning.**
- Promote community awareness about the problems of design of buildings, equipment, transportation, and workplace accidents that contribute to falls.
- Connect the client/family with community resources, neighbors, and friends **to assist elderly or handicapped individuals in providing such things as structural maintenance and clearing of snow, gravel, or ice from walks and steps.**

Documentation Focus

Assessment/Reassessment

- Individual risk factors noting current physical findings (e.g., signs of injury—bruises, cuts; anemia, fatigue; use of alcohol, drugs, and prescription medications)
- Client's/caregiver's understanding of individual risks and safety concerns

Planning

- Plan of care and who is involved in planning
- Teaching plan

Implementation/Evaluation

- Individual responses to interventions, teaching, and actions performed
- Specific actions and changes that are made
- Attainment or progress toward desired outcomes
- Modifications to plan of care

Discharge Planning

- Long-term plans for discharge needs, lifestyle, and home setting and community changes, and who is responsible for actions to be taken
- Specific referrals made

Sample Nursing Outcomes & Interventions Classifications (NOC/NIC)

NOC—Fall Prevention Behavior
NIC—Fall Prevention

Information that appears in brackets has been added by the authors to clarify and enhance the use of nursing diagnoses.

dysfunctional FAMILY PROCESSES

[Diagnostic Division: Social Interaction]

Definition: Psychosocial, spiritual, and physiological functions of the family unit are chronically disorganized, which leads to conflict, denial of problems, resistance to change, ineffective problem-solving, and a series of self-perpetuating crises.

Related Factors

Substance abuse
Family history of substance abuse; resistance to treatment
Ineffective coping strategies; insufficient problem-solving skills
Biochemical influences; genetic predisposition to substance abuse; addictive personality

Defining Characteristics

Subjective

Feelings

Anxiety, tension, distress; low self-esteem; worthlessness; lingering resentment
Anger; frustration; shame; embarrassment; hurt; unhappiness; guilt
Emotional isolation; loneliness; powerlessness; insecurity; hopelessness; rejection
Taking responsibility for substance abuser's behavior; vulnerability; mistrust
Depression; hostility; fear; confusion; dissatisfaction; loss
Feeling different from others; feeling unloved, misunderstood
Emotionally controled by others; loss of identity
Abandonment; confuses love and pity; moodiness; failure

Roles and Relationships

Family denial; deterioration in family relationships; disturbance in family dynamics; ineffective communication with partner; intimacy dysfunction
Change in role function; disrupted family roles; inconsistent parenting; perceived insufficient parental support; chronic family problems
Insufficient relationship skills; insufficient cohesiveness; disrupted family rituals

---

Information that appears in brackets has been added by the authors to clarify and enhance the use of nursing diagnoses.

Pattern of rejection; economically disadvantaged; neglect of obligation to family member

Objective

Feelings

Repressed emotions
Surgical procedure

Roles and Relationships

Closed communication system
Conflict between partners; diminished ability of family members to relate to each other for mutual growth and maturation
Insufficient family respect for individuality or autonomy of its members

Behavioral

Substance abuse; nicotine addiction
Enabling substance use pattern; insufficient knowledge about substance abuse
Special occasions centered on substance use
Rationalization; denial of problems; refusal to get help; inability to accept or receive help appropriately
Inappropriate anger expression; blaming; criticizing; verbal abuse of children, partner, or parent
Lying; broken promises; unreliable behavior; manipulation; dependency
Inability to express or accept a wide range of feelings; difficulty with intimate relationship; decrease in physical contact
Harsh self-judgment; difficulty having fun; self-blaming; social isolation; complicated grieving; seeking of approval or affirmation
Ineffective communication skills; controlling, contradictory, or paradoxical communication pattern; power struggles
Insufficient problem-solving skills; conflict avoidance; orientation favors tension relief rather than goal attainment; agitation; escalating conflict; chaos
Alteration in concentration; disturbance in academic performance in children; failure to accomplish developmental tasks; difficulty with life-cycle transition
Inability to meet the emotional, security, or spiritual needs of its members
Inability to adapt to change; immaturity; stress-related physical illnesses; inability to deal constructively with traumatic experiences

---

Information that appears in brackets has been added by the authors to clarify and enhance the use of nursing diagnoses.

Desired Outcomes/Evaluation Criteria—Family Will:

- Verbalize understanding of dynamics of codependence.
- Participate in individual/family treatment programs.
- Identify ineffective coping behaviors and consequences of choices and actions.
- Demonstrate and plan for necessary lifestyle changes.
- Take action to change self-destructive behaviors and alter behaviors that contribute to client's drinking or substance use.
- Demonstrate improvement in parenting skills.

Actions/Interventions

Nursing Priority No. 1.

To assess contributing factors/underlying problem(s):

- Assess the current level of functioning of family members.
- Ascertain the family's understanding of the current situation; note the results of previous involvement in treatment.
- Review family history, explore roles of family members and circumstances involving substance use.
- Determine history of accidents or violent behaviors within family and safety issues.
- Discuss current and past methods of coping. **This may help to identify methods that would be useful in the current situation.**
- Determine extent and understanding of enabling behaviors being evidenced by family members.
- Identify sabotage behaviors of family members. **Issues of secondary gain (conscious or unconscious) may impede recovery.**
- Note presence and extent of behaviors of family, client, and self that might be "too helpful," such as frequent requests for help, excuses for not following through on agreed-on behaviors, feelings of anger or irritation with others. **Enabling behaviors can complicate acceptance and resolution of problem.**

Nursing Priority No. 2.

To assist family to change destructive behaviors:

- Obtain mutual agreement on behaviors and responsibilities for nurse and client. **This maximizes understanding of what is expected of each individual.**

Information that appears in brackets has been added by the authors to clarify and enhance the use of nursing diagnoses.

- Confront and examine denial and sabotage behaviors used by family members. **This helps individuals recognize and move beyond blocks to recovery.**
- Discuss use of anger, rationalization, and/or projection and ways in which these interfere with problem resolution.
- Encourage the family to deal with anger **to prevent escalation to violence.** Problem-solve concerns.
- Determine family strengths, areas for growth, and individual/family successes.
- Remain nonjudgmental in approach to family members and to member who uses alcohol/drugs.
- Provide information regarding the effects of addiction on mood/personality of the involved person. **This helps family members understand and cope with negative behaviors without being judgmental or reacting angrily.**
- Distinguish between destructive aspects of enabling behavior and genuine motivation to aid the user.
- Identify use of manipulative behaviors and discuss ways to avoid or prevent these situations. **Manipulation has the goal of controlling others; when family members accept self-responsibility and commit to stop using it, new healthy behaviors will ensue.**

Nursing Priority No. 3.

To promote wellness (Teaching/Discharge Considerations):

- Provide factual information to the client/family about the effects of addictive behaviors on the family and what to expect after discharge.
- Provide information about enabling behavior, **an addictive disease characteristic for both user and nonuser who are codependent.**
- Discuss the importance of restructuring life activities, work/leisure relationships. **Previous lifestyle/relationships supported substance use, requiring change to prevent relapse.**
- Encourage the family to refocus celebrations excluding alcohol use where indicated **to reduce risk of relapse.**
- Provide support for family members; encourage participation in group work. **Involvement in a group provides information about how others are dealing with problems, provides role models, and gives the individual an opportunity to practice new healthy skills.**
- Encourage involvement with, and refer to, self-help groups (e.g., Al-Anon, Alateen, Narcotics Anonymous, or family

---

Information that appears in brackets has been added by the authors to clarify and enhance the use of nursing diagnoses.

therapy groups) **to provide ongoing support and assist with problem-solving.**
- Provide bibliotherapy as appropriate.
- In addition, refer to NDs interrupted Family Processes; compromised/disabled family Coping, as appropriate.

Documentation Focus

Assessment/Reassessment
- Assessment findings, including history of substance(s) that have been used and family risk factors and safety concerns
- Family composition and involvement
- Results of prior treatment involvement

Planning
- Plan of care and who is involved in planning
- Teaching plan

Implementation/Evaluation
- Responses of family members to treatment, teaching, and actions performed
- Attainment or progress toward desired outcome(s)
- Modifications to plan of care

Discharge Planning
- Long-term needs, who is responsible for actions to be taken
- Specific referrals made

Sample Nursing Outcomes & Interventions Classifications (NOC/NIC)
NOC—Family Functioning
NIC—Substance Use Treatment

interrupted FAMILY PROCESSES

[Diagnostic Division: Social Interactions]

Definition: Change in family relationships and/or functioning.

Related Factors

Situational transition or crisis
Developmental transition or crisis

Information that appears in brackets has been added by the authors to clarify and enhance the use of nursing diagnoses.

Shift in health status of a family member
Shift in family roles; power shift among family members
Alteration in family finances
Change in family social status, or interaction with community

Defining Characteristics

Subjective

Changes in relationship pattern; alteration in family satisfaction
Alteration in availability for affective responsiveness; decrease in mutual support; decrease in available emotional support; alteration in intimacy
Changes in expression of conflict with, or isolation from, community resources

Objective

Assigned tasks change; ineffective task completion; alteration in participation for problem-solving; change in participation for decision-making
Change in communication pattern; alteration in family conflict resolution; power alliance changes
Change in stress-reduction behavior; change in somatization

Desired Outcomes/Evaluation Criteria—Family Will:

- Express feelings freely and appropriately.
- Demonstrate individual involvement in problem-solving processes directed at appropriate solutions for the situation or crisis.
- Direct energies in a purposeful manner to plan for resolution of the crisis.
- Verbalize understanding of condition, treatment regimen, and prognosis.
- Encourage and allow affected member to handle situation in own way, progressing toward independence.

Actions/Interventions

Nursing Priority No. 1.

To assess individual situation for causative/contributing factors:

- Determine pathophysiology, illness/trauma, or developmental crisis present.

Information that appears in brackets has been added by the authors to clarify and enhance the use of nursing diagnoses.

- Identify family developmental stage (e.g., marriage, birth of a child, children leaving home). **This provides a baseline for establishing a plan of care.**
- Note components and availability of the family: parent(s), children, male/female, and extended family.
- Observe patterns of communication in the family. Are feelings expressed? Freely? Who talks to whom? Who makes decisions? For whom? Who visits? When? What is the interaction between family members? **This identifies weakness/areas of concern to be addressed as well as strengths that can be used for resolution of the problem.**
- Assess boundaries of family members. Do members share family identity and have little sense of individuality? Do they seem emotionally distant and not connected with one another? **Answers to these questions help identify specific problems needing to be addressed.**
- Ascertain role expectations of family members. Who is the ill member (e.g., nurturer, provider)? How does the illness affect the roles of others?
- Identify "family rules"; for example, how adult concerns (finances, illness, etc.) are kept from the children.
- Determine effectiveness of parenting skills and parents' expectations.
- Note energy direction. Are efforts at resolution/problem-solving purposeful or scattered?
- Listen for expressions of despair or helplessness (e.g., "I don't know what to do") **to note degree of distress and inability to handle what is happening.**
- Note cultural and/or religious factors **that may affect perceptions/expectations of family members.**
- Assess availability and use of support systems outside of the family.

Nursing Priority No. 2.

To assist family to deal with situation/crisis:

- Deal with family members in a warm, caring, and respectful way.
- Acknowledge difficulties and realities of the situation. **This reinforces that some degree of conflict is to be expected and can be used to promote growth.**
- Encourage expressions of anger. Avoid taking comments personally as the client is usually angry at the situation over which he or she has little or no control. **This maintains boundaries between nurse and family.**

Information that appears in brackets has been added by the authors to clarify and enhance the use of nursing diagnoses.

- Stress the importance of continuous, open dialogue between family members **to facilitate ongoing problem-solving.**
- Provide information, as necessary, in verbal and written formats. Reinforce as necessary.
- Assist the family to identify and encourage their use of previously successful coping behaviors.
- Recommend contact by family members on a regular, frequent basis.
- Arrange for and encourage family participation in multidisciplinary team conference or group therapy, as appropriate.
- Involve the family in social support and community activities of their interest and choice.

Nursing Priority No. 3.

To promote wellness (Teaching/Discharge Considerations):

- Encourage the use of stress-management techniques (e.g., appropriate expression of feelings, relaxation exercises).
- Provide educational materials and information **to assist family members in resolution of current crisis.**
- Refer to classes (e.g., parent effectiveness, specific disease/disability support groups, self-help groups, clergy, psychological counseling, and family therapy), as indicated.
- Assist the family with identifying situations that may lead to fear or anxiety. (Refer to NDs Fear; Anxiety.)
- Involve the family in planning for future and mutual goal setting. **This promotes commitment to goals/continuation of plan.**
- Identify community agencies (e.g., Meals on Wheels, visiting nurse, trauma support group, American Cancer Society, or Veterans Administration) for both immediate and long-term support.

Documentation Focus

Assessment/Reassessment

- Assessment findings, including family composition, developmental stage of family, and role expectations
- Family communication patterns

Planning

- Plan of care, specific interventions, and who is involved in planning
- Teaching plan

Information that appears in brackets has been added by the authors to clarify and enhance the use of nursing diagnoses.

Implementation/Evaluation

- Each individual's response to interventions, teaching, and actions performed
- Attainment or progress toward desired outcome(s)
- Modifications to plan of care

Discharge Planning

- Long-term needs, noting who is responsible for actions to be taken
- Specific referrals made

Sample Nursing Outcomes & Interventions Classifications (NOC/NIC)

NOC—Family Functioning
NIC—Family Process Maintenance

readiness for enhanced FAMILY PROCESSES

[Diagnostic Division: Social Interaction]

Definition: A pattern of family functioning that is sufficient to support the well-being of family members and can be strengthened.

Defining Characteristics

Subjective

Expresses desire to enhance:

Family dynamics
Communication pattern
Interdependence with community
Energy level of family to support activities of daily living
Family adaptation to change
Growth/safety of family members
Family resilience
Respect for family members
Maintenance of boundaries between family members
Balance between autonomy and cohesiveness

Information that appears in brackets has been added by the authors to clarify and enhance the use of nursing diagnoses.

  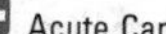 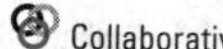 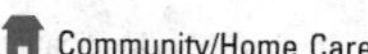 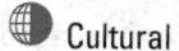

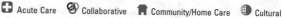

Desired Outcomes/Evaluation Criteria—Client Will:

- Express feelings freely and appropriately.
- Verbalize understanding of desire for enhanced family dynamics.
- Demonstrate individual involvement in problem-solving to improve family communications.
- Acknowledge awareness of and respect for boundaries of family members.

Actions/Interventions

Nursing Priority No. 1.

To determine status of family:

- Determine family composition: parent(s), children, male/female, and extended family. **Many family forms exist in society today, such as biological, nuclear, single parent, step family, communal, and same-sex couple or family. A better way to determine a family may be to determine the attribute of affection, strong emotional ties, a sense of belonging, and durability of membership.**
- Identify participating members of family and how they define family. **This establishes members of the family who need to be directly involved/taken into consideration when developing a plan of care to improve family functioning.**
- ∞ Note the stage of family development (e.g., single, young adult, newly married, family with young children, family with adolescents, grown children, or later in life).
- Ascertain motivation and expectations for change.
- Observe patterns of communication in the family. Are feelings expressed? Freely? Who talks to whom? Who makes decisions? For whom? Who visits? When? What is the interaction between family members? **This identifies possible weaknesses to be addressed, as well as strengths that can be used for improving family communication.**
- Assess boundaries of family members. Do members share family identity and have little sense of individuality? Do they seem emotionally connected with one another? **Individuals need to respect one another, and boundaries need to be clear so family members are free to be responsible for themselves.**

Information that appears in brackets has been added by the authors to clarify and enhance the use of nursing diagnoses.

- Identify "family rules" that are accepted in the family. **Families interact in certain ways over time and develop patterns of behavior that are accepted as the way "we behave" in this family. "Functional family" rules are constructive and promote the needs of all family members.**
- Note energy direction. **Efforts at problem-solving and resolution of different opinions may be purposeful or may be scattered and ineffective.**
- Determine cultural and/or religious factors influencing family interactions. **Expectations related to socioeconomic beliefs may be different in various cultures. For instance, traditional views of marriage and family life may be strongly influenced by Roman Catholicism in Italian-American and Latino-American families. In some cultures, the father is considered the authority figure and the mother is the homemaker. These beliefs may change with stressors or circumstances (e.g., financial, loss or gain of a family member, personal growth).**
- Note the health of married individuals. **Recent reports have determined that marriage increases life expectancy by as much as 5 years.**

Nursing Priority No. 2.

To assist the family to improve interactions:

- Establish nurse-family relationship. **This promotes a warm, caring atmosphere in which family members can share thoughts, ideas, and feelings openly and nonjudgmentally.**
- Acknowledge realities, and possible difficulties, of the individual situation. **This reinforces that some degree of conflict is to be expected in family interactions that can be used to promote growth.**
- Stress the importance of continuous, open dialogue between family members. **This facilitates an ongoing expression of open, honest feelings and opinions and effective problem-solving.**
- Assist the family to identify and encourage use of previously successful coping behaviors. **This promotes recognition of previous successes and confidence in own abilities to learn and improve family interactions.**
- Acknowledge differences among family members with open dialogue about how these differences have occurred. **This conveys an acceptance of these differences among**

Information that appears in brackets has been added by the authors to clarify and enhance the use of nursing diagnoses.

individuals and helps to look at how they can be used to strengthen the family.
- Identify effective parenting skills already being used and additional ways of handling difficult behaviors. **This allows individual family members to realize that some of what has been done already has been helpful and encourages them to learn new skills to manage family interactions in a more effective manner.**

Nursing Priority No. 3.
To promote optimum well-being:
- Discuss and encourage use of and participation in stress-management techniques. **Relaxation exercises, visualization, and similar skills can be useful for promoting reduction of anxiety and ability to manage stress that occurs in their lives.**
- Encourage participation in learning role-reversal activities. **This helps individuals to gain insight and understanding of other person's feelings and perspective/point of view.**
- Involve family members in setting goals and planning for the future. **When individuals are involved in the decision making, they are more committed to carrying out a plan to enhance family interactions as life goes on.**
- Provide educational materials and information. **This enhances learning to assist in developing positive relationships among family members.**
- Assist family members in identifying situations that may create problems and lead to stress/anxiety. **Thinking ahead can help individuals anticipate helpful actions to handle/prevent conflict and untoward consequences.**
- Refer to classes/support groups, as appropriate. **Family effectiveness, self-help, psychology, and religious affiliations can provide role models and new information to enhance family interactions.**

Documentation Focus

Assessment/Reassessment
- Assessment findings, including family composition, developmental stage of family, and role expectations
- Cultural or religious values and beliefs regarding family and family functioning

Information that appears in brackets has been added by the authors to clarify and enhance the use of nursing diagnoses.

- Family communication patterns
- Motivation and expectations for change

Planning
- Plan of care, specific interventions, and who is involved in planning
- Educational plan

Implementation/Evaluation
- Each individual's response to interventions, teaching, and actions performed
- Attainment or progress toward desired outcome(s)
- Modifications to lifestyle
- Changes in treatment plan

Discharge Planning
- Long-term needs, noting who is responsible for actions to be taken
- Specific referrals made

Sample Nursing Outcomes & Interventions Classifications (NOC/NIC)

NOC—Family Social Climate
NIC—Family Support

FATIGUE

[Diagnostic Division: Activity/Rest]

Definition: An overwhelming sustained sense of exhaustion and decreased capacity for physical and mental work at the usual level.

Related Factors

Stressors; anxiety; depression
Nonstimulating lifestyle; negative life event; occupational demands (e.g., shift work, high level of activity, stress)
Environmental barrier (e.g., ambient noise, daylight/darkness exposure, ambient temperature/humidity, unfamiliar setting)
Increase in physical exertion; sleep deprivation

Information that appears in brackets has been added by the authors to clarify and enhance the use of nursing diagnoses.

Physiological condition (e.g., pregnancy, disease, anemia); malnutrition
Physical deconditioning
Altered body chemistry (e.g., medications, drug withdrawal, chemotherapy)

Defining Characteristics

Subjective

Insufficient energy; impaired ability to maintain usual routines or usual physical activity
Tiredness; nonrestorative sleep pattern (i.e., due to caregiver responsibilities, parenting practices, sleep partner)
Guilt about difficulty maintaining responsibilities
Alteration in libido
Increase in physical symptoms, rest requirements

Objective

Lethargy; listlessness; drowsiness
Alteration in concentration
Disinterest in surroundings; introspection
Ineffective role performance

Desired Outcomes/Evaluation Criteria—Client Will:

- Report improved sense of energy.
- Identify basis of fatigue and individual areas of control.
- Perform activities of daily living and participate in desired activities at level of ability.
- Participate in recommended treatment program.

Actions/Interventions

Nursing Priority No. 1.

To assess causative/contributing factors:

- Identify the presence of physical and/or psychological conditions (e.g., pregnancy; infectious processes; blood loss, anemia; connective tissue disorders [e.g., multiple sclerosis (MS), lupus]; trauma, chronic pain syndromes [e.g., arthritis]; cardiopulmonary disorders; cancer and cancer treatments; hepatitis; AIDS; major depressive disorder; anxiety states; substance use or abuse). **Important information can be**

Information that appears in brackets has been added by the authors to clarify and enhance the use of nursing diagnoses.

obtained from knowing if fatigue is a result of an underlying condition or disease process (acute or chronic), whether an exacerbating or remitting condition is in exacerbation, and/or whether fatigue has been present over a long time without any identifiable cause.

- Note diagnosis or possibility of chronic fatigue syndrome (CFS), also sometimes called chronic fatigue immune dysfunction syndrome (CFIDS). **Defining Characteristics listed above indicate that this fatigue far exceeds feeling tired after a busy day. Because no direct tests help in diagnosis of CFS, it is one of exclusion. CSF has been defined as a distinct disorder (affecting children and adults) characterized by chronic (often relapsing, but always debilitating) fatigue, lasting for at least 6 months (often for much longer), causing impairments in overall physical and mental functioning and without an apparent etiology.**
- ∞ Note age, gender, and developmental stage. **Some studies show a prevalence of fatigue more often in females than males; it most often occurs in adolescent girls and in young to middle-aged adults, but the condition may be present in any person at any age.**
- Review medication regimen/use. **Certain medications, including prescription (especially beta-adrenergic blockers, chemotherapy), over-the-counter drugs, herbal supplements, and combinations of drugs and/or substances, are known to cause and/or exacerbate fatigue.**
- Ascertain the client's belief about what is causing the fatigue.
- Assess vital signs **to evaluate fluid status and cardiopulmonary response to activity.**
- Determine the presence/degree of sleep disturbances. **Fatigue can be a consequence of, and/or exacerbated by, sleep deprivation.**
- Note recent lifestyle changes, including conflicts (e.g., expanded responsibilities, demands of others, job-related conflicts); maturational issues (e.g., adolescent with an eating disorder); and developmental issues (e.g., new parenthood, loss of spouse/SO).
- Assess psychological and personality factors that may affect reports of fatigue level.
- Evaluate aspect of "learned helplessness" that may be manifested by giving up. **This can perpetuate a cycle of fatigue, impaired functioning, and increased anxiety and fatigue.**

Information that appears in brackets has been added by the authors to clarify and enhance the use of nursing diagnoses.

Nursing Priority No. 2.

To determine degree of fatigue/impact on life:

- Obtain client/SO descriptions of fatigue (i.e., lacking energy or strength, tiredness, weakness lasting over length of time). Note the presence of additional concerns (e.g., irritability, lack of concentration, difficulty making decisions, problems with leisure, and relationship difficulties) **to assist in evaluating the impact on the client's life.**
- Ask the client to rate fatigue (using a 0 to 10 or similar numerical scale) and its effects on the ability to participate in desired activities. **Fatigue may vary in intensity and is often accompanied by irritability, lack of concentration, difficulty making decisions, problems with leisure, and relationship difficulties that can add to stress level and aggravate sleep problems.**
- Discuss lifestyle changes or limitations imposed by fatigue state.
- Interview parent/caregiver regarding specific changes observed in child or elder client. **These individuals may not be able to verbalize feelings or relate meaningful information.**
- Note daily energy patterns (i.e., peaks and valleys). **This is helpful in determining pattern/timing of activity.**
- Measure the physiological response to activity (e.g., changes in blood pressure or heart and respiratory rate).
- Evaluate the need for individual assistance or assistive devices.
- Review the availability and current use of support systems and resources.
- Perform, or review results of, testing, such as the Multidimensional Assessment of Fatigue (MAF); Piper Fatigue Scale (PFS); Global Fatigue Index (GFI), as appropriate. **Can help determine manifestation, intensity, duration, and emotional meaning of fatigue.**

Nursing Priority No. 3.

To assist client to cope with fatigue and manage within individual limits of ability:

- Accept the reality of client reports of fatigue and do not underestimate effect on client's quality of life. **For example, clients with MS are prone to more frequent and severe fatigue following minimal energy expenditure and require a longer recovery period than is usual; postpolio clients**

Information that appears in brackets has been added by the authors to clarify and enhance the use of nursing diagnoses.

often display a cumulative effect if they fail to pace themselves and rest when early signs of fatigue develop.

- Establish realistic activity goals with the client and encourage forward movement. **This enhances the commitment to promoting optimal outcomes.**
- Plan interventions to allow individually adequate rest periods. Schedule activities for periods when the client has the most energy **to maximize participation.**
- Involve the client/SO(s) in schedule planning.
- Encourage the client to do whatever possible (e.g., self-care, sit up in chair, go for walk, interact with family, or play a game). Increase activity level, as tolerated.
- Instruct in methods to conserve energy:

  Sit instead of stand during daily care and other activities.
  Carry several small loads instead of one large load.
  Combine and simplify activities.
  Take frequent, short breaks during activities.
  Delegate tasks.
  Ask for and accept assistance.
  Say "No" or "Later."
  Plan steps of activity before beginning so that all needed materials are at hand.

- Encourage the use of assistive devices (e.g., wheeled walker, handicap parking spot, elevator, backpack for carrying objects), as needed, **to extend active time/conserve energy for other tasks.**
- Assist with self-care needs; keep the bed in a low position and keep travelways clear of furniture; assist with ambulation, as indicated.
- Avoid or limit exposure to temperature and humidity extremes, **which can negatively impact energy level.**
- Provide diversional activities. Avoid both overstimulation and understimulation (cognitive and sensory). **Participating in pleasurable activities can refocus energy and diminish feelings of unhappiness, sluggishness, and worthlessness that can accompany fatigue.**
- Discuss routines to promote restful sleep. (Refer to ND Insomnia.)
- Encourage nutritionally dense, easy-to-prepare-and-consume foods, and avoidance of caffeine and high-sugar foods and beverages **to promote energy.**
- Instruct in/implement stress-management skills of visualization, relaxation, and biofeedback, when appropriate.
- Refer to comprehensive rehabilitation program, physical and occupational therapy for programmed daily exercises and ac-

Information that appears in brackets has been added by the authors to clarify and enhance the use of nursing diagnoses.

tivities **to improve stamina, strength, and muscle tone and to enhance sense of well-being.**

Nursing Priority No. 4.

To promote wellness (Teaching/Discharge Considerations):

- Discuss therapy regimen relating to individual causative factors (e.g., physical and/or psychological illnesses) and help the client/SO(s) to understand relationship of fatigue to illness.
- Assist client/SO(s) to develop plan for activity and exercise within individual ability. Stress necessity of allowing sufficient time to finish activities.
- Instruct the client in ways to monitor responses to activity and significant signs/symptoms **that indicate the need to alter activity level.**
- Promote overall health measures (e.g., nutrition, adequate fluid intake, and appropriate vitamin and iron supplementation).
- Provide supplemental oxygen, as indicated. **The presence of anemia and hypoxemia reduces oxygen available for cellular uptake and contributes to fatigue.**
- Encourage the client to develop assertiveness skills, to prioritize goals and activities, to learn to delegate duties or tasks, or to say "No." Discuss burnout syndrome, when appropriate, and actions client can take to change individual situation.
- Assist the client to identify appropriate coping behaviors. **This promotes a sense of control and improves self-esteem.**
- Identify support groups and community resources.
- Refer to counseling or psychotherapy, as indicated.
- Identify resources to assist with routine needs (e.g., Meals on Wheels, homemaker or housekeeper services, yard care).

Documentation Focus

Assessment/Reassessment

- Manifestations of fatigue and other assessment findings
- Degree of impairment and effect on lifestyle
- Expectations of client/SO(s) relative to individual abilities and specific condition

Planning

- Plan of care, specific interventions, and who is involved in the planning
- Teaching plan

Information that appears in brackets has been added by the authors to clarify and enhance the use of nursing diagnoses.

Implementation/Evaluation

- Client's response to interventions, teaching, and actions performed
- Attainment or progress toward desired outcome(s)
- Modifications to plan of care

Discharge Planning

- Discharge needs/plan, actions to be taken, and who is responsible
- Specific referrals made

Sample Nursing Outcomes & Interventions Classifications (NOC/NIC)

NOC—Endurance
NIC—Energy Management

FEAR

[Diagnostic Division: Ego Integrity]

Definition: Response to perceived threat that is consciously recognized as a danger.

Related Factors

Innate response to stimuli (e.g., sudden noise, height); innate releasing mechanism to external stimuli (e.g., neurotransmitters); phobic stimulus
Learned response [e.g., conditioning, modeling from others]
Unfamiliar setting
Separation from support system
Language barrier; sensory deficit (e.g., visual, hearing)

Defining Characteristics

Subjective

Apprehensiveness; excitedness; decrease in self-assurance; increase in tension; jitteriness; nausea
Feeling alarm, dread, fear, terror, panic

Cognitive

Identifies object of fear; stimulus believed to be a threat

Physiological

Anorexia; fatigue; dry mouth; dyspnea; [palpitations]

Information that appears in brackets has been added by the authors to clarify and enhance the use of nursing diagnoses.

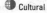

Objective

Vomiting; muscle tension; pallor; increase in blood pressure; pupil dilation

Cognitive

Decrease in productivity, learning ability, or problem-solving ability

Behaviors

Increase in alertness; avoidance behaviors; attack behaviors; impulsiveness; focus narrowed to the source of fear

Physiological

Increased pulse; diarrhea; increase in respiratory rate; change in physiological response (e.g., blood pressure, heart rate, respiratory rate, oxygen saturation and end-tidal CO_2); increase in perspiration

Desired Outcomes/Evaluation Criteria—Client Will:

- Acknowledge and discuss fears, recognizing healthy versus unhealthy fears.
- Verbalize accurate knowledge of and sense of safety related to current situation.
- Demonstrate understanding through use of effective coping behaviors (e.g., problem-solving) and resources.
- Display lessened fear as evidenced by appropriate range of feelings and relief of signs/symptoms (specific to client).

Actions/Interventions

Nursing Priority No. 1.

To assess degree of fear and reality of threat perceived by the client:

- Ascertain client's/SO's perception of what is occurring and how this affects life. **Fear is a defensive mechanism in protecting oneself, but if left unchecked, it can become disabling to the client's life.**
- ∞ Determine the client's age and developmental level. **This helps in understanding usual or typical fears experienced by individuals (e.g., toddler often has different fears than adolescent or older person suffering with dementia being removed from home/usual living situation).**
- Note ability to concentrate, level of attention, degree of incapacitation (e.g., "frozen with fear," inability to engage in necessary activities). **This is indicative of extent of anxiety**

Information that appears in brackets has been added by the authors to clarify and enhance the use of nursing diagnoses.

or fear related to what is happening and need for specific interventions to reduce physiological reactions. The presence of a severe reaction (panic or phobias) requires more intensive intervention.

- Compare verbal and nonverbal responses **to note congruencies or misperceptions of the situation. The client may be able to verbalize what he or she is afraid of, if asked, providing opportunity to address actual fears.**
- Be alert to signs of denial or depression. **Depression may be associated with fear that interferes with productive life and daily activities.**
- Identify sensory deficits that may be present, such as vision or hearing impairment. **These affect sensory reception and interpretation of the environment. The inability to correctly sense and perceive stimuli leads to misunderstanding, increasing fear.**
- Investigate the client's reports of subjective experiences, which could be indicative of delusions/hallucinations, **to help determine the client's interpretation of surroundings and/or stimuli.**
- Be alert to and evaluate potential for violence.
- Measure vital signs and physiological responses to the situation. **Fear and acute anxiety can both involve sympathetic arousal (e.g., increased heart rate, respirations, and blood pressure hyperalertness; diuresis; dilation of skeletal blood vessels; constriction of gut blood vessels, and a surge of catecholamine release).**
- Assess family dynamics. **Actions and responses of family members may exacerbate or soothe fears of the client; conversely, if the client is immersed in illness, whether from crisis or fear, it can take a toll on the family/involved others.** Refer to other NDs, such as interrupted Family Processes; readiness for enhanced family Coping; compromised or disabled family Coping; Anxiety.

Nursing Priority No. 2.

To assist client/SO(s) in dealing with fear/situation:

- Stay with the client or make arrangements to have someone else be there. **Providing the client with usual or desired support persons can diminish feelings of fear.**
- Discuss the client's perceptions and fearful feelings. Active-listen the client's concerns. **This promotes an atmosphere of caring and permits explanation or correction of misperceptions.**

Information that appears in brackets has been added by the authors to clarify and enhance the use of nursing diagnoses.

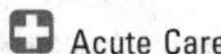

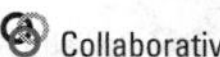

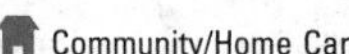

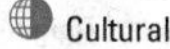

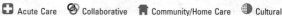

- Provide information in verbal and written forms. Speak in simple sentences and concrete terms. **This facilitates understanding and retention of information.**
- Acknowledge normalcy of fear, pain, and despair, and give "permission" to express feelings appropriately and freely. **This promotes an attitude of caring and opens the door for discussion about feelings and/or addressing reality of situation.**
- Provide an opportunity for questions and answer honestly. **This enhances sense of trust and nurse-client relationship.**
- ∞ Provide presence and physical contact (e.g., hugging, refocusing attention, or rocking a child), as appropriate, when painful procedures are anticipated **to soothe fears and provide assurance.**
- Modify procedures, if possible (e.g., substitute oral for intramuscular medications, combine blood draws, or use finger stick method) **to limit the degree of stress and avoid overwhelming a fearful individual.**
- ∞ Manage environmental factors, such as loud noises, harsh lighting, changing person's location without knowledge of family/SO(s), strangers in care area, unfamiliar people, and high traffic flow, **which can cause or exacerbate stress, especially to very young or to older individuals.**
- Present objective information, when available, and allow the client to use it freely. Avoid arguing about the client's perceptions of the situation. **Limits conflicts when the fear response may impair rational thinking.**
- Promote client control, where possible, and help the client identify and accept those things over which control is not possible. **This strengthens the internal locus of control.**
- Provide touch, Therapeutic Touch, massage, and other adjunctive therapies as indicated. **This aids in meeting basic human need, decreasing sense of isolation, and assisting the client to feel less anxious. Note: Therapeutic Touch requires the nurse to have specific knowledge and experience to use the hands to correct energy field disturbances by redirecting human energies to help or heal.**
- Encourage contact with a peer who has successfully dealt with a similarly fearful situation. **This provides a role model, and the client is more likely to believe others who have had similar experience(s).**

Nursing Priority No. 3.

To assist client in learning to use own responses for problem-solving:

Information that appears in brackets has been added by the authors to clarify and enhance the use of nursing diagnoses.

- Acknowledge usefulness of fear for taking care of self.
- Explain the relationship between disease and symptoms, if appropriate. **Providing accurate information promotes understanding of why the symptoms occur, allaying anxiety about them.**
- Identify the client's responsibility for the solutions while reinforcing that the nurse will be available for help if desired or needed. **This enhances the sense of control.**
- Determine internal and external resources for assistance (e.g., awareness and use of effective coping skills in the past; SOs who are available for support).
- Explain procedures within the level of the client's ability to understand and handle being aware of how much information the client wants **to prevent confusion or information overload.**
- Explain the relationship between disease and symptoms, if appropriate.
- Review the use of antianxiety medications and reinforce use as prescribed.

Nursing Priority No. 4.

To promote wellness (Teaching/Discharge Considerations):

- Support planning for dealing with reality. **This assists in identifying areas in which control can be exercised and those in which control is not possible, thus enabling the client to handle fearful situations/feelings.**
- Instruct in the use of relaxation or visualization and guided imagery skills. **This promotes the release of endorphins and aids in developing an internal locus of control, reducing fear and anxiety. This may enhance coping skills, allowing the body to go about its work of healing.**
- Encourage regular physical activity within limits of ability. Refer to a physical therapist to develop an exercise program to meet individual needs. **This provides a healthy outlet for energy generated by fearful feelings and promotes relaxation.**
- Provide for and deal with sensory deficits in an appropriate manner (e.g., speak clearly and distinctly, use touch carefully, as indicated by situation).
- Refer to pastoral care, mental health care providers, support groups, community agencies and organizations, as indicated. **This provides information, ongoing assistance to meet individual needs, and an opportunity for dis-**

Information that appears in brackets has been added by the authors to clarify and enhance the use of nursing diagnoses.

cussing concerns and obtaining further care when indicated.

Documentation Focus

Assessment/Reassessment

- Assessment findings, noting individual factors contributing to current situation, source of fear
- Manifestations of fear

Planning

- Plan of care and who is involved in the planning
- Teaching plan

Implementation/Evaluation

- Client's responses to treatment plan, interventions, and actions performed
- Attainment or progress toward desired outcome(s)
- Modifications to plan of care

Discharge Planning

- Long-term needs and who is responsible for actions to be taken
- Specific referrals made

Sample Nursing Outcomes & Interventions Classifications (NOC/NIC)

NOC—Fear Self-Control
NIC—Anxiety Reduction

ineffective infant FEEDING PATTERN

[Diagnostic Division: Food/Fluid]

Definition: Impaired ability of an infant to suck or coordinate the suck/swallow response resulting in inadequate oral nutrition for metabolic needs.

Related Factors

Prematurity
Neurological delay or impairment (e.g., positive EEG, head trauma, seizure disorder)

Information that appears in brackets has been added by the authors to clarify and enhance the use of nursing diagnoses.

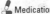

Oral hypersensitivity
Prolonged nil by mouth (NPO)
Otopharyngeal defect

Defining Characteristics

Subjective

[Caregiver reports infant's inability to achieve effective suck]

Objective

Inability to initiate or sustain effective suck
Inability to coordinate sucking, swallowing, and breathing

Desired Outcomes/Evaluation Criteria—Client Will:

- Display adequate output as measured by sufficient number of wet diapers daily.
- Demonstrate appropriate weight gain.
- Be free of aspiration.

Actions/Interventions

Nursing Priority No. 1.

To identify contributing factors/degree of impaired function:

- Assess infant's suck, swallow, and gag reflexes. **This provides a comparative baseline and is useful in determining an appropriate feeding method.**
- Note developmental age, structural abnormalities (e.g., cleft lip/palate), and mechanical barriers (e.g., endotrachial tube and ventilator).
- Determine level of consciousness, neurological impairment, seizure activity, and presence of pain.
- Observe parent/infant interactions **to determine level of bonding and comfort that could impact stress level during feeding activity.**
- Note type and scheduling of medications, **which could cause sedative effect and impair feeding activity.**
- Compare birth and current weight and length measurements **to note progress.**
- Assess signs of stress when feeding (e.g., tachypnea, cyanosis, fatigue, or lethargy).
- Note the presence of behaviors indicating continued hunger after feeding.

Information that appears in brackets has been added by the authors to clarify and enhance the use of nursing diagnoses.

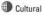

Nursing Priority No. 2.

To promote adequate infant intake:

- Determine appropriate method for feeding (e.g., special nipple or feeding device, gavage or enteral tube feeding) and choice of breast milk or formula to meet infant needs.
- Review early infant feeding cues (e.g., rooting, lip smacking, sucking fingers or hand) versus late cue of crying. **Early recognition of infant hunger promotes timely/more rewarding feeding experience for infant and mother.**
- Demonstrate techniques and procedures for feeding. Note proper positioning of infant, "latching-on" techniques, rate of delivery of feeding, and frequency of burping. (Refer to ND ineffective Breastfeeding, as appropriate.)
- Limit duration of feeding to maximum of 30 min based on infant's response (e.g., signs of fatigue) **to balance energy expenditure with nutrient intake.**
- Monitor caregiver's efforts. Provide feedback and assistance, as indicated. **This enhances learning and encourages the continuation of efforts.**
- Refer nursing mother to lactation specialist for assistance and support in dealing with unresolved issues (e.g., teaching infant to suck).
- Emphasize the importance of a calm, relaxed environment during feeding **to reduce detrimental stimuli and enhance mother's and infant's focus on feeding activity.**
- Adjust frequency and amount of feeding according to infant's response. **This prevents stress associated with under- or overfeeding.**
- Advance diet, adding solids or thickening agent, as appropriate for age and infant needs.
- Alternate feeding techniques (e.g., nipple and gavage) according to infant's ability and level of fatigue.
- Alter medication/feeding schedules, as indicated, **to minimize sedative effects and have infant in alert state.**

Nursing Priority No. 3.

To promote wellness (Teaching/Discharge Considerations):

- Encourage kangaroo care, placing infant skin-to-skin upright, tummy down, on mother's or father's chest. **Skin-to-skin care increases bonding and may promote stable heart rate, temperature, and respiration in infant.**
- Instruct caregiver in techniques to prevent or alleviate aspiration.
- Discuss anticipated growth and development goals for infant, corresponding caloric needs.

Information that appears in brackets has been added by the authors to clarify and enhance the use of nursing diagnoses.

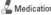

- Suggest monitoring infant's weight and nutrient intake periodically.
- Recommend participation in classes, as indicated (e.g., first aid, infant CPR).
- Refer to support groups (e.g., La Leche League, parenting support groups, stress reduction, or other community resources, as indicated).
- Provide bibliotherapy and appropriate Web sites for further information.

Documentation Focus

Assessment/Reassessment

- Type and route of feeding, interferences to feeding and reactions
- Infant's measurements

Planning

- Plan of care, specific interventions, and who is involved in planning
- Teaching plan

Implementation/Evaluation

- Infant's response to interventions (e.g., amount of intake, weight gain, response to feeding) and actions performed
- Caregiver's involvement in infant care, participation in activities, response to teaching
- Attainment of or progress toward desired outcome(s)
- Modifications to plan of care

Discharge Planning

- Long-term needs, referrals made, and who is responsible for follow-up actions

Sample Nursing Outcomes & Interventions Classifications (NOC/NIC)

NOC—Swallowing Status: Oral Phase
NIC—Swallowing Therapy

readiness for enhanced FLUID BALANCE

[Diagnostic Division: Food/Fluid]

Definition: A pattern of equilibrium between the fluid volume and chemical composition of body fluids which can be strengthened.

Information that appears in brackets has been added by the authors to clarify and enhance the use of nursing diagnoses.

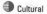

Defining Characteristics

Subjective

Expresses desire to enhance fluid balance

Desired Outcomes/Evaluation Criteria—Client Will:

- Maintain fluid volume at a functional level as indicated by adequate urinary output, stable vital signs, moist mucous membranes, and good skin turgor.
- Demonstrate behaviors to monitor fluid balance.
- Be free of thirst.
- Be free of evidence of fluid overload (e.g., absence of edema and adventitious lung sounds).

Actions/Interventions

Nursing Priority No. 1.

To determine potential for fluid imbalance and ways that client is managing:

- Note the presence of factors with potential for fluid imbalance: (1) diagnoses or disease processes (e.g., hyperglycemia, ulcerative colitis, chronic obstructive pulmonary disease [COPD], burns, cirrhosis of the liver, vomiting, diarrhea, or hemorrhage), or situations (e.g., diuretic therapy, hot or humid climate, prolonged exercise, getting overheated or feverish, diuretic effect of caffeine and alcohol) that may lead to deficits; or (2) conditions or situations potentiating fluid excess (e.g., renal failure, cardiac failure, stroke, cerebral lesions, renal or adrenal insufficiency, psychogenic polydipsia, acute stress, surgical procedures, use of anesthesia, or excessive or rapid infusion of IV fluids). **Body fluid balance is regulated by intake (food and fluid), output (kidney, gastrointestinal [GI] tract, skin, and lungs), and regulatory hormonal mechanisms. Balance is maintained within a relatively narrow margin and can be easily disrupted by multiple factors.**
- ∞ Determine potential effects of age and developmental stage. **Elderly individuals have less body water than younger adults, and more potential for functional and environmental issues that affect their ability to manage fluid intake. Infants and children have a relatively higher percentage of total body water and metabolic rate and are often less able than adults to manage their fluid intake.**

Information that appears in brackets has been added by the authors to clarify and enhance the use of nursing diagnoses.

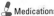

- Evaluate factors that could impact the client's ability to manage fluid balance. **Persons with impaired mobility, diminished vision, or who are confined to bed cannot as easily meet their own needs and may be reluctant to ask for assistance. Persons whose work environment is restrictive or outside may also have greater challenges in meeting fluid needs.**
- Assess vital signs (e.g., temperature, blood pressure, and heart rate), skin and mucous membrane moisture, and urine output. Weigh, as indicated. **These are predictors of fluid balance that should be in the client's usual range in a healthy state.**

Nursing Priority No. 2.

To prevent occurrence of imbalance:

- Monitor input and output (I&O) (e.g., frequency of voids or diaper changes), as appropriate, being aware of insensible losses (e.g., diaphoresis in hot environment, use of oxygen, or permanent tracheostomy), and "hidden sources" of intake (e.g., foods high in water content) **to ensure an accurate picture of fluid status.**
- Weigh the client regularly, and compare with recent weight history. **This is useful in early recognition of water retention or unexplained losses.**
- Establish and review with client individual fluid needs and replacement schedule. Make sure the client has access to fluids at all times. Teach an elderly person to drink when not thirsty and to drink small amounts frequently, rather than large amounts infrequently. **This enhances the likelihood of cooperation with meeting therapeutic goals. Note: Thirst declines with aging, but hydration needs do not.**
- Encourage regular oral intake (e.g., fluids between meals, additional fluids during hot weather or when exercising) **to maximize intake and maintain fluid balance.**
- Discuss judicious use of medications, as indicated (e.g., antiemetics, antidiarrheals, antipyretics, diuretics). **Medications may be indicated to prevent fluid imbalance if individual becomes sick.**

Nursing Priority No. 3.

To promote optimum wellness:

- Discuss client's individual conditions and factors that could cause occurrence of fluid imbalance, as individually appropriate (such as prevention of hyperglycemic episodes) **so that client/SO can take corrective action.**

Information that appears in brackets has been added by the authors to clarify and enhance the use of nursing diagnoses.

- Identify and instruct in ways to meet specific fluid needs (e.g., client could carry water bottle when going to sports events or measure specific 24-hr fluid portions if restrictions apply) **to manage fluid intake over time.**
- Instruct the client/SO(s) in how to measure blood pressure and record I&O, if needed for home management. **This provides the means of monitoring status and adjusting therapy to meet changing needs.**
- Establish a regular schedule for weighing **to help monitor changes in fluid status.**
- Identify actions (if any) the client may take to correct imbalance. **This encourages responsibility for self-care.**
- Review any dietary needs or restrictions and safe substitutes for salt, as appropriate. **This helps prevent fluid retention/edema formation.**
- Review or instruct in medication regimen and administration, and discuss potential for interactions/side effects that could disrupt fluid balance.
- Instruct in signs and symptoms indicating a need for immediate/further evaluation and follow-up care **to prevent complications and/or allow for early intervention.**

Documentation Focus

Assessment/Reassessment

- Individual findings, including factors affecting ability to manage (regulate) body fluids
- I&O, fluid balance, changes in weight, and vital signs

Planning

- Plan of care and who is involved in the planning
- Teaching plan

Implementation/Evaluation

- Client's responses to treatment, teaching, and actions performed
- Attainment or progress toward desired outcome(s)
- Modifications to plan of care

Discharge Planning

- Long-term needs, noting who is responsible for actions to be taken
- Specific referrals made

Information that appears in brackets has been added by the authors to clarify and enhance the use of nursing diagnoses.

Sample Nursing Outcomes & Interventions Classifications (NOC/NIC)

NOC—Fluid Balance
NIC—Fluid Monitoring

[deficient hyper/hypotonic FLUID VOLUME]

[Diagnostic Division: Food/Fluid]

Definition: Decreased intravascular, interstitial, and/or intracellular fluid. This refers to dehydration with changes in sodium.

NOTE: NANDA has restricted deficient Fluid Volume to address only isotonic dehydration. For client needs related to dehydration associated with alterations in sodium, the authors have provided this second diagnostic label.

Related Factors

[Hypertonic dehydration: uncontrolled diabetes mellitus/insipidus, hyperosmolar hyperglycemic state (HHS), increased intake of hypertonic fluids/IV therapy, inability to respond to thirst reflex, inadequate free water supplementation (high-osmolarity enteral feeding formulas), renal insufficiency or failure]

[Hypotonic dehydration: chronic illness, malnutrition, excessive use of hypotonic IV solutions (e.g., D5W), renal insufficiency]

Defining Characteristics

Subjective

[Reports of fatigue, nervousness, exhaustion]
[Thirst]

Objective

[Increased urine output, dilute urine (initially) and/or decreased output/oliguria]
[Weight loss]
[Decreased venous filling; hypotension (postural)]
[Increased pulse rate; decreased pulse volume and pressure]

Information that appears in brackets has been added by the authors to clarify and enhance the use of nursing diagnoses.

[Decreased skin turgor; dry skin/mucous membranes]
[Increased body temperature]
[Change in mental status (e.g., confusion)]
[Hemoconcentration; altered serum sodium]

Desired Outcomes/Evaluation Criteria—Client Will:

- Maintain fluid volume at a functional level, as evidenced by individually adequate urinary output, stable vital signs, moist mucous membranes, good skin turgor.
- Verbalize understanding of causative factors and purpose of individual therapeutic interventions and medications.
- Demonstrate behaviors to monitor and correct deficit, as indicated, when condition is chronic.

Actions/Interventions

Nursing Priority No. 1.

To assess causative/precipitating factors:

- Note possible conditions or processes that may lead to deficits: (1) fluid loss (e.g., diarrhea, vomiting, excessive sweating; heat stroke; diabetic ketoacidosis; burns, other draining wounds; gastrointestinal obstruction; salt-wasting diuretics; rapid breathing or mechanical ventilation; surgical drains); (2) limited intake (e.g., sore throat or mouth; client dependent on others for eating or drinking; NPO status); (3) fluid shifts (e.g., ascites, effusions, burns, sepsis); and (4) environmental factors (e.g., isolation, restraints, malfunctioning air conditioning, exposure to extreme heat).
- ∞ Determine effects of age. Obtain weight and measure subcutaneous fat and muscle mass **to ascertain total body water [TBW], which is approximately 60% of adult's weight and 75% of infant's weight. Very young and extremely elderly individuals are quickly affected by fluid volume deficit and are least able to express need.**
- Evaluate nutritional status, noting current intake, weight changes, problems with oral intake, use of supplements/tube feedings, **factors that can negatively affect fluid intake (e.g., impaired mentation, nausea, wired jaws, immobility, insufficient time for meals, lack of finances restricting availability of food).**
- Collaborate with physician to identify or characterize the nature of fluid and electrolyte imbalance(s). **Dehydration is often categorized according to serum sodium concentration.**

Information that appears in brackets has been added by the authors to clarify and enhance the use of nursing diagnoses.

Hypernatremic (also called "hypertonic dehydration" when relatively less sodium than water is lost) and hyponatremic (or hypotonic dehydration when relatively less water than sodium is lost) can both cause neurological complications, and thus may be more dangerous.

- Be aware of the difference between signs of **hypovolemia** (e.g., poor skin turgor, dizziness on standing, lethargy, delayed capillary refill, sunken eyeballs, fever, weight loss, little or no urine output) and signs of **dehydration** (e.g., lethargy, weakness, irritability, nausea, vomiting, and hyperreflexia, potentially progressing to coma) **which are symptoms of the effect of elevated sodium (hypernatremia) on the central nervous system.**
- Review client's medications, including prescription, over-the-counter (OTC) drugs, herbs, and nutritional supplements **to identify medications that can alter fluid and electrolyte balance. These may include diuretics, vasodilators, beta blockers, aldosterone inhibitors, angiotensin-converting enzyme (ACE) blockers, and medications that can cause syndrome of inappropriate secretion of antidiuretic hormone (e.g., phenothiazides, vasopressin, some antineoplastic drugs).**

Nursing Priority No. 2.

To evaluate degree of fluid deficit:

- Obtain history of usual pattern of fluid intake and recent alterations. **Intake may be reduced because of current physical or environmental issues (e.g., swallowing problems, vomiting, severe heat wave with inadequate fluid replacement); or a behavior pattern (e.g., elderly person refuses to drink water trying to control incontinence).**
- Assess vital signs, including temperature (often elevated), pulse (may be elevated), and respirations. Note the strength of peripheral pulses.
- Measure blood pressure (may be low) with the client lying, sitting, and standing, when possible, and monitor invasive hemodynamic parameters, as indicated.
- Note presence of physical signs (e.g., dry mucous membranes, poor skin turgor, or delayed capillary refill).
- Note change in usual mentation, behavior, or functional abilities (e.g., confusion, falling, loss of ability to carry out usual activities, lethargy, or dizziness). **These signs indicate sufficient dehydration to cause poor cerebral perfusion and/or electrolyte imbalance.**

Information that appears in brackets has been added by the authors to clarify and enhance the use of nursing diagnoses.

- Observe and measure urinary output hourly or for 24 hr as indicated. Note color **(may be dark because of concentration)** and specific gravity **(high number associated with dehydration with usual range being 1.010 to 1.025).**
- Review laboratory data (e.g., Hb/Hct; electrolytes [sodium, potassium, chloride, bicarbonate]; BUN; creatinine; total protein/albumin) **to evaluate the body's response to fluid loss and to determine replacement needs.**

Nursing Priority No. 3.

To correct/replace fluid losses to reverse pathophysiological mechanisms:

- Assist with treatment of underlying conditions causing or contributing to dehydration and electrolyte imbalances.
- Administer fluids and electrolytes, as indicated. **Fluids used for replacement depend on (1) the type of dehydration present (e.g., hypertonic or hypotonic) and (2) the degree of deficit determined by age, weight, and type of condition causing the deficit.**
- Establish 24-hr replacement needs and routes to be used (e.g., IV, PO, enteral feedings). **Steady rehydration over time prevents peaks and valleys in fluid level.**
- Engage client, family, and all caregivers in fluid management plan. **Everyone is responsible for the prevention or treatment of dehydration and should be involved in the planning and provision of adequate fluid on a daily basis.**
- Limit intake of alcohol and caffeinated beverages, **which tend to exert a diuretic effect.**
- Provide nutritionally balanced diet and/or enteral feedings (avoiding use of hyperosmolar or excessively high-protein formulas) and provide an adequate amount of free water with feedings.
- Maintain accurate intake and output (I&O), calculate 24-hr fluid balance, and weigh regularly (daily, in unstable client) **in order to monitor and document trends. Note: A 1-pound weight loss reflects fluid loss of about 500 mL in an adult.**

Nursing Priority No. 4.

To promote comfort and safety:

- Change position frequently. Bathe infrequently, using mild cleanser or soap, and provide optimal skin care with suitable emollients **to maintain skin integrity and prevent excessive dryness.**

Information that appears in brackets has been added by the authors to clarify and enhance the use of nursing diagnoses.

- Provide frequent oral and eye care **to prevent injury from dryness.** Refer to NDs impaired oral Mucous Membranes, and risk for Dry Eye.
- Change position frequently **to reduce pressure on fragile, dehydrated skin and tissues.**
- Provide for safety measures when client is confused. (Refer to NDs acute Confusion, chronic Confusion for additional interventions.)
- Replace electrolytes, as ordered.
- Administer or discontinue medications, as indicated, **when disease process or medications are contributing to dehydration.**

Nursing Priority No. 5.

To promote wellness (Teaching/Discharge Considerations):

- Discuss factors related to occurrence of deficit as individually appropriate. **Early identification of risk factors can decrease occurrence and severity of complications associated with hypovolemia.**
- Recommend drinking more water when exercising or engaging in physical exertion, or during hot weather. Suggest carrying a water bottle when away from home as appropriate.
- Identify and instruct in ways to meet specific fluid and nutritional needs.
- Offer fluids on a regular basis to infants, young children, and the elderly, **who may not sense/or be able to report thirst.**
- Instruct client/SO(s) in how to monitor color of urine (**dark urine equates with concentration and dehydration**), and/or how to measure and record I&O (**may include weighing or counting diapers in infant/toddler**) as indicated.
- Review and instruct in medication regimen and administration. Emphasize the need for reporting suspected drug interactions/side effects to healthcare provider. **This facilitates timely intervention to prevent or reduce complications.**
- Instruct in signs and symptoms indicating need for emergent or further evaluation and follow-up.

Documentation Focus

Assessment/Reassessment

- Individual findings, including factors affecting ability to manage (regulate) body fluids and degree of deficit
- I&O, fluid balance, changes in weight, urine specific gravity, and vital signs
- Results of diagnostic testing and laboratory studies

Information that appears in brackets has been added by the authors to clarify and enhance the use of nursing diagnoses.

Planning

- Plan of care and who is involved in the planning
- Teaching plan

Implementation/Evaluation

- Client's responses to treatment, teaching, and actions performed
- Attainment or progress toward desired outcome(s)
- Modifications to plan of care

Discharge Planning

- Long-term needs, noting who is responsible for actions to be taken
- Specific referrals made

Sample Nursing Outcomes & Interventions Classifications (NOC/NIC)

NOC—Fluid Balance
NIC—Fluid/Electrolyte Management

deficient [isotonic] FLUID VOLUME

[Diagnostic Division: Food/Fluid]

Definition: Decreased intravascular, interstitial, and/or intracellular fluid. This refers to dehydration, water loss alone without a change in sodium.

NOTE: This diagnosis has been structured to address isotonic dehydration (hypovolemia) excluding states in which changes in sodium occur. For client needs related to dehydration associated with alterations in sodium, refer to [deficient hyper/hypotonic Fluid Volume].

Related Factors

Active fluid volume loss [e.g., hemorrhage, gastric intubation, acute or prolonged diarrhea, wounds, abdominal cancer; burns, fistulas, ascites (third spacing); use of hyperosmotic radiopaque contrast agents]

Compromised regulatory mechanisms [e.g., fever, thermoregulatory response, renal tubule damage]

Information that appears in brackets has been added by the authors to clarify and enhance the use of nursing diagnoses.

Defining Characteristics

Subjective

Thirst
Weakness

Objective

Alteration in mental status
Alteration in skin or tongue turgor; dry skin and mucous membranes
Decrease in blood pressure; decrease in pulse pressure and volume; decrease in venous filling
Decrease in urine output
Increase in body temperature and heart rate
Increase in hematacrit and urine concentration
Sudden weight loss

Desired Outcomes/Evaluation Criteria—Client Will:

- Maintain fluid volume at a functional level as evidenced by individually adequate urinary output with normal specific gravity, stable vital signs, moist mucous membranes, good skin turgor and prompt capillary refill, resolution of edema.
- Verbalize understanding of causative factors and purpose of individual therapeutic interventions and medications.
- Demonstrate behaviors to monitor and correct deficit, as indicated.

Actions/Interventions

Nursing Priority No. 1.

To assess causative/precipitating factors:

- Identify relevant diagnoses **that may create a fluid volume depletion (decreased intravascular plasma volume, such as might occur with rapid blood loss or hemorrhage from trauma; or vascular, pregnancy complication, or gastrointestinal [GI] bleeding disorders); significant fluid (other than blood) loss such as might occur with severe gastroenteritis with vomiting and diarrhea; or extensive burns.**
- Note the presence of other factors (e.g., laryngectomy or tracheostomy tubes, drainage from wounds and fistulas or suction devices; water deprivation or fluid restrictions; decreased level of consciousness; dialysis; hot/humid climate, prolonged

Information that appears in brackets has been added by the authors to clarify and enhance the use of nursing diagnoses.

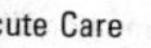

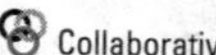

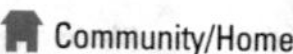

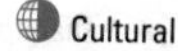

exercise; increased metabolic rate secondary to fever; increased caffeine or alcohol) **that may contribute to a lack of fluid intake or loss of fluid by various routes.**

- Determine the effects of age, gender. weight, subcutaneous fat, and muscle mass **(influence total body water [TBW], which is approximately 60% of an adult's weight and 75% of an infant's weight). Elderly individuals are at higher risk because of decreasing response and effectiveness of compensatory mechanisms. Infants and children have a relatively high percentage of total body water, are sensitive to loss, and are less able to control their fluid intake.**
- Prepare for and assist with diagnostic evaluations (e.g., imaging studies, x-rays) **to locate source of bleeding or cause for hypovolemia.**

Nursing Priority No. 2.

To evaluate degree of fluid deficit:

- Estimate or measure traumatic or procedural fluid losses and note possible routes of insensible fluid losses. Determine customary and current weight. **These factors are used to determine degree of volume depletion and method of fluid replacement.**
- Assess vital signs, noting low blood pressure—severe hypotension, rapid heart beat, and thready peripheral pulses. **These changes in vital signs are associated with fluid volume loss and/or hypovolemia. Note: In an acute, life-threatening hemorrhage state, cold, pale, moist skin may be noted reflecting body compensatory mechanisms to profound hypovolemia.**
- Observe/measure urinary output (hourly/24-hr totals). Note the color **(may be dark greenish brown because of concentration)** and specific gravity **(a number higher than 1.25 is associated with dehydration, with usual range being 1.010–1.025).**
- Note change in usual mentation, behavior, and functional abilities (e.g., confusion, falling, loss of ability to carry out usual activities, lethargy, and dizziness). **These signs indicate sufficient dehydration to cause poor cerebral perfusion or can reflect the effects of electrolyte imbalance. In a hypovolemic shock state, mentation changes rapidly and client may present in coma.**
- Note complaints and physical signs associated with dehydration (e.g., scanty, concentrated urine; lack of tears when crying [infant, child]; dry, sticky mucous membranes; lack of

Information that appears in brackets has been added by the authors to clarify and enhance the use of nursing diagnoses.

sweating; delayed capillary refill; poor skin turgor; confusion; sleepiness; lethargy; muscle weakness; dizziness or light-headedness; headache).

- Measure abdominal girth when ascites or third spacing of fluid occurs. Assess for peripheral edema formation.
- Review laboratory data (e.g., hemoglobin [Hb]/Hct, prothrombin time, activated partial thromboplastin time [aPTT]; electrolytes [sodium, potassium, chloride, bicarbonate] and glucose; blood urea nitrogen [BUN], creatinine [Cr]) **to evaluate the body's response to bleeding/other fluid loss and to determine replacement needs. Note: In isotonic dehydration, electrolyte levels may be lower, but concentration ratios remain near normal.**

Nursing Priority No. 3.

To correct/replace losses to reverse pathophysiological mechanisms:

- Control blood loss (e.g., gastric lavage with room temperature or cool saline solution, drug administration) and prepare for surgical intervention.
- Stop fluid loss (e.g., administer medication to stop vomiting/diarrhea, fever).
- Administer fluids and electrolytes (e.g., blood, isotonic sodium chloride solution, lactated Ringer's solution, albumin, fresh frozen plasma, dextran, and hetastarch).
- Establish 24-hr fluid replacement needs and routes to be used. **This prevents peaks and valleys in fluid level.**
- Note client preferences regarding fluids and foods with high fluid content.
- Keep fluids within the client's reach and encourage frequent intake, as appropriate.
- Control humidity and ambient air temperature, as appropriate, especially when major burns are present; or increase or decrease in presence of fever. Reduce bedding and clothes; provide tepid sponge bath. Assist with hypothermia, when ordered, **to reduce high fever and elevated metabolic rate.** (Refer to ND Hyperthermia.)
- Maintain accurate input and output (I&O) and weigh daily. Monitor urine specific gravity.
- Monitor vital signs (lying/sitting/standing) and invasive hemodynamic parameters, as indicated (e.g., CVP, pulmonary artery pressure/pulmonary capillary wedge pressure).

Information that appears in brackets has been added by the authors to clarify and enhance the use of nursing diagnoses.

Nursing Priority No. 4.

To promote comfort and safety:

- Change position frequently **to reduce pressure on fragile skin and tissues.**
- Bathe every other day; provide optimal skin care with emollients.
- Provide frequent oral as well as eye care **to prevent injury from dryness.**
- Change dressings frequently and use adjunct appliances as indicated, for draining wounds **to protect skin and monitor losses for replacement needs.**
- Provide for safety measures when the client is confused.
- Administer medications (e.g., antiemetics, antidiarrheals **to limit gastric or intestinal losses**; antipyretics **to reduce fever**). (Refer to NDs Diarrhea, Hyperthermia for additional interventions.)
- Observe for sudden or marked elevation of blood pressure, restlessness, moist cough, dyspnea, basilar crackles, and frothy sputum. **Too rapid a correction of fluid deficit may compromise the cardiopulmonary system, causing fluid overload and edema, especially if colloids are used in initial fluid resuscitation.**

Nursing Priority No. 5.

To promote wellness (Teaching/Discharge Considerations):

- Discuss factors related to occurrence of fluid deficit as individually appropriate (e.g., reason for hemorrhage, potential for dehydration in children with fever or diarrhea, inadequate fluid replacement when performing strenuous work or exercise, living in hot climate, improper use of diuretics) **to reduce risk of recurrence.**
- Identify actions (if any) the client can take to prevent or correct deficiencies.
- Instruct the client/SO(s) in how to monitor the color of urine **(dark urine equates with concentration and dehydration)** or how to measure and record I&O (may include weighing or counting diapers in infant/toddler).
- Review medications and interactions and side effects, especially medications that can cause or exacerbate fluid loss (e.g., diuretics, laxatives), and those indicated to prevent fluid loss (e.g., antidiarrheals or anticoagulants).
- Discuss signs/symptoms indicating need for emergent or further evaluation and follow-up. **This promotes timely intervention.**

Information that appears in brackets has been added by the authors to clarify and enhance the use of nursing diagnoses.

Documentation Focus

Assessment/Reassessment

- Assessment findings, including degree of deficit and current sources of fluid intake
- I&O, fluid balance, changes in weight, presence of edema, urine specific gravity, and vital signs
- Results of diagnostic studies

Planning

- Plan of care and who is involved in planning
- Teaching plan

Implementation/Evaluation

- Client's responses to interventions, teaching, and actions performed
- Attainment or progress toward desired outcome(s)
- Modifications to plan of care

Discharge Planning

- Long-term needs, plan for correction, and who is responsible for actions to be taken
- Specific referrals made

Sample Nursing Outcomes & Interventions Classifications (NOC/NIC)

NOC—Hydration
NIC—Hypovolemia Management

excess **FLUID VOLUME**

[Diagnostic Division: Food/Fluid]

Definition: Increased isotonic fluid retention.

Related Factors

Compromised regulatory mechanism [e.g., syndrome of inappropriate antidiuretic hormone (SIADH) or decreased plasma proteins]
Excessive fluid intake
Excessive sodium intake

Information that appears in brackets has been added by the authors to clarify and enhance the use of nursing diagnoses.

 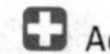  Acute Care 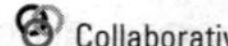 Collaborative 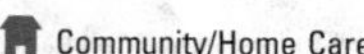 Community/Home Care 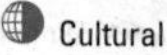 Cultural

Defining Characteristics

Subjective

Orthopnea; paroxysmal nocturnal dyspnea
Anxiety

Objective

Edema; anasarca; weight gain over short period of time
Intake exceeds output; oliguria
Adventitious breath sounds; alteration in respiratory pattern; dyspnea
Pulmonary congestion; pleural effusion; alteration in pulmonary artery pressure (PAP)
Alteration in blood pressure
Increase in central venous pressure (CVP); jugular vein distention; positive hepatojugular reflex; hepatomegaly
Presence of S_3 heart sound
Alteration in mental status; restlessness
Decrease in hemoglobin or hematocrit; azotemia; electrolyte imbalance; alteration in urine specific gravity

Desired Outcomes/Evaluation Criteria—Client Will:

- Stabilize fluid volume as evidenced by balanced input and output (I&O), vital signs within client's normal limits, stable weight, and free of signs of edema.
- Verbalize understanding of individual dietary and fluid restrictions.
- Demonstrate behaviors to monitor fluid status and reduce recurrence of fluid excess.
- List signs that require further evaluation.

Actions/Interventions

Nursing Priority No. 1.

To assess causative/precipitating factors:

- Note the presence of medical conditions or situations (e.g., heart failure, chronic kidney disease, renal or adrenal insufficiency, excessive or rapid infusion of IV fluids, cerebral lesions, psychogenic polydipsia, acute stress, anesthesia, surgical procedures, or decreased or loss of serum proteins) **that can contribute to excess fluid intake or retention.**
- Determine or estimate the amount of fluid intake from all sources: oral, IV, enteral or parenteral feedings, ventilator,

Information that appears in brackets has been added by the authors to clarify and enhance the use of nursing diagnoses.

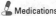

and so forth. **Note: A severely malnourished client can experience significant fluid shifts and electrolyte imbalances after nutritional support is initiated.**

- Review nutritional issues (e.g., intake of sodium, potassium, and protein). **Imbalances in these areas are associated with fluid imbalances.**

Nursing Priority No. 2.

To evaluate degree of excess:

- Compare current weight with admission and/or previously stated weight. Weigh daily or on a regular schedule, as indicated. **This provides a comparative baseline and evaluates the effectiveness of therapies. Note: Volume overload can occur over weeks to months in clients with unrecognized renal failure where lean muscle mass is lost and fluid overload occurs with relatively little change in weight.**
- Measure vital signs and invasive hemodynamic parameters (e.g., central venous pressure [CVP], pulmonary artery pressure [PAP], pulmonary capillary wedge pressure [PCWP]) when indicated. **Pressures may be high because of excess fluid volume or low if cardiac failure is occurring.**
- Note the presence of tachycardia, irregular rhythms. Auscultate heart tones for S_3 and ventricular gallop rhythm. **These signs are suggestive of heart failure, which results in decreased cardiac output and tissue hypoxia.**
- Auscultate breath sounds **for the presence of crackles, congestion.**
- Record the occurrence of exertional breathlessness, dyspnea at rest, or paroxysmal nocturnal dyspnea. **These may be an indication of pulmonary congestion and potential of developing pulmonary edema that can interfere with oxygen–carbon dioxide exchange at the capillary level.**
- Assess for the presence of neck vein distention, hepatojugular reflux.
- Note the presence of edema (puffy eyelids, dependent swelling of ankles and feet if ambulatory or up in chair; sacrum and posterior thighs when recumbent), anasarca. **Heart failure and renal failure are associated with dependent edema because of hydrostatic pressures, with dependent edema being a defining characteristic for excess fluid.**
- Measure abdominal girth **for changes that may indicate increasing fluid retention/edema.**
- Measure and record I&O accurately. Include "hidden" fluids (e.g., IV antibiotic additives, liquid medications, ice chips).

Information that appears in brackets has been added by the authors to clarify and enhance the use of nursing diagnoses.

- Emphasize the need for mobility, frequent position changes, and early/ongoing ambulation **to prevent stasis and reduce risk of tissue injury.**
- Identify "danger" signs requiring notification of healthcare provider **to ensure timely evaluation/intervention.**

Documentation Focus

Assessment/Reassessment

- Assessment findings, noting existing conditions contributing to and degree of fluid retention (vital signs; amount, presence, and location of edema; and weight changes)
- I&O, fluid balance
- Results of laboratory tests and diagnostic studies

Planning

- Plan of care and who is involved in the planning
- Teaching plan

Implementation/Evaluation

- Response to interventions, teaching, and actions performed
- Attainment or progress toward desired outcome(s)
- Modifications to plan of care

Discharge Planning

- Long-range needs, noting who is responsible for actions to be taken

Sample Nursing Outcomes & Interventions Classifications (NOC/NIC)

NOC—Fluid Overload Severity
NIC—Hypervolemia Management

risk for deficient FLUID VOLUME

[Diagnostic Division: Food/Fluid]

Definition: Vulnerable to experiencing decreased intravascular, interstitial, and/or intracellular fluid volumes, which may compromise health.

Risk Factors

Active fluid volume loss; excessive fluid loss through normal routes [e.g., diarrhea]

Information that appears in brackets has been added by the authors to clarify and enhance the use of nursing diagnoses.

Barrier to accessing fluid; deviations affecting intake or absorption
Extremes of age or weight
Factors influencing fluid needs [e.g., hypermetabolic state]
Fluid loss through abnormal routes [e.g., indwelling tubes]; compromised regulatory mechanism
Insufficient knowledge about fluid needs
Pharmaceutical agent [e.g., diuretics]

NOTE: A risk diagnosis is not evidenced by signs and symptoms as the problem has not occurred; rather, nursing interventions are directed at prevention.

Desired Outcomes/Evaluation Criteria—Client/Caregiver Will:

- Identify individual risk factors and appropriate interventions.
- Maintain fluid volume at a functional level as evidenced by individually adequate urinary output with normal specific gravity, stable vital signs, moist mucous membranes, good skin turgor, and prompt capillary refill.
- Demonstrate behaviors or lifestyle changes to prevent development of fluid volume deficit.

Actions/Interventions

Nursing Priority No. 1.

To assess causative/contributing factors:

- Note possible conditions or processes that may lead to deficits: (1) fluid loss (e.g., fever, diarrhea, vomiting, excessive sweating; heat stroke; diabetic ketoacidosis; burns, other draining wounds; gastrointestinal obstruction; salt-wasting diuretics; rapid breathing, mechanical ventilation; surgical drains); (2) limited intake (e.g., sore throat or mouth; client dependent on others for eating and drinking; nothing-by-mouth [NPO] status); (3) fluid shifts (e.g., ascites, effusions, burns, sepsis); and (4) environmental factors (e.g., isolation, restraints, malfunctioning air conditioning, exposure to extreme heat).
- Note the client's level of consciousness and mentation **to evaluate the ability to express needs.**
- ∞ Determine effects of age. **Very young and extremely elderly individuals are quickly affected by fluid volume deficit and are least able to express need. For example, elderly people often have a decreased thirst reflex and/or may not be**

Information that appears in brackets has been added by the authors to clarify and enhance the use of nursing diagnoses.

aware of water needs. Infants, young children, and other nonverbal persons cannot describe thirst.

- Assess an older client's "hydration habits" **to determine the best approach if the client has potential for dehydration. Note: A recent study identified four categories of nursing home residents: (1) can drink (the client is functionally capable of consuming fluids, but does not for any number of reasons); (2) cannot drink (frailty or dysphagia makes this client incapable of consuming fluids safely); (3) will not drink (client may fear incontinence or may have never in life consumed many fluids); and (4) end of life.**
- Evaluate nutritional status, noting current intake and type of diet (e.g., client is NPO or is on a restricted diet). Note problems (e.g., impaired mentation, nausea, fever, facial injuries, immobility, and insufficient time for intake) **that can negatively affect fluid intake.**
- Review the client's medications, including prescription, over-the-counter drugs, herbs, and nutritional supplements, **to identify medications that can alter fluid and electrolyte balance. These may include diuretics, vasodilators, beta blockers, aldosterone inhibitors, angiotensin-converting enzyme (ACE) blockers, and medications that can cause syndrome of inappropriate secretion of antidiuretic hormone (e.g., phenothiazines, vasopressin, some antineoplastic drugs).**
- Review laboratory data (e.g., hemoglobin [Hb]/hematocrit [Hct], osmolality, electrolytes [e.g., sodium and potassium], blood urea nitrogen/creatine [BUN/Cr]) **to evaluate fluid and electrolyte status. Note: Isotonic dehydration results from a balanced loss of water and electrolytes.**

Nursing Priority No. 2.

To prevent occurrence of deficit:

- Compare current fluid intake to fluid goal. Monitor intake and output (I&O) balance, if indicated, being aware of changes in intake or output, as well as insensible losses **to ensure an accurate picture of fluid status.**
- Assess skin and oral mucous membranes **for signs of dehydration, such as dry skin and mucous membranes, poor skin turgor, delayed capillary refill, and flat neck veins.**
- Monitor vital signs for changes (e.g., orthostatic hypotension, tachycardia, or fever) **that may cause or be the effect of dehydration.**
- Weigh the client and compare with recent weight history. Perform serial weights to determine trends.

Information that appears in brackets has been added by the authors to clarify and enhance the use of nursing diagnoses.

- Review laboratory data (e.g., hemoglobin [Hb]/hematocrit [Hct], osmolality, electrolytes [e.g., sodium and potassium], blood urea nitrogen [BUN]/creatinine [Cr]) as indicated **to evaluate fluid and electrolyte status.**
- Offer a variety of fluids and water-rich foods, and make them available throughout the day, if the client is able to take oral fluids. Assist/remind the client to drink, as needed. Determine individual fluid needs and establish replacement over 24 hr **to increase the client's daily fluid intake.**
- Administer medications as appropriate (e.g., antiemetics, antidiarrheals, or antipyretics) **to stop or limit fluid losses.**
- Provide nutritionally balanced diet and/or enteral feedings, when indicated (avoiding use of hyperosmolar or excessively high-protein formulas), and provide an adequate amount of free water with feedings.
- Provide supplemental IV fluids as indicated.
- Review diet orders to remove any nonessential fluid and salt restrictions.

Encourage oral intake:

Provide water and other fluid needs to a minimum amount daily (up to 2.5 L/day or amount determined by healthcare provider for client's age, weight, and condition).

Offer fluids between meals and regularly throughout the day.

Provide fluids in a manageable cup, bottle, or with drinking straw.

Allow for adequate time for eating and drinking at meals.

Ensure that immobile or restrained client is assisted.

Encourage a variety of fluids in small frequent offerings, attempting to incorporate the client's preferred beverages and temperature (e.g., iced or hot).

Limit fluids that tend to exert a diuretic effect (e.g., caffeine or alcohol).

Promote intake of high-water-content foods (e.g., popsicles, gelatin, soup, eggnog, and watermelon) and/or electrolyte replacement drinks (e.g., SmartWater, Gatorade, or Pedialyte), as appropriate.

Nursing Priority No. 3.

To promote wellness (Teaching/Discharge Considerations):

- Discuss individual risk factors, potential problems, and specific interventions **to reduce risk of injury and dehydration (e.g., proper clothing and bedding and increased fluid intake for infants and elderly during hot weather, use of**

Information that appears in brackets has been added by the authors to clarify and enhance the use of nursing diagnoses.

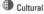

room cooler or fan for comfortable ambient environment, fluid replacement options and schedule).

- Review appropriate use of medications **that have potential for causing or exacerbating dehydration.**
- Encourage the client/caregiver to maintain a diary of fluid intake, number and amount of voidings, and estimate of other fluid losses (e.g., wounds or liquid stools), as necessary **to determine replacement needs.**
- Engage client, family, and all caregivers in a fluid management plan. **This enhances cooperation with the regimen and achievement of goals.**
- Refer to NDs [deficient hyper/hypotonic Fluid Volume]; deficient [isotonic] Fluid Volume.

Documentation Focus

Assessment/Reassessment

- Individual findings, including individual risk factors influencing fluid needs or requirements
- Baseline weight, vital signs
- Results of laboratory tests
- Specific client fluid needs and preferences

Planning

- Plan of care and who is involved in planning
- Teaching plan

Implementation/Evaluation

- Responses to interventions, teaching, and actions performed
- Attainment or progress toward desired outcome(s)
- Modifications to plan of care

Discharge Planning

- Individual long-term needs, noting who is responsible for actions to be taken
- Specific referrals made

Sample Nursing Outcomes & Interventions Classifications (NOC/NIC)

NOC—Fluid Balance
NIC—Fluid Monitoring

Information that appears in brackets has been added by the authors to clarify and enhance the use of nursing diagnoses.

risk for imbalanced FLUID VOLUME

[Diagnostic Division: Food/Fluid]

Definition: Vulnerable to a decrease, increase, or rapid shift from one to the other of intravascular, interstitial, and/or intracellular fluid which may compromise health. This refers to body fluid loss, gain, or both.

Risk Factors

Intestinal obstruction
Pancreatitis; ascites
Burns; sepsis
Trauma
Treatment regimen; apheresis

NOTE: A risk diagnosis is not evidenced by signs and symptoms, as the problem has not occurred; rather, nursing interventions are directed at prevention.

Desired Outcomes/Evaluation Criteria—Client Will:

- Demonstrate adequate fluid balance as evidenced by stable vital signs, palpable pulses of good quality, normal skin turgor, moist mucous membranes, individual appropriate urinary output, lack of excessive weight fluctuation (loss or gain), and no edema present.

Actions/Interventions

Nursing Priority No. 1.

To determine risk/contributing factors:

- Note the presence of conditions (e.g., diabetes insipidus; hyperosmolar nonketotic syndrome; intestinal obstruction; pancreatitis, sepsis; heart, kidney, or liver failure) **associated with fluid imbalance.**
- Note current treatment modalities including (1) major invasive procedures (e.g., surgery or dialysis); (2) use or overuse of certain medications (e.g., heparin or diuretics), (3) use of IV fluids without a delivery device; (4) plasmapheresis (aka apheresis) therapy. **These modalities can cause/exacerbate**

Information that appears in brackets has been added by the authors to clarify and enhance the use of nursing diagnoses.

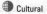

fluid imbalances, and must be monitored for complications.

- Note the client's age, current level of hydration, and mentation. **This provides information regarding the ability to tolerate fluctuations in fluid level and risk for creating or failing to respond to a problem.**
- Review laboratory data and chest x-ray **to determine changes indicative of electrolyte and/or fluid status.**

Nursing Priority No. 2.

To prevent fluctuations/imbalances in fluid levels:

- Measure and record intake:

  Include all sources (e.g., oral, IV, antibiotic additives, liquids with medications).
- Measure and record output:

  Monitor urine output hourly or as needed. Report urine output less than 30 mL/hr or 0.5 mL/kg/hr, **because this may indicate deficient fluid volume or cardiac or kidney failure.**

  Observe the color of all excretions **to evaluate for bleeding.**

  Measure or estimate the amount of liquid stool; weigh diapers or continence pads, when indicated.

  Inspect dressing(s), weigh dressings, estimate blood loss in surgical sponges, count dressings or pads saturated per hour. **Note: Small losses can be life-threatening to pediatric clients.**

  Measure emesis and output from drainage devices (e.g., gastric, wound, or chest).

  Estimate or calculate insensible fluid losses **to include in replacement calculations.**

  Calculate 24-hr fluid balance (intake more than output or output more than intake).
- Weigh daily, or as indicated, and evaluate changes as they relate to fluid status. **This provides for early detection and prompt intervention as needed.**
- Auscultate blood pressure; calculate pulse pressure. **Pulse pressure widens before systolic blood pressure drops in response to fluid loss.**
- Monitor vital sign responses to activities. **Blood pressure and heart and respiratory rate often increase initially when either fluid deficit or excess is present.**
- Assess for clinical signs of dehydration (e.g., hypotension, dry skin and mucous membranes, or delayed capillary refill) or

---

Information that appears in brackets has been added by the authors to clarify and enhance the use of nursing diagnoses.

fluid excess (e.g., peripheral/dependent edema, adventitious breath sounds, or distended neck veins).

- Note increased lethargy, hypotension, and muscle cramping. **Electrolyte imbalances (e.g., sodium, potassium, magnesium, or calcium) may be present.**
- Establish fluid oral intake, incorporating beverage preferences when possible.
- Maintain fluid and sodium restrictions, when needed.
- Administer IV fluids, as prescribed, using infusion pumps **to deliver fluids accurately and at desired rates to prevent either underfusion or overinfusion.**
- Assist with treatment of conditions resulting in deficit. Prepare for procedures (e.g., surgery for trauma, cold lavage for bleeding ulcer, etc.) and/or use of specific fluids or medications **to prevent dehydration, fluid volume depletion.**

  Refer to NDs [deficient hyper/hypotonic Fluid Volume] and deficient [isotonic] Fluid Volume, for additional interventions.

- Assist with the treatment of conditions associated with fluid excess. Prepare for procedures (e.g., dialysis, ultrafiltration, pacemaker, or cardiac assist device) and/or use of specific drugs (e.g., antihypertensives, cardiotonics, or diuretics) **to correct fluid overload situation.**

  Refer to ND excess Fluid Volume for additional interventions.

Nursing Priority No. 3.

To promote wellness (Teaching/Discharge Considerations):

- Engage the client, family, and all caregivers in a fluid management plan. **This enhances cooperation with the regimen and achievement of goals.**
- Discuss individual risk factors or potential problems and specific interventions **to prevent or limit fluid imbalance and complications.**
- Instruct the client/SO in how to measure blood pressure and record I/O as appropriate.
- Review and instruct in medications or nutritional regimen (e.g., enteral or parenteral) **to alert to potential complications and ways to manage.**
- Identify signs and symptoms indicating the need for prompt evaluation or follow-up by the primary healthcare provider **for timely intervention and correction.**

Information that appears in brackets has been added by the authors to clarify and enhance the use of nursing diagnoses.

Documentation Focus

Assessment/Reassessment

- Individual findings, including individual factors influencing fluid needs/requirements
- Baseline weight, vital signs
- Results of laboratory test and diagnostic studies
- Specific client preferences for fluids

Planning

- Plan of care and who is involved in planning
- Teaching plan

Implementation/Evaluation

- Responses to interventions, teaching, and actions performed
- Attainment or progress toward desired outcome(s)
- Modifications to plan of care

Discharge Planning

- Individual long-term needs, noting who is responsible for actions to be taken
- Specific referrals made

Sample Nursing Outcomes & Interventions Classifications (NOC/NIC)

NOC—Fluid Balance
NIC—Fluid Monitoring

FRAIL ELDERLY SYNDROME and risk for FRAIL ELDERLY SYNDROME

[Diagnostic Division: Safety]

Definition: Frail Elderly Syndrome: Dynamic state of unstable equilibrium that affects the older individual experiencing deterioration of one or more domain of health (physical, functional, psychological, or social) and leads to increased susceptibility to adverse health effects, in particular, disability.

Definition: risk for Frail Elderly Syndrome: Vulnerable to a dynamic state of unstable equilibrium that affects the older individual experiencing deterioration of one or more domain of health (physical, functional, psychological, or social) and leads to increased susceptibility to adverse health effects, in particular, disability.

Information that appears in brackets has been added by the authors to clarify and enhance the use of nursing diagnoses.

Related Factors (Frail Elderly Syndrome)

Alteration in cognitive functioning; psychiatric disorder
Chronic illness; prolonged hospitalization
Malnutrition; sarcopenia; sarcopenic obesity
History of falls
Living alone
Sedentary lifestyle

Risk Factors (risk for Frail Elderly Syndrome)

Activity intolerance; average daily physical activity is less than recommended for gender and age; decrease in energy; exhaustion; sedentary lifestyle
Age >70 years; female gender; ethnicity other than Caucasian
Alteration in cognitive functioning
Anorexia; malnutrition; decrease in serum 25-hydroxy vitamin D concentration
Anxiety; depression; sadness
Chronic illness; prolonged hospitalization
Decrease in muscle strength; muscle weakness; walking 15 feet requires >6 seconds (4 meters >5 secconds)
Fear of falling; history of falls
Impaired balance or mobility; immobility
Sensory deficit (e.g., visual, hearing)
Sarcopenia; unintentional weight loss of 25% body weight over one year; unintentional weight loss > 10 pounds (>4.5 Kg) in one year
Obesity; sarcopenic obesity
Endocrine regulatory dysfunction (e.g., glucose intolerance, increase in IGF-1, androgen, DHEA, and cortisol)
Suppressed inflammatory response (e.g., IL-6, CRP); altered clotting process (e.g., factor VII, D-dimers)
Constricted life space; economically disadvantaged; low educational level
Insufficient social support; living alone; social isolation
Social vulnerability (e.g., disempowerment, decreased life control)

NOTE: A risk diagnosis is not evidenced by signs and symptoms, as the problem has not occurred; rather, nursing interventions are directed at prevention.

Information that appears in brackets has been added by the authors to clarify and enhance the use of nursing diagnoses.

Defining Characteristics (Frail Elderly Syndrome)

Author Note: NANDA-I has defined a syndrome as "a clinical judgment concerning a specific cluster of nursing diagnoses [NDs] that occur together and are best addressed together and through similar interventions" (Herdman, 2014). Defining Characteristics contain these ND titles.

Subjective

Activity intolerance
Fatigue
Hopelessness

Objective

Bathing, dressing, feeding, or toileting self-care deficit
Decreased cardiac output
Imbalanced nutrition: less than body requirements
Impaired memory
Impaired physical mobility; impaired walking
Social isolation

Desired Outcomes/Evaluation Criteria—Client/Caregiver Will:

- Acknowledge the presence of factors affecting well-being.
- Identify corrective/adaptive measures for individual situation.
- Demonstrate behaviors/lifestyle changes necessary to enhance functional status.

Client Will:

Look to the future, expressing a sense of control.

Actions/Interventions

Refer to NDs Activity Intolerance; risk-prone Health Behavior; chronic Confusion; ineffective Coping; impaired Dentition; risk for Falls; Grieving; Loneliness; imbalanced Nutrition: less than body requirements; Relocation Stress Syndrome; Self-Care Deficit (specify); chronic low Self-Esteem; risk for Spiritual Distress; ineffective Health Management, as appropriate, for additional relevant interventions.

Information that appears in brackets has been added by the authors to clarify and enhance the use of nursing diagnoses.

Nursing Priority No. 1.

To identify causative/contributing **or risk** factors:

- Identify the presence of "frailty syndrome (FS)." **This is demonstrated in an elderly person by three or more symptoms together: unintentional weight loss (10 or more pounds within the past year), muscle loss and weakness, a feeling of fatigue, slow walking speed, and low levels of physical activity. Note: The presence of FS is a predictor for hospitalization, disability, decreasing mobility, falls, and even death.**
- Note the individual's age and gender. **Chances of frailty rise after age 85. Women are more likely than men to be frail, possibly because women typically start out with less muscle mass than men.**
- Note the presence of physical complaints (e.g., fatigue/exhaustion, unintentional weight loss, muscle weakness, slow walking, inability to participate in usual physical activities) and the presence of conditions (e.g., heart disease, undetected diabetes mellitus, dementia, stroke, renal failure, long-term period of being bedridden, or terminal conditions). **Note: These factors associated with frailty may or may not be recognized by the client, but may be reported or documented by others.**
- Evaluate the medication regimen. **Medications that cause electrolyte imbalances (e.g., diuretics) can exacerbate weakness. Drugs that slow reaction time (e.g., sedatives and antidepressants) can interfere with balance and coordination, as can alcohol.**
- Determine nutritional status. **Malnutrition (e.g., weight loss, laboratory abnormalities, and identified micronutrient deficiencies) and factors contributing to failure to eat (e.g., chronic nausea, loss of appetite, no access to food or cooking, poorly fitting dentures, no one with whom to share meals, depression, and financial problems) greatly impact health status and quality of life.**
- Assess the client's physical and cognitive status **to identify tolerance for activity and/or self-care.**
- Note the client's living situation (e.g., lives alone or lives in a facility). **This helps identify environmental risk factors such as risk for falls, problem with food shopping or preparation, depression, and so on.**
- Evaluate the client's level of adaptive behavior and client/caregiver knowledge and skills about health maintenance, environment, and safety **in order to instruct, intervene, and refer appropriately.**

Information that appears in brackets has been added by the authors to clarify and enhance the use of nursing diagnoses.

- Review with the client/SO previous and current life situations, including role changes, multiple losses (e.g., death of loved ones, change in living arrangements, finances, and independence), social isolation, and grieving **to identify psychological stressors that may be affecting the current situation.**
- Ascertain safety of the home environment and persons providing care **to identify the potential for/presence of neglectful or abusive situations and/or need for referrals.**

Nursing Priority No. 2.

To assess degree of impairment:

- Collaborate with multidisciplinary team to determine the severity of the client's limitations. **Testing may occur over a period of time to identify functional and/or nutritional deficits, and may include blood work, physical therapy evaluation, and nutritional studies. Note: Studies have associated certain laboratory indicators with frailty, including (but not limited to) anemia, inflammation, and clotting factors.**
- Perform nutritional screening and/or refer for comprehensive nutritional assessment. **Studies show that a person may have weight and muscle loss (sarcopenia) or weight gain/obesity with muscle function impairment and loss of strength (sarcopenic obesity).**

Nursing Priority No. 3.

To assist client to achieve **or maintain** general well-being:

- Assist with treatment of underlying comorbid medical, functional, cognitive, or psychiatric conditions **that could positively influence the current situation (e.g., resolution of infection, treating anemia, addressing brain injury, delirium, social isolation, or depression).**
- Develop a plan of action with the client/caregiver **to meet immediate needs for nutrition, safety, and self-care and facilitate implementation of actions.**
- Administer medications as appropriate. **Studies show that optimized management of congestive heart failure and chronic pulmonary disease, or improved glycemic control of diabetes results in improved health status, fewer hospitalizations, and reductions in the physical declines associated with the frailty syndrome.**
- Refer to dietitian or nutritionist **to assist in planning meals to meet client's specific nutritional needs (e.g., calories, proteins, vitamins, micronutrients), taste, and abilities.**

Information that appears in brackets has been added by the authors to clarify and enhance the use of nursing diagnoses.

(Refer to ND imbalanced Nutrition: less than body requirements for additional interventions.)

- Refer to physical and/or occupational therapist as indicated **to improve physical strength, endurance, and stamina. Note: Studies have supported that exercises (e.g., chair aerobics, stretching, resistance training, walking, Tai chi) can improve balance, muscle, and core strength, promoting physical function and endurance, and reducing the risk of falls.**
- Discuss individual concerns about feelings of loss/loneliness and the relationship between these feelings and a current decline in well-being. Note desire or willingness to change situation. **Motivation or lack thereof can impede—or facilitate—achieving desired outcomes.**
- Explore mental strengths and successful coping skills the individual has previously used and apply to current situation. Refine or develop new strategies, as appropriate. **Incorporating these into problem-solving builds on past successes.**
- Assist the client to develop goals for dealing with life or illness situation. Involve the SO in long-range planning. **This promotes commitment to goals and plan, thereby maximizing outcomes.**

Nursing Priority No. 4.

To promote wellness **and reduce risks** (Teaching/Discharge Considerations):

- Assist client/SO(s) to identify and/or access useful community resources (e.g., support groups, Meals on Wheels, social worker, home care or assistive care, placement services). **This enhances coping, assists with problem-solving, and may reduce risks to client and caregiver.**
- Encourage the client to talk about positive aspects of life and to keep as physically active as possible **to reduce the effects of dispiritedness (e.g., "feeling low," sense of being unimportant, disconnected).**
- Promote socialization within individual limitations **to provide additional stimulation and reduce sense of isolation.**
- Offer opportunities to discuss life goals and support the client/SO in setting/attaining new goals for this time in his or her life **to enhance hope for the future.**
- Help the client explore reasons for living or begin to deal with end-of-life issues and provide support for grieving. **This enhances hope and sense of control, providing opportunity for client to take charge of his or her own future.**

Information that appears in brackets has been added by the authors to clarify and enhance the use of nursing diagnoses.

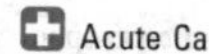

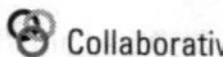

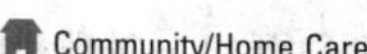

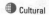

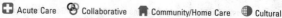

- Assist the client/SO/family to understand that frailty commonly occurs near the end of life and cannot always be reversed.
- Discuss appropriateness of and refer to palliative services or hospice care, as indicated.
- Refer to pastoral care, counseling, or psychotherapy **for grief work or other issues as needed.**

Documentation Focus

Assessment/Reassessment

- Individual findings, including current weight, dietary pattern, food and eating, perceptions of self, motivation for loss, support and feedback from SOs
- Perception of losses or life changes
- Ability to perform ADLs, participate in care, meet own needs
- Motivation for change, support and feedback from SO(s)

Planning

- Plan of care, specific interventions, and who is involved in planning
- Teaching plan

Implementation/Evaluation

- Responses to interventions and actions performed, general well-being, weekly weight
- Attainment or progress toward desired outcome(s)
- Modifications to plan of care

Discharge Planning

- Long-term needs and who is responsible for actions to be taken
- Community resources and support groups
- Specific referrals made

impaired GAS EXCHANGE

[Diagnostic Division: Respiration]

Definition: Excess or deficit in oxygenation and/or carbon dioxide elimination at the alveolar-capillary membrane. [This may be an entity of its own, but it also may be an end result of other pathology with an interrelatedness between airway clearance and/or breathing pattern problems.]

Information that appears in brackets has been added by the authors to clarify and enhance the use of nursing diagnoses.

Related Factors

Ventilation-perfusion imbalance [as in altered blood flow, such as pulmonary embolus or increased vascular resistance; heart failure; hypovolemic shock]

Alveolar-capillary membrane changes [e.g., acute respiratory distress syndrome; chronic conditions, such as restrictive/obstructive lung disease, pneumoconiosis, asbestosis or silicosis]

[Altered oxygen supply (e.g., altitude sickness)]

[Altered oxygen-carrying capacity of blood (e.g., sickle cell or other anemia, carbon monoxide poisoning)]

Defining Characteristics

Subjective

Dyspnea
Visual disturbance
Headache upon awakening
[Sense of impending doom]

Objective

Confusion
Restlessness; irritability
Somnolence

Abnormal arterial blood gases (ABGs)/arterial pH; hypoxia/hypoxemia; hypercapnia; decrease in carbon dioxide (CO_2) level

Cyanosis; abnormal skin color (e.g., pale, dusky, cyanosis)

Abnormal breathing pattern (e.g., rate, rhythm, depth); nasal flaring

Tachycardia; [dysrhythmias]
Diaphoresis
[Polycythemia]

Desired Outcomes/Evaluation Criteria—Client Will:

- Demonstrate improved ventilation and adequate oxygenation of tissues by ABGs within client's usual parameters and absence of symptoms of respiratory distress (as noted in Defining Characteristics).
- Verbalize understanding of causative factors and appropriate interventions.

Information that appears in brackets has been added by the authors to clarify and enhance the use of nursing diagnoses.

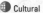

- Participate in treatment regimen (e.g., breathing exercises, effective coughing, use of oxygen) within level of ability or situation.

Actions/Interventions

Nursing Priority No. 1.

To assess causative/contributing factors:

- Note the presence of factors listed in Related Factors. Refer to NDs ineffective Airway Clearance; ineffective Breathing Pattern, as appropriate. **Gas exchange problems can be related to multiple factors, including anemias, anesthesia, surgical procedures, high altitude, allergic response, altered level of consciousness, anxiety, fear, aspiration, decreased lung compliance, excessive or thick secretions, immobility, infection, medication and drug toxicity or overdose, neuromuscular impairment of breathing pattern, pain, and smoking.**

Nursing Priority No. 2.

To evaluate degree of compromise:

- Note respiratory rate, depth, use of accessory muscles, pursed-lip breathing; areas of pallor/cyanosis, such as peripheral (nailbeds) versus central (circumoral) or general duskiness. **This provides insight into the work of breathing and adequacy of alveolar ventilation. Tachypnea is usually present to some degree during illness (especially with fever or upper respiratory infections), but if tachypnea is accompanied by use of accessory muscles of inspiration (e.g., external intercostals), the client may have insufficient muscle strength to sustain the work of breathing.**
- Auscultate breath sounds, note areas of decreased/adventitious breath sounds as well as fremitus. **In this nursing diagnosis, ventilatory effort is insufficient to deliver enough oxygen or to get rid of sufficient amounts of carbon dioxide. Abnormal breath sounds are indicative of numerous problems (e.g., hypoventilation such as might occur with atelectasis or presence of secretions, improper endotracheal (ET) tube placement, or collapsed lung) and must be evaluated for further intervention.**
- Note the character and effectiveness of the cough mechanism. **This affects the ability to clear airways of secretions.**
- Assess level of consciousness and mentation changes. **A decreased level of consciousness can be an indirect mea-**

Information that appears in brackets has been added by the authors to clarify and enhance the use of nursing diagnoses.

surement of impaired oxygenation, but it also impairs one's ability to protect the airway, potentially further adversely affecting oxygenation.

- Note client reports of somnolence, restlessness, and headache on arising. Assess energy level and activity tolerance, noting reports or evidence of fatigue, weakness, and problems with sleep **that are associated with diminished oxygenation.**
- Monitor vital signs and cardiac rhythm. **All vital signs are impacted by changes in oxygenation.**
- Evaluate pulse oximetry and capnography **to determine oxygenation and levels of carbon dioxide retention;** evaluate lung volumes and forced vital capacity **to assess lung mechanics, capacities, and function.**
- Review other pertinent laboratory data (e.g., ABGs, complete blood count (CBC)); chest x-rays.
- Note effect of illness on self-esteem and body image.

Nursing Priority No. 3.

To correct/improve existing deficiencies:

- Elevate the head of the bed and position the client appropriately. **Elevation or upright position facilitates respiratory function by gravity; however, a client in severe distress will seek a position of comfort.**
- Provide airway adjuncts and suction, as indicated, **to clear or maintain open airway, when client is unable to clear secretions, or to improve gas diffusion when client is showing desaturation of oxygen by oximetry or ABGs.**
- Encourage frequent position changes and deep-breathing and coughing exercises. Use incentive spirometer, chest physiotherapy, intermittent positive-pressure breathing, as indicated. **This promotes optimal chest expansion, mobilization of secretions, and oxygen diffusion.**
- Provide supplemental oxygen at lowest concentration indicated by laboratory results and client symptoms or situation.
- Monitor for carbon dioxide narcosis (e.g., change in level of consciousness, changes in O_2 and CO_2 blood gas levels, flushing, decreased respiratory rate, and headaches), **which may occur in a client receiving long-term oxygen therapy.**
- Maintain adequate input and output **for mobilization of secretions,** but avoid fluid overload.
- Use sedation judiciously **to avoid depressant effects on respiratory functioning.**
- Ensure the availability of proper emergency equipment, including ET/tracheostomy set and suction catheters appropriate for age and size of infant, child, or adult.

Information that appears in brackets has been added by the authors to clarify and enhance the use of nursing diagnoses.

- Avoid the use of a face mask in an elderly emaciated client **as oxygen can leak out around the mask because of poor fit, and mask can increase client's agitation.**
- Encourage adequate rest and limit activities to within client tolerance. Promote a calm, restful environment. **This helps limit oxygen needs and consumption.**
- Provide psychological support, and active-listen questions/ concerns **to reduce anxiety.**
- Administer medications as indicated (e.g., inhaled and systemic glucocorticosteroids, antibiotics, bronchodilators, methylxanthines, antitussives/mucolytics, and vasodilators). **Pharmacological agents are varied, specific to the client, but generally used to prevent and control symptoms, reduce frequency and severity of exacerbations, and improve exercise tolerance.**
- Monitor and instruct client in therapeutic and adverse effects as well as interactions of drug therapy.
- Minimize blood loss from procedures (e.g., tests or hemodialysis) **to limit adverse affects of anemia.**
- Assist with procedures as individually indicated (e.g., transfusion, phlebotomy, or bronchoscopy) **to improve respiratory function/oxygen-carrying capacity.**
- Monitor and adjust ventilator settings (e.g., fractional concentration of inspired oxygen, tidal volume, inspiratory/ expiratory ratio, sigh, and positive end-expiratory pressure), as indicated, when mechanical support is being used.
- Keep environment allergen and pollutant free **to reduce irritant effect of dust and chemicals on airways.**

Nursing Priority No. 4.

To promote wellness (Teaching/Discharge Considerations):

- Review risk factors, particularly environmental/employment related, **to promote prevention or management of risk.**
- Discuss implications of smoking related to the illness or condition at each visit. Encourage client and SO(s) to stop smoking; recommend smoking cessation programs **to reduce health risks and/or prevent further decline in lung function.**
- Discuss reasons for allergy testing when indicated.
- Review individual drug regimen and ways of dealing with side effects.
- Instruct in the use of relaxation, stress-reduction techniques, as appropriate.
- Reinforce the need for adequate rest, while encouraging activity and exercise (e.g., upper and lower extremity strength

Information that appears in brackets has been added by the authors to clarify and enhance the use of nursing diagnoses.

and flexibility training, and endurance) **to decrease dyspnea and improve quality of life.**
- Emphasize the importance of nutrition **in improving stamina and reducing the work of breathing.**
- Review oxygen-conserving techniques (e.g., sitting instead of standing to perform tasks; eating small meals; performing slower, purposeful movements).
- Review job description and work activities **to identify need for job modifications or vocational rehabilitation.**
- Discuss home oxygen therapy and safety measures, as indicated, when home oxygen is implemented **to ensure client's safety, especially when used in the very young, fragile elderly, or when cognitive or neuromuscular impairment is present.**
- Identify and refer to specific suppliers for supplemental oxygen/necessary respiratory devices, as well as other individually appropriate resources, such as home care agencies, Meals on Wheels, and so on, **to facilitate independence.**

Documentation Focus

Assessment/Reassessment
- Assessment findings, including respiratory rate, character of breath sounds; frequency, amount, and appearance of secretions; presence of cyanosis; laboratory findings; and mentation level
- Conditions that may interfere with oxygen supply

Planning
- Plan of care, specific interventions, and who is involved in the planning
- Ventilator settings, liters of supplemental oxygen
- Teaching plan

Implementation/Evaluation
- Client's responses to treatment, teaching, and actions performed
- Attainment or progress toward desired outcome(s)
- Modifications to plan of care

Discharge Planning
- Long-term needs, identifying who is responsible for actions to be taken

Information that appears in brackets has been added by the authors to clarify and enhance the use of nursing diagnoses.

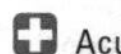
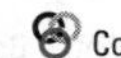
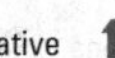
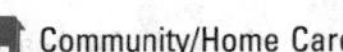
 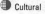

- Community resources for equipment and supplies post discharge
- Specific referrals made

Sample Nursing Outcomes & Interventions Classifications (NOC/NIC)

NOC—Respiratory Status: Gas Exchange
NIC—Respiratory Monitoring

dysfunctional GASTROINTESTINAL MOTILITY and risk for dysfunctional GASTROINTESTINAL MOTILITY

[Diagnostic Division: Elimination]

Definition: dysfunctional Gastrointestinal Motility: Increased, decreased, ineffective, or lack of peristaltic activity within the gastrointestinal system.

Definition: risk for dysfunctional Gastrointestinal Motility: Vulnerable to a decrease in normal frequency of defecation accompanied by difficult or incomplete passage of stool, which may compromise health.

Related Factors (dysfunctional Gastrointestinal Motility)

Aging; prematurity
Anxiety
Enteral feedings; treatment regimen
Food intolerance [e.g., gluten, lactose]; malnutrition
Immobility; sedentary lifestyle
Ingestion of contaminated material (e.g., radioactive, food, water)

Risk Factors

Aging; prematurity
Anxiety; stressors
Change in water source; unsanitary food preparation
Decrease in gastrointestinal circulation; gastroesophageal reflux disease; diabetes mellitus
Eating habit change (e.g., foods, eating times); food intolerance
Immobility; sedentary lifestyle
Pharmaceutical agent
Infection

Information that appears in brackets has been added by the authors to clarify and enhance the use of nursing diagnoses.

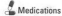

NOTE: A risk diagnosis is not evidenced by signs and symptoms, as the problem has not occurred; rather, nursing interventions are directed at prevention.

Defining Characteristics (dysfunctional Gastrointestinal Motility)

Subjective

Absence of flatus
Abdominal cramping; pain
Diarrhea
Difficulty with defecation
Nausea; regurgitation

Objective

Change in bowel sounds
Abdominal distention
Acceleration of gastric emptying; diarrhea
Increase in gastric residual; bile-colored gastric residual
Hard formed stool
Vomiting

Desired Outcomes/Evaluation Criteria—Client Will:

- Reestablish and maintain normal pattern of bowel functioning.
- Verbalize understanding of causative factors and rationale for treatment regimen.
- Demonstrate appropriate behaviors to assist with resolution of causative factors.

Actions/Interventions

Nursing Priority No. 1.

To assess causative/contributing **or risk** factors:

- Note the presence of conditions (e.g., congestive heart failure, major trauma, chronic conditions, or sepsis) affecting systemic circulation/perfusion **that can result in gastrointestinal (GI) hypoperfusion, and short- and/or long-term gastrointestinal (GI) dysfunction.**
- Determine the presence of disorders causing localized or diffuse reduction in GI blood flow, such as esophageal varices, GI hemorrhage, pancreatitis, or intraperitoneal hemorrhage,

Information that appears in brackets has been added by the authors to clarify and enhance the use of nursing diagnoses.

to identify a client at higher risk for ineffective tissue perfusion.

- Note the presence of chronic/long-term disorders, such as gastrointestinal reflux disease (GERD), hiatal hernia, inflammatory bowel (e.g., ulcerative colitis, Crohn's disease), malabsorption (e.g., dumping syndrome, celiac disease), short-bowel syndrome, as may occur after surgical removal of portions of the small intestine. **These conditions are associated with increased, decreased, or ineffective peristaltic activity.**
- Note the client's age and developmental concerns. **Premature or low-birth-weight neonates are at risk for developing necrotizing enterocolitis (NEC). Children are prone to infections causing gastroenteritis manifested by vomiting and diarrhea. The elderly have problems associated with decreased motility, such as constipation.**
- Note lifestyle (e.g., people who regularly engage in competitive sports such as long-distance running, cycling; persons with poor sanitary living conditions; people who travel to areas with contaminated food or water; overeating or intake of foods associated with gastric distress). **These are issues that can affect gastrointestional function and health.**
- Ascertain whether the client is experiencing anxiety; acute, extreme, or chronic stress; or other psychogenic factors present in a person with emotional or psychiatric disorders (including anorexia/bulimia, etc.) **that can affect interest in eating, and ability to ingest and digest food.**
- Review the client's medication regimen. **Medications (e.g., laxatives, antibiotics, opiates, sedatives, and iron preparations) may cause or exacerbate intestinal issues. In addition, the likelihood of bleeding increases from the use of medications such as nonsteroidal anti-inflammatory agents (NSAIDs), Coumadin, and Plavix.**
- Review laboratory and other diagnostic studies **to evaluate for GI problems, such as bleeding, inflammation, toxicity, and infection; or to help identify masses, dilation/obstruction, abnormal stool and gas patterns, and so forth.**

Nursing Priority No. 2.

To note degree of dysfunction **or risk for** organ involvement:

- Assess vital signs, noting presence of low blood pressure, elevated heart rate, and fever. **This may suggest hypoperfusion or developing sepsis. Fever in the presence of bright red blood in stool may indicate ischemic colitis.**

Information that appears in brackets has been added by the authors to clarify and enhance the use of nursing diagnoses.

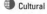

- Ascertain the presence of and characteristics of abdominal pain. **Pain is a common symptom of GI disorders and can vary in location, duration, and intensity. Note: Tension pain caused by organ distention may develop in the presence of bowel obstruction, constipation, or accumulation of pus or fluid. Inflammatory pain is deep and initially poorly localized, caused by irritation of either the visceral or the parietal peritoneum, as in acute appendicitis. Ischemic pain, the most serious type of visceral pain, has sudden onset, is intense, if progressive in severity, and is not relieved by analgesics.**
- Inspect the abdomen, noting contour. **Distention of bowel may indicate accumulation of fluids (salivary, gastric, pancreatic, biliary, and intestinal) and gases formed from bacteria, swallowed air, or any food or fluid the client has consumed.**
- Auscultate abdomen. **Hypoactive bowel sounds may indicate ileus. Hyperactive bowels sounds may indicate early intestinal obstruction or irritable bowel or GI bleeding.**
- Palpate abdomen **to note masses, enlarged organs (such as spleen, liver, or portions of colon); elicitation of pain with touch; and pulsation of aorta.**
- Measure abdominal girth and compare with the client's customary waist size or belt length **to monitor development or progression of distention.**
- Note frequency and characteristics of bowel movements. **Bowel movements by themselves are not necessarily diagnostic, but they need to be considered in total assessment as they may reveal an underlying problem or effect of pathology.**
- Note the presence of nausea, with or without vomiting, and relationship to food intake or other events, if indicated. **History can provide important information about cause (e.g., pregnancy, gastroenteritis, cancers, myocardial infarction, hepatitis, systemic infections, contaminated food, drug toxicity, or eating disorders).**
- Evaluate the client's current nutritional status, noting the ability to ingest and digest food. **Health depends on the intake, digestion, and absorption of nutrients, which both affect and are affected by GI function.**
- Measure intra-abdominal pressure as indicated. **Tissue edema or free fluid collecting in the abdominal cavity leads to intra-abdominal hypertension, which if untreated, can cause abdominal compartment syndrome with end-stage organ failure.**

Information that appears in brackets has been added by the authors to clarify and enhance the use of nursing diagnoses.

Nursing Priority No. 3.

To **reduce risks** or /improve existing dysfunction:

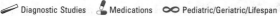

- Collaborate in treatment of underlying conditions **to correct or treat disorders associated with client's current GI dysfunction.**
- Maintain GI rest when indicated—nothing by mouth (NPO), fluids only, or gastric or intestinal decompression **to reduce intestinal bloating and risk of vomiting.**
- Administer prescribed prophylactic medications **to reduce the potential for GI complications such as bleeding, ulceration of stomach mucosa, and viral diarrheas.**
- Administer fluids and electrolytes as indicated **to replace losses and to improve GI circulation and function.**
- Collaborate with dietitian or nutritionist **to provide diet sufficient in nutrients by best possible route—oral, enteral, or parenteral.**
- Emphasize the importance of and assist with early ambulation, especially following surgery, **to stimulate peristalsis and help reduce GI complications associated with immobility.**
- Encourage the client to report changes in nature or intensity of pain, **as this may indicate worsening of condition, requiring more intensive interventions.**
- Encourage relaxation and distraction techniques **if anxiety is suspected to play a role in GI dysfunction.**
- Manage pain with medications as ordered, and nonpharmacological interventions such as positioning, back rub, or heating pad (unless contraindicated) **to enhance muscle relaxation and reduce discomfort.**
- Prepare the client for procedures and surgery, as indicated. **This may require a variety of interventions to treat the problem causing or contributing to severe GI dysfunction.**

Nursing Priority No. 4.

To promote wellness (Teaching/Discharge Considerations):

- Discuss normal variations in bowel patterns **to help alleviate unnecessary concern, initiate planned interventions, or seek timely medical care. This may prevent overuse of laxatives or help the client understand when food, fluid, or drug modifications are needed.**
- Review measures to maintain bowel health:

  Use dietary fiber and/or stool softeners.

  Ensure fluid intake is appropriate to individual.

Information that appears in brackets has been added by the authors to clarify and enhance the use of nursing diagnoses.

Establish or maintain regular bowel evacuation habits, incorporating privacy needs, assistance to bathroom on regular schedule, and so forth, as indicated.

Emphasize the benefits of regular exercise in promoting normal GI function.

- Discuss dietary recommendations with client/SO. **The client may elect to make adaptations in food choices and eating habits to avoid GI complications.**
- Instruct in healthier variations in preparation of foods, as indicated, **when these factors may affect GI health.**
- Recommend maintenance of normal weight, or weight loss if client obese, **to decrease risk associated with GI disorders such as GERD or gallbladder disease.**
- Discuss fluid intake appropriate to individual situation. **Water is necessary to general health and GI function; client may need encouragement to increase intake or to make appropriate fluid choices if intake restricted for certain medical conditions.**
- Collaborate with physician in medication management. **Dose modification, discontinuation of certain drugs (e.g., laxatives, opioids, antidepressants, or iron supplements), or alternative route of administration may be required to reduce risk of GI dysfunction.**
- Emphasize importance of discussing with physician current and new prescribed medications, and/or planned use of certain medications (e.g., NSAIDs, including aspirin; corticosteroids, some over-the-counter (OTC) drugs, and herbal supplements) **that can be harmful to GI mucosa.**
- Encourage discussion of feelings regarding prognosis and long-term effects of condition. **Major or unplanned life changes can strain coping abilities, impairing functioning and jeopardizing relationships, and may even result in depression.**
- Discuss the value of relaxation and distraction techniques or counseling **if anxiety or other emotional/psychiatric issue is suspected to play a role in GI dysfunction.**
- Recommend smoking cessation. **Studies have shown various deleterious short- and long-term effects of smoking on the GI circulation and organs. Smoking is a risk factor for acquiring or exacerbating certain GI disorders such as Crohn's disease.**
- Review foodborne and waterborne illnesses, contamination and hygiene issues, as indicated, and make needed follow-up referrals.

Information that appears in brackets has been added by the authors to clarify and enhance the use of nursing diagnoses.

- Refer to appropriate resources (e.g., Social Services, Public Health Services) **for follow-up if client is at risk for ingestion of contaminated water or food sources or would benefit from teaching concerning food preparation and storage.**
- Recommend and/or refer to physician for vaccines as indicated. **The Centers for Disease Control and Prevention (CDC) make recommendations for travelers and/or persons in high-risk areas or situations in which person might be exposed to contaminated food or water.**
- Refer to NDs bowel Incontinence; Constipation; Diarrhea, for additional interventions.

Documentation Focus

Assessment/Reassessment

- Individual findings, noting specific risk factors; or nature, extent, and duration of problem, effect on independence and lifestyle
- Dietary pattern, recent intake, food intolerances
- Frequency and characteristics of stools
- Characteristics of abdominal tenderness or pain, precipitators, and what relieves pain

Planning

- Plan of care and who is involved in planning
- Teaching plan

Implementation/Evaluation

- Response to interventions, teaching, and actions performed
- Attainment or progress toward desired outcome(s)
- Modifications to plan of care

Discharge Planning

- Long-term needs and who is responsible for actions to be taken
- Available resources, specific referrals made

Sample Nursing Outcomes & Interventions Classifications (NOC/NIC)

NOC—Gastrointestinal Function
NIC—Bowel Management

Information that appears in brackets has been added by the authors to clarify and enhance the use of nursing diagnoses.

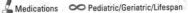

risk for ineffective GASTROINTESTINAL PERFUSION

[Diagnostic Division: Circulation]

Definition: Vulnerable to decrease in gastrointestinal circulation, which may compromise health.

Risk Factors

Abdominal aortic aneurysm; abdominal compartment syndrome
Abnormal prothrombin time (PT); abnormal partial thromboplastin time (PTT); coagulopathy (e.g., sickle sell anemia); anemia; disseminated intravascular coagulopathy; hemodynamic instability
Age > 60 years; female gender
Cerebral vascular accident; vascular disease; diabetes mellitus
Gastrointestinal condition (e.g., ulcer, ischemic colitis or pancreatitis); acute gastrointestinal hemorrhage; gastroesophageal varicies
Impaired liver function (e.g., cirrhosis, hepatitis);
Myocardial infarction; decrease in left ventricular performance
Renal disease (e.g., polycystic kidney, renal artery stenosis, failure)
Smoking
Trauma; treatment regimen

NOTE: A risk diagnosis is not evidenced by signs and symptoms, as the problem has not occurred; rather, nursing interventions are directed at prevention.

Desired Outcomes/Evaluation Criteria—Client Will:

- Demonstrate adequate tissue perfusion as evidenced by active bowel sounds; absence of abdominal pain, nausea, and vomiting
- Verbalize understanding of condition, therapy regimen, side effects of medication, and when to contact healthcare provider.
- Engage in behaviors and lifestyle changes to improve circulation.

Information that appears in brackets has been added by the authors to clarify and enhance the use of nursing diagnoses.

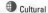

Actions/Interventions

Nursing Priority No. 1.

To identify individual risk factors/needs:

- Note the presence of conditions affecting systemic circulation and perfusion such as heart failure with left ventricular dysfunction, major trauma with blood loss and hypotension, septic shock, and so forth. **Blood loss and hypovolemic or hypotensive shock can result in GI hypoperfusion and bowel ischemia.**
- Determine the presence of disorders such as esophageal varices, pancreatitis; abdominal or chest trauma, increase of intra-abdominal pressure; prior history of bowel obstruction or strangulated hernia, **which could cause local or regional reduction in GI blood flow.**
- Identify client with history of bleeding or coagulation disorders, such as prior GI bleed, coagulopathies; cancer, **to identify risk for potential bleeding problems.**
- ∞ Note the client's age and gender when assessing for impaired GI perfusion **(e.g., studies suggest that risk for GI bleeding increases with age in both sexes, but that risk for abdominal aortic aneurysm is higher in men than in women). Premature or low-birth-weight neonates are at risk for developing necrotizing enterocolitis (NEC).**
- Investigate reports of abdominal pain, noting location, intensity, and duration. **Many disorders can result in abdominal pain, some of which can include conditions affecting GI perfusion such as postprandial abdominal angina due to occlusive mesenteric vascular disease, abdominal compartment syndrome, or other potential perforating disorders such as duodenal or gastric ulcer, or ischemic pancreatitis.**
- Review routine medication regimen (e.g., NSAIDs, Coumadin, low-dose aspirin such as used for prophylaxis in certain cardiovascular conditions, and corticosteroids). **The likelihood of bleeding increases from use of these medications.**
- Note history of smoking, **which can potentiate vasoconstriction; or excessive alcohol use/abuse, which can cause general inflammation of the stomach mucosa and potentiate risk of GI bleeding; or liver involvement and esophageal varices.**
- Auscultate abdomen to evaluate peristaltic activity. **Hypoactive or absent bowel sounds may indicate intraperito-**

Information that appears in brackets has been added by the authors to clarify and enhance the use of nursing diagnoses.

neal injury, bowel perforation, and bleeding. Abdominal bruit can indicate abdominal aortic injury or aneurysm.

- Palpate abdomen for distention, masses, enlarged organs (such as spleen, liver, or portions of colon); elicitation of pain with touch; pulsation of aorta.
- Percuss abdomen for fixed or shifting dullness over regions that normally contain air. **This can indicate accumulated blood or fluid.**
- Measure and monitor progression of abdominal girth as indicated. **This can reflect bowel problems such as obstruction, or organ failure (e.g., heart, liver, or kidney) or organ injury with intra-abdominal fluid and gas accumulation.**
- Note reports of nausea or vomiting accompanied by problems with bowel elimination. **May reflect hypoperfusion of the GI tract, which is particularly vulnerable to even small decreases in circulating volume.**
- Assess the client with severe or prolonged vomiting, or forceful coughing, engaging in lifting or straining activities or childbirth, **which can result in a tear in the esophageal or stomach wall, resulting in hemorrhage.**
- Evaluate stool color and consistency. Test for occult blood, as indicated. **If bleeding is present, stools may be black or "tarry," currant-colored, or bright red. Consistency can range from normal with occult blood to thick liquid stools.**
- Test gastric suction contents for blood when the tube is used to decompress stomach and/or manage vomiting.
- Assess vital signs, noting sustained hypotension, **which can result in hypoperfusion of abdominal organs.**
- Review laboratory and other diagnostic studies (e.g., complete blood count [CBC], bilirubin, liver enzymes, electrolytes, stool guaiac; endoscopy, abdominal ultrasound or computed tomography [CT] scan, aortic angiography, paracentesis) **to identify any conditions or disorders that may affect GI perfusion and function.**
- Measure intra-abdominal pressure as indicated. **Tissue edema or free fluid collecting in the abdominal cavity leads to intra-abdominal hypertension, which if untreated can cause abdominal compartment syndrome with end-stage organ failure.**

Nursing Priority No. 2.

To reduce or correct individual risk factors:

- Collaborate in the treatment of underlying conditions **to correct or treat disorders that could affect GI perfusion.**

Information that appears in brackets has been added by the authors to clarify and enhance the use of nursing diagnoses.

- Administer fluids and electrolytes as indicated **to replace losses and to maintain GI circulation and cellular function.**
- Administer prescribed prophylactic medications in at-risk clients during illness and hospitalization (e.g., anti-emetics, proton pump inhibitors, antihistamines, anticholinergics, and antibiotics) **to reduce the potential for stress-related GI complications.**
- Maintain gastric or intestinal decompression, when indicated; measure output periodically, and note characteristics of drainage.
- Provide small, easily digested food and fluids when oral intake is tolerated.
- Encourage rest after meals **to maximize blood flow to the digestive system.**
- Prepare the client for surgery as indicated, such as gastric resection, bypass graft, or mesenteric endarterectomy.
- Refer to NDs dysfunctional Gastrointestinal Motility; risk for Bleeding; Nausea; imbalanced Nutrition: less than body requirements, for additional interventions.

Nursing Priority No. 3.

To promote wellness (Teaching/Discharge Considerations):

- Discuss individual risk factors (e.g., family history, obesity, age, smoking, hypertension, diabetes, and clotting disorders) and potential outcomes of atherosclerosis (e.g., systemic and peripheral vascular disease conditions), as appropriate. **This is information necessary for the client to make informed choices about remedial risk factors and commit to lifestyle changes.**
- Identify necessary changes in lifestyle and assist client to incorporate disease management into activities of daily living (ADLs).
- Encourage the client to quit smoking, join Smoke-out or other smoking-cessation programs, **to reduce the risk of vasoconstriction compromising GI perfusion.**
- Establish a regular exercise program **to enhance circulation and promote general well-being.**
- Emphasize the importance of routine follow-up and laboratory monitoring as indicated. **This is important for effective disease management and possible changes in therapeutic regimen.**
- Emphasize the importance of discussing with primary care provider current and new prescribed medications, and/or planned use of certain medications (e.g., anticoagulants,

---

Information that appears in brackets has been added by the authors to clarify and enhance the use of nursing diagnoses.

NSAIDs including aspirin; corticosteroids, some over-the-counter drugs, and herbal supplements), **which can be harmful to GI mucosa or cause bleeding.**

Documentation Focus

Assessment/Reassessment

- Individual findings, noting specific risk factors
- Vital signs, adequacy of circulation
- Abdominal assessment, characteristics of emesis or gastric drainage and stools

Planning

- Plan of care and who is involved in planning
- Teaching plan

Implementation/Evaluation

- Response to interventions, teaching, and actions performed
- Attainment or progress toward desired outcome(s)
- Modifications to plan of care

Discharge Planning

- Long-term needs and who is responsible for actions to be taken
- Available resources, specific referrals made

Sample Nursing Outcomes & Interventions Classifications (NOC/NIC)

NOC—Tissue Perfusion: Abdominal Organs
NIC—Surveillance

GRIEVING

[Diagnostic Division: Ego Integrity]

Definition: A normal complex process that includes emotional, physical, spiritual, social, and intellectual responses and behaviors by which individuals, families, and communities incorporate an actual, anticipated, or perceived loss into their daily lives.

Related Factors

Anticipatory loss or loss of significant object (e.g., possession, job, status, home, body part)
Anticipatory loss or death of significant other

Information that appears in brackets has been added by the authors to clarify and enhance the use of nursing diagnoses.

Defining Characteristics

Subjective

Anger; pain; suffering; despair; blaming
Alteration in activity level, sleep pattern, dream patterns
Finding meaning in a loss; personal growth
Guilt about feeling relief

Objective

Detachment; disorganization; psychological distress; panic behavior
Maintaining a connection to the deceased
Alterations in immune or neuroendocrine functioning

Desired Outcomes/Evaluation Criteria—Client/Family Will:

- Identify and express feelings (e.g., sadness, guilt, fear) freely and effectively.
- Acknowledge impact or effect of the grieving process (e.g., physical problems of eating, sleeping) and seek appropriate help.
- Look toward and plan for future, one day at a time.

Community Will:

- Recognize the needs of the citizens, including underserved population.
- Activate or develop a plan to address identified needs.

Actions/Interventions

Nursing Priority No. 1.

To identify causative/contributing factors:

- Determine circumstances of current situation (e.g., sudden death, prolonged fatal illness, or loved one kept alive by extreme medical interventions). **Grief can be anticipatory (e.g., mourning the loss of a loved one's former self before actual death) or actual. Both types of grief can provoke a wide range of intense and often conflicting feelings. Grief also follows losses other than death (e.g., traumatic loss of a limb, loss of home by a tornado, and loss of known self due to brain injury).**
- Evaluate the client's perception of anticipated or actual loss and meaning to him or her: "What are your concerns?" "What are your fears?" "What is your greatest fear?" "How do you see this affecting you or your lifestyle?"

Information that appears in brackets has been added by the authors to clarify and enhance the use of nursing diagnoses.

- Identify cultural or religious beliefs that may impact the sense of loss.
- Ascertain the response of the family/SO(s) to the client's situation and concerns.
- Determine significance of the loss to community (e.g., school bus accident with loss of life, major tornado damage to infrastructure, or financial failure of major employer).

Nursing Priority No. 2.

To determine current response:

- Note emotional responses, such as withdrawal, angry behavior, and crying.
- Observe the client's body language and check out meaning with the client. Note congruency with verbalizations.
- Note cultural and religious expectations that may dictate a client's responses **to assess appropriateness of client's reaction to the situation.**
- Identify problems with eating, activity level, sexual desire, and role performance (e.g., work and parenting). **These are indicators of severity of feelings client is experiencing and the need for specific interventions to address these issues.**
- Determine the impact on general well-being (e.g., increased frequency of minor illnesses or exacerbation of chronic condition).
- Note family communication and interaction patterns.
- Determine availability and use of community resources and support groups.
- Note community plans in place to deal with a major loss (e.g., team of crisis counselors stationed at a school to address the loss of classmates, vocational counselors or retraining programs, or outreach of services from neighboring communities).

Nursing Priority No. 3.

To assist client/community to deal with situation:

- Provide an open environment and a trusting relationship. **This promotes a free discussion of feelings and concerns.**
- Use therapeutic communication skills of active-listening, silence, and acknowledgment. Respect the client's desire/request not to talk.
- Inform children about death or anticipated loss in age-appropriate language. **Providing accurate information about impending loss or change in life situation will help the child begin the mourning process.**

Information that appears in brackets has been added by the authors to clarify and enhance the use of nursing diagnoses.

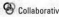

- Provide puppets or play therapy for toddlers and young children. **This may help them more readily express grief and deal with loss.**
- Permit appropriate expressions of anger and fear. Note hostility toward or feelings of abandonment by spiritual power. (Refer to appropriate NDs; e.g., Spiritual Distress.)
- Provide information about the normalcy of individual grief reaction.
- Be honest when answering questions and providing information. **This enhances the sense of trust and nurse-client relationship.**
- Provide assurance to the child that the cause for the situation is not his or her own doing, bearing in mind age and developmental level. **This may lessen the sense of guilt and affirm there is no need to assign blame to self or any family member.**
- Provide hope within the parameters of the specific situation. Refrain from giving false reassurance.
- Review past life experiences and previous loss(es), role changes, and coping skills, noting strengths and successes. **This may be useful in dealing with the current situation and problem solving existing needs.**
- Discuss control issues, such as what is in the power of the individual to change and what is beyond control. **Recognition of these factors helps the client focus energy for maximal benefit and outcome.**
- Incorporate family/SO(s) in problem solving. **This encourages the family to support and assist the client to deal with the situation while meeting the needs of family members.**
- Determine the client's status and role in family (e.g., parent, sibling, or child) and address loss of family member role.
- Instruct in use of visualization and relaxation techniques.
- Use sedatives or tranquilizers with caution. **This may retard passage through the grief process, although short-term use may be beneficial to enhance sleep.**
- Encourage community members or groups to engage in talking about the event or loss and verbalizing feelings. Seek out underserved populations to include in the process.
- Encourage individuals to participate in activities to deal with loss and rebuild community.

Nursing Priority No. 4.

To promote wellness (Teaching/Discharge Considerations):

- Give information that feelings are okay and are to be expressed appropriately. **Expression of feelings can facilitate**

Information that appears in brackets has been added by the authors to clarify and enhance the use of nursing diagnoses.

the grieving process, but destructive behavior can be damaging.

- Provide information that on birthdays, major holidays, at times of significant personal events, or anniversary of loss, client may experience (needs to be prepared for) intense grief reactions. **If these reactions start to disrupt day-to-day functioning, the client may need to seek help.** (Refer to NDs complicated Grieving; ineffective community Coping, as appropriate.)
- Encourage continuation of usual activities or schedule and involvement in appropriate exercise program.
- Identify and promote family and social support systems.
- Discuss and assist with planning for future or funeral, as appropriate.
- Refer to additional resources, such as pastoral care, counseling, psychotherapy, community or organized support groups (including hospice), as indicated, for both client and family/SO(s), **to meet ongoing needs and facilitate grief work.**
- Support community efforts to strengthen, support, or develop a plan to foster recovery and growth.

Documentation Focus

Assessment/Reassessment

- Assessment findings, including client's perception of anticipated loss and signs/symptoms that are being exhibited
- Responses of family/SO(s) or community members, as indicated
- Availability and use of resources

Planning

- Plan of care and who is involved in planning
- Teaching plan

Implementation/Evaluation

- Client's response to interventions, teaching, and actions performed
- Attainment or progress toward desired outcome(s)
- Modifications to plan of care

Discharge Planning

- Long-term needs and who is responsible for actions to be taken
- Specific referrals made

Information that appears in brackets has been added by the authors to clarify and enhance the use of nursing diagnoses.

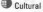

Sample Nursing Outcomes & Interventions Classifications (NOC/NIC)

NOC—Grief Resolution
NIC—Grief Work Facilitation

complicated GRIEVING

[Diagnostic Division: Ego Integrity]

Definition: A disorder that occurs after the death of a significant other, in which the experience of distress accompanying bereavement fails to follow normative expectations and manifests in functional impairment.

Related Factors

Death of significant other
Emotional instability; [loss of significant object (e.g., possessions, job, status, home, parts and processes of body)]
Insufficient social support

Defining Characteristics

Subjective

Anxiety; nonacceptance of a death; persistent painful memories; distress about the deceased person; self-blame
Anger, disbelief, mistrust
Feeling dazed, detachment from others, stunned, of emptiness, shock
Insufficient sense of well-being; fatigue; low levels of intimacy; depression
Yearning for deceased person

Objective

Decrease in functioning in life roles
Excessive stress; separation or traumatic distress
Preoccupation with thoughts about a deceased person; longing/searching for a deceased person
Experiencing symptoms the deceased experienced

Information that appears in brackets has been added by the authors to clarify and enhance the use of nursing diagnoses.

Rumination
Avoidance of grieving

Desired Outcomes/Evaluation Criteria—Client Will:

- Acknowledge presence and impact of dysfunctional situation.
- Demonstrate progress in dealing with stages of grief at own pace.
- Participate in work and self-care activities of daily living (ADLs) as able.
- Verbalize a sense of progress toward grief resolution, hope for the future.

Actions/Interventions

Nursing Priority No. 1.

To determine causative/contributing factors:

- Identify loss that is present. Note circumstances of death, such as sudden or traumatic (e.g., fatal accident, suicide, or homicide), related to socially sensitive issue (e.g., AIDS, suicide, or murder) or associated with unfinished business (e.g., spouse died during time of crisis in marriage; son has not spoken to parent for years). **These situations can sometimes cause the individual to become stuck in grief and unable to move forward with life.**
- Determine significance of the loss to the client (e.g., presence of chronic condition leading to divorce or disruption of family unit and change in lifestyle, financial security).
- Identify cultural or religious beliefs and expectations that may impact or dictate the client's response to loss.
- Ascertain the response of the family/SO(s) to the client's situation (e.g., sympathetic or urging client to "just get over it").

Nursing Priority No. 2.

To determine degree of impairment/dysfunction:

- Observe for cues of sadness (e.g., sighing; faraway look; unkempt appearance; inattention to conversation; somatic complaints, such as exhaustion, headaches).
- Listen to words/communications indicative of renewed or intense grief (e.g., constantly bringing up death or loss even in casual conversation long after event; outbursts of anger at relatively minor events; expressing desire to die), **indicating**

Information that appears in brackets has been added by the authors to clarify and enhance the use of nursing diagnoses.

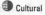

the person is possibly unable to adjust or move on from feelings of severe grief.

- Identify stage of grief being expressed: denial, isolation, anger, bargaining, depression, or acceptance.
- Determine level of functioning and ability to care for self.
- Note availability and use of support systems and community resources.
- Be aware of avoidance behaviors (e.g., anger, withdrawal, long periods of sleeping, or refusing to interact with family; sudden or radical changes in lifestyle; inability to handle everyday responsibilities at home, work, or school; conflict).
- Determine if the client is engaging in reckless or self-destructive behaviors (e.g., substance abuse, heavy drinking, promiscuity, or aggression) **to identify safety issues.**
- Identify cultural factors and ways individual has dealt with previous loss(es) **to put current behavior and responses in context.**
- Refer to mental health providers for specific diagnostic studies and intervention in issues associated with debilitating grief.
- Refer to ND Grieving for additional interventions, as appropriate.

Nursing Priority No. 3.

To assist client to deal appropriately with loss:

- Encourage verbalization without confrontation about realities. **This helps to begin resolution and acceptance.**
- Encourage the client to talk about what he or she chooses and refrain from forcing the client to "face the facts."
- Active-listen feelings and be available for support and assistance. Speak in a soft, caring tone.
- Encourage expression of anger, fear, and anxiety. Refer to appropriate NDs.
- Permit verbalization of anger with acknowledgment of feelings and setting of limits regarding destructive behavior. **This enhances client safety and promotes resolution of the grief process.**
- Acknowledge the reality of feelings of guilt or blame, including hostility toward spiritual power. Do not minimize loss, avoid clichés and easy answers. (Refer to ND Spiritual Distress.) Assist the client to take steps toward resolution.
- Respect the client's needs and wishes for quiet, privacy, talking, or silence.
- Give "permission" to be at this point when the client is depressed.

Information that appears in brackets has been added by the authors to clarify and enhance the use of nursing diagnoses.

- Provide comfort and availability as well as caring for physical needs.
- Reinforce use of previously effective coping skills. Instruct in, or encourage use of, visualization and relaxation techniques.
- Assist SO(s) to cope with client's response and include age-specific interventions. **The family/SO(s) may not understand or be intolerant of client's distress and inadvertently hamper client's progress.**
- Include family/SO(s) in setting realistic goals for meeting needs of family members.
- Encourage family members to participate in support group or family-focused therapy as indicated.
- Use sedatives or tranquilizers with caution **to avoid retarding resolution of grief process.**

Nursing Priority No. 4.

To promote wellness (Teaching/Discharge Considerations):

- Discuss with client/SO(s) healthy ways of dealing with difficult situations.
- Have client identify familial, religious, and cultural factors that have meaning for him or her. **This may help bring loss into perspective and promote grief resolution.**
- Encourage involvement in usual activities, exercise, and socialization within limits of physical ability and psychological state.
- Advocate planning for the future, as appropriate, to individual situation (e.g., staying in own home after death of spouse, returning to sporting activities following traumatic amputation, choice to have another child or to adopt, rebuilding home following a disaster, etc.).
- Refer to other resources (e.g., pastoral care, family counseling, psychotherapy, organized support groups). **This provides additional help, when needed, to resolve situation/continue grief work.**

Documentation Focus

Assessment/Reassessment

- Assessment findings, including meaning of loss to the client, current stage of the grieving process, and responses of family/SO(s)
- Cultural or religious beliefs and expectations
- Availability and use of resources

Information that appears in brackets has been added by the authors to clarify and enhance the use of nursing diagnoses.

Planning

- Plan of care and who is involved in the planning
- Teaching plan

Implementation/Evaluation

- Client's response to interventions, teaching, and actions performed
- Attainment or progress toward desired outcome(s)
- Modifications to plan of care

Discharge Planning

- Long-term needs and who is responsible for actions to be taken
- Specific referrals made

Sample Nursing Outcomes & Interventions Classifications (NOC/NIC)

NOC—Grief Resolution
NIC—Grief Work Facilitation

risk for complicated GRIEVING

[Diagnostic Division: Ego Integrity]

Definition: At risk for a disorder that occurs after the death of a significant other, in which the experience of distress accompanying bereavement fails to follow normative expectations and manifests in functional impairment.

Risk Factors

Death of significant other
Emotional disturbance; [loss of significant object (e.g., possessions, job, status, home, parts and processes of body)]
Insufficient social support

NOTE: A risk diagnosis is not evidenced by signs and symptoms, as the problem has not occurred; rather, nursing interventions are directed at prevention.

Information that appears in brackets has been added by the authors to clarify and enhance the use of nursing diagnoses.

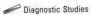

Desired Outcomes/Evaluation Criteria—Client Will:

- Acknowledge awareness of individual factors affecting client in this situation. (See Risk Factors.)
- Identify emotional responses and behaviors occurring after the death or loss.
- Participate in therapy to learn new ways of dealing with anxiety and feelings of inadequacy.
- Discuss meaning of loss to individual/family.
- Verbalize a sense of beginning to deal with grief process.

Actions/Interventions

Nursing Priority No. 1.

To identify risk/contributing factors:

- Determine loss that has occurred and meaning to client. Note whether loss was sudden or expected.
- ∞ Ascertain gestational age of fetus at time of loss or length of life of infant or child. **Death of a child may be more difficult for parents/family to deal with based on individual values and sense of life unlived.**
- Note stage of grief client is experiencing. **Stages of grief may progress in a predictable manner or stages may be random or revisited.**
- Assess the client's ability to manage activities of daily living and period of time since loss has occurred. **Periods of crying, feelings of overwhelming sadness, and loss of appetite and insomnia can occur with grieving; however, when they persist and interfere with normal activities, the client may need additional assistance.**
- Note availability and use of support systems and community resources.
- Identify cultural or religious beliefs and expectations that may impact or dictate client's response to loss.
- Assess status of relationships, marital difficulties, and adjustments to loss.

Nursing Priority No. 2.

To assist client to deal appropriately with loss:

- Discuss meaning of loss to client and active-listen responses without judgment.
- Encourage expression of feelings, including anger, fear, or anxiety. Let the client know that all feelings are okay, while setting limits on destructive behavior.

Information that appears in brackets has been added by the authors to clarify and enhance the use of nursing diagnoses.

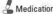

- Respect the client's desire for quiet, privacy, talking, or silence.
- Acknowledge the client's sense of relief or guilt at feeling relief when death follows a long and debilitating course. **Sadness and loss are still there, but the death may be a release, or the client may feel guilty about having a sense of relief.**
- Discuss the circumstances surrounding the death of a fetus or child. Was it sudden or expected? Have other children been lost (multiple miscarriages)? Was a congenital anomaly present? **Repeated losses increase sense of futility and compromise resolution of the grieving process.**
- Meet with both members of the couple **to determine how they are dealing with the loss.**
- Encourage the client/SOs to honor cultural practices through funerals, wakes, sitting shiva, and so forth.
- Assist SO(s)/family to understand and be tolerant of client's feelings and behavior.

Nursing Priority No. 3.

To promote wellness (Teaching/Discharge Considerations):

- Encourage the client/SO(s) to identify healthy coping skills they have used in the past. **These can be used in the current situation to facilitate dealing with grief.**
- Assist in setting goals for meeting needs of client and family members to move beyond the grieving process.
- Suggest resuming involvement in usual activities, exercise, and socialization within physical and psychological abilities.
- Discuss planning for the future, as appropriate to individual situation (e.g., staying in own home after death of spouse, returning to sporting activities following traumatic amputation, choosing to have another child or to adopt, rebuilding home following a disaster).
- Refer to other resources, as needed, such as counseling, psychotherapy, spiritual advisor, or grief support group. **Depending on meaning of the loss, the individual may require ongoing support to work through grief.**

Documentation Focus

Assessment/Reassessment

- Assessment findings, including meaning of loss to the client, current stage of the grieving process, psychological status, and responses of family/SO(s)
- Availability and use of resources

Information that appears in brackets has been added by the authors to clarify and enhance the use of nursing diagnoses.

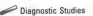

Planning
- Plan of care and who is involved in the planning
- Teaching plan

Implementation/Evaluation
- Client's response to interventions, teaching, and actions performed
- Attainment or progress toward desired outcome(s)
- Modifications to plan of care

Discharge Planning
- Long-term needs and who is responsible for actions to be taken
- Specific referrals made

Sample Nursing Outcomes & Interventions Classifications (NOC/NIC)

NOC—Grief Resolution
NIC—Grief Work Facilitation

risk for disproportionate GROWTH

[Diagnostic Division: Teaching/Learning]

Definition: Vulnerable to growth above the 97th percentile or below the 3rd percentile for age, crossing two percentile channels, which may compromise health.

Risk Factors

Prenatal
Inadequate maternal nutrition; maternal infection; multiple gestation
Substance abuse; exposure to teratogen
Congenital or genetic disorder

Individual
Prematurity
Malnutrition; maladaptive feeding behavior by caregiver, or self-feeding; insatiable appetite; anorexia
Infection; chronic illness
Substance abuse [including anabolic steroids]

Information that appears in brackets has been added by the authors to clarify and enhance the use of nursing diagnoses.

Environmental
Deprivation; economically disadvantaged
Exposure to violence; natural disasters
Exposure to teratogen; lead poisoning

Caregiver
Presence of abuse (e.g., physical, psychological, sexual)
Mental health issue (e.g., depression, psychosis, personality disorder, substance abuse)
Learning disability; alteration in cognitive functioning

> **NOTE:** A risk diagnosis is not evidenced by signs and symptoms, as the problem has not occurred; rather, nursing interventions are directed at prevention.

Desired Outcomes/Evaluation Criteria—Client Will:

- Receive appropriate nutrition as indicated by individual needs.
- Demonstrate weight and growth stabilizing or progress toward age-appropriate size.
- Participate in plan of care as appropriate for age and ability.

Caregiver Will:

- Verbalize understanding of potential for growth delay or deviation and plans for prevention.

Actions/Interventions

Nursing Priority No. 1.

To assess causative/contributing factors:

- Determine factors or condition(s) existing that could contribute to growth deviation as listed in Risk Factors, including familial history of pituitary tumors, Marfan's syndrome, genetic anomalies, use of certain drugs or substances during pregnancy, maternal diabetes or other chronic illness, poverty or inability to attend to nutritional issues, eating disorders, and so forth.
- Identify nature and effectiveness of parenting and caregiving activities. **Inadequate, inconsistent caregiving, unrealistic or insufficient expectations, lack of stimulation, inadequate limit setting; lack of responsiveness indicates problems in parent-child relationship.**

Information that appears in brackets has been added by the authors to clarify and enhance the use of nursing diagnoses.

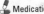

- Note severity and pervasiveness of situation (e.g., individual showing effects of long-term physical or emotional abuse or neglect versus individual experiencing recent-onset situational disruption or inadequate resources during period of crisis or transition).
- Evaluate nutritional status. **Overfeeding or malnutrition (protein and other basic nutrients) on a constant basis prevents child from reaching healthy growth potential, even if no disorder/disease exists.**
- Determine cultural, familial, and societal issues **that may impact the situation (e.g., childhood obesity a risk for American children; parental concern for amount of food intake; expectations for "normal growth").**
- Assess significant stressful events, losses, separation, and environmental changes (e.g., abandonment, divorce, death of parent/sibling, aging, move).
- Assess cognition, awareness, orientation, and behavior of the client and caregiver. **Actions such as withdrawal or aggression and reactions to environment and stimuli provide information for identifying needs and planning care.**
- Active-listen concerns about body size and ability to perform competitively (e.g., sports, body building) **to ascertain the potential for use of anabolic steroids or other drugs.**

Nursing Priority No. 2.

To prevent/limit deviation from growth norms:

- Determine chronological age and where child should be on growth charts **to determine growth expectations.** Note reported losses or alterations in functional level. **This provides a comparative baseline.**
- Note familial factors (e.g., parent's body build and stature) **to help determine individual developmental expectations (e.g., when child should attain a certain weight and height) and how the expectations may be altered by the child's condition.**
- Investigate deviations from normal (e.g., height and weight, head circumference, hand and feet size, facial features). **Deviations can be multifactorial and require varying interventions (e.g., weight deviation only [increased or decreased] may be remedied by changes in nutrition and exercise; other deviations may require in-depth evaluation and long-term treatment).**
- Determine if child's growth is above 97th percentile (very tall and large) for age. **This suggests a need for evaluation for**

Information that appears in brackets has been added by the authors to clarify and enhance the use of nursing diagnoses.

endocrine or other disorders or pituitary tumor (could result in gigantism). Other disorders may be characterized by excessive weight for height (e.g., hypothyroidism, Cushing's syndrome), abnormal sexual maturation, or abnormal body/limb proportions.

- Determine if child's growth is below 3rd percentile (very short and small) for age. **This may require evaluation for failure to thrive related to intrauterine growth retardation, prematurity or very low birth weight, small parents, poor nutrition, stress or trauma, or medical condition (e.g., intestinal disorders with malabsorption, diseases of heart, kidneys, diabetes mellitus). Treatment of the underlying condition may alter or improve the child's growth pattern.**
- Note reports of changes in facial features, joint pain, lethargy, sexual dysfunction, and/or progressive increase in hat, glove, ring, or shoe size in adults, especially after age 40. **The individual should be referred for further evaluation for hyperpituitarism, growth hormone imbalance, or acromegaly.**
- Review the results of studies such as skull and hand x-rays, bone scans (such as computed tomography [CT] or magnetic resonance imaging [MRI]), and chest or abdominal imaging **to determine bone age and extent of bone and soft tissue overgrowth; presence of pituitary or other growth hormone–secreting tumor.** Note laboratory studies (e.g., growth hormone levels, glucose tolerance, thyroid and other endocrine studies, serum transferrin and prealbumin) **to identify pathology.**
- Assist with therapies to treat or correct underlying conditions (e.g., Crohn's disease, cardiac problems, renal disease); endocrine problems (e.g., hyperpituitarism, hypothyroidism, type 1 diabetes mellitus, growth hormone abnormalities); genetic or intrauterine growth retardation; infant feeding problems; and nutritional deficits.
- Include nutritionist and other specialists (e.g., physical and occupational therapist) in developing plan of care. **This is helpful in determining specific dietary needs for growth and weight issues as well as child's issues with foods (e.g., child who is sensory overresponsive may be bothered by food textures; child with posture problems may need to stand to eat, etc.); the child may require assistive devices and appropriate exercise and rehabilitation programs.**
- Determine the need for medications (e.g., appetite stimulants or antidepressants, growth hormones).

Information that appears in brackets has been added by the authors to clarify and enhance the use of nursing diagnoses.

- Monitor growth periodically. **This aids in evaluating the effectiveness of interventions and promotes early identification of need for additional actions.**

Nursing Priority No. 3.

To promote wellness (Teaching/Discharge Considerations):

- Provide information regarding normal growth, as appropriate, including pertinent reference materials and credible Web sites.
- Address caregiver issues (e.g., parental abuse, learning deficiencies, environment of poverty) **that could impact the client's ability to thrive.**
- Recommend involvement in regular exercise or sports medicine program **to enhance muscle tone and strength and appropriate body building.**
- Promote a lifestyle that prevents or limits complications (e.g., management of obesity, hypertension, sensory or perceptual impairments); regular medical follow-up; nutritionally balanced meals; and socialization for age and development **to maintain functional independence and enhance quality of life.**
- Discuss with pregnant women and adolescents consequences of substance use or abuse. **Prevention of growth disturbances depends on many factors but includes the cessation of smoking, alcohol, and many drugs that have the potential for causing central nervous system (CNS) or orthopedic disorders in the fetus.**
- Refer for genetic screening, as appropriate. **There are many reasons for referral, including (and not limited to) positive family history of a genetic disorder (e.g., fragile X syndrome, muscular dystrophy), woman with exposure to toxins or potential teratogenic agents, women older than 35 years at delivery, previous child born with congenital anomalies, history of intrauterine growth retardation, and so forth.**
- Emphasize the importance of periodic reassessment of growth and development (e.g., periodic laboratory studies to monitor hormone levels, bone maturation, and nutritional status). **This aids in evaluating the effectiveness of interventions over time, promotes early identification of need for additional actions, and helps to avoid preventable complications.**
- Identify available community resources, as appropriate (e.g., public health programs, such as Women, Infants, and Children (WIC); medical equipment supplies; nutritionists; substance-abuse programs; specialists in endocrine problems/genetics).

Information that appears in brackets has been added by the authors to clarify and enhance the use of nursing diagnoses.

Documentation Focus

Assessment/Reassessment
- Assessment findings, individual needs, including current growth status, and trends
- Caregiver's understanding of situation and individual role

Planning
- Plan of care and who is involved in the planning
- Teaching plan

Implementation/Evaluation
- Client's responses to interventions, teaching, and actions performed
- Caregiver response to teaching
- Attainment or progress toward desired outcome(s)
- Modifications to plan of care

Discharge Planning
- Identified long-term needs and who is responsible for actions to be taken
- Specific referrals made, sources for assistive devices, educational tools

Sample Nursing Outcomes & Interventions Classifications (NOC/NIC)

NOC—Growth
NIC—Nutritional Monitoring

risk-prone HEALTH BEHAVIOR

[Diagnostic Division: Teaching/Learning]

Definition: Inability to modify lifestyle/behaviors in a manner that improves health status.

Related Factors

Inadequate comprehension; low self-efficacy
Stressors
Smoking; substance abuse
Insufficient social support; economically disadvantaged
Negative attitude toward healthcare

Information that appears in brackets has been added by the authors to clarify and enhance the use of nursing diagnoses.

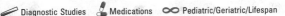

Defining Characteristics

Subjective

Minimization of health status change
Failure to achieve optimal sense of control

Objective

Failure to take action that prevents health problems
Nonacceptance of health status change

Desired Outcomes/Evaluation Criteria—Client Will:

- Demonstrate increasing interest/participation in self-care.
- Develop ability to assume responsibility for personal needs when possible.
- Identify stress situations leading to difficulties in adapting to change in health status and specific actions for dealing with them.
- Initiate lifestyle changes that will permit adaptation to current life situations.
- Identify and use appropriate support systems.

Actions/Interventions

Nursing Priority No. 1.

To assess degree of impaired function:

- Perform a physical and/or psychosocial assessment **to determine the extent of the limitation(s) of the current condition.**
- Listen to the client's perception of inability or reluctance to adapt to situations that are currently occurring.
- Survey (with the client) past and present significant support systems (e.g., family, church, groups, and organizations) **to identify helpful resources.**
- Explore the expressions of emotions signifying impaired adjustment by client/SO(s). **Overwhelming anxiety, fear, anger, worry, and passive or active denial can be experienced by the client who is having difficulty adjusting to change in health, feared diagnosis.**
- ∞ Note the child's interaction with the parent/caregiver. **Development of coping behaviors is limited at this age, and primary caregivers provide support for the child and serve as role models.**

Information that appears in brackets has been added by the authors to clarify and enhance the use of nursing diagnoses.

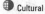

- Determine whether the child displays problems with school performance, withdraws from family or peers, or demonstrates aggressive behavior toward others/self. **These are indicators of poor coping and need for specific interventions to help child deal with own health issues or what is happening in the family.**

Nursing Priority No. 2.

To identify the causative/contributing factors relating to the change in health behavior:

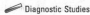

- Listen to the client's perception of the factors leading to the present dilemma, noting onset, duration, presence or absence of physical complaints, and social withdrawal. **The client may benefit from feedback that corrects misperceptions about how life will be with the change in health status.**
- Review previous life situations and role changes with client **to determine effects of prior experiences and coping skills used.**
- Note substance use/abuse (e.g., smoking, alcohol, prescription medications, or street drugs) **that may be used as a coping mechanism, exacerbate health problem, or impair client's comprehension of situation.**
- Identify possible cultural beliefs or values influencing a client's response to change. **Different cultures deal with change of health issues in different ways.**
- Assess affective climate within family system and how it determines family members' response to adjustment to major health challenge. **Families who are high-strung and nervous may interfere with the client's dealing with illness in a rational manner, while those who are more sedate and phlegmatic may be more helpful to the client in accepting the current circumstances.**
- Determine lack of or inability to use available resources. **The high degree of anxiety that usually accompanies a major lifestyle change often interferes with the ability to deal with problems created by the change or loss. Helping the client learn to use these resources enables him or her to take control of his or her own illness.**
- Review available documentation and resources to determine actual life experiences (e.g., medical records, statements by SO[s], consultants' notes). **In situations of great stress, physical and/or emotional, the client may not accurately assess occurrences leading to the present situation.**

Information that appears in brackets has been added by the authors to clarify and enhance the use of nursing diagnoses.

Nursing Priority No. 3.

To assist client in coping/dealing with impairment:

- Organize a team conference (including client and ancillary services) **to focus on contributing factors affecting adjustment and plan for management of the situation.**
- Explain disease process or causative factors and prognosis as appropriate, promote questioning, and provide written and other resource materials. **This enhances understanding, clarifies information, and provides an opportunity to review information at the individual's leisure.**
- Acknowledge client's efforts to adjust: "Have done your best." **This lessens feelings of blame, guilt, or defensive response.**
- Share information with adolescent's peers with permission as indicated when illness/injury affects body image. **Peers are the primary support for this age group.**
- Use therapeutic communication skills (active-listening, acknowledgment, silence, and I-statements). **This promotes an open relationship in which the client can explore possibilities and solutions for changing a lifestyle situation.**
- Discuss/evaluate resources that have been useful to the client in adapting to changes in other life situations. **Vocational rehabilitation, employment experiences, and psychosocial support services may be useful in the current situation.**
- Develop a plan of action with the client to meet immediate needs (e.g., physical safety and hygiene, emotional support of professionals and SO[s]) and assist in implementation of the plan. **This provides a starting point to deal with the current situation for moving ahead with plan and for evaluation of progress.**
- Explore previously used coping skills and application to current situation. Refine or develop new strategies, as appropriate. **This identifies the strengths that may be used to facilitate adaptation to change or loss that has occurred.**
- Identify and problem-solve with the client frustration in daily health-related care. **Focusing on smaller factors of concern gives the individual the ability to perceive impaired function from a less-threatening perspective, a one-step-at-a-time concept.**
- Involve SO(s) in long-range planning for emotional, psychological, physical, and social needs. **Change that is occurring when illness is long term or permanent indicates that lifestyle changes will need to be dealt with on an ongoing basis.**

Information that appears in brackets has been added by the authors to clarify and enhance the use of nursing diagnoses.

Nursing Priority No. 4.

To promote wellness (Teaching/Discharge Considerations):

- Identify strengths the client perceives in current life situation. Keep focus on the present, **as unknowns of the future may be too overwhelming.**
- Refer to other resources in the long-range plan of care. **Long-term assistance may include such elements as home care, transportation alternatives, occupational therapy, or vocational rehabilitation that may be useful for making indicated changes in life, assisting with adjustment to new situation.**
- Assist client/SO(s) to see appropriate alternatives and potential changes in locus of control.
- Assist SO(s) to learn methods for managing present needs. (Refer to NDs specific to client's deficits.)
- Pace and time learning sessions **to meet client's needs.** Provide feedback during and after learning experiences (e.g., self-catheterization, range-of-motion exercises, wound care, therapeutic communication) **to enhance retention, skill, and confidence.**

Documentation Focus

Assessment/Reassessment

- Reasons for, and degree of, impaired adaptation
- Client's/SO's perception of the situation
- Effect of behavior on health status/condition

Planning

- Plan for adjustments and interventions for achieving the plan and who is involved
- Teaching plan

Implementation/Evaluation

- Client responses to the interventions, teaching, and actions performed
- Attainment or progress toward desired outcome(s)
- Modifications to plan of care

Discharge Planning

- Long-term needs and who is responsible for actions to be taken
- Specific referrals made

Information that appears in brackets has been added by the authors to clarify and enhance the use of nursing diagnoses.

Sample Nursing Outcomes & Interventions Classifications (NOC/NIC)

NOC—Acceptance: Health Status
NIC—Coping Enhancement

deficient community HEALTH

[Diagnostic Division: Teaching/Learning]

Definition: Presence of one or more health problems or factors that deter wellness or increase the risk of health problems experienced by an aggregate.

Related Factors

Insufficient access to healthcare providers; insufficient resources (e.g., financial, social, knowledge)
Insufficient community experts
Inadequate program budget, outcome data, or evaluation plan
Inadequate social support or consumer satisfaction with program

Defining Characteristics

Subjective

[Community members or agencies verbalize overburdening of resources or inability to meet therapeutic needs of all members.]

Objective

Risk of hospitalization experienced by aggregates or populations
Risk of physiological or psychological states experienced by aggregates or populations
Health problem experienced by aggregates or populations
Program unavailable to enhance wellness of an aggregate or population
Program unavailable to prevent, reduce, or eliminate health problem(s) of an aggregate or population

Desired Outcomes/Evaluation Criteria—Community Will:

- Identify both strengths and limitations affecting community treatment programs for meeting health-related goals.

Information that appears in brackets has been added by the authors to clarify and enhance the use of nursing diagnoses.

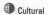

- Participate in problem-solving of factors interfering with regulating and integrating community programs.
- Develop plans to address identified community health needs.

Actions/Interventions

Nursing Priority No. 1.

To identify causative/precipitating factors:

- Evaluate healthcare providers' understanding, terminology, and practice policies relating to community (populations and aggregate). **Population-based practice considers the broad determinants of health, such as income/social status, housing, nutrition, employment/working conditions, social support networks, education, neighborhood safety/violence issues, physical environment, personal health practices and coping skills, cultural customs and values, and community capacity to support family and economic growth.**
- Investigate health problems, unexpected outbreaks or acceleration of illness, and health hazards in the community. **Identifying specific problems allows for population-based interventions emphasizing primary prevention, promoting health, and preventing problems before they occur. Current available resources provide a starting point to determine needs of the community and plan for future needs.**
- Evaluate strengths and limitations of community healthcare resources for wellness, illness, or sequelae of illness. **Knowledge of currently available resources and ease of access provide a starting point to determine needs of the community and plan for future needs.**
- Note reports from members of the community regarding ineffective or inadequate community functioning.
- Determine areas of conflict among members of community. **Cultural or religious beliefs, values, social mores, and lack of a shared vision may limit dialogue or creative problem-solving if not addressed.**
- Ascertain effect of related factors on community. **Issues of safety, poor air quality, lack of education or information, and lack of sufficient healthcare facilities affect citizens and how they view their community—whether it is a healthy, positive environment in which to live or lacks adequate healthcare or safety resources.**
- Determine knowledge and understanding of treatment regimen.
- Note use of resources available to community for developing and funding programs.

Information that appears in brackets has been added by the authors to clarify and enhance the use of nursing diagnoses.

Nursing Priority No. 2.

To assist community to develop strategies to improve community functioning/management:

- Foster cooperative spirit of community without negating individuality of members/groups. **As individuals feel valued and respected, they are more willing to work together with others to develop plan for identifying and improving healthcare for the community.**
- Involve the community in determining and prioritizing healthcare goals **to facilitate the planning process.**
- Plan together with community health and social agencies **to problem-solve solutions to identified and anticipated problems and needs.**
- Identify specific populations at risk or underserved **to actively involve them in the process.**
- Create teaching plan, form speakers' bureau **to disseminate information to community members regarding value of treatment and preventive programs.**
- Network with others involved in educating healthcare providers and healthcare consumers regarding community needs. Present information in a culturally appropriate manner. **Disseminating information to community members regarding value of treatment or preventive programs helps people know and understand the importance of these actions and be willing to support the programs.**

Nursing Priority No. 3.

To promote wellness (Teaching/Discharge Considerations):

- Assist the community to develop a plan for continuing assessment of community needs and the functioning and effectiveness of the plan. **This promotes a proactive approach in planning for the future and continuation of efforts to improve healthy behaviors and necessary services.**
- Encourage the community to form partnerships within the community and between the community and the larger society **to aid in long-term planning for anticipated or projected needs and concerns.**

Documentation Focus

Assessment/Reassessment

- Assessment findings, including members' perceptions of community problems, healthcare resources
- Community use of available resources

Information that appears in brackets has been added by the authors to clarify and enhance the use of nursing diagnoses.

Planning
- Plan of care and who is involved in planning
- Teaching plan

Implementation/Evaluation
- Community's response to plan, teaching, and interventions performed
- Attainment or progress toward desired outcome(s)
- Modifications to plan of care

Discharge Planning
- Long-term goals and who is responsible for actions to be taken
- Specific referrals made

Sample Nursing Outcomes & Interventions Classifications (NOC/NIC)

NOC—Community Competence
NIC—Community Health Development

ineffective HEALTH MAINTENANCE

[Diagnostic Division: Safety]

Definition: Inability to identify, manage, and/or seek out help to maintain health.

This diagnosis contains components of other NDs. We suggest subsuming health maintenance interventions under the "basic" nursing diagnosis when a single causative factor is identified (e.g., deficient Knowledge [specify]; ineffective Health Management; chronic Confusion; impaired verbal Communication; ineffective Coping; compromised family Coping; risk for delayed Development).

Related Factors

Ineffective communication skills
Unachieved developmental tasks
Alteration in cognitive functioning; impaired decision-making
Perceptual impairment
Decrease in gross or fine motor skills
Ineffective coping strategies; complicated grieving; spiritual distress
Insufficient resources (e.g., financial, social, knowledge)

Information that appears in brackets has been added by the authors to clarify and enhance the use of nursing diagnoses.

Defining Characteristics

Objective

Insufficient knowledge about basic health practices
Absence of interest in improving health behaviors; pattern of lack of health-seeking behavior
Absence of adaptive behaviors to environmental changes
Insufficient social support

Desired Outcomes/Evaluation Criteria—Client Will:

- Identify necessary health maintenance activities.
- Verbalize understanding of factors contributing to current situation.
- Assume responsibility for own healthcare needs within level of ability.
- Adopt lifestyle changes supporting individual healthcare goals.

SO/Caregiver Will:

- Verbalize the ability to cope adequately with existing situation, provide support/monitoring as indicated.

Actions/Interventions

Nursing Priority No. 1.

To assess causative/contributing factors:

- Recognize differing perceptions regarding health issues between healthcare providers and clients. Explore ways to partner. **Awareness that healthcare provider's goals may not be the same as client's goals can provide opportunities to explore and communicate. If left undone, the door is open for frustration on both sides, affecting client care experience and/or perceived outcome of care.**
- Identify health practices and beliefs in client's personal and family history, including health values, religious or cultural beliefs, and expectations regarding healthcare. **Clients and healthcare providers do not always view a health risk in the same way. The client may not view current situation as a problem or may be unaware of routine health maintenance practices and needs.**
- Note the client's age (e.g., very young or elderly); cognitive, emotional, physical, and developmental status; and level of dependence and independence. **The client's status may**

Information that appears in brackets has been added by the authors to clarify and enhance the use of nursing diagnoses.

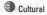

range from complete dependence (dysfunctional) to partial or relative independence and determines type of interventions/support needed.

- Determine whether impairment is an acute or sudden onset situation, progressive illness, long-term health problem, or exacerbation or complication of chronic illness. **This requires more intensive or long-lasting support and interventions with progressive or chronic conditions.**
- Evaluate medication regimen and also for substance use or abuse (e.g., alcohol or other drugs). **This can affect the client's understanding of information or desire and ability to help self.**
- Ascertain recent changes in lifestyle (e.g., widowed man who has no skills for taking care of his own/family's health needs; loss of independence; changing support systems).
- Note the setting where the client lives (e.g., long-term/other residential care facility, rural versus urban setting; homebound, homeless). **Socioeconomic status and geographic location contribute to an individual's ability to achieve or maintain good health.**
- Note desire and level of ability to meet health maintenance needs, as well as self-care activities of daily living (ADLs).
- Determine level of adaptive behavior, knowledge, and skills about health maintenance, environment, and safety. **This determines the beginning point for planning and interventions to assist the client in addressing needs.**
- Assess the client's ability and desire to learn. Determine barriers to learning (e.g., cannot read, speaks or understands different language than is used in the present setting, is overcome with grief or stress, has no interest in subject).
- Assess communication skills and ability or need for interpreter. Identify support person requesting or willing to accept information. **The ability to understand is essential to identification of needs and planning care. The information may need to be provided to another individual if the client is unable to comprehend.**
- Note the client's use of professional services and resources (e.g., appropriate or inappropriate/nonexistent).

Nursing Priority No. 2.

To assist client/caregiver(s) to maintain and manage desired health practices:

- Discuss with client/SO(s) beliefs about health and reasons for not following prescribed plan of care. **This determines the client's view of current situation and potential for change.**

Information that appears in brackets has been added by the authors to clarify and enhance the use of nursing diagnoses.

- Evaluate environment **to note individual adaptation needs.**
- Develop plan with client/SO(s) for self-care. **This allows for incorporating existing disabilities with client's/SO's desires and ability to adapt and organize care activities.**
- Involve comprehensive specialty health teams when indicated (e.g., pulmonary, psychiatric, enterostomal, IV therapy, nutritional support, substance abuse counselors).
- Provide anticipatory guidance **to maintain and manage effective health practices during periods of wellness, and identify ways the client can adapt when progressive illness/long-term health problems occur.**
- Encourage socialization and personal involvement **to enhance support system, provide pleasant stimuli, and prevent permanent regression.**
- Provide for communication and coordination between the healthcare facility team and community healthcare providers **to provide continuation of care.**
- Monitor adherence to prescribed medical regimen **to problem-solve difficulties in adherence and alter the plan of care, as needed.**

Nursing Priority No. 3.

To promote wellness (Teaching/Discharge Considerations):

- Provide information about individual healthcare needs, using the client's/SO's preferred learning style (e.g., pictures, words, video, Internet) **to assist the client in understanding his or her own situation and enhance interest/involvement in meeting own health needs.**
- Limit the amount of information presented at one time, especially when dealing with the elderly or cognitively or developmentally impaired client. Present new material through self-paced instruction when possible. **This allows the client time to process and store new information.**
- Help the client/SO(s) develop realistic healthcare goals. Provide a written copy to those involved in the planning process **for future reference and revision, as appropriate.**
- Assist the client/SO(s) to develop stress management skills.
- Identify ways to adapt things in current circumstances **to meet the client's changing needs and abilities and environmental concerns.**
- Identify signs and symptoms requiring further medical screening, evaluation, and follow-up care.
- Make referral, as needed, for community support services (e.g., homemaker/home attendant, meals-on-wheels, skilled nursing care, well-baby clinic, senior citizen healthcare activ-

---

Information that appears in brackets has been added by the authors to clarify and enhance the use of nursing diagnoses.

ities). **The client may need additional assistance to maintain self-sufficiency.**

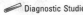

- Refer to social services, as indicated, **for assistance with financial, housing, or legal concerns (e.g., conservatorship).**
- Refer to support groups, as appropriate (e.g., senior citizens, Salvation Army shelter, homeless clinic, Alcoholics or Narcotics Anonymous).
- Arrange for hospice service for client with terminal illness **to help client and family deal with end-of-life issues in a positive manner.**

Documentation Focus

Assessment/Reassessment

- Assessment findings, including individual abilities; family involvement; support factors, and availability of resources
- Cultural or religious beliefs and healthcare values

Planning

- Plan of care and who is involved in planning
- Teaching plan

Implementation/Evaluation

- Responses of client/SO(s) to plan, specific interventions, teaching, and actions performed
- Attainment or progress toward desired outcome(s)
- Modifications to plan of care

Discharge Planning

- Long-range needs and who is responsible for actions to be taken
- Specific referrals made

Sample Nursing Outcomes & Interventions Classifications (NOC/NIC)

NOC—Health Promoting Behavior
NIC—Health System Guidance

ineffective HEALTH MANAGEMENT

[Diagnostic Division: Teaching/Learning]

Definition: Pattern of regulating and integrating into daily living a therapeutic regimen for the treatment of illness and its sequelae that is unsatisfactory for meeting specific health goals.

Information that appears in brackets has been added by the authors to clarify and enhance the use of nursing diagnoses.

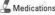

Related Factors

Complexity of healthcare system or therapeutic regimen
Decisional conflicts
Economically disadvantaged
Excessive demands; family conflict
Family pattern of healthcare
Inadequate number of cues to action
Insufficient knowledge of therapeutic regimen
Perceived seriousness of condition, susceptibility, benefit, or barrier
Powerlessness
Insufficient social support

Defining Characteristics

Subjective

Difficulty with prescribed regimens

Objective

Failure to include treatment regimen in daily living, or to take action to reduce risk factors
Ineffective choices in daily living for meeting health goal
Unexpected acceleration of illness symptoms

Desired Outcomes/Evaluation Criteria—Client Will:

- Verbalize acceptance of need and desire to change actions to achieve agreed-on health goals.
- Verbalize understanding of factors or blocks involved in individual situation.
- Participate in problem-solving of factors interfering with integration of therapeutic regimen.
- Demonstrate behaviors and changes in lifestyle necessary to maintain therapeutic regimen.
- Identify and use available resources.

Actions/Interventions

Nursing Priority No. 1.

To identify causative/contributing factors:

- Determine whether the client has acute or chronic illness; if chronic, note whether more than one condition is present at the same time and assess the complexity of care needs. **These**

Information that appears in brackets has been added by the authors to clarify and enhance the use of nursing diagnoses.

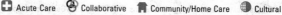

 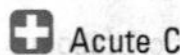 Acute Care 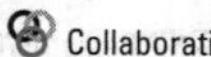 Collaborative 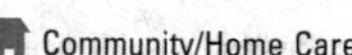 Community/Home Care  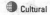 Cultural

factors affect how the client views and manages self-care. The client may be overwhelmed, in denial, depressed, or have complications exacerbating care needs.

- Ascertain the client's knowledge and understanding of condition and treatment needs **so that he or she can make informed decisions about managing self-care. This provides a baseline so planning care can begin where the client is in relation to condition or illness and current regimen.**
- Determine the client's/family's health goals and patterns of healthcare.
- Identify health practices and beliefs in the client's personal and family history, including health values, religious or cultural beliefs, and expectations regarding healthcare. **The client may not view his or her current situation as a problem or be unaware of health management needs. Expectations of others may dictate the client's adaptation to the situation and willingness to modify life.**
- Identify client locus of control. **Those with an internal locus of control (e.g., expressions of responsibility for self and ability to control outcomes, such as "I didn't quit smoking") are more likely to take charge of the situation; individuals with an external locus of control (e.g., expressions of lack of control over self and environment, such as, "What bad luck to get lung cancer") may perceive difficulties as beyond his or her control and will look to others to solve his or her problems.**
- Identify individual perceptions and expectations of treatment regimen. **This may reveal misinformation, unrealistic expectations, or other factors that may be interfering with the client's willingness to follow a therapeutic regimen.**
- Review complexity of treatment regimen (e.g., number of expected tasks, such as taking medication several times/day; visiting multiple healthcare providers with treatment or follow-up appointments; abundant, often conflicting, information sources). Evaluate how difficult tasks might be for client (e.g., must stop smoking or must follow strict dialysis diet even when feeling well and manage limitations while remaining active in life roles). **These factors are often involved in lack of participation in treatment plan.**
- Note availability and use of resources for assistance, caregiving, and respite care. **The client may not have, be aware of, or know how to access resources that may be available.**

Nursing Priority No. 2.

To assist client/SO(s) to develop strategies to improve management of therapeutic regimen:

Information that appears in brackets has been added by the authors to clarify and enhance the use of nursing diagnoses.

- Use therapeutic communication skills **to assist client to problem-solve solution(s).**
- Explore client involvement in or lack of mutual goal setting.
- Use the client's locus of control to develop an individual plan to adapt to regimen. **Encourage the client with internal control to take control of his or her own care; for those with external control, begin with small tasks and add, as tolerated.**
- Identify steps necessary to reach desired goal(s). **Specifying steps to take requires discussion and the use of critical-thinking skills to determine how to best reach the agreed-on goals.**
- Contract with the client for participation in care.
- Accept the client's evaluation of own strengths and limitations while working together to improve abilities. State belief in client's ability to cope and/or adapt to situation. **Individuals may minimize own strengths and exaggerate limitations when faced with the difficulties of a chronic illness. Stating your belief in positive terms lets the client hear someone else's evaluation and begin to accept that he or she can manage the situation.**
- Provide positive reinforcement for efforts **to encourage continuation of desired behaviors.**
- Provide information and encourage the client to seek out resources on his or her own. Reinforce previous instructions and rationale, using a variety of learning modalities, including role-playing, demonstration, and written materials. **Incorporating multiple modalities promotes retention of information. Developing the client's skill at finding his or her own information encourages self-sufficiency and sense of self-worth.**

Nursing Priority No. 3.

To promote wellness (Teaching/Discharge Considerations):

- Emphasize the importance of client knowledge and understanding of the need for treatment or medication as well as consequences of actions and choices.
- Promote client/caregiver/SO(s) participation in planning and evaluating process. **This enhances commitment to the plan and promotes competent self-management, optimizing outcomes.**
- Assist the client to develop strategies for monitoring symptoms and response to therapeutic regimen. **This promotes early recognition of changes, allowing a proactive response.**
- Mobilize support systems, including family/SO(s), social services, and financial assistance. **Success of a therapeutic reg-**

Information that appears in brackets has been added by the authors to clarify and enhance the use of nursing diagnoses.

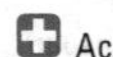  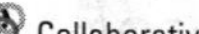 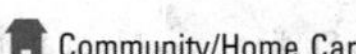 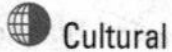

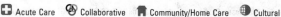

imen is enhanced by using support systems effectively, avoiding or reducing stress and worry of dealing with unresolved problems.

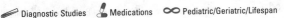

- Refer to counseling or therapy (group and individual), as indicated.
- Identify home- and community-based nursing services **for assessment, follow-up care, and education in the client's home.**

Documentation Focus

Assessment/Reassessment

- Findings, including underlying dynamics of individual situation, client's perception of problem or needs, locus of control
- Cultural values, religious beliefs
- Family involvement and needs
- Individual strengths and limitations
- Availability and use of resources

Planning

- Plan of care and who is involved in planning
- Teaching plan

Implementation/Evaluation

- Response to interventions, teaching, and actions performed
- Attainment or progress toward desired outcome(s)
- Modifications to plan of care

Discharge Planning

- Long-term needs and who is responsible for actions to be taken
- Available resources, specific referrals made

Sample Nursing Outcomes & Interventions Classifications (NOC/NIC)

NOC—Treatment Behavior: Illness or Injury
NIC—Self-Modification Assistance

ineffective family HEALTH MANAGEMENT

[Diagnostic Division: Teaching/Learning]

Definition: A pattern of regulating and integrating into family processes a program for the treatment of illness and its sequelae that is unsatisfactory for meeting specific health goals.

Information that appears in brackets has been added by the authors to clarify and enhance the use of nursing diagnoses.

Related Factors

Complexity of therapeutic regimen, or healthcare system
Decisional conflict
Economically disadvantaged
Family conflicts

Defining Characteristics

Subjective

Difficulty with prescribed regimen

Objective

Inappropriate family activities for meeting health goal
Acceleration of illness symptoms of a family member
Failure to take action to reduce risk factors; decrease in attention to illness

Desired Outcomes/Evaluation Criteria—Family Will:

- Identify individual factors affecting regulation/integration of treatment program.
- Participate in problem-solving of factors.
- Verbalize acceptance of need or desire to change actions to achieve agreed-on outcomes or health goals.
- Demonstrate behaviors and changes in lifestyle necessary to maintain therapeutic regimen.

Actions/Interventions

Nursing Priority No. 1.

To identify causative/precipitating factors:

- Ascertain family's perception of efforts to date.
- Evaluate family functioning and activities—looking at frequency and effectiveness of family communication, promotion of autonomy, adaptation to meet changing needs, health of home environment and lifestyle, problem-solving abilities, and ties to community. **Understanding the family and the context in which it lives allows for more personalized support of the family and choosing coping strategies in partnership with the family to meet individualized goals.**
- Note family health goals and agreement of individual members. **The presence of conflict interferes with problem-solving.**

Information that appears in brackets has been added by the authors to clarify and enhance the use of nursing diagnoses.

- Determine understanding of and value of the treatment regimen to the family.
- Identify cultural values or religious beliefs affecting view of situation and willingness to make necessary changes.
- Identify availability and use of resources.

Nursing Priority No. 2.

To assist family to develop strategies to improve management of therapeutic regimen:

- Provide family-centered education addressing management of condition/chronic illness and incorporation of strategies into family's lifestyle. **This helps the family to make informed decisions and see the connection between illness and treatment; it also facilitates treatment adherence and improved client outcomes.**
- Assist family members to recognize inappropriate family activities. Help the members identify both togetherness and individual needs and behavior **so that effective interactions can be enhanced and perpetuated.**
- Make a plan jointly with family members to deal with the complexity of the healthcare regimen or system and other related factors. **This enhances commitment to the plan, optimizing outcomes.**
- Identify community resources, as needed, using the three strategies of education, problem-solving, and resource linking **to address specific deficits.**

Nursing Priority No. 3.

To promote wellness as related to future health of family members:

- Help the family identify criteria to promote ongoing self-evaluation of situation and effectiveness and family progress. **This provides an opportunity to be proactive in meeting needs.**
- Make referrals to and/or jointly plan with other health, social, and community resources. **Problems are often multifaceted, requiring involvement of numerous providers and agencies.**
- Encourage involvement in disease/condition support groups. **Family resiliency is gained through contact with other families dealing with similar challenges.**
- Provide a contact person or case manager for one-to-one assistance, as needed, **to coordinate care, provide support, assist with problem-solving, and so forth.**
- Refer to NDs caregiver Role Strain; ineffective Health Management, as indicated.

Information that appears in brackets has been added by the authors to clarify and enhance the use of nursing diagnoses.

Documentation Focus

Assessment/Reassessment

- Individual findings, including nature of problem and degree of impairment; family values, health goals, and level of participation and commitment of family members
- Cultural values, religious beliefs
- Availability and use of resources

Planning

- Plan of care and who is involved in planning
- Teaching plan

Implementation/Evaluation

- Response to interventions, teaching, and actions performed
- Attainment or progress toward desired outcome(s)
- Modifications of plan of care

Discharge Planning

- Long-term needs, plan for meeting, and who is responsible for actions
- Specific referrals made

Sample Nursing Outcomes & Interventions Classifications (NOC/NIC)

NOC—Family Health Status
NIC—Family Involvement Promotion

readiness for enhanced HEALTH MANAGEMENT

[Diagnostic Division: Teaching/Learning]

Definition: A pattern of regulating and integrating into daily living a therapeutic regimen for treatment of illness and its sequelae, which can be strengthened.

Defining Characteristics

Subjective

Expresses desire to enhance management of illness, symptoms, or risk factors
Expresses desire to enhance management of prescribed regimens
Expresses desire to enhance immunization/vaccination status

Information that appears in brackets has been added by the authors to clarify and enhance the use of nursing diagnoses.

Expresses desire to enhance choices of daily living for meeting goals

Desired Outcomes/Evaluation Criteria—Client Will:

- Assume responsibility for managing treatment regimen.
- Demonstrate proactive management by anticipating and planning for eventualities of condition or potential complications.
- Identify and use additional resources as appropriate.
- Remain free of preventable complications, progression of illness and sequelae.

Actions/Interventions

Nursing Priority No. 1.

To determine motivation for continued growth:

- Ascertain the client's beliefs about health and his/her ability to maintain health. **Belief in the ability to accomplish desired action is predictive of performance.**
- Determine the client's current health status and perception of possible threats to health.
- Verify the client's level of knowledge and understanding of therapeutic regimen. Note specific health goals and what measures the client has been using to achieve his/her goals. **This provides an opportunity to ensure accuracy and completeness of knowledge base for future learning.**
- Determine source(s) the client uses when seeking health information and what is done with this information (e.g., incorporated into self-management or used as basis for seeking healthcare). **The manner in which people access and use healthcare information varies widely, with variables including age, race/culture, location, literacy, and computer use.**
- Active-listen concerns to identify underlying issues (e.g., physical or emotional stressors, external factors such as environmental pollutants or other hazards) **that could impact the client's ability to control his or her own health.**
- Determine the influence of cultural beliefs on the client/caregiver(s) participation in the regimen. **These factors influence the way people view health issues and management.**
- Identify the individual's expectations of long-term treatment needs and anticipated changes.
- Determine the resources presently used by the client **to note whether changes can be arranged (e.g., increased hours of**

Information that appears in brackets has been added by the authors to clarify and enhance the use of nursing diagnoses.

home care assistance; access to case manager to support complex or long-term program).

Nursing Priority No. 2.

To assist client/significant other (SO)(s) to develop plan to meet individual needs:

- Acknowledge the client's strengths in present health management and build on in planning for future.
- Identify steps necessary to reach desired health goal(s). **Understanding the process enhances commitment and the likelihood of achieving the goals.**
- Explore with the client/SO(s) areas of health over which each individual has control, and discuss barriers to healthy practices (e.g., chooses fast food instead of cooking for one; lack of time or access to convenient facility or safe environment in which to exercise). **This identifies actions the individual can take to plan for improving health practices.**
- Accept the client's evaluation of own strengths and limitations while working together to improve abilities. **This promotes a sense of self-esteem and confidence to continue efforts.**
- Incorporate the client's cultural values or religious beliefs that support attainment of health goals.
- Provide information and bibliotherapy. Help the client/SO(s) identify and evaluate resources they can access on their own. **When referencing the Internet or nontraditional, unproven resources, the individual must exercise some restraint and determine the reliability of the source and information provided before acting on it.**
- Acknowledge individual efforts and capabilities to reinforce movement toward attainment of desired outcomes. **This provides positive reinforcement encouraging continued progress toward desired goals.**

Nursing Priority No. 3.

To promote optimum wellness:

- Promote client/caregiver choices and involvement in planning for and implementing added tasks and responsibilities. **Knowing that he or she can make his or her own choices promotes commitment to program and enhances the probability that the client will follow through with change.**
- Encourage the use of exercise, relaxation skills, yoga, meditation, visualization, and guided imagery **to assist in the management of stress and promote general health and wellbeing.**

Information that appears in brackets has been added by the authors to clarify and enhance the use of nursing diagnoses.

- Assist in implementing strategies for monitoring progress and responses to the therapeutic regimen. **This promotes proactive problem-solving.**
- Identify additional community resources/support groups (e.g., nutritionist/weight control program or smoking cessation program). **This provides further opportunities for role modeling, skill training, anticipatory problem-solving, and so forth.**
- Instruct in individually appropriate wellness behaviors such as breast self-examination and mammogram, testicular self-examination and prostate examination, immunizations and flu shots, and regular medical and dental examinations.

Documentation Focus

Assessment/Reassessment

- Findings, including dynamics of individual situation
- Individual strengths, additional needs
- Cultural values, religious beliefs

Planning

- Plan of care and who is involved in planning
- Teaching plan

Implementation/Evaluation

- Response to interventions, teaching, and actions performed
- Attainment or progress toward desired outcome(s)
- Modifications to plan of care

Discharge Planning

- Short- and long-term needs and who is responsible for actions
- Available resources, specific referrals made

Sample Nursing Outcomes & Interventions Classifications (NOC/NIC)

NOC—Adherence Behavior
NIC—Health System Guidance

impaired HOME MAINTENANCE

[Diagnostic Division: Safety]

Definition: Inability to independently maintain a safe growth-promoting immediate environment.

Information that appears in brackets has been added by the authors to clarify and enhance the use of nursing diagnoses.

Related Factors

Condition impacting ability to maintain home (e.g., disease; illness; injury)
Illness/injury impacting ability to maintain home
Alteration in cognitive functioning
Insufficient role model, support system
Insufficient knowledge of home maintenance, neighborhood resources

Defining Characteristics

Subjective

Difficulty maintaining a comfortable [safe] environment
Request for assistance with home maintenance
Excessive family responsibilities
Financial crisis (e.g., debt, insufficient finances)

Objective

Unsanitary environment
Pattern of disease or infection caused by unhygienic conditions
Insufficient equipment for maintaining home; insufficient cooking equipment, clothing, or linen

Desired Outcomes/Evaluation Criteria—Client/Caregiver Will:

- Identify individual factors related to difficulty in maintaining a safe environment.
- Verbalize plan to eliminate health and safety hazards.
- Adopt behaviors reflecting lifestyle changes to create and sustain a healthy, growth-promoting environment.
- Demonstrate appropriate, effective use of resources.

Actions/Interventions

Nursing Priority No. 1.

To assess causative/contributing factors:

- Identify the presence of, or potential for, physical or mental conditions (e.g., advanced age, chronic illnesses, brain/other traumatic injuries; severe depression or other mental illness; multiple persons in one home incapable of handling home tasks) **that compromise the client's/SO's functional abilities in taking care of the home.**
- Note the presence of personal and/or environmental factors (e.g., family member with multiple care tasks; addition of fam-

Information that appears in brackets has been added by the authors to clarify and enhance the use of nursing diagnoses.

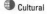

ily member(s) [e.g., new baby, or ill parent moving in]; substance abuse; poverty/inadequate financial resources; absence of family/support systems; lifestyle of self-neglect; client comfortable with home environment, has no desire for change) **that can contribute to neglect of home cleanliness or repair.**

- Determine problem in household and degree of discomfort and unsafe conditions noted by client/SO(s). **Safety problems may be obvious (e.g., lack of heat or water; unsanitary rooms), while other problems may be more subtle and difficult to manage (e.g., lack of finances for home repair; or lack of knowledge about food storage or rodent control).**
- Assess the client's/SO's level of cognitive, emotional, or physical functioning **to ascertain needs and capabilities in handling tasks of home management.**
- Identify a lack of interest, knowledge, or misinformation **to determine the need for health education/home safety program or other intervention.**
- Discuss the home environment or perform a home visit, as appropriate, **to determine the ability to care for self and to identify potential health and safety hazards.**
- Identify support systems available to client/SO(s) **to determine needs and initiate referrals (e.g., companionship, daily care, household cleaning or homemaking, or running errands).**
- Determine financial resources to meet needs of individual situation.

Nursing Priority No. 2.

To help client/SO(s) create/maintain a safe, growth-promoting environment:

- Coordinate planning with multidisciplinary team, as appropriate.
- Discuss home environment or perform home visit as indicated **to determine the client's ability to care for self, to identify potential health and safety hazards, and to determine adaptations that may be needed (e.g., wheelchair-accessible doors and hallways, safety bars in bathroom, safe place for child play, clean water available, working cook stove or microwave, and secured screens on windows).**
- Assist the client/SO(s) to develop a plan for maintaining a clean, healthful environment (e.g., sharing of household tasks and repairs between family members, contract services, exterminators, and trash removal).
- Educate and assist the client/family to address lifestyle adjustments that may be required, such as personal/home hy-

Information that appears in brackets has been added by the authors to clarify and enhance the use of nursing diagnoses.

giene practices, elimination of substance abuse or unsafe smoking habits; proper food storage, stress management; and so forth. **Individuals may not be aware of the impact of these factors on their health or welfare or they may be overwhelmed and in need of specific assistance for varying periods of time.**

- Assist the client/SO(s) to identify and acquire necessary equipment (e.g., lifts, commode chair, safety grab bars, cleaning supplies, or structural adaptations) **to meet individual needs.**
- Identify resources available for appropriate assistance (e.g., visiting nurse, budget counseling, homemaker, meals-on-wheels, physical or occupational therapy, or social services).
- Discuss options for financial assistance with housing needs. **The client may be able to stay in home with minimal assistance or may need significant assistance over a wide range of possibilities, including removal from the home.**

Nursing Priority No. 3.

To promote wellness (Teaching/Discharge Considerations):

- Evaluate the client at each community contact or before facility discharge **to determine if home maintenance needs are ongoing in order to initiate appropriate referrals.**
- Discuss environmental hazards **that may negatively affect health or ability to perform desired activities.**
- Develop long-term plan for taking care of environmental needs (e.g., assistive personnel to clean house, do laundry; trash removal; and pest control services).
- Identify ways to access and use community resources and support systems (e.g., extended family, neighbors).
- Refer to NDs deficient Knowledge [Learning Need (specify)]; Self-Care Deficit [specify]; ineffective Coping; compromised family Coping; Caregiver Role Strain; risk for Injury.

Documentation Focus

Assessment/Reassessment

- Assessment findings include individual and environmental factors
- Availability and use of support systems

Planning

- Plan of care and who is involved in planning; support systems and community resources identified
- Teaching plan

Information that appears in brackets has been added by the authors to clarify and enhance the use of nursing diagnoses.

Implementation/Evaluation

- Client's/SO's responses to interventions, teaching, and actions performed
- Attainment or progress toward desired outcome(s)
- Modifications to plan of care

Discharge Planning

- Long-term needs and who is responsible for actions to be taken
- Specific referrals made, equipment needs/resources

Sample Nursing Outcomes & Interventions Classifications (NOC/NIC)

NOC—Self-Care: Instrumental Activities of Daily Living (IADL)
NIC—Home Maintenance Assistance

HOPELESSNESS

[Diagnostic Division: Ego Integrity]

Definition: Subjective state in which an individual sees limited or no alternatives or personal choices available and is unable to mobilize energy on own behalf.

Related Factors

Prolonged activity restriction; social isolation
Deteriorating physiological condition
Chronic stress; history of abandonment
Loss of belief in spiritual power or transcendent values

Defining Characteristics

Subjective

Despondent verbal cues (e.g., "I can't," sighing); [believes things will not change]

Objective

Passivity; decrease in verbalization
Decrease in affect, appetite, or response to stimuli
Decrease in initiative; inadequate involvement in care
Alteration in sleep pattern
Turning away from speaker; shrugging in response to speaker; poor eye contact

---

Information that appears in brackets has been added by the authors to clarify and enhance the use of nursing diagnoses.

Desired Outcomes/Evaluation Criteria—Client Will:

- Recognize and verbalize feelings.
- Identify and use coping mechanisms to counteract feelings of hopelessness.
- Involve self in and control (within limits of the individual situation) own self-care and activities of daily living.
- Set progressive short-term goals that develop and sustain behavioral changes and foster positive outlook.
- Participate in diversional activities of own choice.

Actions/Interventions

Nursing Priority No. 1.

To identify causative/contributing factors:

- Review familial and social history and physiological history for problems, such as history of poor coping abilities, disorder of familial relating patterns, emotional problems, recent or long-term illness of client or family member, or multiple social and/or physiological traumas to individual or family members.
- Note current familial, social, or physical situation of client (e.g., newly diagnosed with chronic or terminal disease, lack of support system, recent job loss, loss of spiritual or religious faith, recent multiple traumas, alcoholism or other substance abuse).
- Identify cultural or spiritual values **that can impact beliefs in his or her own ability to change situation.**
- Determine coping behaviors and defense mechanisms displayed.
- Discuss the problem of alcohol or drug abuse. **The client may feel hopeless, believing behavior is impossible to stop.**
- Determine suicidal thoughts and if the client has a plan. **Hopelessness is a symptom of suicidal ideation.**

Nursing Priority No. 2.

To assess level of hopelessness:

- Note behaviors indicative of hopelessness. (Refer to Defining Characteristics.)
- Determine coping behaviors previously used and the client's perception of effectiveness then and now.
- Evaluate and discuss the use of defense mechanisms (useful or not), such as increased sleeping, use of drugs (including alcohol), illness behaviors, eating disorders, denial, forgetful-

---

Information that appears in brackets has been added by the authors to clarify and enhance the use of nursing diagnoses.

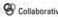

ness, daydreaming, ineffectual organizational efforts, exploiting own goal setting, or regression.

Nursing Priority No. 3.

To assist client to identify feelings and to begin to cope with problems as perceived by the client:

- Establish a therapeutic and facilitative relationship showing positive regard for the client. **The client may then feel safe to disclose feelings and feel understood and listened to.**
- Complete Beck's Depression Scale. Explain all tests and procedures. Involve the client in planning a schedule for care. Answer questions truthfully. **This enhances trust and therapeutic relationship, enabling the client to talk freely about concerns.**
- Discuss initial signs of hopelessness (e.g., procrastination, increasing need for sleep, decreased physical activity, and withdrawal from social or familial activities).
- Encourage the client to verbalize and explore feelings and perceptions (e.g., anger, helplessness, powerlessness, confusion, despondency, isolation, grief).
- Provide an opportunity for children to "play out" feelings (e.g., puppets or art for preschooler, peer discussions for adolescents). **This provides insight into perceptions and may give direction for coping strategies.**
- Engage teens in discussions and arrange to do activities with them. **Parents can make a difference in their children's lives by being with them, discussing sensitive topics, and going different places with them.**
- Express hope to client and encourage SO(s) and other health team members to do so. **The client may not identify the positives in his or her own situation.**
- Assist the client to identify short-term goals. Encourage activities to achieve goals; facilitate contingency planning. **This promotes dealing with the situation in manageable steps, enhancing chances for success and sense of control.**
- Discuss current options and list actions that may be taken to gain some control of the situation. Correct misconceptions expressed by the client.
- Endeavor to prevent situations that might lead to feelings of isolation or lack of control in the client's perception.
- Promote client control in establishing time, place, and frequency of therapy sessions. Involve family members in the therapy situation, as appropriate.
- Help the client recognize areas in which he or she has control versus those that are not within his or her control.

Information that appears in brackets has been added by the authors to clarify and enhance the use of nursing diagnoses.

- Encourage risk taking in situations in which the client can succeed.
- Help the client begin to develop coping mechanisms that can be learned and used effectively **to counteract hopelessness.**
- Encourage structured and controlled increase in physical activity. **This enhances the sense of well-being.**
- Demonstrate and encourage use of relaxation exercises, guided imagery.
- Discuss safe use of prescribed antidepressants, including expected effects, adverse side effects, and interactions with other drugs.

Nursing Priority No. 4.

To promote wellness (Teaching/Discharge Considerations):

- Provide positive feedback for actions taken to deal with and overcome feelings of hopelessness. **This encourages continuation of desired behaviors.**
- Assist the client/family to become aware of factors/situations leading to feelings of hopelessness. **This provides an opportunity to avoid/modify the situation.**
- Facilitate the client's incorporation of personal loss. **This enhances grief work and promotes resolution of feelings.**
- Encourage the client/family to develop support systems in the immediate community.
- Help the client to become aware of, nurture, and expand spiritual self. (Refer to ND Spiritual Distress.)
- Introduce the client into a support group before the individual therapy is terminated **for continuation of therapeutic process.**
- Stress the need for continued monitoring of medication regimen by healthcare provider.
- Refer to other resources for assistance, as indicated (e.g., clinical nurse specialist, psychiatrist, social services, spiritual advisor, Alcoholics or Narcotics Anonymous, Al-Anon or Alateen).

Documentation Focus

Assessment/Reassessment

- Assessment findings, including degree of impairment, use of coping skills, and support systems

Planning

- Plan of care and who is involved in planning
- Teaching plan

Information that appears in brackets has been added by the authors to clarify and enhance the use of nursing diagnoses.

Implementation/Evaluation
- Responses to interventions, teaching, and actions performed
- Attainment or progress toward desired outcome(s)
- Modifications to plan of care

Discharge Planning
- Identified long-term needs, client's goals for change and who is responsible for actions to be taken
- Specific referrals made

Sample Nursing Outcomes & Interventions Classifications (NOC/NIC)

NOC—Depression Self-Control
NIC—Hope Inspiration

readiness for enhanced HOPE

[Diagnostic Division: Ego Integrity]

Definition: A pattern of expectations and desires for mobilizing energy on one's own behalf, which can be strengthened.

Defining Characteristics

Subjective
Expresses desire to enhance hope; belief in possibilities; congruency of expectation with goal; ability to set achievable goals; problem-solving to meet goals
Expresses desire to enhance sense of meaning in life; connectedness with others; spirituality

Desired Outcomes/Evaluation Criteria—Client Will:
- Identify and verbalize feelings related to expectations and desires.
- Verbalize belief in possibilities for the future.
- Discuss current situation and desire to enhance hope.
- Set short-term goals that will lead to behavioral changes to meet desire for enhanced hope.

Information that appears in brackets has been added by the authors to clarify and enhance the use of nursing diagnoses.

Actions/Interventions

Nursing Priority No. 1.

To determine needs and desire for improvement:

- Review familial and social history to identify past situations (e.g., illness, emotional conflicts, alcoholism) that have led to decision to improve life.
- Determine current physical condition of client/significant other (SO)(s). **The treatment regimen can influence the ability to promote positive feelings of hope.**
- Ascertain the client's perception of current state and expectations/goals for the future (e.g., general well-being, prosperity, independence).
- Identify spiritual beliefs and cultural values that influence sense of hope and connectedness and give meaning to life.
- Note degree of involvement in activities and relationships with others. **Superficial interactions with others can limit sense of connectedness and reduce enjoyment of relationships.**
- Determine level of commitment and expectations for change and congruency of expectations with desires.

Nursing Priority No. 2.

To assist client to achieve goals and strengthen sense of hope:

- Establish a therapeutic relationship, showing positive regard and sense of hope for the client. **Enhances feelings of worth and comfort, inspiring client to continue pursuit of goals.**
- Help the client recognize areas that are in his or her control versus those that are not. **To be most effective, the client needs to expend energy in those areas where he or she has control/can make changes and let the others go.**
- Assist the client to develop manageable short-term goals.
- Identify activities to achieve goals and facilitate contingency planning. **This helps the client deal with the situation in manageable steps, enhancing chances for success and sense of control.**
- Explore interrelatedness of unresolved emotions, anxieties, fears, and guilt. **This provides an opportunity to address issues that may be limiting the individual's ability to improve his or her life situation.**

Information that appears in brackets has been added by the authors to clarify and enhance the use of nursing diagnoses.

- Assist the client to acknowledge current coping behaviors and defense mechanisms that are not helping the client move toward goals. **This allows the client to focus on coping mechanisms that are more successful in problem-solving.**
- Encourage the client to concentrate on progress not perfection. **If the client can accept that perfection is difficult and generally not the focus—rather, achieving the desired goal is the focus—then he or she may be able to view his or her own accomplishments with pride.**
- Involve the client in care and explain all procedures thoroughly, answering questions truthfully. **This enhances trust and relationship, promoting hope for a positive outcome.**
- Express hope to client and encourage SO(s) and other health team members to do so. **This enhances the client's sense of hope and belief in the possibility of a positive outcome.**
- Identify ways to strengthen a sense of interconnectedness or harmony with others **to support sense of belonging and connection that promotes feelings of wholeness and hopefulness.**

Nursing Priority No. 3.

To promote optimum wellness:

- Demonstrate and encourage the use of relaxation techniques, guided imagery, and meditation activities.
- Provide positive feedback for actions taken to improve problem-solving skills and for setting achievable goals. **This acknowledges the client's efforts and reinforces gains.**
- Explore how beliefs give meaning and value to daily living. **As the client's understanding of these issues improves, hope for the future is strengthened.**
- Encourage life-review by the client **to acknowledge his or her own successes, identify opportunity for change, and clarify meaning in life.**
- Identify ways for the client to express and strengthen spirituality. **There are many options for enhancing spirituality through connectedness with self/others (e.g., volunteering, mentoring, involvement in religious activities).** (Refer to ND readiness for enhanced Spiritual Well-Being.)
- Encourage the client to join groups with similar or new interests. **Expanding knowledge and making friendships with new people will broaden horizons for the individual.**
- Refer to community resources and support groups, spiritual advisor, as indicated.

Information that appears in brackets has been added by the authors to clarify and enhance the use of nursing diagnoses.

Documentation Focus

Assessment/Reassessment
- Assessment findings, including client's perceptions of current situation, relationships, sense of desire for enhancing life
- Motivation and expectations for improvement

Planning
- Plan of care and who is involved in planning
- Teaching plan

Implementation/Evaluation
- Responses to interventions, teaching, and actions performed
- Attainment or progress toward desired outcome(s)
- Modifications to plan of care

Discharge Planning
- Long-term needs and goals for change, and who is responsible for actions to be taken
- Specific referrals made

Sample Nursing Outcomes & Interventions Classifications (NOC/NIC)

NOC—Hope
NIC—Hope Inspiration

risk for compromised HUMAN DIGNITY

[Diagnostic Division: Ego Integrity]

Definition: Vulnerable for perceived loss of respect and honor, which may compromise health.

Risk Factors

Loss of control over body function; exposure of the body
Humiliation; invasion of privacy
Disclosure of confidential information; stigmatization
Dehumanizing treatment; intrusion by clinician
Insufficient comprehension of health information
Little decision-making experience
Cultural incongruence

Information that appears in brackets has been added by the authors to clarify and enhance the use of nursing diagnoses.

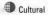

Desired Outcomes/Evaluation Criteria—Client Will:

- Verbalize awareness of specific problem.
- Identify positive ways to deal with situation.
- Demonstrate problem-solving skills.
- Express desire to increase participation in decision-making process.
- Express sense of dignity in situation.

Actions/Interventions

Nursing Priority No. 1.

To evaluate source/degree of risk:

- Determine the client's perceptions and specific factors that could lead to a sense of loss of dignity. **Human dignity is a totality of the individual's uniqueness—mind, body, and spirit.**
- Note labels or terms used by staff or friends/family that stigmatize the client. **Human dignity is threatened by insensitivity, as well as inadequate healthcare and lack of client participation in care decisions.**
- Ascertain cultural beliefs and values and degree of importance to the client. **Some individuals cling to their basic culture, especially during times of stress, which may result in conflict with current circumstances.**
- Identify healthcare goals and expectations. **This clarifies the client's (or significant other's [SO's]/family's) vision, provides a framework for planning care, and identifies possible conflicts.**
- Note the availability of family/friends for support and encouragement. **The client may manage difficult circumstances better when support of family and friends surrounds the individual.**

Nursing Priority No. 2.

To assist client/caregiver to reduce or correct individual risk factors:

- Ask the client by what name he or she would like to be called. **A person's name is important to his or her identity and recognizes one's individuality. Many older people prefer to be addressed in a formal manner (e.g., Mr. or Mrs.).**
- Active-listen feelings and be available for support and assistance, as desired, **so the client can discover underlying reasons for feelings and seek solutions to problems.**

Information that appears in brackets has been added by the authors to clarify and enhance the use of nursing diagnoses.

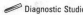

- Provide for privacy when discussing sensitive or personal issues. **This demonstrates respect for the client and promotes a sense of a safe environment for free exchange of thoughts and feelings.**
- Encourage the family/SO(s) to treat the client with respect and understanding, especially when the client is older and may be irritable and difficult to deal with. **Everyone should be treated with respect and dignity regardless of individual ability/frailty.**
- Use understandable terms when talking to the client/family about the medical condition, procedures, and treatments (component of informed consent). **Most laypeople do not understand medical terms and may be hesitant to ask what is meant.**
- Respect the client's needs and wishes for quiet, privacy, talking, or silence.
- Include the client and family in decision making, especially regarding end-of-life issues. **This helps individuals feel respected and valued, and that they are participants in the care process.**
- Protect the client's privacy when providing personal care or during procedures. Assure the client is covered adequately when care is being given **to prevent unnecessary exposure/embarrassment and preserve the client's dignity.**
- Involve the facility/local ethics committee, as appropriate, **to facilitate mediation and resolution of issues.**

Nursing Priority No. 3.

To promote wellness (Teaching/Discharge Considerations):

- Discuss the client's rights as an individual. **Hospitals and other care settings have a Patient's Bill of Rights, and a broader view of human dignity is stated in the U.S. Constitution.**
- Discuss and assist with planning for the future, taking into account the client's desires and rights.
- Incorporate identified familial, religious, and cultural factors that have meaning for the client.
- Refer to other resources (e.g., pastoral care, counseling, organized support groups, classes), as appropriate.

Documentation Focus

Assessment/Reassessment

- Assessment findings, including individual risk factors, client's perceptions, and concerns about involvement in care

Information that appears in brackets has been added by the authors to clarify and enhance the use of nursing diagnoses.

- Individual cultural and religious beliefs, values, healthcare goals
- Responses and involvement of family/SO(s)

Planning
- Plan of care and who is involved in planning
- Teaching plan

Implementation/Evaluation
- Client's response to interventions, teaching, and actions performed
- Attainment or progress toward desired outcome(s)
- Modifications to plan of care

Discharge Planning
- Long-term needs and who is responsible for actions to be taken
- Specific referrals made

Sample Nursing Outcomes & Interventions Classifications (NOC/NIC)

NOC—Client Satisfaction: Protection of Rights
NIC—Cultural Brokerage

HYPERTHERMIA

[Diagnostic Division: Safety]

Definition: Core body temperature above the normal diurnal range due to failure of thermoregulation.

Related Factors

Decreased sweat response; dehydration; vigorous activity
High environmental temperature; inappropriate clothing;
Illness; increase in metabolic rate; ischemia; sepsis
Pharmaceutical agent
Trauma

Defining Characteristics

Objective

Abnormal posturing; convulsion, seizure
Flushed skin; skin warm to touch; vasodilation

Information that appears in brackets has been added by the authors to clarify and enhance the use of nursing diagnoses.

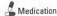

Hypotension; tachycardia; tachypnea; apnea
Irritability; lethargy; stupor; coma
Infant does not maintain suck

Desired Outcomes/Evaluation Criteria—Client Will:

- Maintain core temperature within normal range.
- Be free of complications such as irreversible brain or neurological damage, acute renal failure.
- Identify underlying cause or contributing factors and importance of treatment, as well as signs/symptoms requiring further evaluation or intervention.
- Demonstrate behaviors to monitor and promote normothermia.
- Be free of seizure activity.

Actions/Interventions

Nursing Priority No. 1.

To assess causative/contributing factors:

- Identify underlying cause. **These factors can include (1) *excessive heat production,* such as occurs with strenuous exercise, fever, shivering, tremors, convulsions, hyperthyroid state, infection or sepsis; malignant hyperpyrexia, heatstroke, use of sympathomimetic drugs; (2) *impaired heat dissipation,* such as occurs with heatstroke, dermatological diseases, burns, inability to perspire such as occurs with spinal cord injury and certain medications (e.g., diuretics, sedatives, certain heart and blood pressure medications); and (3) *loss of thermoregulation,* such as may occur in infections, brain lesions, drug overdose.**
- ∞ Note chronological and developmental age of client. **Children are more susceptible to heatstroke; elderly or impaired individuals may not be able to recognize and/or act on symptoms of hyperthermia.**

Nursing Priority No. 2.

To evaluate effects/degree of hyperthermia:

- Monitor core temperature by appropriate route (e.g., tympanic, rectal). Note the presence of temperature elevation (> 98.6°F [37°C]) or fever (100.4°F [38°C]). **Rectal and tympanic temperatures most closely approximate core temperature; however, abdominal temperature monitoring may be done in the premature neonate.**

Information that appears in brackets has been added by the authors to clarify and enhance the use of nursing diagnoses.

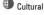

- Assess neurological responses, noting the level of consciousness and orientation, reaction to stimuli, reaction of pupils, and presence of posturing or seizures.
- Monitor blood pressure and invasive hemodynamic parameters if available (e.g., mean arterial pressure [MAP], central venous pressure [CVP]; pulmonary arterial pressure [PAP], pulmonary capillary wedge pressure [PCWP]). **Central hypertension or postural hypotension can occur.**
- Monitor heart rate and rhythm. **Dysrhythmias and electrocardiogram (ECG) changes are common due to electrolyte imbalance, dehydration, specific action of catecholamines, and direct effects of hyperthermia on blood and cardiac tissue.**
- Monitor respirations. **Hyperventilation may initially be present, but ventilatory effort may eventually be impaired by seizures or hypermetabolic state (shock and acidosis).**
- Auscultate breath sounds, noting adventitious sounds such as crackles (rales).
- Monitor and record all sources of fluid loss such as urine **(oliguria and/or renal failure may occur due to hypotension, dehydration, shock, and tissue necrosis);** vomiting and diarrhea; wounds, fistulas; and insensible losses, **which can potentiate fluid and electrolyte losses.**
- Note the presence or absence of sweating as the body attempts to increase heat loss by evaporation, conduction, and diffusion. **Evaporation is decreased by environmental factors of high humidity and high ambient temperature, as well as body factors producing loss of ability to sweat or sweat gland dysfunction (e.g., spinal cord transection, cystic fibrosis, dehydration, vasoconstriction).**
- Monitor laboratory studies, such as arterial blood gas (ABGs), electrolytes, and cardiac and liver enzymes **(may reveal tissue degeneration)**; glucose; urinalysis **(myoglobinuria, proteinuria, and hemoglobinuria can occur as products of tissue necrosis)**; and coagulation profile **(for presence of disseminated intravascular coagulation [DIC]).**

Nursing Priority No. 3.

To assist with measures to reduce body temperature/restore normal body/organ function:

- Administer antipyretics, orally or rectally (e.g., ibuprofen, acetaminophen), as ordered. Refrain from use of aspirin products in children **(may cause Reye's syndrome or liver failure)** or individuals with a clotting disorder or receiving anticoagulant therapy.

Information that appears in brackets has been added by the authors to clarify and enhance the use of nursing diagnoses.

- Promote surface cooling by means of undressing **(heat loss by radiation and conduction);** cool environment and/or fans **(heat loss by convection);** cool, tepid sponge baths or immersion (**heat loss by evaporation and conduction);** or local ice packs, especially in groin and axillae **(areas of high blood flow). Note:** In pediatric clients, tepid water is preferred. **Alcohol sponge baths are contraindicated because they increase peripheral vascular constriction and central nervous system (CNS) depression; cold water sponges or immersion can increase shivering, producing heat.**
- Monitor use of hypothermia blanket and wrap extremities with bath towels **to minimize shivering.** Turn off hypothermia blanket when core temperature is within 1 to 3 degrees of desired temperature **to allow for downward drift.**
- Administer medications (e.g., chlorpromazine or diazepam), as ordered, **to control shivering and seizures.**
- Assist with internal cooling methods to treat malignant hyperthermia **to promote rapid core cooling.**
- Promote client safety (e.g., maintain patent airway; padded side rails; skin protection from cold, such as when hypothermia blanket is used; observation of equipment safety measures).
- Provide supplemental oxygen **to offset increased oxygen demands and consumption.**
- Administer medications, as indicated, **to treat underlying cause,** such as antibiotics **(for infection),** dantrolene **(for malignant hyperthermia),** or beta-adrenergic blockers **(for thyroid storm).**
- Administer replacement fluids and electrolytes **to support circulating volume and tissue perfusion.**
- Maintain bedrest **to reduce metabolic demands and oxygen consumption.**
- Provide high-calorie diet, enteral or parenteral nutrition **to meet increased metabolic demands.**

Nursing Priority No. 4.

To promote wellness (Teaching/Discharge Considerations):

- Instruct the parents in how to measure the child's temperature, at what body temperature to give antipyretic medications, and what symptoms to report to the physician. **Fever may be treated at home to relieve the general discomfort and lethargy associated with fever. Fever is reportable, however, especially in infants or very young children with or without other symptoms and in older children or adults if it is unresponsive to antipyretics and fluids, because it often accompanies a treatable infection (viral or bacterial).**

Information that appears in brackets has been added by the authors to clarify and enhance the use of nursing diagnoses.

- Review specific risk factor or cause, such as (1) underlying conditions (hyperthyroidism, dehydration, neurological diseases, nausea, vomiting, sepsis); (2) use of certain medications (diuretics, blood pressure medications, alcohol or other drugs [cocaine, amphetamines]); (3) environmental factors (exercise or labor in hot environment, lack of air conditioning, lack of acclimatization); (4) reaction to anesthesia (malignant hyperthermia); or (5) other risk factors (salt or water depletion, elderly living alone).
- Identify those factors that the client can control (if any), such as (1) treating underlying disease process (e.g., thyroid control medication), (2) protecting oneself from excessive exposure to environmental heat (e.g., proper clothing, restriction of activity, scheduling outings during cooler part of day, use of fans/air-conditioning where possible), and (3) understanding family traits (e.g., malignant hyperthermia reaction to anesthesia is often familial).
- ∞ Instruct families/caregivers (of young children, persons who are outdoors in very hot climate, elderly living alone) in the dangers of heat exhaustion and heatstroke and ways to manage hot environments. Caution parents to avoid leaving young children in an unattended car, emphasizing the extreme hazard to the child in a very short period of time **to prevent heat injury and death.**
- Discuss the importance of adequate fluid intake **to prevent dehydration.**
- Review signs/symptoms of hyperthermia (e.g., flushed skin, increased body temperature, increased respiratory and heart rate, fainting, loss of consciousness, seizures). **This indicates a need for prompt intervention.**
- Recommend avoidance of hot tubs and saunas, as appropriate **(e.g., clients with multiple sclerosis and cardiac conditions; during pregnancy, as the high temperature may affect fetal development or increase cardiac workload).**
- ∞ Identify community resources, especially for elderly clients, to address specific needs **(e.g., provision of fans for individual use, location of cooling rooms—usually in a community center—during heat waves, daily telephone contact to assess wellness).**

Documentation Focus

Assessment/Reassessment

- Temperature and other assessment findings, including vital signs and state of mentation

Information that appears in brackets has been added by the authors to clarify and enhance the use of nursing diagnoses.

Planning
- Plan of care, specific interventions, and who is involved in the planning
- Teaching plan

Implementation/Evaluation
- Responses to interventions, teaching, and actions performed
- Attainment or progress toward desired outcome(s)
- Modifications to plan of care

Discharge Planning
- Referrals that are made, those responsible for actions to be taken

Sample Nursing Outcomes & Interventions Classifications (NOC/NIC)

NOC—Thermoregulation
NIC—Temperature Regulation

HYPOTHERMIA and risk for HYPOTHERMIA

[Diagnostic Division: Safety]

Definition: Hypothermia: Core body temperature below the normal diurnal range due to failure of thermoregulation.

Definition: risk for Hypothermia: Vulnerable to a failure of thermoregulation that may result in a core body temperature below the normal diurnal range, which may compromise health.

Related Factors (Hypothermia)

Alcohol consumption
Economically disadvantaged
Extremes of age or weight
Insufficient clothing

Information that appears in brackets has been added by the authors to clarify and enhance the use of nursing diagnoses.

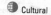

Heat transfer (e.g., conduction, convection, evaporation, radiation)
Insufficient knowledge of hypothermia prevention
Malnutrition; decrease in metabolic rate; insufficient supply of subcutaneous fat; inactivity
Pharmaceutical agent, [drug overdose]
Trauma; damage to hypothalamus; radiation

Neonates

High risk or unplanned out-of-hospital birth
Delay in breastfeeding
Early bathing of newborn
Immature stratum corneum
Increased body surface area to weight ratio
Increase in oxygen demand; increase in pulmonary vascular resistance (PVR); ineffective vascular control
Insufficient nonshivering thermogenesis

Risk Factors (risk for Hypothermia)

Alcohol consumption
Economically disadvantaged
Extremes of age or weight
Heat transfer (e.g., conduction, convection, evaporation, radiation)
Insufficient caregiver knowledge of hypothermia prevention
Low environmental temperature; inactivity; insufficient clothing
Malnutrition; insufficient supply of subcutaneous fat
Pharmaceutical agent
Trauma; damage to hypothalamus; radiation

Children and Adults: Accidental

Mild hypothermia, core temperature approaching 95°F (35°C)
Moderate hypothermia, core temperature approaching 89.6°F (32°C)
Severe hypothermia, core temperature approaching 86°F (30°C)

Children and Adults: Injured Patients

Hypothermia, core temperature approaching 95°F (35°C)
Severe hypothermia, core temperature approaching 89.6°F (32°C)

Information that appears in brackets has been added by the authors to clarify and enhance the use of nursing diagnoses.

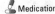

Neonates

Grade 1 hypothermia, core temperature approaching 97.7°F (36.5°C)
Grade 2 hypothermia, core temperature approaching 96.8°F (36°C)
Grade 3 hypothermia, core temperature approaching 95°F (35°C)
Grade 4 hypothermia, core temperature approaching 93.2°F (34°C)
Decrease in metabolic rate; increase in oxygen demand; increase in pulmonary vascular resistance (PVR); ineffective vascular control
Delay in breastfeeding
Early bathing of newborn
High-risk or unplanned-out-of-hospital birth
Immature stratum corneum
Increased body surface area to weight ratio
Ineffective nonshivering thermogenesis

> **NOTE:** A risk diagnosis is not evidenced by signs and symptoms as the problem has not occurred; rather, nursing interventions are directed at prevention.

Defining Characteristics (Hypothermia only)

Objective

Acrocyanosis, cyanotic nail beds; peripheral vasoconstriction; hypoxia
Bradycardia; tachycardia
Decrease in blood glucose level; hypoglycemia
Increase in metabolic rate; increase in oxygen consumption
Shivering; piloerection
Skin cool to touch; slow capillary refill

Accidental Low Body Temperature in Children and Adults

Mild hypothermia, core temperature 89.6°F–95°F (32°C–35°C)
Moderate hypothermia, core temperature 86°F–89.6°F (30°C–32°C)
Severe hypothermia, core temperature 86°F (<30°C)

Injured Adults and Children

Hypothermia, core temperature 95°F (<35°C)
Severe hypothermia, core temperature 89.6°F (<32°C)

Information that appears in brackets has been added by the authors to clarify and enhance the use of nursing diagnoses.

Neonates

Grade 1 hypothermia, core temperature 96.8°F–97.7°F (36°C–36.5°C)

Grade 2 hypothermia, core temperature 95°F–96.6°F (35°C–35.9°C)

Grade 3 hypothermia, core temperature 93.2°F–94.8°F (34°C–34.9°C)

Grade 4 hypothermia, core temperature 93.2°F (<34°C)

Infant with insufficient energy to maintain sucking; or with insufficient weight gain (<30 g/d)

Irritability

Jaundice, pallor

Respiratory distress; metabolic acidosis

Bradycardia; tachycardia

Decrease in blood glucose level; hypoglycemia

Increase in metabolic rate; increase in oxygen consumption

Shivering; piloerection

Skin cool to touch; slow capillary refill

Desired Outcomes/Evaluation Criteria—Client Will:

- Display core temperature within normal range.
- Be free of complications, such as cardiac failure, respiratory infection or failure, thromboembolic phenomena.
- Identify underlying cause or contributing factors that are within client control.
- Verbalize understanding of specific interventions to prevent hypothermia.
- Demonstrate behaviors to monitor and promote normothermia.

Caregiver Will:

- Maintain a safe environment.
- Identify underlying cause or contributing factors that are within caregiver control.
- Verbalize an understanding of specific interventions to prevent hypothermia.
- Demonstrate behaviors to monitor and promote normothermia.

Actions/Interventions

Nursing Priority No. 1.

To assess causative/contributing or risk factors:

Information that appears in brackets has been added by the authors to clarify and enhance the use of nursing diagnoses.

- Note underlying cause, for example, **(1) *decreased heat production,* such as occurs with hypopituitary, hypoadrenal and hypothyroid conditions, hypoglycemia and neuromuscular inefficiencies seen in extremes of age; (2) *increased heat loss,* such as occurs with exposure to cold weather, winter outdoor activities; cold water drenching or immersion, improper clothing, shelter, or food for conditions; vasodilation from medications, drugs, or poisons; skin-surface problems such as burns or psoriasis; fluid losses, dehydration; surgery, open wounds, exposed skin or viscera; multiple rapid infusions of cold solutions or transfusions of banked blood; overtreatment of hyperthermia; or (3) *impaired thermoregulation.* Hypothalamus failure might occur with central nervous system (CNS) trauma or tumor; intracranial bleeding or stroke; toxicological and metabolic disorders; or Parkinson's disease, multiple sclerosis (MS).**
- Note contributing or risk factors, such as age of client (e.g., premature neonate, child, elderly person); concurrent or coexisting medical problems (e.g., brainstem injury, CNS trauma, near drowning, sepsis, hypothyroidism); other factors (e.g., alcohol or other drug use or abuse; homelessness); living conditions; or relationship status (e.g., mentally impaired client alone).

Nursing Priority No. 2.

To prevent hypothermia **(risk for Hypothermia)**:

- Maintain a warm ambient environment, especially in facility settings (e.g., operating room, delivery room, bath areas, etc.).
- Wear appropriate warm clothing (layers plus appropriate outwear, shoes, socks, and boots) in cold weather. Make sure children and frail elderly are well wrapped up when outdoors and have limited time exposures.
- Heed severe cold weather warnings, staying inside when possible.
- Carry cold weather, blankets, emergency gear, and extra batteries for cell phones in car in event of winter storms.
- Remove wet clothing and bedding promptly.
- Add extra clothing and warmed blankets.
- Increase physical activity if possible.
- Eat and drink (warm drinks) regularly when outside during cold weather. Avoid alcohol.

Information that appears in brackets has been added by the authors to clarify and enhance the use of nursing diagnoses.

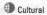

- For newborns: Dry newborn with a clean, soft, warm towel. Wrap the baby in layers. Ensure the head is well covered. Keep the baby by the side of the mother and/or use skin-to-skin contact with the mother. Postpone the first bath.

Nursing Priority No. 3.

To prevent a further decrease in body temperature **(Hypothermia)**:

Mild-to-moderate hypothermia:

- Remove wet clothing and bedding.
- Add layers of clothing, and wrap in warm blankets.
- Increase physical activity if possible.
- Provide warm liquids after shivering stops if client is alert and can swallow.
- Provide warm, nutrient-dense food (carbohydrates, proteins, and fats) and fluids (hot sweet liquids are easily digestible and absorbable).
- Avoid alcohol, caffeine, and tobacco **to prevent vasodilation, diuresis, or vasoconstriction, respectively.**
- Place in warm ambient temperature environment and protect from drafts; provide external heat sources.
- Provide barriers to heat loss, as well as active rewarming for newborns, especially preterm and/or low-birth-weight infants, monitoring temperature closely. **Measures might include the use of protective hats, open radiant warmer or Isolette, and/or heating blanket.**

Severe hypothermia:

- Remove the client from causative or contributing factors.
- Dry the skin, cover with blankets, and provide shelter with warm ambient temperature; use radiant lights.
- Provide heat to trunk, not to extremities, initially. Avoid the use of heat lamps or hot water bottles. **Surface re-warming can result in rewarming shock due to surface vasodilation.**
- Keep the individual lying down. Avoid jarring **(can trigger an abnormal heart rhythm).**

Nursing Priority No. 4.

To evaluate effects of hypothermia (**Hypothermia**):

- Measure the core temperature with a low-register thermometer (measuring below 94°F [34.4°C]).
- Assess respiratory effort (**rate and tidal volume are reduced when metabolic rate decreases and respiratory acidosis occurs**).

Information that appears in brackets has been added by the authors to clarify and enhance the use of nursing diagnoses.

- Auscultate lungs, noting adventitious sounds. **Pulmonary edema, respiratory infection, and pulmonary embolus are possible complications of hypothermia.**
- Monitor heart rate and rhythm. **Cold stress reduces pacemaker function, and bradycardia (unresponsive to atropine), atrial fibrillation, atrioventricular blocks, and ventricular tachycardia can occur. Ventricular fibrillation occurs most frequently when core temperature is 82°F (27.7°C) or below.**
- Monitor blood pressure, noting hypotension. **This can occur due to vasoconstriction and shunting of fluids as a result of cold injury effect on capillary permeability.**
- Measure urine output. **Oliguria and renal failure can occur due to low flow state and/or following hypothermic osmotic diuresis.**
- Note CNS effects (e.g., mood changes, sluggish thinking, amnesia, complete obtundation); and peripheral CNS effects (e.g., paralysis—87.7°F [30.9°C]; dilated pupils—below 86°F [30°C]; flat electroencephalogram [EEG]—68°F [20°C]).
- Monitor laboratory studies, such as arterial blood gas (ABGs) **(respiratory and metabolic acidosis);** electrolytes; complete blood count (CBC) **(increased hematocrit, decreased white blood cell count);** cardiac enzymes **(myocardial infarct may occur owing to electrolyte imbalance, cold-stress catecholamine release, hypoxia, or acidosis);** coagulation profile; glucose; and pharmacological profile **(for possible cumulative drug effects).**

Nursing Priority No. 5.

To restore normal body temperature/organ function **(Hypothermia):**

- Assist with measures to normalize core temperature, such as warmed IV solutions and warm solution lavage of body cavities (gastric, peritoneal, bladder) or cardiopulmonary bypass, if indicated.
- Rewarm no faster than 1 to 2 degrees per hour **to avoid sudden vasodilation, increased metabolic demands on heart, and hypotension (rewarming shock).**
- Assist with surface warming by means of heated blankets, warm environment or radiant heater, electronic heating/cooling devices. Cover head, neck, and thorax. Leave extremities uncovered, as appropriate, **to maintain peripheral vaso-**

Information that appears in brackets has been added by the authors to clarify and enhance the use of nursing diagnoses.

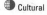

constriction. Refrain from instituting surface rewarming prior to core rewarming in severe hypothermia **as it may cause afterdrop of temperature by shunting cold blood back to the heart in addition to rewarming shock as a result of surface vasodilation.**

- Protect the skin and tissues by repositioning, applying lotion or lubricants, and avoiding direct contact with heating appliance or blanket. **Impaired circulation can result in severe tissue damage.**
- Keep client quiet; handle gently **to reduce the potential for fibrillation in a cold heart.**
- Provide CPR, as necessary, with compressions initially at one-half the normal heart rate **(severe hypothermia causes slowed conduction, and a cold heart may be unresponsive to medications, pacing, and defibrillation).**
- Maintain patent airway. Assist with intubation and mechanical ventilation, if indicated.
- Provide heated, humidified oxygen when used.
- Turn off warming blanket when temperature is within 1 to 3 degrees of desired temperature **to avoid hyperthermia situation.**
- Administer IV fluids with caution **to prevent overload as the vascular bed expands (a cold heart is slow to compensate for increased volume).**
- Avoid vigorous drug therapy. **As rewarming occurs, organ function returns, correcting endocrine abnormalities, and tissues become more receptive to the effects of drugs previously administered.**
- Perform range-of-motion exercises, provide sequential compression devices (SCDs), reposition, encourage coughing and deep-breathing exercises, avoid restrictive clothing or restraints **to reduce effects of circulatory stasis.**
- Provide well-balanced, high-calorie diet or feedings **to replenish glycogen stores and nutritional balance.**

Nursing Priority No. 6.

To promote wellness (Teaching/Discharge Considerations)**(Hypothermia and risk for Hypothermia)**:

- Review specific risk factors or causes of hypothermia. Note that hypothermia can be *accidental* or *intentional* (such as occurs when induced-hypothermia therapy is used after cardiac arrest or brain injury), requiring interventions to protect client from adverse effects.
- Discuss signs/symptoms of early hypothermia (e.g., changes in mentation, poor judgment, somnolence, impaired coordi-

Information that appears in brackets has been added by the authors to clarify and enhance the use of nursing diagnoses.

nation, slurred speech) **to facilitate recognition of problem and timely intervention.**
- Identify factors that client can control (if any), such as protection from environment/adequate heat in home; layering clothing and blankets; minimizing heat loss from head with hat/scarf; appropriate cold weather clothing; avoidance of alcohol/other drugs if anticipating exposure to cold; potential risk for future hypersensitivity to cold; and so forth.
- Identify assistive community resources, as indicated (e.g., social services, emergency shelters, clothing suppliers, food bank, public service company, financial resources). **Individual/SO may be in need of numerous resources if hypothermia was associated with inadequate housing, homelessness, or malnutrition.**

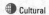

Documentation Focus

Assessment/Reassessment
- Findings, noting degree of system involvement, respiratory rate, ECG pattern, capillary refill, and level of mentation
- Graph temperature

Planning
- Plan of care and who is involved in planning
- Teaching plan

Implementation/Evaluation
- Responses to interventions, teaching, and actions performed
- Attainment or progress toward desired outcome(s)
- Modifications to plan of care

Discharge Planning
- Long-term needs, identifying who is responsible for each action

Sample Nursing Outcomes & Interventions Classifications (NOC/NIC)

NOC—Thermoregulation
NIC—Hypothermia Treatment

Information that appears in brackets has been added by the authors to clarify and enhance the use of nursing diagnoses.

risk for perioperative **HYPOTHERMIA**

[Diagnostic Division: Safety]

Definition: Vulnerable to an inadvertent drop in core body temperature below 36°C/96.8°F occurring one hour before to 24 hours after surgery, which may compromise health.

Risk Factors

American Society of Anesthesiologists (ASA) Physical Status classification score > 1
Cardiovascular complications
Combined regional and general anesthesia
Diabetic neuropathy
Heat transfer (e.g., high volume of unwarmed infusion, unwarmed irrigation > 20 liters)
Low body weight
Low environmental temperature
Low preoperative temperature (<36°C/96.8°F)
Surgical procedure

NOTE: A risk diagnosis is not evidenced by signs and symptoms as the problem has not occurred; rather, nursing interventions are directed at prevention.

Desired Outcomes/Evaluation Criteria—Client Will:

- Display core temperature within normal range.
- Be free of complications such as cardiac failure, respiratory infection or failure, thromboembolic phenomena, and delayed healing.

Caregiver Will:

Identify client condition/situations that may lead to problems with temperature regulation.
Engage in protective actions to control body temperature.

Actions/Interventions

Nursing Priority No. 1.

To identify risk factors affecting current situation:

Information that appears in brackets has been added by the authors to clarify and enhance the use of nursing diagnoses.

- Ascertain the type of surgical procedure the client is having. **This helps in identifying elements of risk. For example, some procedures carry a higher risk of hypothermia (e.g., laparoscopic abdominal procedure with carbon dioxide insufflation; extensive surgical procedure of any sort with prolonged exposure of body surfaces and long period of anesthesia).**
- Assess client conditions/comorbidites (e.g., diabetes, impaired skin and tissue integrity, respiratory, cardiac, vascular, or neurologic disorders) **that may place the client at a higher risk for perioperative complications, including hypothermia.**
- ∞ Note the client's body type and age. **Very thin, malnourished, or dehydrated individuals, as well as the very young or elderly are more susceptible to perioperative hypothermia.**
- Note the client's medication regimen. **Medications including some vasodilators, antipsychotics, and sedatives can impair the body's ability to regulate its temperature.**

Nursing Priority No. 2.

To maintain appropriate body temperature/prevent hypothermia complications:

- Measure the client's temperature preoperatively, and confirm that continuous monitoring of temperature is occurring during the procedure. Report a preoperative temperature below the ideal range to the surgical team/anesthesiologist.
- Implement preventive warming techniques (e.g., blankets from warmer in holding area; forced-air warming, warm IV and irrigation fluids) in the operating room: **(Evidence supports commencement of active warming preoperatively and monitoring it throughout the intraoperative period.)**

  Consider administering warmed IV fluids. **AORN states, "warming IV fluids to near 37°C (98.6°F) prevents heat loss from the administration of cold IV fluids and should be considered as an adjunct to skin surface warming."**

  Use heated blankets from warming cabinet, if needed. **While easy to use and effective, blankets on top of the client can limit access to the surgical site. Also, adding too many layers of warmed cotton blankets is ineffective in raising the patient's body temperature.**

  Use conductive warming devices, such as **an electrical resistive/conductive device that warms from under-**

Information that appears in brackets has been added by the authors to clarify and enhance the use of nursing diagnoses.

neath the client's body; therefore, blankets need not be placed on top, allowing for greater surgical access.

Provide forced air warming blanket. **Heat transfer results from the movement of warm air across the surface of the patient's skin, which allows more heat to be transferred at a lower temperature than with the use of other devices.**

Use warm water garment or mattress. **Circulating water garments and energy transfer pads warm about 50% better than forced air, because they warm both over and under the body.**

Increase the operating room temperature, as indicated. **Optimal operating room temperatures are currently thought to be no less than 68°F (20°C) to reduce the risk of hypothermia complications while still providing a comfortable environment for scrubbed personnel under surgical lights. Recovery room temperatures of 68°F to 75°F (20°C to 24°C) may be ideal for rewarming the client.**

Documentation Focus

Assessment/Reassessment

- Findings, noting degree of system involvement
- Graph temperature

Planning

- Plan of care

Implementation/Evaluation

- Responses to interventions and actions performed
- Attainment of desired outcome(s)
- Modifications to plan of care

Sample Nursing Outcomes & Interventions Classifications (NOC/NIC)

NOC—Risk Control: Hypothermia
NIC—Temperature Regulation: Intraoperative

Information that appears in brackets has been added by the authors to clarify and enhance the use of nursing diagnoses.

ineffective IMPULSE CONTROL

[Diagnostic Division: Ego Integrity]

Definition: A pattern of performing rapid, unplanned reactions to internal or external stimuli without regard for the negative consequences of these reactions to the impulsive individual or to others.

Related Factors

Anger; denial; delusion
Insomnia; fatigue
Chronic low self-esteem; disturbed body image; hopelessness
Stress vulnerability; environment that might cause irritation, frustration
Ineffective coping; codependency
Smoker; substance abuse
Economically disadvantage
Social isolation; suicidal feelings
Compunction [i.e., feeling of uneasiness about rightness of action]; unpleasant physical symptoms
Organic brain disorders; disorder of cognition, development, mood, personality

Defining Characteristics

Subjective

Inability to save money or regulate finances
Asking personal questions of others despite their discomfort

Objective

Acting without thinking
Sensation seeking; sexual promiscuity
Sharing personal details inappropriately; too familiar with strangers
Irritability; temper outbursts; violence
Pathological gambling

Desired Outcomes/Evaluation Criteria—Client Will:

- Acknowledge problem with impulse control.
- Identify feelings that precede desire to engage in impulsive actions.

Information that appears in brackets has been added by the authors to clarify and enhance the use of nursing diagnoses.

- Verbalize desire to learn new ways of controlling impulsive behavior.
- Participate in anger management therapy.

Actions/Interventions

Nursing Priority No. 1.

To assess causative/contributing factors:

- Investigate causes/individual factors that may be involved in the client's situation. **Current theory suggests unbalanced neurotransmitters in the brain may be a cause as well as hormone imbalances implicated in violent and aggressive behavior. Brain injuries/tumors may also result in poor impulse control.**
- Explore the individual's inability to control actions. **Healthy people are aware of an impulse and are able to make a decision about following the urge or not. The key differentiation between healthy impulsiveness and an impulse disorder is the negative consequences that follow.**
- Note negative consequences incurred by client's impulsive actions such as repeat detentions or suspensions from school, loss of employment, financial ruin, arrests/convictions, or civil litigation. **Those with lack of control engage in the behavior even if the individual knows that there will be a negative consequence.**
- Ascertain the degree of anxiety the client experiences when having an impulse to act on the desire. **Not acting on the impulse creates intense anxiety or arousal in the individual. Engaging in the behavior produces a release of the anxiety and possibly pleasure or gratification. This may be followed by remorse, regret, or, conversely, satisfaction.**
- Identify behaviors indicative of attention deficit disorder for further evaluation by therapeutic team.

Nursing Priority No. 2.

To assist client to develop strategies to manage impulsive behaviors:

- Collaborate with treatment of underlying conditions, when possible. **Individuals with impulsive control disorders do not necessarily present for treatment. Those with kleptomania, fire starters, and compulsive gamblers usually come to the attention of court authorities and may be referred for mental health services.**

Information that appears in brackets has been added by the authors to clarify and enhance the use of nursing diagnoses.

- Encourage the client to make the decision to change and set personally achievable goals.
- Have the client identify negative consequences of behavior by expressing his or her own feelings and anxieties regarding the adverse impact on his or her life. **This helps the individual begin to understand problems of impulsive behavior.**
- Help the client take responsibility and control in the situation. **Recognizing his or her own control over impulsive behavior can help the client begin to manage problems.**
- Develop a treatment plan for a child with attention deficit-hyperactivity disorder (ADHD) in conjunction with the parents and the physician. **Medications and behavioral therapy can be helpful, along with monitoring the child and setting goals that are realistic and achievable.**
- Organize a routine schedule for the child with Autism spectrum disorder. **Deficits in cognitive functioning make it difficult for the child to see the big picture, process information, see the consequences of an action, and understand the concept of time.**
- Plan for problem with "melt-downs," tantrums, or rage in children with Autism spectrum disorder. **These children do not recognize feelings, and parents/caregivers need to maintain a calm manner and remove the child in a nonpunitive calming fashion. The child who is acting out may need to go to a safe room where he or she can regain control.**
- Discuss the issue of hypersexuality.
- Determine the use of medications. **No specific medications have been approved by the U.S. Food and Drug Administration for use with impulse control disorders; however, some medications such as selective serotonin reuptake inhibitor (SSRI) antidepressants are being used successfully.**

Nursing Priority No. 3.

To promote wellness (Teaching/Discharge Considerations):

- Involve the client in cognitive/behavioral therapy. **Having the client identify behavioral patterns that result in negative consequences/harmful effects allows the individual to recognize these situations and use techniques that facilitate self-restraint.**
- Discuss the use of exposure therapy. **This helps the client build up a tolerance for the trigger situation while using self-control.**
- Encourage the client to become involved in group or community activities. **This provides opportunity to learn new social skills and feel better about self.**

Information that appears in brackets has been added by the authors to clarify and enhance the use of nursing diagnoses.

Documentation Focus

Assessment/Reassessment

- Individual findings, including type of situation involved in client's loss of control
- Negative consequences incurred due to behavior
- Client awareness of consequences of actions

Planning

- Plan of care, specific interventions, and who is involved in planning
- Individual teaching plan

Implementation/Evaluation

- Responses to interventions, teaching and actions performed
- Attainment or progress toward desired outcome(s)
- Any modifications to plan of care

Discharge Planning

- Long-term needs and who is responsible for actions to be taken
- Specific referrals made

Sample Nursing Outcomes & Interventions Classifications (NOC/NIC)

NOC—Impulse Self-Control
NIC—Impulse Control Training

bowel INCONTINENCE

[Diagnostic Division: Elimination]

Definition: Change in normal bowel habits characterized by involuntary passage of stool.

Related Factors

Abnormal increase in abdominal or intestinal pressure
Alteration in cognitive functioning; stressors
Chronic diarrhea; impaction; incomplete emptying of the bowel
Colorectal lesion; dysfunctional or abnormal rectal sphincter; impaired reservoir capacity; upper or lower motor nerve damage
Deficient dietary habits

Information that appears in brackets has been added by the authors to clarify and enhance the use of nursing diagnoses.

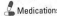

Difficulty in toileting self-care
Environmental factor (e.g., inaccessible bathroom)
Generalized decline in muscle tone; immobility
Pharmaceutical agent; laxative abuse

Defining Characteristics

Subjective

Inability to expel formed stool despite recognition of rectal fullness
Bowel urgency; inability to delay defecation
Inability to recognize rectal fullness

Objective

Constant passage of soft stool
Fecal staining of clothing, bedding
Fecal odor
Reddened perianal skin
Does not recognize or inattention to urge to defecate

Desired Outcomes/Evaluation Criteria—Client Will:

- Verbalize understanding of causative and controlling factors.
- Identify individually appropriate interventions.
- Participate in therapeutic regimen to control incontinence.
- Establish/maintain as regular a pattern of bowel functioning as possible.

Actions/Interventions

Nursing Priority No. 1.

To assess causative/contributing factors:

- Determine the type of bowel incontinence present, as possible **(1) loss of anal sphincter control (such as might occur with sphincter trauma); (2) stool seepage (as may result from fistulas or prolapse); or (3) poor bowel control (as might occur with inflammatory bowel disease, following intestinal surgery; chronic constipation with weakening musculature; laxative abuse, parasitic infection, and toxins).**
- Determine historical aspects of incontinence with preceding/precipitating events. **Common factors include (1) structural changes in the sphincter muscle (e.g., hemorrhoids, rectal prolapse; prostate, anal, or gynecological surgery; vaginal delivery; inadequate repair of obstetric sphincter disrup-**

Information that appears in brackets has been added by the authors to clarify and enhance the use of nursing diagnoses.

 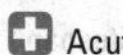 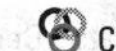 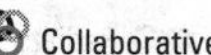 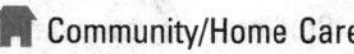 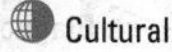

tion); (2) injuries to sensory nerves (e.g., spinal cord injury, multiple sclerosis); major trauma; stroke, tumor, radiation therapy; (3) strong-urge or severe prolonged diarrhea (e.g., ulcerative colitis, Crohn's disease, infectious diarrhea); (4) dementia (e.g., acute or chronic cognitive impairment, not necessarily related to sphincter control); (5) result of toxins (e.g., salmonella); (6) aging, particularly in menopausal women; and (7) effects of improper diet or type and rate of enteral feedings.**

- Note the client's age and gender. **Bowel incontinence is more common in children, women of childbearing age, and elderly adults (difficulty responding to urge in a timely manner, problems walking or undoing zippers, decrease of maximum squeeze pressure); more common in boys than girls, but more common in elderly women than elderly men.**
- Review medication regimen (e.g., sedatives/hypnotics, narcotics, muscle relaxants, antacids). **Many medications and their side effects or interactions can increase the potential for bowel problems.**
- Review results of diagnostic studies (e.g., abdominal x-rays, colon endoscopy/other imaging, complete blood count, serum chemistries, stool for blood [guaiac]), as appropriate.
- Palpate abdomen **for distention, masses, and tenderness.**

Nursing Priority No. 2.

To determine current pattern of elimination:

- Ascertain timing and characteristic aspects of incontinent occurrence, noting preceding or precipitating events. **This helps to identify patterns or worsening trends. Interventions are different for sudden acute accident than for chronic long-term incontinence problems.**
- Note stool characteristics including consistency (may be liquid, hard formed, or hard at first and then soft), amount (may be a small amount of liquid or entire solid bowel movement), and frequency. **Characteristics provide information that can help differentiate the type of incontinence present and provide comparative baseline for response to interventions.**
- Encourage the client/significant other (SO) to record times at which incontinence occurs **to note relationship to meals, activity, medications, or client's behavior.**
- Auscultate abdomen **for presence, location, and characteristics of bowel sounds.**

Information that appears in brackets has been added by the authors to clarify and enhance the use of nursing diagnoses.

Nursing Priority No. 3.

To promote control/management of incontinence:

- Assist in the treatment of causative/contributing factors (e.g., as listed in the Related Factors and Defining Characteristics).
- Establish bowel program in client requiring constant bowel care, with predictable time for defecation efforts; use suppositories and/or digital stimulation when indicated. Maintain daily program initially. Progress to alternate days dependent on usual pattern or amount of stool.
- Establish a toileting program where possible (e.g., take client to the bathroom, or place on commode or bedpan at specified intervals, taking into consideration individual needs and incontinence patterns) **to maximize success of program and preserve client's comfort and self-esteem.**
- Encourage and instruct client/caregiver in providing diet high in bulk/fiber and adequate fluids (minimum of 2,000 mL/day if cardiac or renal conditions allow). Encourage warm fluids after meals.
- Identify and eliminate problem foods **to avoid diarrhea, constipation, and gas formation.**
- Administer stool softeners, fiber-filled agents, or bulk formers as indicated.
- Adjust enteral feedings and/or change formula, as indicated, **to reduce diarrhea effect.**
- Provide pericare with frequent gentle cleansing and use of emollients **to avoid perineal excoriation.**
- Promote exercise program, as individually able, **to increase muscle tone/strength, including perineal muscles.**
- Provide incontinence aids/pads until control is obtained. **Note:** Incontinence pads should be changed frequently **to reduce incidence of skin rashes/breakdown.**
- Demonstrate techniques (e.g., contracting abdominal muscles, leaning forward on commode, manual compression) **to increase intra-abdominal pressure during defecation,** and left to right abdominal massage **to stimulate peristalsis.**
- Refer to ND Diarrhea if incontinence is due to uncontrolled diarrhea; refer to ND Constipation if incontinence is due to impaction.

Nursing Priority No. 4.

To promote wellness (Teaching/Discharge Considerations):

- Review and encourage continuation of successful interventions as individually identified.

Information that appears in brackets has been added by the authors to clarify and enhance the use of nursing diagnoses.

- Instruct in use of suppositories or stool softeners, if indicated, **to stimulate timed defecation.**
- Identify foods (e.g., daily bran muffins, prunes) **that promote soft stool consistency and bowel regularity.**
- Provide emotional support to client and SO(s), especially when condition is long term or chronic. **This enhances coping with the difficult situation.**
- Encourage scheduling of social activities within time frame of bowel program, as indicated (e.g., avoid a 4-hr excursion if bowel program requires toileting every 3 hr and facilities will not be available), **to maximize social functioning and success of bowel program.**
- Refer the client/caregivers to outside resources when condition is long term or chronic **to obtain care assistance and emotional support and respite.**

Documentation Focus

Assessment/Reassessment

- Current and previous pattern of elimination, physical findings, character of stool, actions tried

Planning

- Plan of care and who is involved in planning
- Teaching plan

Implementation/Evaluation

- Client's/caregiver's responses to interventions, teaching, and actions performed
- Changes in pattern of elimination, characteristics of stool
- Attainment or progress toward desired outcome(s)
- Modifications to plan of care

Discharge Planning

- Identified long-term needs, noting who is responsible for each action
- Specific bowel program at time of discharge

Sample Nursing Outcomes & Interventions Classifications (NOC/NIC)

NOC—Bowel Continence
NIC—Bowel Incontinence Care

Information that appears in brackets has been added by the authors to clarify and enhance the use of nursing diagnoses.

functional urinary INCONTINENCE

[Diagnostic Division: Elimination]

Definition: Inability of usually continent person to reach the toilet in time to avoid unintentional loss of urine.

Related Factors

Alteration in environmental factor
Neuromuscular impairment
Weakened supporting pelvic structure
Impaired vision
Psychological disorder; alteration in cognitive functioning; [reluctance to call for assistance or use bedpan]

Defining Characteristics

Subjective

Sensation of need to void

Objective

Voiding prior to reaching toilet; time between sensation of urge and ability to reach toilet is too short
Completely empties bladder
Early morning urinary incontinence

Desired Outcomes/Evaluation Criteria—Client/Caregiver Will:

- Verbalize understanding of condition and identify interventions to prevent incontinence.
- Alter environment to accommodate individual needs.
- Report voiding in individually appropriate amounts.
- Urinate at acceptable times and places.

Actions/Interventions

Nursing Priority No. 1.

To assess causative/contributing factors:

- ∞ Identify or differentiate client with functional incontinence (e.g., bladder and urethra are functioning normally, but client either cannot get to toilet or fails to recognize need to urinate in time to get to the toilet) from other types of incontinence.

Information that appears in brackets has been added by the authors to clarify and enhance the use of nursing diagnoses.

Many of these causes are transient and reversible but can often occur in elderly hospitalized client.

- Evaluate cognition. **Delirium or acute confusion or psychiatric illness can affect mental status, orientation to place, recognition of urge to void, and/or its significance.**
- Note presence and type of functional impairments (e.g., poor eyesight, mobility problems, dexterity problems, self-care deficits) **that can hinder ability to get to bathroom.**
- Identify environmental conditions that interfere with timely access to bathroom or successful toileting process. **Unfamiliar surroundings, poor lighting, improperly fitted chair walker, low toilet seat, absence of safety bars, and travel distance to toilet may affect self-care ability.**
- Determine if the client is voluntarily postponing urination. **Often the demands of the work setting (e.g., restrictions on bathroom breaks, heavy workload, and inability to find time for bathroom breaks) make it difficult for individuals to go to the bathroom when the need arises, resulting in incontinence.**
- Review medical history for conditions known to increase urine output or alter bladder tone. **For example, diabetes mellitus, prolapsed bladder, and multiple sclerosis can affect frequency of urination and ability to hold urine until individual can reach the bathroom.**
- Note use of medications or agents that can increase urine formation. **Diuretics, alcohol, and caffeine are several substances that can increase amount and frequency of voiding.**
- Test urine for the presence of glucose. **Hyperglycemia can cause polyuria and overdistention of the bladder, resulting in problems with continence.**

Nursing Priority No. 2.

To assess degree of interference/disability:

- Determine frequency and timing of continent and incontinent voids. Note time of day or night when incontinence occurs, as well as timing issues (e.g., difference between the time it takes to get to bathroom and remove clothing and involuntary loss of urine). **Information will be used to plan program to manage incontinence.**
- Ascertain effect on client's lifestyle (including socialization and sexuality) and self-esteem. **Individuals with incontinence problems are often embarrassed, withdraw from so-**

Information that appears in brackets has been added by the authors to clarify and enhance the use of nursing diagnoses.

cial activities and relationships, and hesitate to discuss the problem—even with their healthcare provider.

Nursing Priority No. 3.

To assist in treating/preventing incontinence:

- Remind the client to void when needed and schedule voiding times **to reduce incontinence episodes and promote comfort for client who ambulates slowly because of physical limitations or who has cognitive decline.**
- Administer prescribed diuretics in the morning **to lessen nighttime voidings.**
- Reduce or eliminate the use of hypnotics, if possible, **as client may be too sedated to recognize or respond to urge to void.**
- Provide means of summoning assistance (e.g., call light or bell) and respond immediately to summons. **This enables the client to obtain toileting help, as needed. Quick response to summons can promote continence.**
- Use night-lights. **An elderly person may become confused upon arising and be unable to locate the bathroom in the dark. Lighting will facilitate access, reducing the possibility of accidents.**
- Provide cues, such as adequate room lighting, signs, color coding of door, **to assist the client who is disoriented to find the bathroom.**
- Remove throw rugs and excess furniture in travel path to the bathroom.
- Provide a raised toilet seat or easily accessible bedside commode, urinal, or bedpan, as indicated. **This facilitates toileting when an individual has difficulty with movement.**
- Adapt clothes for quick removal, for example, Velcro fasteners, full skirts, crotchless panties, suspenders or elastic waists instead of belts on pants. **This facilitates toileting once the urge to void is noted.**
- Assist the client to assume a normal anatomic position **for ease of complete bladder emptying.**
- Schedule voiding for every 2 to 3 hr. Encourage the client to resist ignoring the urge to urinate or have a bowel movement. **Emptying the bladder on a regular schedule or when feeling an urge reduces the risk for incontinence. Since the urge to void may be difficult to differentiate from the urge to defecate, advise the client to respond to the urge.**
- Restrict fluid intake 2 to 3 hr before bedtime **to reduce nighttime voidings.**

Information that appears in brackets has been added by the authors to clarify and enhance the use of nursing diagnoses.

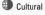

- Include physical/occupational therapist in determining ways to alter environment and identifying appropriate assistive devices to meet the client's individual needs.
- Refer to urologist or continence specialist as indicated for interventions such as pelvic floor strengthening exercises, biofeedback techniques, and vaginal weight training. **This may be useful/needed to meet individual needs of client.**

Nursing Priority No. 4.

To promote wellness (Teaching/Discharge Considerations):

- Discuss with client/SO(s) need for prompted and scheduled voidings **to manage continence when the client is unable to respond immediately to the urge to void.**
- Suggest limiting intake of coffee, tea, and alcohol **because of diuretic effect and impact on voiding pattern.**
- Maintain positive regard **to reduce embarrassment associated with incontinence, need for assistance, or use of bedpan.**
- Promote participation in developing a long-term plan of care. **This encourages involvement in follow-through of plan, thus increasing possibility of success and confidence in own ability to manage program.**
- Refer to NDs reflex urinary Incontinence; stress urinary Incontinence; urge urinary Incontinence.

Documentation Focus

Assessment/Reassessment

- Current elimination pattern and assessment findings
- Effect on lifestyle and self-esteem

Planning

- Plan of care and who is involved in planning
- Teaching plan

Implementation/Evaluation

- Response to interventions, teaching, and actions performed
- Attainment or progress toward desired outcome(s)
- Modifications to plan of care

Discharge Planning

- Long-term needs and who is responsible for actions to be taken
- Specific referrals made

Information that appears in brackets has been added by the authors to clarify and enhance the use of nursing diagnoses.

Sample Nursing Outcomes & Interventions Classifications (NOC/NIC)

NOC—Urinary Continence
NIC—Prompted Voiding

overflow urinary INCONTINENCE

[Diagnostic Division: Elimination]

Definition: Involuntary loss of urine associated with overdistention of the bladder.

Related Factors

Bladder outlet obstruction; fecal impaction
Urethral obstruction; severe pelvic prolapse
Detrusor external sphincter dyssynergia; detrusor hypocontractility
Treatment regimen [e.g., side effects of medications]

Defining Characteristics

Subjective

Involuntary leakage of small volume of urine
Nocturia

Objective

Bladder distention
High postvoid residual volume

Desired Outcomes/Evaluation Criteria—Client Will:

- Verbalize understanding of causative factors and appropriate interventions for individual situation.
- Demonstrate techniques or behaviors to alleviate or prevent overflow incontinence.
- Void in sufficient amounts with no palpable bladder distention; experience no post-void residuals greater than 50 mL; have no dribbling or overflow.

Information that appears in brackets has been added by the authors to clarify and enhance the use of nursing diagnoses.

Actions/Interventions

Nursing Priority No. 1.

To assess causative/contributing factors:

- Review the client's history for (1) bladder outlet obstruction (e.g., prostatic hypertrophy, urethral stricture, urinary stones or tumors); (2) nonfunctioning detrusor muscle (i.e., sensory or motor paralytic bladder due to underlying neurological disease); or (3) atonic bladder that has lost its muscular tone (i.e., chronic overdistention) **to identify potential for or presence of conditions associated with overflow incontinence.**
- Note the client's age and gender. **Urinary incontinence due to overflow bladder is more common in men because of the prevalence of obstructive prostate gland enlargement. However, age and sex are not factors in other conditions affecting overflow bladder incontinence, such as nerve damage from diseases such as diabetes, alcoholism, Parkinson's disease, multiple sclerosis, or spina bifida.**
- Review medication regimen **for drugs that can cause or exacerbate retention and overflow incontinence (e.g., anticholinergic agents, calcium channel blockers, psychotropics, anesthesia, opiates, sedatives, alpha- and beta-adrenergic blockers, antihistamines, and neuroleptics).**

Nursing Priority No. 2.

To determine degree of interference/disability:

- Note client reports of symptoms common to overflow incontinence, such as:

  Feeling no need to urinate, while simultaneously losing urine; frequent leaking or dribbling

  Feeling the urge to urinate, but not being able to do so

  Feeling as though the bladder is never completely empty

  Passing a dribbling stream of urine, even after spending a long time at the toilet

  Frequently getting up at night to urinate
- Prepare for and assist with urodynamic testing (e.g., uroflowmetry **to assess urine speed and volume;** cystometrogram **to measure bladder pressure and volume;** bladder scan **to measure retention and/or postvoid residual;** leak point pressure).

Nursing Priority No. 3.

To assist in treating/preventing overflow incontinence:

- Collaborate in the treatment of underlying conditions (e.g., medications or surgery for prostatic hypertrophy or severe pelvic prolapse; use of medication, such as terazosin, to relax

Information that appears in brackets has been added by the authors to clarify and enhance the use of nursing diagnoses.

urinary sphincter; altering dose or discontinuing medications contributing to retention). **If the underlying cause of the overflow problem can be treated or eliminated, the client may be able to return to a normal voiding pattern.**

- Collaborate with the physician regarding the client's medications (e.g., anticholinergics, antidepressants, antipsychotics, sedatives, narcotics, and alpha-adrenergic blockers) **that could be discontinued or altered to reduce/limit their effects on cognition, and/or innervation and function of the bladder.**
- Administer medications, as indicated. **For some men with an enlarged prostate, treatment with a alpha-adrenergic blocker (e.g., doxazosin [Cardura], tamulosin [Flomax]) can help relax the muscle at the base of the urethra and allow urine to pass from the bladder.**
- Assess the client for constipation and/or fecal impaction. Administer stool softeners, laxatives, enema, or other treatments, as indicated. **Chronic constipation is a factor in weakening muscles that control urination. Fecal impaction can be a cause of urinary retention and overflow incontinence, especially in elderly clients.**
- Demonstrate/instruct client/significant other (SO)(s) in the use of gentle massage over bladder (Credé's maneuver). **This may facilitate bladder emptying when the cause is detrusor weakness.**
- Implement intermittent or continuous catheterization. **Short-term use may be required while acute conditions are treated (e.g., infection, surgery for enlarged prostate); long-term use is required for permanent conditions (e.g., spinal cord injuries [SCIs] or other neuromuscular conditions resulting in permanent bladder dysfunction).**

Nursing Priority No. 4.

To promote wellness (Teaching/Discharge Considerations):

- Identify and continue the client's successful self-management of incontinence, where possible. **Continuation of successful strategies can reduce the risk of recurrence/failure of continence.**
- Establish a regular schedule for bladder emptying whether voiding or using catheter.
- Emphasize the need for adequate fluid intake, including the use of acidifying fruit juices or ingestion of vitamin C **to discourage bacterial growth and stone formation.**

Information that appears in brackets has been added by the authors to clarify and enhance the use of nursing diagnoses.

- Instruct the client/SO(s) in clean intermittent self-catheterization (CISC) techniques.
- Review signs/symptoms of complications requiring prompt medical evaluation/intervention.

Documentation Focus

Assessment/Reassessment

- Current elimination pattern and effect on lifestyle and sleep pattern

Planning

- Plan of care and who is involved in planning
- Teaching plan

Implementation/Evaluation

- Response to interventions, teaching, and actions performed
- Attainment or progress toward desired outcome(s)
- Modifications to plan of care

Discharge Planning

- Long-term needs and who is responsible for actions to be taken
- Specific referrals made

Sample Nursing Outcomes & Interventions Classifications (NOC/NIC)

NOC—Urinary Continence
NIC—Urinary Incontinence Care

reflex urinary INCONTINENCE

[Diagnostic Division: Elimination]

Definition: Involuntary loss of urine at somewhat predictable intervals when a specific bladder volume is reached.

Related Factors

Tissue damage [e.g., due to radiation cystitis, radical pelvic surgery]
Neurological impairment above level of sacral or pontine micturition center

Information that appears in brackets has been added by the authors to clarify and enhance the use of nursing diagnoses.

Defining Characteristics

Subjective

Absence of sensation of bladder fullness, urge to void, or of voiding sensation

Sensation of urgency to void without voluntary inhibition of bladder contraction

Sensation of bladder fullness

Objective

Predictable pattern of voiding

Inability to voluntarily inhibit or initiate voiding

Incomplete emptying of bladder with [brain] lesion above pontine micturition center

Desired Outcomes/Evaluation Criteria—Client Will:

- Verbalize understanding of condition or contributing factors.
- Establish bladder regimen appropriate for individual situation.
- Demonstrate behaviors or techniques to manage condition and prevent complications.

Actions/Interventions

Nursing Priority No. 1.

To assess degree of interference/disability:

- Note condition or disease process as listed in Related Factors (e.g., pelvic cancer, radiation, or surgery; central nervous system [CNS] disorders, stroke, multiple sclerosis [MS], Parkinson's disease, diabetes with bladder neuropathy, spinal cord injuries, and brain tumors resulting in neurogenic bladder [either hypnotic or spastic]; interstitial cystitis [IC]) **affecting bladder storage, emptying, and control. Note: Causes of reflex incontinence are often mixed, for example, most people with reflex incontinence experience symptoms of urinary frequency, urgency, and nocturia. In this situation, the bladder empties urine as it fills.**
- Ascertain whether the client experiences any sense of bladder fullness or awareness of incontinence. **Individuals with reflex incontinence have little, if any, awareness of need to void. Loss of sensation of bladder filling can result in overfilling, inadequate emptying (retention), and dribbling.**

Information that appears in brackets has been added by the authors to clarify and enhance the use of nursing diagnoses.

(Refer to NDs acute/chronic Urinary Retention; overflow urinary Incontinence.)

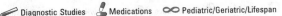

- Review voiding diary, if available, or record frequency and time of urination. Compare timing of voidings, particularly in relation to certain factors (e.g., liquid intake or medications). **This aids in targeting interventions to meet individual situation.**
- Measure amount of each voiding during assessment phase **because incontinence often occurs once a specific bladder volume is achieved.**
- Determine postvoid residual (via bladder scan) in client with incomplete emptying or on scheduled catheterization **to evaluate for urinary retention when attempting toilet training, to establish schedule for intermittent catheterization, and to avoid unnecessary catheterization. Note: Often the bladder is not completely emptied because there is no voluntary control of the bladder.**
- Evaluate the client's ability to manipulate or use a urinary collection device or catheter **to determine long-term need for assistance.**
- Refer to urologist or appropriate specialist for testing of bladder capacity, muscle fibers, and sphincter control. **Urinalysis, ultrasound, radiographs, and urine flowmetry are standard to measure urine flow. A urodynamic evaluation measuring bladder capacity, pressure, and rate of urinary flow may also be indicated.**

Nursing Priority No. 2.

To assist in managing incontinence:

- Evaluate the client's ability to manipulate or use a urinary collection device or catheter. **The type and degree of neurological impairment (i.e., spinal cord injury, MS, dementia) may interfere with the client's ability to be self-sufficient.**
- Collaborate in the treatment of underlying cause or management of reflex incontinence. **Of all the types of urinary incontinence, reflex incontinence probably is the most difficult to treat; however, this condition may be treated with medications, neuromodulation (electrical stimulation of specific nerves to influence the nerve circuit that controls urination), bladder surgery, or indwelling bladder catheters.**
- Involve client/SO/caregiver in developing a plan of care to address specific needs.

Information that appears in brackets has been added by the authors to clarify and enhance the use of nursing diagnoses.

- Encourage a minimum of 1,500 to 2,000 mL of fluid intake daily. **This reduces the risk of bladder and kidney infection/stone formation and may reduce symptoms of IC when caused by concentrated urine.**
- Remind the client or assist to toilet before the expected time of incontinence **in an attempt to stimulate the reflexes for voiding.**
- Engage in bladder retraining program as appropriate. **Suppression of urgency and progressive small increases in intervals between voiding may help reduce urinary frequency in clients with IC.**
- Set alarm to awaken during the night, if necessary, to maintain catheterization schedule or use external catheter or external collection device, as appropriate. **Developing a regular time to empty the bladder will prevent urinary retention or overflow incontinence during the night.**
- Implement continuous catheterization or intermittent self-catheterization using small-lumen straight catheter, if condition indicates, **to prevent bladder overdistention and detrusor muscle damage.**
- Evaluate the effectiveness of medication when used.

Nursing Priority No. 3.

To promote wellness (Teaching/Discharge Considerations):

- Encourage continuation of a regularly timed bladder program **to limit overdistention and related complications.**
- Suggest the use of incontinence pads/pants during the day and with social contact, if appropriate. **Depending on the client's activity level, amount of urine loss, manual dexterity, and cognitive ability, these devices provide security and comfort and protect the skin and clothing from urine leakage, reduce odor, and are generally unnoticeable under clothing.**
- Emphasize the importance of perineal care following voiding and frequent changing of incontinence pads, if used, **to maintain cleanliness and prevent skin irritation or breakdown and odor.**
- Stress the importance of perineal care following voiding and frequent changing of incontinence pads, if used.
- Encourage limited intake of coffee, tea, and alcohol **because of diuretic effect, which may affect predictability of voiding pattern,** or avoidance of citrus, artificial sweeteners, tomatoes, spicy foods, as well as caffeine, **which can cause flare-ups/exacerbate symptoms of IC.**

Information that appears in brackets has been added by the authors to clarify and enhance the use of nursing diagnoses.

- Instruct in proper care of catheter and cleaning techniques when used **to reduce risk of infection.**
- Review signs/symptoms of urinary complications and need for timely medical follow-up care.

Documentation Focus

Assessment/Reassessment

- Individual findings including degree of disability and effect on lifestyle
- Availability of resources or support person

Planning

- Plan of care and who is involved in planning
- Teaching plan

Implementation/Evaluation

- Responses to treatment plan, interventions, and actions performed
- Attainment or progress toward desired outcome(s)
- Modifications to plan of care

Discharge Planning

- Long-term needs and who is responsible for actions to be taken
- Available resources, equipment needs and sources

Sample Nursing Outcomes & Interventions Classifications (NOC/NIC)

NOC—Urinary Continence
NIC—Urinary Incontinence Care

stress urinary INCONTINENCE

[Diagnostic Division: Elimination]

Definition: Sudden leakage of urine with activities that increase intra-abdominal pressure.

Related Factors

Degenerative changes in pelvic muscles; weak pelvic muscles
Increase in intra-abdominal pressure [e.g., obesity, gravid uterus]
Intrinsic urethral sphincter deficiency

Information that appears in brackets has been added by the authors to clarify and enhance the use of nursing diagnoses.

Defining Characteristics

Subjective

Involuntary leakage of small volume of urine (e.g., with sneezing, laughing, coughing, on exertion; in the absence of detrusor contraction or an overdistended bladder)

Objective

Involuntary leakage of small volume of urine in the absence of detrusor contraction or an overdistended bladder

Desired Outcomes/Evaluation Criteria—Client Will:

- Verbalize understanding of condition and interventions for bladder conditioning.
- Demonstrate behaviors or techniques to strengthen pelvic floor musculature.
- Remain continent even with increased intra-abdominal pressure.

Actions/Interventions

Nursing Priority No. 1.

To assess causative/contributing factors:

- Identify physiological causes of increased intra-abdominal pressure (e.g., obesity, gravid uterus, repeated heavy lifting); contributing history such as multiple births; bladder or pelvic trauma, fractures; surgery (e.g., radical prostatectomy, bladder or other pelvic surgeries that may damage sphincter muscles); and participation in high-impact athletic or military field activities (particularly women). **Identification of specifics of individual situation provides for developing an accurate plan of care.**
- Assess for urine loss (usually small amount) with coughing, sneezing, or sports activities; relaxed pelvic musculature and support, noting inability to start or stop stream while voiding, bulging of perineum when bearing down.
- ∞ Note the client's gender and age. **The majority of clients with stress urinary incontinence are women, although men who undergo surgical prostatectomy may also experience it. Although pregnancy and childbirth is a known cause in younger women, stress incontinence is also common in older women, possibly related to loss of estrogen and weakened muscles in the pelvic organs.**

Information that appears in brackets has been added by the authors to clarify and enhance the use of nursing diagnoses.

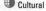

- Review the client's medications (e.g., alpha-blockers, angiotensin-converting enzyme [ACE] inhibitors, loop diuretics) **for those that may cause or exacerbate stress incontinence. Note: The urge incontinence effect with these agents is usually transient.**
- Assess for mixed incontinence (consisting of two or more kinds of incontinence), noting whether bladder irritability, reduced bladder capacity, or voluntary overdistention is present. **The most common combinations are urge with stress incontinence and urge or stress with functional incontinence. These impact treatment choices.** (Refer to NDs urge and reflex urinary Incontinence; [acute/chronic] Urinary Retention.)

Nursing Priority No. 2.

To assess degree of interference/disability:

- Observe voiding patterns, time and amount voided, and stimulus provoking incontinence. Review voiding diary, if available.
- Prepare for, and assist with, appropriate testing. **Diagnosing urinary incontinence often requires comprehensive evaluation (e.g., measuring bladder filling and capacity, bladder scan, leak-point pressure, rate of urinary flow, pelvic ultrasound, cystogram/other scans) to differentiate stress incontinence from other types.**
- Determine effect on lifestyle (including daily activities, participation in sports or exercise and recreation, socialization, sexuality) and self-esteem. **Untreated incontinence can have emotional and physical consequences. The client may limit or abstain from sports or recreational activities. Urinary tract infections, skin rashes, and sores can occur. Self-esteem is affected, and the client may suffer from depression and withdraw from social functions.**
- Ascertain methods of self-management (e.g., regularly timed voiding, limiting liquid intake, using undergarment protection).
- Perform bladder scan to determine postvoid residuals as indicated. **The presence of volumes greater than 200 mL (or 150 mL in elder clients) suggests incomplete emptying of the bladder, requiring further evaluation.**

Nursing Priority No. 3.

To assist in treating/preventing incontinence:

- Assist with medical treatment of underlying urological condition, as indicated. **Stress incontinence may be treated with**

Information that appears in brackets has been added by the authors to clarify and enhance the use of nursing diagnoses.

surgical intervention (e.g., bladder neck suspension, pubovaginal sling to reposition bladder and strengthen pelvic musculature; or prostate surgery) or nonsurgical therapies (e.g., behavioral modification, pelvic muscle exercises, medications, use of pessary, vaginal cones; electrical stimulation; biofeedback).

- Suggest and implement self-help techniques:

  Keep a voiding diary, as indicated. **The use of a frequency/volume chart is helpful in bladder training.**

  Practice timed voidings (e.g., every 3 hr during the day) **to keep the bladder relatively empty.**

  Extend time between voidings to 3- to 4-hr intervals. **This may improve bladder capacity and retention time.**

  Void before physical exertion, such as exercise/sports activities, heavy lifting, **to reduce potential for incontinence.**

  Encourage weight loss, as indicated, **to reduce pressure on pelvic organs.**

  Suggest limiting use of coffee, tea, and alcohol **because of diuretic effect.**

  Recommend regular pelvic floor–strengthening exercises (Kegel exercises). **These exercises involve tightening the muscles of the pelvic floor and need to be done numerous times throughout the day.**

  Suggest starting and stopping stream two or three times during voiding **to isolate muscles involved in voiding process for exercise training.**

  Incorporate bent-knee sit-ups into exercise program **to increase abdominal muscle tone.**

- Administer medications, as indicated, such as midodrine (ProAmatine); oxybutynin (Ditropan); tolterodine (Detrol); solifenacin (Vesicare). **Medication may improve bladder tone and capacity and increase effectiveness of bladder sphincter and proximal urethra contractions.**

Nursing Priority No. 4.

To promote wellness (Teaching/Discharge Considerations):

- Discuss participation in incontinence management for activities such as heavy lifting and impact aerobics **that increase intra-abdominal pressure.** Substitute swimming, bicycling, or low-impact exercise.
- Refer to weight-loss program or support group **when obesity is a contributing factor.**
- Suggest the use of incontinence pads or briefs, as needed. Consider the client's activity level, amount of urine loss, physical size, manual dexterity, and cognitive ability **to de-**

Information that appears in brackets has been added by the authors to clarify and enhance the use of nursing diagnoses.

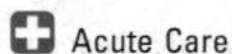

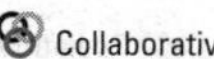

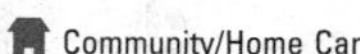

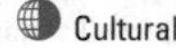

termine specific product choices best suited to individual situation and needs.

- Emphasize the importance of perineal care following voiding and frequent changing of incontinence pads **to prevent incontinence-associated dermatitis and infection.** Recommend application of oil-based emollient **to protect skin from irritation.**

Documentation Focus

Assessment/Reassessment

- Individual findings including pattern of incontinence and physical factors present
- Effect on lifestyle and self-esteem
- Client understanding of condition

Planning

- Plan of care and who is involved in the planning
- Teaching plan

Implementation/Evaluation

- Responses to interventions, teaching, actions performed, and changes that are identified
- Attainment or progress toward desired outcome(s)
- Modifications to plan of care

Discharge Planning

- Long-term needs and who is responsible for specific actions
- Specific referrals made

Sample Nursing Outcomes & Interventions Classifications (NOC/NIC)

NOC—Urinary Continence
NIC—Pelvic Muscle Exercise

Information that appears in brackets has been added by the authors to clarify and enhance the use of nursing diagnoses.

urge urinary INCONTINENCE and risk for urge urinary INCONTINENCE

[Diagnostic Division: Elimination]

Definition: urge urinary Incontinence: Involuntary passage of urine occurring soon after a strong sense of urgency to void.

Definition: risk for urge urinary Incontinence: Vulnerable to involuntary passage of urine occurring soon after a strong sensation of urgency to void, which may compromise health.

Related and Risk Factors

Decrease in bladder capacity
Bladder infection; atrophic urethritis or vaginitis
Alcohol consumption; caffeine intake; [increased fluid intake]
Treatment regimen [e.g., diuretic use]
Fecal impaction
Detrusor hyperactivity with impaired bladder contractility

NOTE: A risk diagnosis is not evidenced by signs and symptoms as the problem has not occurred; rather, nursing interventions are directed at prevention.

Defining Characteristics (urge urinary Incontinence)

Subjective

Urinary urgency; involuntary loss of urine with bladder contractions or spasms
Inability to reach toilet in time to avoid urine loss

Desired Outcomes/Evaluation Criteria—Client Will:

- Identify individual risk factors and appropriate interventions.
- Verbalize understanding of condition.
- Demonstrate behaviors or techniques to control or correct situation.
- Report increase in interval between urge and involuntary loss of urine.
- Void every 3 to 4 hours in individually appropriate amounts.

Information that appears in brackets has been added by the authors to clarify and enhance the use of nursing diagnoses.

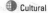

Actions/Interventions

Nursing Priority No. 1.

To assess causative/contributing **or risk** factors:

- Note the presence of conditions often associated with urgent voiding (e.g., urinary tract infection; pregnancy; pelvic or gynecological surgery; prostatitis or prostate surgery; obesity; bladder tumors or stones; nerve damage from conditions such as diabetes, stroke, Parkinson's disease, multiple sclerosis; certain cancers, including bladder and prostate; recent or lengthy use of indwelling urinary catheter) **affecting bladder capacity; pelvic, bladder, or urethral musculature tone; and/or innervation.**
- Ask the client about urgency (more than just normal desire to void). **Urgency (also called overactive bladder [OAB]) is a sudden, compelling need to void that is difficult to defer and may be accompanied by leaking or urge incontinence.**
- Note factors that may affect the ability to respond to urge to void in a timely manner (e.g., impaired mobility, debilitation, sensory or perceptual impairments). **Impaired mobility, use of sedation, or cognitive impairments may result in the client failing to recognize the need to void or moving too slowly to make it to the bathroom, with subsequent loss of urine.**
- Determine the use of or presence of bladder irritants. **A significant intake of alcohol, caffeine, acidic, or spicy food and fluids can result in increased output or urge symptoms and contribute to the possibility of incontinence.**
- Review the client's medications and substance use (e.g., diuretics, antipsychotic agents, sedatives, caffeine, alcohol) **for agents that increase urine production or exert a bladder irritant effect.**
- Assess for signs and symptoms of bladder infection (e.g., cloudy, odorous urine; burning pain with voiding; bacteriuria) **associated with acute, painful urgency symptoms.**
- Prepare for and assist with appropriate testing (e.g., prevoid or postvoid bladder scanning; pelvic examination for strictures; impaired perineal sensation or musculature; urinalysis; uroflowmetry voiding pressures; cystoscopy; cystometrogram) **to determine anatomical and functional status of bladder and urethra.**
- Assess for concomitant stress or functional incontinence. **Older women often have a mix of stress and urge incontinence, while individuals with dementia or disabling neurological disorders tend to have urge and functional**

Information that appears in brackets has been added by the authors to clarify and enhance the use of nursing diagnoses.

incontinence. (Refer to NDs stress/functional urinary Incontinence for additional interventions.)

Nursing Priority No. 2.

To assess degree of interference/disability (urge urinary Incontinence):

- Record frequency of voiding during a typical 24-hr period.
- Discuss degree of urgency and length of warning time between initial urge and loss of urine. **Overactivity or irritability shortens the length of time between urge and urine loss and helps clarify the type of incontinence.**
- Ascertain if the client experiences triggers (e.g., sound of running water, putting hands in water, seeing a restroom sign, "key-in-the-lock" syndrome).
- Measure the amount of urine voided, especially noting amounts less than 100 mL or greater than 550 mL. **Bladder capacity may be impaired or bladder contractions facilitating emptying may be ineffective.** (Refer to ND [acute/chronic] Urinary Retention.)
- Ascertain effect on lifestyle (including daily activities, socialization, sexuality) and self-esteem. **There is a considerable impact on the quality of life of individuals with an incontinence problem, affecting socialization and view of themselves as sexual beings and sense of self-esteem.**

Nursing Priority No. 3.

To assist in preventing/managing incontinence:

- Ascertain the client's awareness and concerns about developing problem and whether lifestyle might be affected (e.g., daily living activities, socialization, sexual patterns).
- Collaborate in treating underlying cause and/or managing urge symptoms. **Urgency symptoms may resolve with treatment of medical problem (e.g., infection, recovery from surgery, childbirth, or pelvic trauma) or may be resistant to resolution (e.g., incontinence associated with neurogenic bladder).**
- Administer medications as indicated (e.g., antibiotic for urinary tract infection, or antimuscarinics [oxybutynin (Ditropan), tolterodine (Detrol), solifenacin (Vesicare)]) **to reduce voiding frequency and urgency by blocking overactive detrusor contractions.**
- Provide assistance or devices, as indicated, for the client who is mobility impaired (e.g., provide means of summoning assistance; place bedside commode, urinal, or bedpan within client's reach).

Information that appears in brackets has been added by the authors to clarify and enhance the use of nursing diagnoses.

- Offer assistance to cognitively impaired client (e.g., prompt client, or take to bathroom on regularly timed schedule) **to reduce the frequency of incontinence episodes and promote comfort.**
- Recommend lifestyle changes:

  Adjust fluid intake to 1,500 to 2,000 mL/day, if client is prone to ingesting too much fluid. Regulate liquid intake at prescheduled times (with and between meals) and limit fluids 2 to 3 hr prior to bedtime **to promote predictable voiding pattern and limit nocturia.**

  Modify foods and fluids as indicated (e.g., reduce caffeine, citrus juices, spicy foods, etc.) **to reduce bladder irritation.**

  Manage bowel elimination **to prevent urinary problems associated with constipation or fecal impaction.**
- Encourage the client to participate in behavioral interventions, if able:

  Establish voiding schedule (habit and bladder training) based on the client's usual voiding pattern and gradually increase time interval.

  Recommend consciously delaying voiding by using distraction (e.g., slow deep breaths); making self-statements (e.g., "I can wait"); and contracting pelvic muscles when exposed to triggers, which are **behavioral techniques for urge suppression.**

  Encourage regular pelvic floor strengthening exercises or Kegel exercises as indicated by specific condition.

  Instruct the client to tighten pelvic floor muscles before arising from bed. **This helps prevent loss of urine as abdominal pressure changes.**

  Suggest starting and stopping stream two or more times during voiding **to isolate muscles involved in voiding process for exercise training.**
- Refer to specialists or treatment program, as indicated, for additional and specialized interventions (e.g., biofeedback, use of vaginal cones, electronic stimulation therapy, possible surgical interventions).

Nursing Priority No. 4.

To promote wellness (Teaching/Discharge Considerations):

- Provide information to client/significant other (SO)(s) about potential for urge incontinence (also called overactive bladder [OAB]) and lifestyle measures to prevent or limit incontinence.

Information that appears in brackets has been added by the authors to clarify and enhance the use of nursing diagnoses.

- Encourage comfort measures (e.g., use of incontinence pads or undergarments, wearing loose-fitting or especially adapted clothing) **to prepare for and manage urge incontinence symptoms over the long term and enhance sense of security and confidence in abilities to be socially active.**
- Emphasize the importance of regular perineal care **to reduce risk of ascending infection and incontinence-related dermatitis.**
- Identify signs/symptoms indicating urinary complications and need for timely medical follow-up care.

Documentation Focus

Assessment/Reassessment

- Individual findings, including specific risk factors and pattern of voiding or incontinence effect on lifestyle, and self-esteem

Planning

- Plan of care, specific interventions, and who is involved in planning
- Teaching plan

Implementation/Evaluation

- Response to interventions, teaching, and actions performed
- Attainment or progress toward desired outcome(s)
- Modifications to plan of care

Discharge Planning

- Discharge needs and who is responsible for actions to be taken
- Specific referrals made

Sample Nursing Outcomes & Interventions Classifications (NOC/NIC)

NOC—Urinary Continence
NIC—Urinary Bladder Training

risk for **INFECTION**

[Diagnostic Division: Safety]

Definition: Vulnerable to invasion and multiplication of pathogenic organisms, which may compromise health.

Information that appears in brackets has been added by the authors to clarify and enhance the use of nursing diagnoses.

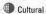

Risk Factors

Chronic illness (e,g., diabetes mellitus)
Inadequate vaccination
Insufficient knowledge to avoid exposure to pathogens
Inadequate Primary Defenses:
Alteration in peristalsis
Alteration in pH of secretions; status of body fluids
Alteration in skin integrity
Decrease in ciliary action
Premature or prolonged rupture of amniotic membrane
Smoking
Inadequate Secondary Defenses:
Decrease in hemoglobin; leukopenia, suppressed inflammatory response (e.g., interleukin-6 [IL-6], C-reactive protein [CRP]); immunosuppression
Inadequate vaccination
Increased Environmental Exposure to Pathogens:
Exposure to disease outbreak
[Exposure to multiple healthcare workers, multiple care settings]

NOTE: A risk diagnosis is not evidenced by signs and symptoms, as the problem has not occurred; rather, nursing interventions are directed at prevention.

Desired Outcomes/Evaluation Criteria—Client Will:

- Verbalize understanding of individual causative or risk factor(s).
- Identify interventions to prevent or reduce risk of infection.
- Demonstrate techniques, lifestyle changes to promote safe environment.
- Achieve timely wound healing; be free of purulent drainage or erythema; be afebrile.

Actions/Interventions

Nursing Priority No. 1.

To assess causative/contributing factors:

- Assess for presence of host-specific factors that affect immunity:

∞ Extremes of age. **Newborns and the elderly are more susceptible to disease and infection than the general population.**

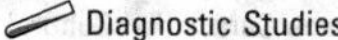

Information that appears in brackets has been added by the authors to clarify and enhance the use of nursing diagnoses.

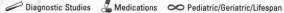

Presence of underlying disease. **The client may have a disease that directly impacts the immune system (e.g., cancer, AIDS, autoimmune disorder) or may be weakened by prolonged disease conditions (e.g., diabetes, kidney disease, heart failure) or their treatments.**

Certain treatment settings/modalities. **The client in acute care/critical care setting and/or on mechanical ventilation may have a prolonged exposure to risk factors for infection, including problems with breathing and circulation, gastrointestinal (GI) motility disorders, and use of analgesics and sedatives, causing a higher rate of acquired infections.**

Lifestyle. **Personal habits or living situations such as persons sharing close quarters and/or equipment (e.g., college dorm, group home, long-term care facility, day care, correctional facility); persons/groups with inadequate vaccination protection; IV drug use and shared needles; and unprotected sex can increase susceptibility to infections.**

Nutritional status. **Malnutrition weakens the immune system; and elevated serum glucose levels (e.g., administration of total parenteral nutrition [TPN] or poorly controlled diabetes) provide growth media for pathogens.**

Trauma. **Loss of skin and tissue integrity; invasive diagnostic procedures or surgery; premature rupture of amniotic membrane; urinary catheterizations; parenteral injection; sharps; and needle sticks are common paths of pathogen entry.**

Certain medications. **Steroids and chemotherapeutic agents directly affect the immune system. Long-term or improper antibiotic treatment can disrupt the body's normal flora and result in increased susceptibility to antibiotic-resistant organisms.**

Presence or absence of immunity. **Natural immunity may be acquired as a result of development of antibodies to a specific agent following infection, preventing recurrence of specific disease (e.g., chicken pox). Active immunization (via vaccination, e.g., measles, polio) and passive immunization (e.g., antitoxin or immunoglobulin administration) can prevent certain communicable diseases.**

Environmental exposure. **This may be accidental or intentional. Exposure can occur in different ways such as use**

Information that appears in brackets has been added by the authors to clarify and enhance the use of nursing diagnoses.

of specific microorganisms (in laboratories, biotechnological industries, or acts of bioterrorism). Accidental exposures can result from exposure to contaminants arising from commonplace processes (e.g., wastewater recycling), or through animal contact (e.g., agriculture, animal food processing); and through contact with humans (e.g., healthcare, education, mass transit, close contact living, etc.)

- Observe at-risk client for:

  Changes in skin color and warmth at insertion sites of invasive lines, sutures, surgical incisions, wounds **that could be signs of developing localized infection**

  Changes in mental status, skin warmth and color, heart and respiratory rate **that could be signs of developing systemic infection**;

  Changes in color and/or odor of secretions (e.g., sputum); drainage (e.g.,wound drains or invasive tubes); and excretions (e.g., urine) **that could indicate onset of infection.**

- Obtain appropriate tissue or fluid specimens for observation and culture and sensitivities testing.
- Refer to NDs: risk for Aspiration, risk for urinary tract Injury; risk for impaired oral Mucous Membranes; risk for impaired Skin or Tissue Integrity for related assessments and interventions.

Nursing Priority No. 2.

To reduce/correct existing risk factors:

- Practice and emphasize constant and proper hand hygiene by all caregivers between therapies and clients. Wear gloves when appropriate to minimize contamination of hands, and discard after each client. Wash hands after glove removal. Instruct the client/significant other (SO)/visitors to wash hands, as indicated, as this is **a first-line defense against healthcare-associated infections (HAIs).**
- Provide clean, well-ventilated environment (may require turning off central air-conditioning and opening window for good ventilation; room with negative air pressure, etc.).
- Monitor the client's visitors and caregivers for respiratory illnesses. Ask sick visitors to leave client area or offer masks and tissues to client or visitors who are coughing or sneezing **to limit exposures, thus reducing cross-contamination.**
- Post visual alerts in healthcare settings instructing clients/SO(s) to inform healthcare providers if they have symptoms of respiratory infections or influenza-like symptoms.

Information that appears in brackets has been added by the authors to clarify and enhance the use of nursing diagnoses.

- Provide for isolation, as indicated (e.g., contact, droplet, and airborne precautions). Educate staff in infection control procedures. **This reduces the risk of cross-contamination.**
- Emphasize proper use of personal protective equipment (PPE) by staff and visitors, as dictated by agency policy **for particular exposure risk (e.g., airborne, droplet, splash risk), including mask or respiratory filter of appropriate particulate regulator, gowns, aprons, head covers, face shields, and protective eyewear.**
- Perform or instruct in daily mouth care. Include use of antiseptic mouthwash for individuals in acute or long-term care settings **at high risk for nosocomial or HAIs.**
- Recommend routine or preoperative body shower or scrubs, when indicated (e.g., orthopedic, plastic surgery), **to reduce bacterial colonization.**
- Maintain sterile technique for all invasive procedures (e.g., IV, urinary catheter, pulmonary suctioning).
- Fill bubbling humidifiers and nebulizers with *sterile* water, not distilled or tap water. Avoid use of room-air humidifiers unless unit is sterilized daily and filled with sterile water.
- Assist with weaning from mechanical ventilator as soon as possible **to reduce risk of ventilator-associated pneumonia (VAP).**
- Choose a proper vascular access device based on anticipated treatment duration and solution/medication to be infused and best available aseptic insertion techniques.
- Change surgical or other wound dressings, as indicated, using proper technique for changing/disposing of contaminated materials.
- Cleanse incisions and insertion sites per facility protocol with appropriate antimicrobial topical or solution **to reduce the potential for catheter-related bloodstream infections, and to prevent the growth of bacteria.**
- Separate touching surfaces when skin is excoriated, such as in herpes zoster. Use gloves when caring for open lesions **to minimize auto-inoculation or transmission of viral diseases (e.g., herpes simplex virus, hepatitis, AIDS).**
- Cover perineal and pelvic region dressings or casts with plastic when using bedpan **to prevent contamination.**
- Encourage early ambulation, deep breathing, coughing, position changes, and early removal of endotracheal (ET) tube or nasal or oral feeding tubes **for mobilization of respiratory secretions and prevention of aspiration/respiratory infections.**

Information that appears in brackets has been added by the authors to clarify and enhance the use of nursing diagnoses.

- Assist with medical procedures (e.g., wound or joint aspiration, incision and drainage of abscess, bronchoscopy), as indicated.
- Administer/monitor medication regimen (e.g., antimicrobials, drip infusion into osteomyelitis, subeschar clysis, topical antibiotics) and note the client's response **to determine effectiveness of therapy or presence of side effects.**
- Administer prophylactic antibiotics and immunizations, as indicated.
- Encourage parents of sick children to keep them away from childcare settings and school until afebrile for 24 hr.
- Encourage or assist with use of adjuncts (e.g., respiratory aids, such as incentive spirometry) **to prevent pneumonia.**
- Maintain adequate hydration, stand or sit to void, and catheterize, if necessary, **to avoid bladder distention and urinary stasis.**
- Provide regular urinary catheter and perineal care. **This reduces the risk of ascending urinary tract infection.**

Nursing Priority No. 3.

To promote wellness (Teaching/Discharge Considerations):

- Review individual nutritional needs, appropriate exercise program, and need for rest.
- Instruct the client/SO(s) in techniques to protect the integrity of the skin, care for lesions, and prevention of spread of infection.
- Emphasize the necessity of taking antivirals or antibiotics, as directed (e.g., dosage and length of therapy). **Premature discontinuation of treatment when client begins to feel well may result in return of infection and potentiation of drug-resistant strains.**
- Discuss the importance of not taking antibiotics or using "left-over" drugs unless specifically instructed by healthcare provider. **Inappropriate use can lead to development of drug-resistant strains or secondary infections.**
- Discuss the role of smoking in respiratory infections.
- Promote safer-sex practices and report sexual contacts of infected individuals **to prevent the spread of HIV and other sexually transmitted infections (STIs).**
- Provide information and involve the client in appropriate community and national education programs **to increase awareness of and prevention of communicable diseases.**
- Discuss precautions with the client engaged in international travel, and refer for immunizations **to reduce incidence and transmission of global infections.**

Information that appears in brackets has been added by the authors to clarify and enhance the use of nursing diagnoses.

- Promote childhood immunization program. Encourage adults to obtain/update immunizations as appropriate.
- Include information in preoperative teaching about ways to reduce the potential for postoperative infection (e.g., respiratory measures to prevent pneumonia, wound and dressing care, avoidance of others with infection).
- Review the use of prophylactic antibiotics if appropriate (e.g., prior to dental work for clients with history of immunosuppressive conditions, rheumatic fever, or valvular heart disease).
- Encourage contacting healthcare provider for prophylactic therapies, as indicated, following exposure to individuals with infectious disease (e.g., tuberculosis, hepatitis, influenza).
- Identify resources available to the individual (e.g., substance abuse rehabilitation or needle exchange program, as appropriate; free condoms).
- Refer to NDs risk for Disuse Syndrome; impaired Home Maintenance; ineffective Health Maintenance.

Documentation Focus

Assessment/Reassessment

- Individual risk factors, including recent or current antibiotic therapy
- Wound and/or insertion sites, character of drainage or body secretions
- Signs and symptoms of infectious process

Planning

- Plan of care, specific interventions, and who is involved in planning
- Teaching plan

Implementation/Evaluation

- Responses to interventions, teaching, and actions performed
- Attainment or progress toward desired outcome(s)
- Modifications to plan of care

Discharge Planning

- Discharge needs, referrals made, and who is responsible for actions to be taken
- Specific referrals made

Information that appears in brackets has been added by the authors to clarify and enhance the use of nursing diagnoses.

Sample Nursing Outcomes & Interventions Classifications (NOC/NIC)

NOC—Knowledge: Infection Management
NIC—Infection Protection

risk for INJURY

[Diagnostic Division: Safety]

Definition: Vulnerable to physical damage due to environmental conditions interacting with the individual's adaptive and defensive resources, which may compromise health.

Risk Factors

Internal

Abnormal blood profile [e.g., leukocytosis/leukopenia, altered clotting factors, thrombocytopenia, sickle cell, thalassemia, decreased hemoglobin]; immune/autoimmune dysfunction; biochemical dysfunction
Alteration in affective orientation; effector dysfunction
Alteration in sensation (resulting from spinal cord injury, diabetes mellitus, etc,)
Extremes of age
Impaired primary defense mechanisms (e.g., broken skin); tissue hypoxia; malnutrition

External

Alteration in cognitive or psychomotor functioning
Compromised nutritional source (e.g., vitamins, food types)
Exposure to pathogen or toxic chemical [pollutants, poisons, drugs, pharmaceutical agents, alcohol, nicotine]
Immunization level within community; nosocomial agent
Physical barrier (e.g., design, structure, and arrangement of community, building, equipment); unsafe mode of transport

NOTE: A risk diagnosis is not evidenced by signs and symptoms, as the problem has not occurred; rather, nursing interventions are directed at prevention.

Information that appears in brackets has been added by the authors to clarify and enhance the use of nursing diagnoses.

Desired Outcomes/Evaluation Criteria—Client/Caregivers Will:

- Be free of injury.
- Verbalize understanding of individual factors that contribute to possibility of injury.
- Demonstrate behaviors, lifestyle changes to reduce risk factors and protect self from injury.
- Modify environment as indicated to enhance safety.

Actions/Interventions

In reviewing this ND, it is apparent there is much overlap with other diagnoses. We have chosen to present generalized interventions. Although there are commonalities to injury situations, we suggest that the reader refer to other primary diagnoses as indicated, such as risk for Bleeding; risk for acute Confusion; chronic Confusion; risk for Contamination; risk for Falls; ineffective Health Maintenance; impaired Home Maintenance; risk for Infection; impaired physical Mobility; impaired/risk for impaired Parenting; ineffective Protection; risk for Poisoning; impaired/risk for impaired Skin/Tissue Integrity; Rape-Trauma Syndrome; risk for Pressure Ulcer; ineffective peripheral Tissue Perfusion; risk for Trauma; risk for self- and other-directed Violence; Wandering for additional interventions.

Nursing Priority No. 1.

To evaluate degree/source of risk inherent in the individual situation:

- Perform thorough assessments regarding safety issues when planning for client care and/or preparing for discharge from care. **Failure to accurately assess and intervene or refer these issues can place the client at needless risk and creates negligence issues for the healthcare practitioner. Note: Research has identified 30 safe practices that evidence shows can work to reduce or prevent adverse events and medical errors regarding client safety, including (and not limited to) adequate numbers of nursing personnel; evaluating each person upon admission, and regularly thereafter, for the risk of developing pressure ulcers; employing clinically appropriate strategies to prevent malnutrition; vaccinating healthcare workers against influenza to protect both them and clients; and standardizing methods for labeling, packaging, and storing medications.**

Information that appears in brackets has been added by the authors to clarify and enhance the use of nursing diagnoses.

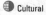

- Ascertain knowledge of safety needs, injury prevention, and motivation to prevent injury in home, community, and work settings.
- ∞ Note the client's age, gender, developmental stage, decision-making ability, and level of cognition/competence. **These affect the client's ability to protect self and/or others, and influence choice of interventions and teaching.**
- ∞ Review expectations caregivers have of children, cognitively impaired, and/or elderly family members.
- Assess mood, coping abilities, personality styles (e.g., temperament, aggression, impulsive behavior, level of self-esteem) **that may result in carelessness or increased risk taking without consideration of consequences.**
- Assess client's muscle strength and gross and fine motor coordination **to identify risk for falls. Note: The frequency of falls increases with age and frailty level. Risk factors for falls lie in four categories: (1) biological, (2) behavioral, (3) environmental, and (4) socioeconomic. In each of these areas, some risk factors can be modified to decrease fall risk.**
- Note socioeconomic status and availability and use of resources.
- Evaluate the individual's emotional and behavioral response to violence in environmental surroundings (e.g., home, neighborhood, peer group, media). **This may affect the client's view of and regard for own/others' safety.**
- Determine the potential for abusive behavior by family members/significant other (SO)(s)/peers.
- Observe for signs of injury and age (current, recent, and past such as old or new bruises, history of fractures, frequent absences from school or work) **to determine need for evaluation of intentional injury or abuse in client relationship or living environment.**

Nursing Priority No. 2.

✚ To assist client/caregiver to reduce or correct individual risk factors:

- Provide healthcare within a culture of safety (e.g., adherence to nursing standards of care and facility safe-care policies) **to prevent errors resulting in client injury, promote client safety, and model safety behaviors for client/SO(s):**

Information that appears in brackets has been added by the authors to clarify and enhance the use of nursing diagnoses.

Adhere to measures to prevent blood clots, especially in client with abnormal blood profile; surgical procedures, immobility.

Practice hand hygiene at all times, and device safety when client has IV lines and catheters **to prevent nosocomial infections and potential for bloodborne pathogens.**

Administer medications and infusions using "6 rights" system (right client, right medication, right route, right dose, right time, right documentation).

Inform and educate client/SO regarding all treatments and medications.

Monitor the environment for potentially unsafe conditions or hazards and modify as needed.

- Prevent falls:

Orient or reorient client to environment, as needed.

Place confused elderly client or young child near the nurses' station **to provide for frequent observation.**

Instruct the client/SO to request assistance, as needed; make sure call light is within reach and client knows how to operate.

Utilize bed/chair alarms **that alert when client is trying to get up alone.**

Maintain bed or chair in lowest position with wheels locked. Provide netted bed for agitated clients with traumatic brain injury.

Provide seat raisers for chairs, use stand-assist, repositioning, or lifting devices as indicated **to prevent injury to both client and care providers.**

Ensure that all floors are clear of tripping hazards and that pathway to bathroom is unobstructed and properly lighted.

Place assistive devices (e.g., walker, cane, glasses, hearing aid) within reach, and ascertain that the client is using them appropriately.

Safety-lock exit and stairwell doors **when the client can wander away.**

Avoid the use of restraints as much as possible when the client is confused. **Restraints can increase the client's agitation and risk of entrapment and death.**

- Develop plan of care with family to meet client's and SO's individual needs.
- Provide information regarding disease or condition(s) that may result in increased risk of injury (e.g., weakness, dementia, head injury, immunosuppression, use of multiple medica-

---

Information that appears in brackets has been added by the authors to clarify and enhance the use of nursing diagnoses.

tions, use of alcohol or other drugs, exposure to environmental chemicals or other hazards).

- Identify interventions and safety devices **to promote safe physical environment and individual safety.**
- Refer to physical or occupational therapist, as appropriate, **to identify high-risk tasks, conduct site visits; select, create, and modify equipment or assistive devices; and provide education about body mechanics and musculoskeletal injuries, in addition to providing therapies as indicated.**
- Demonstrate and encourage the use of techniques to reduce or manage stress and vent emotions, such as anger, hostility.
- Review consequences of previously determined risk factors that client is reluctant to modify. **Many consequences could occur (e.g., oral cancer in teenager using smokeless tobacco, fetal alcohol syndrome or neonatal addiction in prenatal woman using drugs, fall related to failure to use assistive equipment, toddler getting into medicine cabinet, binge drinking while skiing, health and legal implications of illicit drug use).**
- Discuss the importance of self-monitoring of condition or emotions **that can contribute to occurrence of injury (e.g., fatigue, anger, irritability).**
- Encourage participation in self-help programs, such as assertiveness training, positive self-image, **to enhance self-esteem and sense of self-worth.**
- Perform home assessment and identify safety issues such as:

  Locking up medications and poisonous substances
  Using window grates or locks; and safety gates at top and bottom of stairs
  Installing handrails, ramps, bathtub safety tapes
  Using electrical outlet covers or lockouts
  Locking exterior doors
  Removing matches, smoking materials, and knobs from the stove
  Properly placing lights, alarms (e.g., fire, carbon monoxide, and intruder) and fire extinguishers
  Discussing safe use of oxygen
  Obtaining medical alert device or home monitoring service
- Review specific employment concerns or worksite issues and needs (e.g., ergonomic chairs and workstations; properly fitted safety equipment, footwear; regular use of safety glasses or goggles and ear protectors; safe storage of hazardous substances; number of hours worked per shift/week).

Information that appears in brackets has been added by the authors to clarify and enhance the use of nursing diagnoses.

- Discuss the need for and sources of supervision (e.g., before- and after-school programs, elder day care).
- Discuss concerns about childcare, discipline practices.
- Encourage participation in self-help programs, such as assertiveness training, anger management, positive self-image.

Nursing Priority No. 3.

To promote wellness (Teaching/Discharge Considerations):

- Identify individual needs and resources for safety education such as First Aid/CPR classes, babysitter class, water or gun safety, smoking cessation, substance abuse program, weight and exercise management, and industry and community safety courses.
- Provide telephone numbers and other contact numbers, as individually indicated (e.g., doctor, 911, poison control, police, lifeline, hazardous materials handler).
- Refer to other resources, as indicated (e.g., counseling, psychotherapy, budget counseling, parenting classes).
- Provide bibliotherapy or written resources **for later review and self-paced learning.**
- Promote community education programs geared to increasing awareness of safety measures and resources available to the individual. **Many evidence-based programs are being implemented nationally to promote safe environments for children, adolescents, and adults (e.g., correct use of child safety seats, home hazard information, firearm safety, fall prevention, CPR and First Aid; education about bullying, Internet safety issues; suicide prevention; use of helmets when riding bicycles or skateboarding; drowning prevention; substance abuse, intimate partner violence, and anger management).**
- Promote community awareness about the problems of design of buildings, equipment, transportation, and workplace practices that contribute to accidents.
- Identify community resources/neighbors/friends to assist elderly/handicapped individuals in providing such things as structural maintenance and removal of snow and ice from walks and steps.

Documentation Focus

Assessment/Reassessment

- Individual risk factors, noting current physical findings (e.g., bruises, cuts)

Information that appears in brackets has been added by the authors to clarify and enhance the use of nursing diagnoses.

- Client's/caregiver's understanding of individual risks and safety concerns
- Availability and use of resources

Planning

- Plan of care and who is involved in planning
- Teaching plan

Implementation/Evaluation

- Individual responses to interventions, teaching, and actions performed
- Specific actions and changes that are made
- Attainment or progress toward desired outcome(s)
- Modifications to plan of care

Discharge Planning

- Long-range plans for discharge needs, lifestyle and community changes, and who is responsible for actions to be taken
- Specific referrals made

Sample Nursing Outcomes & Interventions Classifications (NOC/NIC)

NOC—Safety Behavior: Personal
NIC—Surveillance: Safety

risk for corneal INJURY

[Diagnostic Division: Safety]

Definition: Vulnerable to infection or inflammatory lesion in the corneal tissue that can affect superficial or deep layers, which may compromise health.

Risk Factors

Blinking <5 times per minute
Exposure of the eyeball; periorbital edema
Glasgow Coma Scale score <7
Pharmaceutical agent
Prolonged hospitalization
Use of supplemental oxygen; intubation; mechanical ventilation; tracheostomy

Information that appears in brackets has been added by the authors to clarify and enhance the use of nursing diagnoses.

NOTE: A risk diagnosis is not evidenced by signs and symptoms, as the problem has not occurred; rather, nursing interventions are directed at prevention.

Desired Outcomes/Evaluation Criteria—Client/Caregiver Will:

- Identify/monitor personal risk factors.
- Engage in risk control strategies.

Caregiver Will:

- Be free of discomfort or damage to corneal tissues.

Actions/Interventions

Nursing Priority No. 1.

To identify causative/precipitating factors related to risk:

- Obtain history of eye conditions when assessing client concerns overall. Listen for reports of eye pain, foreign body sensation, light sensitivity (photophobia), and blurred vision. **These symptoms can be associated with corneal injury and, if present, require further evaluation and possible treatment.**
- Note the presence of conditions (e.g., recent neurological event, facial trauma or burns; use of contact lenses, failure to use safety glasses in high-risk employment situation) or treatment environments (e.g., intubated client on mechanical ventilation; use of therapeutic hypothermia; sedated, anesthetized, or obtunded client with absent blink reflex) **to identify client at high risk for corneal injury. Note: Mercieca et al. found that 75% of sedated/paralyzed patients on mechanical ventilation in the intensive care unit (ICU) have incomplete closure of the eyelids (lagophthalmos), predisposing them to corneal dryness and inflammation.**
- Obtain a history of events from client/others when trauma (e.g., facial blunt force trauma, car crash with airbag deployment, accidental or intentional gunshot wounds; accidents with fireworks or hot metal) has occurred. **Eye injury (including corneal abrasions and lacerations) may not be immediately discovered but should be suspected.**
- Evaluate current drug regimen, noting pharmaceutical agents (e.g., topical drugs and preservatives in eyedrops; beta blockers, antihistimines, phenothiazides; diuretics, steroids, sedatives, neuromuscular blocking agents) **which can contribute**

Information that appears in brackets has been added by the authors to clarify and enhance the use of nursing diagnoses.

to dry eye, thereby increasing risk of corneal inflammation or injury in high-risk clients.

Nursing Priority No. 2.

To promote eye health/comfort:

- Refer for diagnostic evaluation and interventions as indicated. **Standard eye exam, and visual acuity testing may be performed, and other diagnostic studies (e.g., radiography, computed tomography [CT], or magnetic resonance imaging [MRI] may be indicated to locate foreign bodies or associated orbital, cranial, or facial trauma).**
- Assist in/refer for treatment of underlying conditions that might be affecting corneal health.
- Perform routine assessment of eyes and preventive interventions in critically ill client:
  - Evaluate the client's ability to maintain eyelid closure on a daily basis and as needed.
  - Perform actions to maintain eyelid closure in a client who cannot do it for self (e.g., taping).
  - Perform eye care (e.g., cleaning with saline-soaked gauze, and administration of eye-specific lubricant, where indicated).
  - Observe for developing complications.
- Refer for medical assessment and intervention, as indicated.
- Ascertain that the client undergoing anesthesia has proper eye protection (e.g., lubricant, eyelids taped, goggles) especially when placed in prone position. **The cornea is easily abraded because of reduced lacrimation during anesthesia or if face masks are improperly applied. In some positions, such as prone, a significant amount of pressure can be applied to the eyes.**

Nursing Priority No. 3.

To promote wellness (Teaching/Discharge Criteria):

- Instruct high-risk client/caregivers in self-management interventions **to prevent corneal inflammation symptoms:**
  - Avoid rubbing eyes with fingers or harsh cloths.
  - Protect eyes from blowing air or oxygen; discuss benefit of redirecting airflow.
  - Wear protective eyewear in situations or sports where objects may fly into eyes or face.
  - Wear protective eyewear that gives 180-degree protection while using a grinding wheel or hammering on metal.
  - Wear sunglasses that block ultraviolet radiation when in bright sunlight or under sunlamps.

Information that appears in brackets has been added by the authors to clarify and enhance the use of nursing diagnoses.

Follow prescribed wear time for contact lenses.

Add moisture to indoor air, especially in winter. **Reduce corneal irritation associated with dryness.**

Blink repeatedly for a few seconds at intervals when using the computer for any length of time **to prevent dryness and help spread tears evenly over eye.**

- Instruct in use of eyedrops or ointments as indicated **to prevent inflammation/infection, or to protect corneal surface.**
- Refer to appropriate healthcare provider concerning glasses, contact lenses, or other safety eyewear and offer information about suppliers.

Documentation Focus

Assessment/Reassessment

- Individual risk factors identified
- Client concerns or difficulty making and following through with plan

Planning

- Plan of care and who is involved in planning
- Teaching plan

Implementation/Evaluation

- Response to interventions, teaching, and actions performed
- Attainment or progress toward outcomes

Discharge Planning

- Referrals to other resources
- Long-term need and who is responsible for actions

Sample Nursing Outcomes & Interventions Classifications (NOC/NIC)

NOC—Dry Eye Severity
NIC—Eye Care

risk for urinary tract INJURY

[Diagnostic Division: Safety]

Definition: Vulnerable to damage of the urinary tract structures from use of catheters, which may compromise health.

Information that appears in brackets has been added by the authors to clarify and enhance the use of nursing diagnoses.

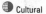

Risk Factors

Condition preventing ability to secure catheter (e.g., burn, trauma, amputation)
Long-term use of urinary catheters; multiple catheterizations
Retention balloon inflated to ≥30 ml
Use of large caliber urinary catheter

NOTE: A risk diagnosis is not evidenced by signs and symptoms, as the problem has not occurred; rather, nursing interventions are directed at prevention.

Desired Outcomes/Evaluation Criteria—Client Will:

- Be free of injury.

Client/Caregivers Will:

- Verbalize an understanding of individual factors that contribute to the possibility of injury.
- Demonstrate behaviors, lifestyle changes to reduce risk factors and protect from injury.

Actions/Interventions

Nursing Priority No. 1.

To assess causative/contributing factors:

- Identify conditions potentially affecting client need for/response to catheterization (e.g., acute illness, presence of infection, surgery, trauma including skin and tissue problems; chronic illness, including neurological conditions with paralysis or weakness; prolonged immobility; acute or chronic confusion, dementia, sedation, or use of multiple medications affecting mental acuity). **These conditions could require indwelling catheter for varying lengths of time with attendant potential for complications. Risk factors include longer duration of catheterization, bacterial colonization of the drainage bag, errors in catheter care, catheterization late in the hospital course, and immunocompromised or debilitated states.**
- Determine type of catheterization client is likely to require. **The client might require one-time or intermittent long-term single catheterization for any number of reasons (e.g., relief of acute urinary retention, management of voiding issues associated with multiple sclerosis or spinal cord injury). Indwelling urinary catheters are generally**

Information that appears in brackets has been added by the authors to clarify and enhance the use of nursing diagnoses.

used when longer-term urinary management issues are expected.

- Note age, developmental level, decision-making ability, level of cognition, competence, and independence. **These determine the client's/significant other's (SO) ability to attend to safety issues, and influences choice of interventions or teaching about catheterization.**
- Check for allergies to latex, and select appropriate catheter (e.g., coated). **Latex allergic reactions are implicated in the development of urethritis and urethral stricture or anaphylaxis.**

Nursing Priority No. 2.

To reduce potential for complications:

- Avoid catheterization when possible. Refer to NDs pertaining to impaired urinary Elimination and Incontinence for related interventions. **Studies have shown that urinary catheters often are placed unnecessarily, remain in use without physician awareness, and are not removed promptly when no longer needed.**
- Perform catheterization using best practices:

  Use strict aseptic technique when inserting indwelling catheter (clean technique may be implemented for long-term intermittent catheterization). **Note: The Centers for Disease Control and Prevention (CDC) 2009 recommend using aseptic technique and sterile equipment in the acute care setting, but clean (i.e., nonsterile) technique is acceptable and more practical in the community care setting for patients requiring chronic intermittent catheterization.**

  Select the smallest-bore catheter possible that will allow for adequate drainage, using size guidelines. **Appropriate catheter size helps reduce the likelihood of bladder spasm. Adult sizes are typically 14 Fr or 16 Fr. Guidelines are available for each pediatric age group from neonate (5-6 Fr.) to adolescent (10, 12, 14 Fr).**

  Inflate the balloon, using the correct amount of sterile liquid (usually 10 cc but check actual balloon size). **Balloon size is relevant to levels of bladder irritation. Although balloons are thin walled to reduce irritation to the bladder, it is still important to use the smallest size possible, usually with a 5- to 10-mL capacity.**

  Refrain from inflating the balloon without first establishing urine flow. **This assures that the catheter has been cor-**

Information that appears in brackets has been added by the authors to clarify and enhance the use of nursing diagnoses.

rectly inserted into the bladder. Note: If the balloon is opened before the catheter is completely inserted into the bladder, bleeding, damage, and even rupture of the urethra can occur.

Secure catheter to thigh or abdomen, as indicated. Inspect the skin underneath the securement device with each reapplication to monitor for irritation or dermatitis. **There are many reasons for this intervention, including (1) reducing bladder irritability/spasms; (2) preventing meatal erosion or inflammation; (3) managing discomfort related to catheter movement and traction; (4) preventing inadvertent migration of balloon from bladder into urethra or accidental removal of catheter; (5) avoiding obstruction of urine flow secondary to catheter kinking; and (6) preventing retention of urine; and risk for catheter-associated urinary tract infection (CAUTI).**

Position the collection bag level **to facilitate gravity drainage of the bladder and to prevent reflux of urine into the bladder.**

Perform an ongoing evaluation of catheter function and monitor color and characteristics of urine **to assess for developing complications. A properly maintained closed-drainage system and unobstructed urine flow are essential for prevention of urinary tract infection (UTI).**

- Ascertain if the client is experiencing discomfort or pain (e.g., bladder spasms). **Bladder spasms are distressing but are usually self-limiting when procedure is followed (e.g., proper size and insertion of catheter, as well as appropriate size and inflation of balloon).**

Nursing Priority No. 3.

To promote wellness (Teaching/Discharge Instructions):

- Review individual needs regarding catheter self-management with client/SO **to reduce the risk of complications:**

  Always wash hands before and after handling the catheter.

  Make sure that urine is flowing out of the catheter into the collection bag.

  Keep the urine collection bag below the level of the bladder.

  Make sure that catheter tubing does not get twisted or kinked.

  Check for inflammation or signs of infection (e.g., pus or irritated, swollen, red, or tender skin) in the area around the catheter.

Information that appears in brackets has been added by the authors to clarify and enhance the use of nursing diagnoses.

Clean the area around the catheter twice a day using soap and water. Dry with a clean towel afterward.

Avoid applying powder or lotion to the skin around the catheter.

Refrain tugging or pulling on the catheter.

Follow physician instructions regarding catheter cleaning and/or replacement (if long-term indwelling).

Follow physician instructions regarding frequency of catheterization (if intermittent).

- Instruct client/caregiver in techniques to protect the integrity of the skin. Refer to NDs, risk for impaired Skin/Tissue Integrity, risk for Pressure Ulcer for related interventions.
- Instruct client/caregiver in reportable problems, such as leaking, sediment in urine, absence of urine, presence of pain, and so on.
- Identify resources available to the individual (e.g., substance abuse or rehabilitation, or needle-exchange program as appropriate; available or free condoms).

Documentation Focus

Assessment/Reassessment

- Individual risk factors, noting current physical findings
- Client's/caregiver's understanding of individual risks and safety concerns

Planning

- Plan of care and who is involved in planning
- Teaching plan

Implementation/Evaluation

- Individual responses to interventions, teaching, and actions performed
- Specific actions and changes that are made
- Attainment or progress toward desired outcome(s)
- Modifications to plan of care

Discharge Planning

- Long-term plans for discharge needs, lifestyle changes, and who is responsible for actions to be taken
- Specific referrals made

Sample Nursing Outcomes & Interventions Classifications (NOC/NIC)

NOC—Physical Injury Severity
NIC—Urinary Catheterization

Information that appears in brackets has been added by the authors to clarify and enhance the use of nursing diagnoses.

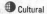

INSOMNIA

[Diagnostic Division: Activity/Rest]

Definition: A disruption in amount and quality of sleep that impairs functioning

Related Factors

Alcohol consumption; pharmaceutical agent; hormonal change
Stressors; depression; fear; anxiety; grieving
Inadequate sleep hygiene; frequent naps
Average daily physical activity is less than recommended for gender and age
Physical discomfort
Environmental barrier (e.g., ambient noise, daylight/darkness exposure, ambient temperature/humidity, unfamiliar setting)

Defining Characteristics

Subjective

Difficulty initiating or maintaining sleep; early awaking; alteration in sleep pattern
Dissatisfaction with sleep; nonrestorative sleep pattern (e.g., due to caregiver responsibilities, parenting practices, sleep partner)
Sleep disturbance producing next-day consequences; insufficient energy
Decrease in quality of life; compromised health status
Increase in accidents

Objective

Alteration in concentration
Alteration in mood/affect
Increase in absenteeism

Desired Outcomes/Evaluation Criteria—Client Will:

- Verbalize understanding of sleep impairment.
- Identify individually appropriate interventions to promote sleep.
- Adjust lifestyle to accommodate chronobiological rhythms.
- Report improvement in sleep-rest pattern.
- Report increased sense of well-being and feeling rested.

Information that appears in brackets has been added by the authors to clarify and enhance the use of nursing diagnoses.

Actions/Interventions

Nursing Priority No. 1.

To identify causative/contributing factors:

- Identify presence of Related Factors such as chronic pain, arthritis, dyspnea, movement disorders, dementia, obesity, pregnancy, menopause, psychiatric disorders; metabolic diseases (e.g., hyperthyroidism, diabetes); prescribed and over-the-counter (OTC) drugs; alcohol, stimulant, or other recreational drug use; circadian rhythm disorders (e.g., shift work, jet lag); environmental factors (e.g., noise, no control over thermostat, uncomfortable bed); major life stressors (e.g., grief, loss, finances) **that can contribute to insomnia.**
- Note age **(high percentage of elderly individuals are affected by sleep problems). Two primary sleep disorders that increase with age are sleep apnea (SA) and periodic limb movements in sleep (PLMS).**
- Observe parent-infant interaction and provision of emotional support. Note mother's sleep-wake pattern. **Lack of knowledge of infant cues or problem relationships may create tension interfering with sleep. Structured sleep routines based on adult schedules may not meet child's needs.**
- Ascertain presence and frequency of enuresis, incontinence, or need for frequent nighttime voidings, **interrupting sleep.**
- Review psychological assessment, noting individual and personality characteristics **if anxiety disorders or depression could be affecting sleep.**
- Determine recent traumatic events in client's life (e.g., death in family, loss of job). **Physical and emotional trauma often affects client's sleep patterns and quality for a short period of time. This disruption can become long term and require more intensive assessment and intervention.**
- Review client's medications, including prescription drugs (e.g., beta-blockers, sedative antidepressants, sedative neuroleptics; bronchodilators, weight-loss drugs, thyroid preparations), OTC products, and herbals **to determine if adjustments may be needed (such as change in dose or time medication is taken) or if a different medication may be needed.**
- Evaluate the use of caffeine and alcoholic beverages. **These may interfere with falling asleep or duration and quality of sleep (overindulgence interferes with rapid eye movement [REM] sleep).**
- Assist with diagnostic testing (e.g., polysomnography; daytime multiple sleep latency testing; Actigraphy; full-night

Information that appears in brackets has been added by the authors to clarify and enhance the use of nursing diagnoses.

sleep studies) **to determine cause and type of sleep disturbance.**

Nursing Priority No. 2.

To evaluate sleep pattern and dysfunction(s):

- Review sleep diary (where available); observe and/or obtain feedback from client/SO(s) regarding client's sleep problems, usual bedtime, rituals and routines, number of hours of sleep, time of arising, and environmental needs **to determine usual sleep pattern and provide comparative baseline.**
- Listen to subjective reports of sleep quality (e.g., client never feels rested, or feels excessively sleepy during day).
- Identify circumstances that interrupt sleep and the frequency at which they occur.
- Determine the client's/SO's expectations of adequate sleep. **This provides an opportunity to address misconceptions or unrealistic expectations.**
- Investigate whether the client snores and in what position(s) this occurs **to determine if further evaluation is needed to rule out obstructive SA.**
- Note alteration of habitual sleep time, such as change of work pattern, rotating shifts, and change in normal bedtime (hospitalization). **This helps identify circumstances that are known to interrupt sleep patterns, resulting in mental and physical fatigue, affecting concentration, interest, energy, and appetite.**
- Observe physical signs of fatigue (e.g., restlessness, hand tremors, thick speech).
- Develop a chronological chart **to determine peak performance rhythm.**

Nursing Priority No. 3.

To assist the client to establish optimal sleep/rest patterns:

- Collaborate in the treatment of underlying medical and psychiatric problems (e.g., obstructive SA, pain, gastroesophageal reflux disease [GERD], lower urinary tract infection [UTI]/prostatic hypertrophy; depression, bipolar disorder; complicated grief).
- Arrange care to provide for uninterrupted periods for rest, especially allowing for longer periods of sleep at night when possible. Do as much care as possible without waking the client.
- Explain necessity of disturbances for monitoring vital signs and/or other care when client is hospitalized.

Information that appears in brackets has been added by the authors to clarify and enhance the use of nursing diagnoses.

- Provide a quiet environment and comfort measures (e.g., back rub, washing hands/face, cleaning and straightening sheets) in preparation for sleep.
- Discuss and implement effective age-appropriate bedtime rituals (e.g., going to bed at same time each night, drinking warm milk, rocking, story reading, cuddling, favorite blanket or toy) **to enhance the client's relaxation, reinforce that bed is a place to sleep, and promote sense of security for child or confused elder.**
- Recommend limiting intake of chocolate and caffeinated or alcoholic beverages, especially prior to bedtime.
- Limit fluid intake in evening if nocturia is a problem **to reduce the need for nighttime elimination.**
- Explore other sleep aids (e.g., warm bath, light protein snack before bedtime; soothing music, etc.). **Nonpharmaceutical aids may enhance falling asleep free of concern of medication side effects such as morning hangover or drug dependence.**
- Administer pain medications (if required) 1 hr before sleep **to relieve discomfort and take maximum advantage of sedative effect.**
- Monitor effects of drug regimen—amphetamines or stimulants (e.g., methylphenidate [Ritalin] used in narcolepsy).
- Use barbiturates and/or other sleeping medications sparingly. **Research indicates long-term use of these medications, especially in the absence of cognitive behavioral therapy (CBT), can actually induce sleep disturbances.**
- Encourage routine use of continuous positive airway pressure (CPAP) therapy, when indicated, **to obtain optimal benefit of treatment for SA.**
- Develop behavioral program for insomnia, such as:

  Establishing and maintaining a regular sleeping time and waking-up time

  Thinking relaxing thoughts when in bed

  Not napping in the daytime

  Exercising daily, but not immediately before bedtime

  Avoiding heavy meals at bedtime

  Using bed only for sleeping or sex

  Wearing comfortable, loose-fitting clothing to bed and participating in relaxing activity until sleepy

  Not reading or watching TV in bed

  Getting out of bed if not asleep in 15 to 30 min

  Getting up the same time each day—even on weekends and days off

  Getting adequate exposure to bright light during day

Information that appears in brackets has been added by the authors to clarify and enhance the use of nursing diagnoses.

Individually tailoring stress reduction program, music therapy, relaxation routine

- Administer and monitor effects of prescribed medications to promote sleep (e.g., *benzodiazapines,* such as zolpiden [Ambien], zaleplon [Sonata], eszopiclone [Lunesta]; *antidepressants,* such as trazadone [Desyrel], nefazodone [Serzone]; *melatonin agonists,* such as ramelteon [Rozerem]). **While most are effective in the short term, many lose effectiveness over time. The client may have adverse side effects or develop tolerance and misuse the drug. Many drug regimens are most effective when combined with CBT, in which the client can be weaned off medications at some point.**
- Refer to sleep specialist, as indicated or desired. **Follow-up evaluation or intervention may be needed when insomnia is seriously impacting the client's quality of life, productivity, and safety (e.g., on the job, at home, on the road).**

Nursing Priority No. 4.

To promote wellness (Teaching/Discharge Considerations):

- Assure the client that occasional sleeplessness should not threaten health. **Worrying about not sleeping can perpetuate or exacerbate the problem.**
- Assist the client to develop an individual program of relaxation. Demonstrate techniques (e.g., biofeedback, self-hypnosis, visualization, progressive muscle relaxation).
- Encourage participation in regular exercise program during the day **to aid in stress control and release of energy. Note: Exercise at bedtime may stimulate rather than relax client and actually interfere with sleep.**
- Recommend inclusion of bedtime snack (e.g., milk or mild juice, crackers, protein source such as cheese/peanut butter) in dietary program **to reduce sleep interference from hunger or hypoglycemia.**
- Provide for the child's (or impaired individual's) sleep time safety (e.g., infant placed on back, bedrails or bed in low position, nonplastic sheets).
- Investigate the use of aids to block out light and noise, such as sleep mask, darkening shades or curtains, earplugs, monotonous sounds such as low-level background noise (white noise).
- Participate in a program to "reset" the body's sleep clock (chronotherapy) **when the client has delayed-sleep-onset insomnia.**

Information that appears in brackets has been added by the authors to clarify and enhance the use of nursing diagnoses.

- Assist the individual to develop schedules that take advantage of peak performance times as identified in chronobiological chart.
- Recommend midmorning nap if one is required. **Napping, especially in the afternoon, can disrupt normal sleep patterns.**
- Assist the client to deal with the grieving process when loss has occurred. (Refer to ND Grieving.)

Documentation Focus

Assessment/Reassessment

- Assessment findings, including specifics of sleep pattern (current and past) and effects on lifestyle and level of functioning
- Medications or interventions used, previous therapies tried

Planning

- Plan of care and who is involved in planning
- Teaching plan

Implementation/Evaluation

- Client's response to interventions, teaching, and actions performed
- Attainment or progress toward desired outcome(s)
- Modifications to plan of care

Discharge Planning

- Long-term needs and who is responsible for actions to be taken
- Specific referrals made

Sample Nursing Outcomes & Interventions Classifications (NOC/NIC)

NOC—Sleep
NIC—Sleep Enhancement

Information that appears in brackets has been added by the authors to clarify and enhance the use of nursing diagnoses.

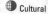

neonatal JAUNDICE and risk for neonatal JAUNDICE

[Diagnostic Division: Safety]

Definition: neonatal Jaundice: The yellow-orange tint of the neonate's skin and mucous membranes that occurs after 24 hours of life as a result of unconjugated bilirubin in the circulation.

Definition: risk for neonatal Jaundice: Vulnerable to the yellow-orange tint of the neonate's skin and mucous membranes that occurs after 24 hours of life as a result of unconjugated bilirubin in the circulation, which may compromise health.

Related Factors

Age < 7 days
Deficient feeding pattern
Unintentional weight loss [more than 7% to 8% in breastfeeding newborn; 15% in term infant]
Delay in meconium passage
Infant experiences difficulty making the transition to extrauterine life

Risk Factors

Age <7 days; prematurity
Feeding pattern not well established
Abnormal weight loss (more than 7% to 8% in breastfeeding newborn; 15% in nonbreastfeeding newborn)
Delay in meconium passage
Infant experiences difficulty making the transition to extrauterine life

NOTE: A risk diagnosis is not evidenced by signs and symptoms, as the problem has not occurred; rather nursing interventions are directed at prevention.

Defining Characteristics (neonatal Jaundice)

Objective

Yellow-orange skin color; yellow sclera, mucous membranes
Bruised skin

Information that appears in brackets has been added by the authors to clarify and enhance the use of nursing diagnoses.

Abnormal blood profile [e.g., hemolysis; total serum bilirubin more than 2 mg/dL; total serum bilirubin in the high-risk range on age in hour-specific nomogram]

Desired Outcomes/Evaluation Criteria—Infant Will:

- Display decreasing bilirubin levels with resolution of jaundice.
- Be free of central nervous system (CNS) involvement or complications associated with therapeutic regimen.

Parent/Caregiver Will:

- Verbalize an understanding of cause, treatment, and possible outcomes of hyperbilirubinemia.
- Demonstrate appropriate care of infant.

Actions/Interventions

Nursing Priority No. 1.

To assess causative/contributing **or risk** factors:

- Determine infant and maternal blood groups and blood types. **ABO incompatibilities affect 20% of all pregnancies.**
- Note gender, race, and place of birth. **The risk of developing jaundice is higher in males, infants of East Asian or American Indian descent, and those living at high altitudes.**
- Review intrapartal record for specific risk factors, such as low birth weight (LBW) or intrauterine growth retardation (IUGR), prematurity, abnormal metabolic processes, vascular injuries, abnormal circulation, sepsis, or polycythemia. **The risk of significant neonatal jaundice is increased in LBW or premature infants, presence of congenital infection, or maternal diabetes.**
- Note the use of instruments or vacuum extractor for delivery. Assess the infant for the presence of birth trauma, cephalohematoma, and excessive ecchymosis or petechiae. **Resorption of blood trapped in fetal scalp tissue and excessive hemolysis may increase the amount of bilirubin being released.**
- Review the infant's condition at birth, noting the need for resuscitation or evidence of excessive ecchymosis or petechiae, cold stress, asphyxia, or acidosis. **Asphyxia and acidosis reduce affinity of bilirubin to albumin, increasing**

Information that appears in brackets has been added by the authors to clarify and enhance the use of nursing diagnoses.

the amount of unbound circulating (indirect) bilirubin, which may cross the blood-brain barrier, causing CNS toxicity.

- Evaluate maternal and prenatal nutritional levels; note possible neonatal hypoproteinemia, especially in a preterm infant. **One gram of albumin carries 16 mg of unconjugated bilirubin; therefore, lack of sufficient albumin (hypoproteinemia) in the newborn increases the risk of jaundice.**
- Assess the infant for signs of hypoglycemia such as jitteriness, irritability, and lethargy. Obtain heel stick glucose levels as indicated. **Hypoglycemia necessitates the use of fat stores for energy-releasing fatty acids, which compete with bilirubin for binding sites on albumin.**
- Determine successful initiation and adequacy of breastfeeding. **Poor caloric intake and dehydration associated with ineffective breastfeeding increase the risk of developing hyperbilirubinemia.**
- Evaluate the infant for pallor, edema, or hepatosplenomegaly. **These signs may be associated with hydrops fetalis, Rh incompatibility, and in-utero hemolysis of fetal red blood cells (RBCs).**
- Evaluate for jaundice in natural light, noting sclera and oral mucosa, yellowing of skin immediately after blanching, and specific body parts involved. Assess oral mucosa, posterior portion of hard palate, and conjunctival sacs in dark-skinned newborns.
- Note the infant's age at onset of jaundice. This aids in differentiating the type of jaundice (i.e., physiological, breast milk induced, or pathological). **Physiological jaundice usually appears between the second and third days of life, breast milk jaundice between the fourth and seventh days of life, and pathological jaundice occurs within the first 24 hr of life, or when the total serum bilirubin level rises by more than 5 mg/dL per day.**

Nursing Priority No. 2.

To evaluate degree of compromise/**prevent complications**:

- Review laboratory studies including total serum bilirubin and albumin levels, hemoglobin and hematocrit, and reticulocyte count.
- Calculate plasma bilirubin-albumin binding capacity. **This aids in determining the risk of kernicterus and treatment needs.**
- Assess the infant for progression of signs and behavioral changes associated with bilirubin toxicity. **Early-stage tox-**

Information that appears in brackets has been added by the authors to clarify and enhance the use of nursing diagnoses.

icity involves neuro-depression-lethargy, poor feeding, high-pitched cry, diminished or absent reflexes; late-stage toxicity signs may include hypotonia, neuro-hyperreflexia-twitching, convulsions, opisthotonos, and fever.

- Evaluate the appearance of skin and urine, noting brownish-black color. **An uncommon side effect of phototherapy involves exaggerated pigment changes (bronze baby syndrome) that may last for 2 to 4 months but are not associated with harmful sequelae.**

Nursing Priority No. 3.

To **prevent onset or** correct hyperbilirubinemia:

- Keep the infant warm and dry; monitor skin and core temperature frequently. **This prevents cold stress and the release of fatty acids that compete for binding sites on albumin, thus increasing the level of freely circulating bilirubin.**
- Initiate early oral feedings within 4 to 6 hr following birth, especially if infant is to be breastfed. **This establishes proper intestinal flora necessary for reduction of bilirubin to urobilinogen and decreases reabsorption of bilirubin from bowel.**
- Encourage frequent breastfeeding—8 to 12 times per day. Assist the mother with pumping of breasts as needed **to maintain milk production.**
- Administer small amounts of breast milk substitute (L-aspartic acid or enzymatically hydrolyzed casein [EHC]) for 24 to 48 hr if indicated. **The use of feeding additives is under investigation for inhibition of beta-glucuronidase leading to increased fecal excretion of bilirubin; results have been mixed.**
- Apply transcutaneous jaundice meter. **This provides noninvasive screening of jaundice.**
- Initiate phototherapy per protocol, using fluorescent bulbs placed above the infant or fiberoptic pad or blanket (except for newborns with Rh disease). **This is the primary therapy for neonates with unconjugated hyperbilirubinemia.**
- Apply eye patches, ensuring correct fit during periods of phototherapy, to prevent retinal injury. Remove eye covering during feedings or other care activities as appropriate **to provide visual stimulation and interaction with caregivers/parents.**
- Avoid application of lotion or oils to skin of infant receiving phototherapy **to prevent dermal irritation or injury.**

Information that appears in brackets has been added by the authors to clarify and enhance the use of nursing diagnoses.

- Reposition the infant every 2 hr **to ensure that all areas of skin are exposed to bili light when fiberoptic pad or blanket is not used.**
- Cover male groin with small pad **to protect from heat-related injury to testes.**
- Monitor the infant's weight loss, urine output and specific gravity, and fecal water loss from loose stools associated with phototherapy **to determine adequacy of fluid intake.** *Note:* **The infant may sleep for longer periods in conjunction with phototherapy, increasing the risk of dehydration.**
- Administer IV immunoglobulin (IVIG) to neonates with Rh or ABO isoimmunization. **The rate of hemolysis in Rh disease or other cases of immune hemolytic jaundice usually exceeds the rate of bilirubin reduction related to phototherapy. IVIG inhibits antibodies that cause red cell destruction, helping to limit the rise in bilirubin levels.**
- Administer enzyme induction agent (phenobarbital) as appropriate. **This may be used on occasion to stimulate hepatic enzymes to enhance the clearance of bilirubin.**
- Assist with preparation and administration of exchange transfusion. **Exchange transfusions are occasionally required in cases of severe hemolytic anemia unresponsive to other treatment options or in the presence of acute bilirubin encephalopathy as evidenced by hypertonia, arching, retrocollis, opisthotonos, fever, and high-pitched cry.**
- Document events during transfusion, carefully recording amount of blood withdrawn and injected (usually 7 to 20 mL at a time).

Nursing Priority No. 4.

To promote wellness (Teaching/Discharge Considerations):

- Provide information about types of jaundice and pathophysiological factors and future implications of hyperbilirubinemia. **This promotes understanding, corrects misconceptions, and can reduce fear and feelings of guilt.**
- Review means of assessing infant status (feedings, intake and ouptut, stools, temperature, and serial weights if scale available) and monitoring increasing bilirubin levels (e.g., observing blanching of skin over bony prominence or behavior changes), especially if the infant is to be discharged early. *Note:* **Persistence of jaundice in formula-fed infant beyond 2 weeks, or 3 weeks in breastfed infant, requires further evaluation.**

Information that appears in brackets has been added by the authors to clarify and enhance the use of nursing diagnoses.

- Review proper formula preparation/storage and demonstrate feeding techniques, as indicated **to meet nutritional and fluid needs.**
- Refer to lactation specialist **to enhance or reestablish breast-feeding process.**
- Provide parents with 24-hr emergency telephone number and name of contact person, emphasizing importance of reporting increased jaundice or changes in behavior.
- Arrange appropriate referral for home phototherapy program if necessary.
- Provide a written explanation of home phototherapy, safety precautions, and potential problems. **Home phototherapy is recommended only for full-term infants after the first 48 hr of life, if serum bilirubin levels are between 14 and 18 mg/dL, with no increase in direct reacting bilirubin concentration.**
- Make appropriate arrangements for follow-up testing of serum bilirubin at the same laboratory facility. **Treatment is discontinued once serum bilirubin concentrations fall below 14 mg/dL. Untreated or chronic hyperbilirubinemia can lead to permanent damage such as high-pitch hearing loss, cerebral palsy, or developmental difficulties.**
- Discuss possible long-term effects of hyperbilirubinemia and the need for continued assessment and early intervention. **Neurological damage associated with kernicterus includes cerebral palsy, developmental delays, sensory difficulties, delayed speech, poor muscle coordination, learning difficulties, and death.**

Documentation Focus

Assessment/Reassessment

- Assessment findings, risk or related factors
- Adequacy of intake—hydration level, character and number of stools
- Laboratory results and bilirubin trends

Planning

- Plan of care, specific interventions, and who is involved in the planning
- Teaching plan and resources provided

Implementation/Evaluation

- Client's responses to treatment and actions performed
- Parents' understanding of teaching

Information that appears in brackets has been added by the authors to clarify and enhance the use of nursing diagnoses.

  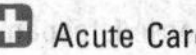 Acute Care 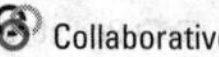 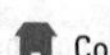 Collaborative 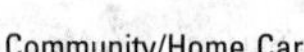 Community/Home Care  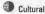 Cultural

- Attainment or progress toward desired outcome(s)
- Modifications to plan of care

Discharge Planning

- Long-range needs, identifying who is responsible for actions to be taken
- Community resources for equipment and supplies post discharge
- Specific referrals made

Sample Nursing Outcomes & Interventions Classifications (NOC/NIC)

NOC—Newborn Adaptation
NIC—Phototherapy: Neonate

deficient KNOWLEDGE [Learning Need] (Specify)

[Diagnostic Division: Teaching/Learning]

Definition: Absence or deficiency of cognitive information related to specific topic.

Related Factors

Insufficient information; insufficient knowledge of resources
Insufficient interest in learning
Misinformation presented by others
Alteration in cognitive functioning or memory
Insufficient interest in learning

Defining Characteristics

Subjective

Insufficient knowledge

Objective

Inaccurate follow-through of instruction or performance on a test or procedure
Inappropriate behavior (e.g., hysterical, hostile, agitated, apathetic)
Development of preventable complication

Information that appears in brackets has been added by the authors to clarify and enhance the use of nursing diagnoses.

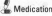

Desired Outcomes/Evaluation Criteria—Client Will:

- Participate in learning process.
- Identify interferences to learning and specific action(s) to deal with them.
- Exhibit increased interest and assume responsibility for own learning by beginning to look for information and ask questions.
- Verbalize understanding of condition, disease process, and treatment.
- Identify relationship of signs/symptoms to the disease process, and correlate symptoms with causative factors.
- Perform necessary procedures correctly, and explain reasons for the actions.
- Initiate necessary lifestyle changes, and participate in treatment regimen.

Actions/Interventions

Nursing Priority No. 1.

To assess readiness to learn and individual learning needs:

- Ascertain level of knowledge, including anticipatory needs.
- Determine the client's ability, readiness, and barriers to learning. **The individual may not be physically, emotionally, or mentally capable at this time.**
- Be alert to signs of avoidance. **The client may need to suffer the consequences of lack of knowledge before he or she is ready to accept information.**
- Identify support individuals/significant other (SO)(s) requiring information (e.g., parent, caregiver, spouse).

Nursing Priority No. 2.

To determine other factors pertinent to the learning process:

- Note personal factors (e.g., age and developmental level, gender, social and cultural influences, religion, life experiences, level of education, and emotional stability).
- Determine blocks to learning: language barriers (e.g., client cannot read; speaks or understands a different language than healthcare provider), physical factors (e.g., cognitive impairment, aphasia, dyslexia), physical stability (e.g., acute illness, activity intolerance), or difficulty of material to be learned.
- Assess the level of the the client's capabilities and the possibilities of the situation. **The SO(s) and/or caregivers may need help to learn.**

Information that appears in brackets has been added by the authors to clarify and enhance the use of nursing diagnoses.

Nursing Priority No. 3.

To assess the client's/SO's motivation:

- Identify motivating factors for the individual (e.g., client needs to stop smoking because of advanced lung cancer or client wants to lose weight because family member died of complications of obesity). **Motivation may be a negative stimulus (e.g., smoking caused lung cancer) or positive (e.g., client wants to promote health and prevent disease).**
- Provide information relevant only to the situation **to prevent overload.**
- Provide positive reinforcement. **This could encourage continuation of efforts.** Avoid the use of negative reinforcers (e.g., criticism, threats).

Nursing Priority No. 4.

To establish priorities in conjunction with client:

- Determine the client's most urgent need from both client's and nurse's viewpoints **(which may differ and require adjustments in teaching plan).**
- Discuss the client's perception of need. Relate the information to the client's personal desires, needs, values, and beliefs **so that the client feels competent and respected.**
- Differentiate "critical" content from "desirable" content. **This identifies information that can be addressed at a later time.**

Nursing Priority No. 5.

To establish the content to be included:

- Identify information that needs to be remembered (cognitive).
- Identify information having to do with emotions, attitudes, and values (affective).
- Identify psychomotor skills that are necessary for learning.

Nursing Priority No. 6.

To develop learner's objectives:

- State objectives clearly in learner's terms **to meet learner's (not instructor's) needs.**
- Identify outcomes (results) to be achieved.
- Recognize level of achievement, time factors, and short- and long-term goals.
- Include the affective goals (e.g., reduction of stress).

Information that appears in brackets has been added by the authors to clarify and enhance the use of nursing diagnoses.

Nursing Priority No. 7.

To identify teaching methods to be used:

- Determine the client's method of accessing information (visual, auditory, kinesthetic, gustatory/olfactory) and include in teaching plan **to facilitate learning or recall.**
- Involve the client/SO(s) by using age-appropriate materials tailored to the client's literacy skills, questions, and dialogue.
- Involve the client/SO(s) with others who have the same problems, needs, or concerns (e.g., group presentations, support groups). **This provides a role model and sharing of information.**
- Provide mutual goal setting and learning contracts. **This clarifies the expectations of teacher and learner.**
- Use team and group teaching as appropriate.

Nursing Priority No. 8.

To facilitate learning:

- Use short, simple sentences and concepts. Repeat and summarize as needed.
- Use gestures and facial expressions that help convey meaning of information.
- Discuss one topic at a time; avoid giving too much information in one session.
- Provide written information or guidelines and self-learning modules for client to refer to as necessary. **This reinforces the learning process and allows the client to proceed at his or her own pace.**
- Pace and time learning sessions and learning activities to individual's needs. Evaluate the effectiveness of learning activities with client.
- Provide an environment that is conducive to learning.
- Be aware of factors related to the teacher in the situation (e.g., vocabulary, dress, style, knowledge of the subject, and ability to impart information effectively).
- Begin with information the client already knows and move to what the client does not know, progressing from simple to complex. **This can arouse interest/limit sense of being overwhelmed.**
- Deal with the client's anxiety or other strong emotions. Present information out of sequence, if necessary, dealing first with material that is most anxiety producing **when the anxiety is interfering with the client's ability to learn.**
- Provide an active role for the client in the learning process. **This promotes a sense of control over the situation and is**

Information that appears in brackets has been added by the authors to clarify and enhance the use of nursing diagnoses.

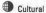

a means for determining that the client is assimilating and using new information.

- Provide for feedback (positive reinforcement) and evaluation of learning and acquisition of skills.
- Be aware of informal teaching and role modeling that takes place on an ongoing basis (e.g., answering specific questions and reinforcing previous teaching during routine care).
- Assist the client to use information in all applicable areas (e.g., situational, environmental, personal).

Nursing Priority No. 9.

To promote wellness (Teaching/Discharge Considerations):

- Provide access information for the contact person **to answer questions and validate information post discharge.**
- Identify available community resources and support groups.
- Provide information about additional learning resources (e.g., bibliography, Web sites, tapes). **This may assist with further learning and promote learning at his or her own pace.**

Documentation Focus

Assessment/Reassessment

- Individual findings including learning style, identified needs, presence of learning blocks (e.g., hostility, inappropriate behavior)

Planning

- Plan for learning, methods to be used, and who is involved in the planning
- Teaching plan

Implementation/Evaluation

- Responses of the client/SO(s) to the learning plan and actions performed; how the learning is demonstrated
- Attainment or progress toward desired outcome(s)
- Modifications to plan of care

Discharge Planning

- Additional learning and referral needs

Sample Nursing Outcomes & Interventions Classifications (NOC/NIC)

NOC—Knowledge: [specify—42 choices]
NIC—Teaching: [specify—30 choices]

Information that appears in brackets has been added by the authors to clarify and enhance the use of nursing diagnoses.

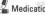

readiness for enhanced **KNOWLEDGE** (specify)

[Diagnostic Division: Teaching/Learning]

Definition: A pattern of cognitive information related to a specific topic, or its acquisition, which can be strengthened.

Defining Characteristics

Subjective

Expresses desire to enhance learning

Desired Outcomes/Evaluation Criteria—Client Will:

- Exhibit responsibility for own learning by seeking answers to questions.
- Verify accuracy of informational resources.
- Verbalize understanding of information gained.
- Use information to develop individual plan to meet healthcare needs and goals.

Actions/Interventions

Nursing Priority No. 1.

To develop plan for learning:

- Verify the client's level of knowledge about a specific topic. **This provides an opportunity to ensure accuracy and completeness of knowledge base for future learning.**
- Determine motivation and expectations for learning. **This provides insight useful in developing goals and identifying information needs.**
- Assist the client to identify learning goals. **This helps to frame or focus content to be learned and provides a measure to evaluate the learning process.**
- Ascertain preferred methods of learning (e.g., auditory, visual, interactive, or "hands-on"). **This identifies the best approaches to facilitate the learning process.**
- Note personal factors (e.g., age/developmental level, gender, social/cultural influences, religion, life experiences, level of education) **that may impact learning style, choice of informational resources.**

Information that appears in brackets has been added by the authors to clarify and enhance the use of nursing diagnoses.

- Determine any challenges to learning: language barriers (e.g., client cannot read, speaks or understands language other than that of care provider, dyslexia); physical factors (e.g., sensory deficits, such as vision or hearing deficits, aphasia); physical stability (e.g., acute illness, activity intolerance); difficulty of material to be learned. **This identifies special needs to be addressed if learning is to be successful.**

Nursing Priority No. 2.

To facilitate learning:

- Identify and provide information in varied formats appropriate to client's learning style (e.g., audiotapes, print materials, videos, classes or seminars, Internet). **Use of multiple formats increases learning and retention of material.**
- Provide information about additional or outside learning resources (e.g., bibliography, pertinent Web sites). **This promotes ongoing learning at the client's own pace.**
- Discuss ways to verify the accuracy of informational resources. **This encourages an independent search for learning opportunities while reducing the likelihood of acting on erroneous or unproven data that could be detrimental to the client's well-being.**
- Identify available community resources/support groups. **This provides additional opportunities for role modeling, skill training, anticipatory problem-solving, and so forth.**
- Be aware of informal teaching and role modeling that takes place on an ongoing basis (e.g., community and peer role models, support group feedback, print advertisements, popular music or videos). **Incongruencies may exist, creating questions and potentially undermining learning process.**

Nursing Priority No. 3.

To enhance optimum wellness:

- Assist the client to identify ways to integrate and use information in all applicable areas (e.g., situational, environmental, personal). **The ability to apply or use information increases the desire to learn and retain information.**
- Encourage the client to journal, keep a log, or graph as appropriate. **This provides an opportunity for self-evaluation of effects of learning, such as better management of chronic condition, reduction of risk factors, and acquisition of new skills.**

Information that appears in brackets has been added by the authors to clarify and enhance the use of nursing diagnoses.

Documentation Focus

Assessment/Reassessment

- Individual findings, including learning style and identified needs, presence of challenges to learning
- Motivation and expectations for learning

Planning

- Plan for learning, methods to be used, and who is involved in the planning
- Educational plan

Implementation/Evaluation

- Responses of the client/SO(s) to the learning plan and actions performed
- How the learning is demonstrated
- Attainment or progress toward desired outcome(s)
- Modifications to lifestyle and treatment plan

Discharge Planning

- Additional learning/referral needs

Sample Nursing Outcomes & Interventions Classifications (NOC/NIC)

NOC—Knowledge: [specify—42 choices]
NIC—Teaching: Individual

LATEX ALLERGY RESPONSE and risk for LATEX ALLERGY RESPONSE

[Diagnostic Division: Safety]

Definition: Latex Allergy Response: A hypersensitive reaction to natural latex rubber products.

Definition: risk for Latex Allergy Response: Vulnerable to a hypersensitivity to natural latex rubber products, which may compromise.

Related Factors (Latex Allergy Response)

Hypersensitivity to natural latex rubber protein

Information that appears in brackets has been added by the authors to clarify and enhance the use of nursing diagnoses.

Risk Factors

History of allergy or latex reaction
Frequent exposure to latex product
Food allergy (e.g., avocado, banana, chestnut, kiwi, peanut, shellfish, mushroom, tropical fruit); allergy to poinsettia plant
Asthma
Multiple surgical procedures; history of surgery during infancy

> **NOTE:** A risk diagnosis is not evidenced by signs and symptoms, as the problem has not occurred; rather, nursing interventions are directed at prevention.

Defining Characteristics (Latex Allergy Response)

Subjective

Life-Threatening Reactions within 1 Hour of Exposure: Chest tightness
Type IV Reactions Occurring ≥1 hour after Exposure: Discomfort reaction to additives (e.g., thiurams and carbamates)
Gastrointestinal Characteristics: Abdominal pain; nausea
Orofacial Characteristics: Itching (e.g., eyes; facial, nasal, oral); nasal congestion
Generalized Characteristics: Generalized discomfort; reports total body warmth

Objective

Life-Threatening Reactions within 1 Hour of Exposure:
Contact urticaria progressing to generalized symptoms
Edema (e.g., lips, throat, tongue, uvula)
Dyspnea; wheezing; bronchospasm; respiratory arrest
Hypotension; syncope; myocardial infarction
Type IV Reactions Occurring ≥1 hour after Exposure:
Eczema; skin irritation and/or redness
Orofacial Characteristics: Erythema (e.g., eyes, facial, nasal); periorbital edema; rhinorrhea, tearing of the eyes
Generalized Characteristics: Skin flushing; generalized edema; restlessness

Desired Outcomes/Evaluation Criteria—Client Will:

- Be free of signs of hypersensitive response.
- Identify and correct potential risk factors in the environment.

Information that appears in brackets has been added by the authors to clarify and enhance the use of nursing diagnoses.

- Verbalize understanding of individual risks and responsibilities in avoiding exposure.
- Identify signs/symptoms requiring prompt intervention.
- Identify resources to assist in promoting a safe environment.

Actions/Interventions

Nursing Priority No. 1.

To assess contributing **and risk** factors:

- Identify persons in high-risk categories such as (1) those with history of certain food allergies (e.g., banana, avocado, chestnut, kiwi, papaya, peach, nectarine); (2) prior allergies, asthma, and skin conditions (e.g., eczema and other dermatitis); (3) those occupationally exposed to latex products (e.g., healthcare workers, police, firefighters, EMTs, food handlers, hairdressers, cleaning staff, factory workers in plants that manufacture latex-containing products); (4) those with neural tube defects (e.g., spina bifida); or (5) those with congenital urological conditions requiring frequent surgeries and/or catheterizations (e.g., extrophy of the bladder). **The most severe reactions tend to occur with latex proteins contacting internal tissues during invasive procedures and when they touch mucous membranes of the mouth, vagina, urethra, or rectum.**
- Question the client regarding latex allergy upon admission to healthcare facility, especially when procedures are anticipated (e.g., laboratory, emergency department, operating room, wound care management, 1-day surgery, dentist). **This is basic safety information to help healthcare providers prevent/prepare for safe environment for client and themselves while providing care.**
- Discuss potential routes of exposure, if indicated (e.g., works where latex is manufactured or latex gloves are used frequently; child was blowing up balloons [may be an acute reaction to the powder]; use of condoms [may affect either partner]; individual requires frequent catheterizations. **Finding the cause of the reaction may be simple or complex but often requires diligent investigation and history-taking from multiple sources.**
- Note positive skin-prick test when client is skin-tested with latex extracts. **This is a sensitive, specific, and rapid test, and should be used with caution in persons with suspected sensitivity as it carries risk of anaphylaxis.**

Information that appears in brackets has been added by the authors to clarify and enhance the use of nursing diagnoses.

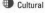

- Perform challenge/patch test, if appropriate, **to identify specific allergens in client with known type IV hypersensitivity.**
- Note response to radioallergosorbent test (RAST) or enzyme-linked assays (ELISA) of latex-specific IgE. **This is performed to measure the quantity of IgE antibodies in serum after exposure to specific antigens and has generally replaced skin tests and provocation tests, which are inconvenient, often painful, and/or hazardous to the client.**

Nursing Priority No. 2. (risk for latex allergy)

To assist in correcting factors that could lead to latex allergy:

- Discuss the necessity of avoiding/limiting latex exposure if sensitivity is suspected.
- Recommend that client/family survey environment and remove any medical or household products containing latex.
- Create latex-safe healthcare environments (e.g., substitute nonlatex products, such as natural rubber gloves, PCV IV tubing, latex-free tape, thermometers, electrodes, oxygen cannulas) **to enhance client safety by reducing exposure.**
- Obtain lists of latex-free products and supplies for client/care provider if appropriate **in order to limit exposure.**
- Ascertain that facilities and/or employers have established policies and procedures **to address safety and reduce risk to workers and clients.**
- Promote good skin care when latex gloves may be preferred for barrier protection in specific disease conditions such as HIV or during surgery. Use powder-free gloves, wash hands immediately after glove removal; refrain from use of oil-based hand cream. **This reduces dermal and respiratory exposure to latex proteins that bind to the powder in gloves.**

Nursing Priority No. 3. (Latex allergy interventions)

To take measures to reduce/limit allergic response/avoid exposure to allergens:

- Ascertain the client's current symptoms, noting the presence of rash, hives, or itching; red, teary eyes; edema; diarrhea; nausea; feeling of faintness **to help identify where the client is along a continuum of reactions so that appropriate treatments can be initiated.**
- Determine time since exposure (e.g., immediate or delayed onset, such as 24 to 48 hr).

Information that appears in brackets has been added by the authors to clarify and enhance the use of nursing diagnoses.

- Assess skin (usually hands but may be anywhere) for dry, crusty, hard bumps, scaling, lesions, and horizontal cracks. **There may be irritant contact dermatitis (the least serious and most common type of hypersensitivity reaction) or allergic contact dermatitis (a delayed-onset and more severe form of skin/other tissue reaction).**
- Assist with the treatment of dermatitis/type IV reaction (e.g., washing affected skin with mild soap and water, possible application of topical steroid ointment, and avoidance of further exposure to latex).
- Monitor closely for signs of systemic reactions (e.g., difficulty breathing or swallowing, wheezing, hoarseness, stridor; hypotension, tremors, chest pain, tachycardia, dysrhythmias; edema of face, eyelids, lips, tongue, and mucous membranes). **This is indicative of anaphylactic reaction and can lead to cardiac arrest.**
- Administer treatment, as appropriate. **If severe/life-threatening reaction occurs, urgent interventions may include antihistamines, epinephrine, IV fluids, corticosteroids, and oxygen and mechanical ventilation, if indicated.**
- Ascertain that latex-safe environment (e.g., surgery/hospital room) and products are available according to recommended guidelines and standards, including equipment and supplies (e.g., powder-free, low-protein latex products and latex-free items such as gloves, syringes, catheters, tubings, tape, thermometers, electrodes, oxygen cannulas, underpads, storage bags, diapers, feeding nipples), as appropriate.
- Educate all care providers in ways to prevent inadvertent exposure (e.g., post latex precaution signs in the client's room, document allergy to latex in chart/client bracelet), and emergency treatment measures should they be needed.
- Notify physicians, colleagues, and medical products suppliers of client's condition (e.g., pharmacy **so that medications can be prepared in a latex-free environment,** home-care oxygen company **to provide latex-free cannulas).**

Nursing Priority No. 4.

To promote wellness (Teaching/Learning):

- Instruct the client/SO(s) to survey and routinely monitor the environment for latex-containing products, and replace as needed.
- Instruct the client and care providers about the potential for sensitivity reactions, how to recognize symptoms of latex allergy (e.g., skin rash; hives; flushing; itching; nasal, eye, or sinus symptoms; asthma; and [rarely] shock).

Information that appears in brackets has been added by the authors to clarify and enhance the use of nursing diagnoses.

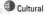

- Identify measures to take if reactions occur.
- Refer to allergist/other physician **for testing, as appropriate.**
- Provide a list of suppliers of products that can replace latex (e.g., rubber grip utensils/toys/hoses, rubber-containing pads, undergarments, carpets, shoe soles, computer mouse pad, erasers, and rubber bands).
- Emphasize the necessity of wearing a medical ID bracelet and informing all new care providers of hypersensitivity **to reduce preventable exposures.**
- Advise the client to be aware of the potential for related food allergies (e.g., bananas, kiwis, melons, tomatoes, avocados, nuts [among others]). **These foods can trigger a latex-like allergic reaction because the proteins in them mimic latex proteins as they break down in the body.**
- Provide worksite review/recommendations to prevent exposure. **Latex allergy can be a disabling occupational disorder. Education about the problem promotes the prevention of allergic reaction, facilitates timely intervention, and helps the nurse to protect clients, latex-sensitive colleagues, and themselves.**
- Refer to resources, including but not limited to ALERT (Allergy to Latex Education & Resource Team, Inc.), Latex Allergy News, Spina Bifida Association, National Institute for Occupational Safety and Health (NIOSH), Kendall's Healthcare Products (Web site), and Hudson RCI (Web site) **for further information about common latex products in the home, latex-free products, and assistance.**

Documentation Focus

Assessment/Reassessment

- Assessment findings, pertinent history of contact with latex products, and frequency of exposure
- Type and extent of symptomatology

Planning

- Plan of care and interventions, and who is involved in planning
- Teaching plan

Implementation/Evaluation

- Response to interventions, teaching, and actions performed
- Attainment or progress toward desired outcome(s)
- Modifications to plan of care

Information that appears in brackets has been added by the authors to clarify and enhance the use of nursing diagnoses.

Discharge Planning

- Discharge needs and referrals made, additional resources available

Sample Nursing Outcomes & Interventions Classifications (NOC/NIC)

NOC—Allergic Response: Systemic
NIC—Latex Precautions

sedentary LIFESTYLE

[Diagnostic Division: Activity/Rest]

Definition: Reports a habit of life that is characterized by a low physical activity level.

Related Factors

Insufficient interest in, motivation, or resources [e.g., time, money, companionship, facilities] for physical activity
Insufficient training for physical exercise
Insufficient knowledge of health benefits associated with physical exercise

Defining Characteristics

Subjective

Preference for activity low in physical activity

Objective

Average daily physical activity is less than recommended for gender and age
Physical deconditioning

Desired Outcomes/Evaluation Criteria—Client Will:

- Verbalize understanding of importance of regular exercise to general well-being.
- Identify necessary precautions or safety concerns and self-monitoring techniques.
- Formulate realistic exercise program with gradual increase in activity.

Information that appears in brackets has been added by the authors to clarify and enhance the use of nursing diagnoses.

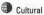

Nursing Priority No. 1.

To assess precipitating/etiological factors:

- Identify conditions that may contribute to immobility or the onset and continuation of inactivity or sedentary lifestyle (e.g., obesity, depression, multiple sclerosis, arthritis, Parkinson's disease, surgery, hemiplegia or paraplegia, chronic pain, brain injury) **that may contribute to immobility or the onset and continuation of inactivity or sedentary lifestyle.**
- Assess the client's age, developmental level, motor skills, ease and capability of movement, posture, and gait. **These determine the type and intensity of needed interventions related to activity.**
- Note emotional and behavioral responses to problems associated with self- or condition-imposed sedentary lifestyle. **Feelings of frustration and powerlessness may impede the attainment of goals.**
- Determine usual exercise and dietary habits, physical limitations, work environment, family dynamics, and available resources.

Nursing Priority No. 2.

To motivate and stimulate client involvement:

- Establish therapeutic relationship acknowledging reality of situation and client's feelings. **Changing a lifelong habit can be difficult, and the client may be feeling discouragement with body and hopelessness (i.e., unable to turn situation around into a positive experience).**
- Ascertain the client's perception of current activity/exercise patterns, impact on life, and cultural expectations of client/others.
- Determine the client's actual ability to participate in exercise or activities, noting attention span, physical limitations and tolerance, level of interest or desire, and safety needs. **Identifies the barriers that need to be addressed.**
- Discuss motivation for change. **Concerns of SO(s) regarding threats to personal health and longevity or acceptance by teen peers may be sufficient to cause the client to initiate change; to sustain change, however, the client must want to change for himself or herself.**
- Review necessity for, and benefits of, regular exercise. **Research confirms that exercise has benefits for the whole body (e.g., can boost energy, enhance coordination, reduce muscle deterioration, improve circulation, lower blood pressure, produce healthier skin and a toned body, and prolong youthful appearance). Exercise has also been**

Information that appears in brackets has been added by the authors to clarify and enhance the use of nursing diagnoses.

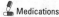

found to boost cardiac fitness in both conditioned and out-of-shape individuals.

- Involve client, SO, parent, or caregiver in developing exercise plan and goals to meet individual needs, desires, and available resources.
- Introduce activities at the client's current level of functioning, progressing to more complex activities, as tolerated.
- Recommend a mix of age- and gender-appropriate activities or stimuli (e.g., movement classes, walking, hiking, jazzercise or other dancing, swimming, biking, skating, bowling, golf, or weight training). **Activities need to be personally meaningful for the client to derive the most enjoyment and to sustain motivation to continue with the program.**
- Encourage a change of scenery (indoors and out, where possible) and periodic changes in the personal environment when the client is confined inside.

Nursing Priority No. 3.

To promote optimal level of function and prevent exercise failure:

- Assist with the treatment of any underlying conditions impacting participation in activities **to maximize function within limitations of the situation.**
- Collaborate with physical medicine specialist or occupational/physical therapist in providing active or passive range-of-motion exercises, isotonic muscle contractions. **Techniques such as gait training, strength training, and exercise to improve balance and coordination can be helpful in rehabilitating the client.**
- Schedule ample time to perform exercise activities balanced with adequate rest periods.
- Provide for safety measures as indicated by individual situation, including environmental management/fall prevention. (Refer to ND risk for Falls.)
- Reevaluate ability/commitment periodically. **Changes in strength/endurance signal readiness for progression of activities or possibly decrease in exercise if overly fatigued. Wavering commitment may require change in types of activities or the addition of a workout buddy to reenergize involvement.**
- Discuss discrepancies in planned and performed activities with the client aware and unaware of observation. Suggest methods for dealing with identified problems. **This may be necessary when the client is using avoidance or controlling behavior or is not aware of his or her own abilities due to anxiety/fear.**

Information that appears in brackets has been added by the authors to clarify and enhance the use of nursing diagnoses.

- Review the importance of adequate intake of fluids, especially during hot weather/strenuous activity.

Nursing Priority No. 4.

To promote wellness (Teaching/Discharge Considerations):

- Educate the client/SO about the benefits of physical activity as it relates to the client's particular situation. **Many studies have shown the health benefits of physical activity in the setting of chronic illness, for example, it increases function in arthritis, improves glycemic control in type 2 diabetes, and can enhance quality of life.**
- Review components of physical fitness: (1) muscle strength and endurance, (2) flexibility, (3) body composition (muscle mass, percentage of body fat), and (4) cardiovascular health. **Fitness routines need to include all elements to attain maximum benefits and prevent deconditioning.**
- Instruct in safety measures as individually indicated (e.g., warm-up and cool-down activities; taking pulse before, during, and after activity; wearing reflective clothing when jogging, placing reflectors on bicycle; locking wheelchair before transfers; judiciously using medications; having supervision as indicated).
- Recommend keeping an activity or exercise log, including physical and psychological responses, changes in weight, endurance, and body mass. **This provides visual evidence of progress or goal attainment and encouragement to continue with program.**
- Encourage the client to involve self in exercise as part of wellness management for the whole person.
- Encourage parents to set a positive example for children by participating in exercise and engaging in an active lifestyle.
- Identify community resources, charity activities, and support groups. **Community walking or hiking trails, sports leagues, and so on, provide free or low-cost options. Activities such as 5K walks for charity, participation in Special Olympics, or age-related competitive games provide goals to work toward.** ***Note:*** **Some individuals may prefer solitary activities; however, most individuals enjoy supportive companionship when exercising.**
- Discuss alternatives for exercise program in changing circumstances (e.g., walking the mall during inclement weather, using exercise facilities at a hotel when traveling, participating in water aerobics at a local swimming pool, joining a gym).
- Promote individual participation in community awareness of problem and discussion of solutions. **Physical inactivity (and**

Information that appears in brackets has been added by the authors to clarify and enhance the use of nursing diagnoses.

associated diseases) is a major public health problem that affects huge numbers of people in all regions of the world. Recognizing the problem and future consequences may empower the global community to develop effective measures to promote physical activity and improve public health.

- Introduce and promote established goals for increasing physical activity, such as Sports, Play, and Active Recreation for Kids (SPARK) and Physician-Based Assessment and Counseling for Exercise (PACE), **to address national concerns about obesity and major barriers to physical activity, such as time constraints, lack of training in physical activity or behavioral change methods, and lack of standard protocols.**

Documentation Focus

Assessment/Reassessment

- Individual findings, including level of function and ability to participate in specific or desired activities
- Motivation for change

Planning

- Plan of care and who is involved in the planning
- Teaching plan

Implementation/Evaluation

- Responses to interventions, teaching, and actions performed
- Attainment or progress toward desired outcome(s)
- Modifications to plan of care

Discharge Planning

- Discharge and long-range needs, noting who is responsible for each action to be taken
- Specific referrals made
- Sources of, and maintenance for, assistive devices

Sample Nursing Outcomes & Interventions Classifications (NOC/NIC)

NOC—Knowledge: Prescribed Activity
NIC—Exercise Promotion

Information that appears in brackets has been added by the authors to clarify and enhance the use of nursing diagnoses.

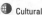

risk for impaired LIVER FUNCTION

[Diagnostic Division: Food/Fluid]

Definition: Vulnerable to a decrease in liver function, which may compromise health.

Risk Factors

Viral infection [e.g., hepatitis A/B/C, Epstein-Barr]; HIV coinfection
Pharmaceutical agent [e.g., acetaminophen, statins]
Substance abuse

NOTE: A risk diagnosis is not evidenced by signs and symptoms, as the problem has not occurred; rather, nursing interventions are directed at prevention.

Desired Outcomes/Evaluation Criteria—Client Will:

- Verbalize understanding of individual risk factors that contribute to possibility of liver damage/failure.
- Demonstrate behaviors, lifestyle changes to reduce risk factors and protect self from injury.
- Be free of signs of liver failure as evidenced by liver function studies within normal levels, and absence of jaundice, hepatic enlargement, or altered mental status.

Actions/Interventions

Nursing Priority No. 1.

To identify individual risk factors/needs:

- Determine the presence of condition(s) as listed in Risk Factors, noting whether problem is acute (e.g., viral hepatitis, acetaminophen overdose) or chronic (e.g., alcoholic hepatitis or cirrhosis). **These influence choice of interventions.**
- Note client history of known/possible exposure to virus, bacteria, or toxins **that can damage the liver:**

  Works in high-risk occupation (e.g., performs tasks that involve contact with blood, blood-contaminated body fluids, other body fluids, or sharps)

  Injects drugs, especially if client shared a needle or received a tattoo or a piercing with an unsterile needle

Information that appears in brackets has been added by the authors to clarify and enhance the use of nursing diagnoses.

Received blood or blood products prior to 1989

Ingested contaminated food or water or experienced poor sanitation practices by food-service workers

Has close contact (e.g., lives with or has sex with infected person or carrier; infant born to infected mother)

Is regularly exposed to toxic chemicals (e.g., carbon tetrachloride cleaning agents, bug spray, paint fumes, and tobacco smoke)

Uses prescription drugs (e.g., sulfonamides, phenothiazines, isoniazid)

Ingests certain herbal remedies or mega doses of vitamins

Uses alcohol with medications (including over-the-counter medications)

Consumes alcohol heavily and/or over long period of time

Ingested acetaminophen (accidentally, as may occur when a client takes too large a dose or has several medications containing acetaminophen over time; or intentionally, as may occur with suicide attempt)

Travels internationally to or immigrates from areas/countries such as Africa, Southeast Asia, Korea, China, Vietnam, Eastern Europe, Mediterranean countries, or the Caribbean.

- Review results of laboratory tests (e.g., abnormal liver function studies, drug toxicity, HVB positive) and other diagnostic studies (e.g., ultrasonography, computed tomography [CT] scanning; magnetic resonance imaging [MRI]) **that indicate the presence of a hepatotoxic condition and the need for medical treatment.**

Nursing Priority No. 2.

To assist client to reduce or correct individual risk factors:

- Assist with medical treatment of underlying condition **to support organ function and minimize liver damage.**
- Educate the client on way(s) to prevent exposure to/incidence of hepatitis infections and limit damage to liver:

Practice safer sex (e.g., avoid multiple-partner sex, wear condoms, avoid sex with partners known to be infected).

Wash hands well after using the bathroom or changing soiled diapers/briefs.

Avoid injecting drugs or sharing needles.

Avoid sharing razors, toothbrushes, or nail clippers.

Make sure needles and inks are sterile for tattooing and body piercing.

Use proper precautions and appropriate protective equipment when working in high-risk occupations, such as healthcare, police and fire departments, emergency services, day-care

Information that appears in brackets has been added by the authors to clarify and enhance the use of nursing diagnoses.

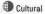

services, and chemical manufacturing, **where one is most at risk for inhalation of toxins, needlesticks, or body fluid exposure.**

Avoid tap water and practice good hygiene and sanitation when traveling internationally.

Use harsh cleansers and aerosol products in well-ventilated room; wear mask and gloves, cover skin, and wash well afterward. **Insecticides and other chemicals can reach the liver through skin and destroy liver cells.**

Obtain vaccinations when appropriate. **Some hepatitis strains (e.g., A and B) are preventable, thus minimizing the risk of liver damage.**

- Emphasize the importance of responsible drinking or avoiding alcohol, when indicated, **to reduce the incidence of cirrhosis or severity of liver damage or failure.**
- Encourage the client with liver dysfunction to avoid fatty foods. **Fat interferes with normal function of liver cells and can cause additional damage and permanent scarring to liver cells when they can no longer regenerate.**
- Encourage smoking cessation. **The additives in cigarettes pose a challenge to the liver by reducing the liver's ability to eliminate toxins.**
- Refer to a nutritionist, as indicated, for dietary needs, including intake of calories, proteins, vitamins, and trace minerals, **to promote healing and limit effects of deficiencies.**
- Discuss safe use and concerns about client's medication regimen (e.g., acetaminophen; NSAIDs; herbal or vitamin supplements; phenobarbitol; cholesterol-lowering drugs, such as "statins"; some antibiotics [e.g., sulfonamides, INH]; certain cardiovascular drugs [e.g., amiodarone, hydralazine]; antidepressants [e.g., tricyclics]) **known to cause hepatotoxicity, either alone or in combination, or in an overdose situation.**
- Identify signs/symptoms that warrant prompt notification of healthcare provider (e.g., increased abdominal girth; rapid weight loss or gain; increased peripheral edema; dyspnea, fever; blood in stool or urine; excess bleeding of any kind; jaundice). **These are indicators of severe liver dysfunction, possible organ failure.**
- Refer to specialist or liver treatment center, as indicated. **Referral may be beneficial for a person with chronic liver disease when decompensating, or a client with hepatitis and other coexisting disease condition (e.g., HIV) or intolerance to treatment due to side effects.**

Information that appears in brackets has been added by the authors to clarify and enhance the use of nursing diagnoses.

Nursing Priority No. 3.

To promote wellness (Teaching/Discharge Considerations):

- Encourage the client routinely taking acetaminophen for pain management to read labels, determine strength of medication, note safe number of doses over 24 hr, become familiar with "hidden" sources of acetaminophen (e.g., Nyquil, Vicodin), and limit alcohol intake **to avoid/limit risk of liver damage.**
- Emphasize the importance of hand hygiene and avoidance of fresh produce, use of bottled water and avoidance of raw meat and seafood **if client is traveling to an area where hepatitis A is endemic or food or waterborne illness is a risk.**
- Instruct in measures including protection from blood and other body fluids, sharps safety, safer sex practices, avoiding needle sharing and body tattoos or piercings **to prevent occupational and nonoccupational exposures to hepatitis.**
- Discuss need and refer for vaccination, as indicated (e.g., healthcare and public safety worker, children under 18, international traveler, recreational drug user, men who have sexual relationships with other men, client with clotting disorders or liver disease, anyone sharing household with an infected person), **to prevent exposure and transmission of blood or body fluid hepatitis and limit risk of liver injury.**
- Discuss appropriateness of prophylactic immunizations. **Although the best way to protect against hepatitis B and C infections is to prevent exposure to viruses, postexposure prophylaxis should be initiated promptly to prevent or limit the severity of the infection.**
- Provide information regarding the availability of gamma globulin, immune serum globulin, HepB immunoglobulin, and HepB vaccine (Recombivax HB, Engerix-B) through the health department or family physician.
- Emphasize the necessity of follow-up care (in client with chronic liver disease) and adherence to therapeutic regimen **to monitor liver function and effectiveness of interventions** and importance of adherence to therapeutic regimen **to prevent or minimize permanent liver damage.**
- Refer to community resources, drug and alcohol treatment program, as indicated.

Documentation Focus

Assessment/Reassessment

- Assessment findings, including individual risk factors
- Results of laboratory tests and diagnostic studies

Information that appears in brackets has been added by the authors to clarify and enhance the use of nursing diagnoses.

Planning
- Plan of care and who is involved in planning
- Teaching plan

Implementation/Evaluation
- Response to interventions, teaching, and actions performed
- Attainment or progress toward desired outcome(s)
- Modifications to plan of care

Discharge Planning
- Long-term needs, plan for follow-up, and who is responsible for actions to be taken
- Specific referrals made

Sample Nursing Outcomes & Interventions Classifications (NOC/NIC)

NOC—Knowledge: Disease Process
NIC—Substance Use Treatment

risk for LONELINESS

[Diagnostic Division: Social Interaction]

Definition: Vulnerable to experiencing discomfort associated with a desire or need for more contact with others, which may compromise health.

Risk Factors

Affectional deprivation
Physical or social isolation
Emotional deprivation

NOTE: A risk diagnosis is not evidenced by signs and symptoms, as the problem has not occurred; rather, nursing interventions are directed at prevention.

Desired Outcomes/Evaluation Criteria—Client Will:

- Identify individual difficulties and ways to address them.
- Engage in social activities.
- Report involvement in interactions and relationship client views as meaningful.

Information that appears in brackets has been added by the authors to clarify and enhance the use of nursing diagnoses.

Parent/Caregiver Will:

- Provide infant/child with consistent and loving caregiving.
- Participate in programs for adolescents and families.

Actions/Interventions

Nursing Priority No. 1.

To identify causative/precipitating factors:

- Differentiate between ordinary loneliness and a state or constant sense of dysphoria. **This influences the type of and intensity of interventions.**
- ∞ Note the client's age and duration of the problem; that is, situational (such as leaving home for college) or chronic. **Adolescents may experience lonely feelings related to the changes that are happening as they become adults. Elderly individuals incur multiple losses associated with aging, loss of spouse, decline in physical health, and changes in roles that intensify feelings of loneliness.**
- Determine degree of distress, tension, anxiety, or restlessness present. Note history of frequent illnesses, accidents, and crises. **Individuals under stress tend to have more illnesses and accidents related to inattention and anxiety.**
- Note the presence and proximity of family/significant other (SO)(s), and whether they are helpful or not. **Loneliness may not be related to being alone, but knowing that family is available can help with planning care. The client may be estranged from other family members or family may not be willing to be involved with client.**
- Discuss with the client whether there is a person or persons in his or her life who can be trustworthy and who will listen with empathy to the feelings that are expressed.
- Determine how the individual perceives and deals with solitude. **The client may see being alone as positive, allowing time to pursue own interests, or may view solitude as sad and long for lost people, lifestyle pattern, or events.**
- ∞ Review issues of separation from parents as a child, loss of SO(s)/spouse. **Early separation from parents often affects the individual as other losses occur throughout life, leading to feelings of inadequacy and inability to deal with current situation.**
- Assess sleep and appetite disturbances and ability to concentrate. **These are indicators of distress related to feelings of loneliness and low self-esteem.**

Information that appears in brackets has been added by the authors to clarify and enhance the use of nursing diagnoses.

- Note expressions of "yearning" for an emotional partnership.
- Assess feelings of loneliness in a client who is receiving palliative/hospice care. **These individuals often feel alienated and lonely as they face the end of their life and may need additional socialization to help them feel valued.**

Nursing Priority No. 2.

To assist client to identify feelings and situations in which he or she experiences loneliness:

- Establish a nurse-client relationship. **The client may feel free to talk about feelings in the context of an empathetic relationship.**
- Discuss individual concerns about feelings of loneliness and relationship between loneliness and lack of SO(s). Note desire and willingness to change situation. **Motivation can impede—or facilitate—achieving desired outcomes.**
- Support expression of negative perceptions of others and note whether the client agrees. **This provides opportunity for the client to clarify reality of the situation and recognize his or her own denial.**
- Accept the client's expressions of loneliness as a primary condition and not necessarily as a symptom of some underlying condition.

Nursing Priority No. 3.

To assist client to become involved:

- Discuss reality versus perceptions of situation.
- ∞ Discuss importance of emotional bonding (attachment) between infants or young children and parents/caregivers when appropriate.
- Involve in classes, such as assertiveness, language and communication, social skills, **to address individual needs and potential for enhanced socialization.**
- Role-play situations **to develop interpersonal skills.**
- Discuss positive health habits, including personal hygiene and exercise activity of client's choosing.
- Identify individual strengths, areas of interest **that provide opportunities for involvement with others.**
- Encourage attendance at support group activities to meet individual needs (e.g., therapy, separation/grief, religious).
- Help the client establish a plan for progressive involvement, beginning with a simple activity (e.g., call an old friend, speak to a neighbor) and leading to more complicated interactions and activities.

Information that appears in brackets has been added by the authors to clarify and enhance the use of nursing diagnoses.

- Provide opportunities for interactions in a supportive environment (e.g., have client accompanied, as in a "buddy system") during initial attempts to socialize. **This helps to reduce stress, provides positive reinforcement, and facilitates a successful outcome.**

Nursing Priority No. 4.

To promote wellness (Teaching/Discharge Considerations):

- Inform the client that loneliness can be overcome. **It is up to the individual to build self-esteem and learn to feel good about self.**
- Encourage involvement in special-interest groups (e.g., computers, gardening club, reading circles, bird watchers) and charitable services (e.g., serving in a soup kitchen, youth groups, animal shelter).
- Suggest volunteering for a church committee or choir; attending community events with friends and family; becoming involved in political issues or campaigns; or enrolling in classes at a local college or continuing education programs. **When the client is willing to become involved in these kinds of activities, the perception of loneliness fades into the background, and even though the individual may still be lonely, the sense of loneliness is not so pervasive.**
- Refer to appropriate counselors for help with relationships or other identified needs.
- Refer to NDs Hopelessness; Anxiety; Social Isolation for related interventions, as appropriate.

Documentation Focus

Assessment/Reassessment

- Assessment findings, including client's perception of problem, availability of resources and support systems
- Client's desire and commitment to change

Planning

- Plan of care and who is involved in planning
- Teaching plan

Implementation/Evaluation

- Response to interventions, teaching, and actions performed
- Attainment or progress toward desired outcome(s)
- Modifications to plan of care

Information that appears in brackets has been added by the authors to clarify and enhance the use of nursing diagnoses.

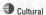

Discharge Planning

- Long-term needs, plan for follow-up, and who is responsible for actions to be taken
- Specific referrals made

Sample Nursing Outcomes & Interventions Classifications (NOC/NIC)

NOC—Loneliness
NIC—Socialization Enhancement

risk for disturbed MATERNAL-FETAL DYAD

[Diagnostic Division: Safety]

Definition: Vulnerable to disruption of the symbiotic maternal-fetal dyad as a result of comorbid or pregnancy-related conditions, which may compromise health.

Risk Factors

Pregnancy complication (e.g., premature rupture of membranes, placenta previa or abruption, multiple gestation)
Compromised fetal oxygen transport (e.g., anemia, [sickle cell anemia], cardiac disease, asthma, hypertension, seizures, premature labor, hemorrhage, etc.)
Alteration in glucose metabolism (e.g., diabetes, steroid use)
Presence of abuse (e.g., physical, psychological, sexual)
Substance abuse
Treatment regimen [e.g., pharmaceutical agents, surgery]

NOTE: A risk diagnosis is not evidenced by signs and symptoms, as the problem has not occurred; rather, nursing interventions are directed at prevention.

Desired Outcomes/Evaluation Criteria—Client Will:

- Verbalize understanding of individual risk factors or condition(s) that may impact pregnancy.
- Engage in necessary alterations in lifestyle and daily activities to manage risks.
- Participate in screening procedures as indicated.

Information that appears in brackets has been added by the authors to clarify and enhance the use of nursing diagnoses.

- Identify signs/symptoms requiring medical evaluation or intervention.
- Display fetal growth within normal limits and carry pregnancy to term.

Actions/Interventions

Nursing Priority No. 1.

To identify individual risk/contributing factors:

- Review history of previous pregnancies for presence of complications, such as premature rupture of membranes (PROM), placenta previa, miscarriage or pregnancy losses due to premature dilation of the cervix, preterm labor or deliveries, previous birth defects, hyperemesis gravidarum, or repeated urinary tract or vaginal infections.
- Obtain history about prenatal screening and amount and timing of care. **Lack of prenatal care can place both mother and fetus at risk.**
- Note conditions potentiating vascular changes/reduced placental circulation (e.g., diabetes, gestational hypertension, cardiac problems, smoking) or those that alter oxygen-carrying capacity (e.g., asthma, anemia, Rh incompatibility, hemorrhage). **Extent of maternal vascular involvement and reduction of oxygen-carrying capacity have a direct influence on uteroplacental circulation and gas exchange.**
- Note maternal age. **Maternal age above 35 years is associated with increased risk of spontaneous abortions, preterm delivery or stillbirths, fetal chromosomal abnormalities and malformations, and intrauterine growth retardation (IUGR). In pregnant adolescents (younger than 15), the most common high-risk conditions include gestational hypertension, anemia, labor dysfunction, cephalopelvic disproportion and low birth weight, and preterm delivery.**
- Ascertain current/past dietary patterns and practices. **Client may be malnourished, obese, or underweight (weight less than 100 lb or over 200 lb); may reveal preconception eating disorders that can have a negative impact on fetal organ development—especially brain tissue in the early weeks of pregnancy.**
- Assess for severe, unremitting nausea and vomiting, especially when it persists after the first trimester (hyperemesis gravidarum). **Hyperemesis gravidarum places the mother at risk for substantial weight loss and fluid and electrolyte imbalances, and exposes the developing fetus to acidotic**

Information that appears in brackets has been added by the authors to clarify and enhance the use of nursing diagnoses.

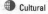

state and malnutrition. Development of hyperemesis gravidarum may require hospitalization.

- Note history of exposure to teratogenic agents, infectious diseases (e.g., tuberculosis, influenza, measles); high-risk occupations; exposure to toxic substances such as lead, organic solvents, carbon monoxide; use of certain over-the-counter or prescription medications; substance use or abuse (including illicit drugs and alcohol).
- Identify family or cultural influences in pregnancy. **Family history may include multiple births or congenital diseases, or generational abuse or lack of support or finances. Cultural background may identify health risks associated with nationality (e.g., sickle cell in people of African descent or Tay-Sachs disease in people of eastern European Jewish ancestry); or religious practices (e.g., exclusion of dairy products, or no maternal immunizations for rubella) that can impact health of mother or fetal development.**
- Review laboratory studies. **Low hemoglobin suggests anemia, which is associated with hypoxia. Blood type and Rh group may reveal incompatibility risks; elevated serum glucose may be seen in gestational diabetes mellitus (GDM); elevated liver function studies suggest hypertensive liver involvement; drop in platelet count may be associated with gestational hypertension and HELLP (hemolysis, elevated liver enzymes, and low platelet) syndrome. Nutritional studies may reveal decreased levels of serum proteins, electrolytes, minerals, or vitamins essential to maternal health and fetal development.**
- Review vaginal, cervical, or rectal cultures and serology results. **May reveal presence of sexually transmitted infections (STIs) or identify active or carrier state of hepatitis, HIV, AIDS.**
- Assist in screening for and identifying genetic or chromosomal disorders. **Disorders such as phenylketonuria (PKU) or sickle cell disease necessitate special treatment to prevent negative effects on fetal growth.**
- Investigate current home situation. **Client may have history of unstable relationship, or inadequate/lack of housing that affects safety as well as general well-being.**

Nursing Priority No. 2.

To monitor maternal/fetal status:

- Weigh client and compare current weight with pregravid weight. Have client record weight between visits.

Information that appears in brackets has been added by the authors to clarify and enhance the use of nursing diagnoses.

Underweight clients are at risk for anemia, inadequate protein and calorie intake, vitamin or mineral deficiencies, and gestational hypertension. Overweight women are at increased risk for development of gestational hypertension, gestational diabetes, and hyperinsulinemia of the fetus.

- Assess fetal heart rate (FHR), noting rate and regularity. Have the client monitor fetal movement daily as indicated. **Tachycardia in a term infant may indicate a compensatory mechanism to reduced oxygen levels and/or presence of sepsis. A reduction in fetal activity occurs before bradycardia.**
- Test urine for presence of ketones. **Indicates inadequate glucose utilization and breakdown of fats for metabolic processes.**
- Provide information and assist with procedures as indicated, for example:

  Amniocentesis: **May be performed for genetic purposes or to assess fetal lung maturity. Spectrophotometric analysis of the fluid may be done to detect bilirubin after 26 weeks' gestation.**

  Ultrasonography: **Assesses gestational age of fetus, detects presence of multiples, or fetal abnormalities. Locates placenta (and amniotic fluid pockets before amniocentesis, if performed), monitors clients at risk for reduced or inadequate placental perfusion (such as adolescents, clients older than 35 years, and clients with diabetes, gestational hypertension, cardiac or kidney disease, anemia, or respiratory disorders).**

  Biophysical profile: **Assesses fetal well-being through ultrasound evaluation to measure amniotic fluid index (AFI), FHR, nonstress test (NST) reactivity, fetal breathing movement, body movement (large limbs), and muscle tone (flexion and extension).**

  Contraction stress test (CST): **A positive CST with late decelerations indicates a high-risk client and fetus with possible reduced uteroplacental reserves.**
- Screen for abuse during pregnancy. **Prenatal abuse is correlated with a low maternal weight gain, infections, anemia, delay in seeking prenatal care until the third trimester, and preterm delivery.**
- Screen for preterm uterine contractions, which may or may not be accompanied by cervical dilatation.

Information that appears in brackets has been added by the authors to clarify and enhance the use of nursing diagnoses.

Nursing Priority No. 3.

To correct/improve maternal/fetal well-being:

- Instruct client in reportable symptoms and monitor for unusual symptoms at each prenatal visit (e.g., vaginal bleeding, headache along with blurred vision and ankle swelling, faintness, persistent vomiting). **Provides opportunity for early intervention in event of developing complications.**
- Assist in treatment of underlying medical condition(s) that have potential for causing maternal or fetal harm.
- Assess perceived impact of complication on client and family members. Encourage verbalization of concerns. **Family stress is amplified in a high-risk pregnancy, where concerns focus on the health of both the client and the fetus. Family is strengthened if all members have a chance to express fears openly and work cooperatively.**
- Facilitate positive adaptation to situation, through Active-listening, acceptance, and problem-solving. **Helps in successful accomplishment of the psychological tasks of pregnancy.**
- Develop dietary plan with client that provides necessary nutrients (calories, protein, vitamins, and minerals) **to create new tissue and to meet increased maternal metabolic needs.**
- Promote fluid intake of at least two quarts of noncaffeinated fluid per day **to prevent dehydration, which may compromise optimal uterine and placental functioning and increase uterine irritability.**
- Encourage client to participate in individually appropriate adaptations and self-care techniques, such as scheduling rest periods two to three times a day, avoiding overexertion or heavy lifting, or maintaining contact with family and daily life if bedrest is required. **Preventive problem-solving promotes participation in own care and enhances self-confidence, sense of control, and client/couple satisfaction.**
- Review medication regimen. **Prepregnancy treatment for chronic conditions may require alteration for maternal and fetal safety.**
- Review availability and use of resources. **Presence or absence of supportive resources can make the difference for the client and family in being able to manage the situation.**
- Administer Rh immunoglobulin (RhIgG) to client at 28 weeks' gestation in Rh-negative clients with Rh-positive partners, or following amniocentesis, if indicated. **RhIgG helps reduce the incidence of maternal isoimmunization in non-**

Information that appears in brackets has been added by the authors to clarify and enhance the use of nursing diagnoses.

sensitized mothers and helps prevent erythroblastosis fetalis and fetal red blood cell (RBC) hemolysis.

- Encourage modified or complete bedrest as indicated. **Activity level may need modification, depending on symptoms of uterine activity, cervical changes, or bleeding. Side-lying position increases renal and placental perfusion, which is effective in preventing supine hypotensive syndrome.**
- Provide supplemental oxygen as appropriate. **Increases the oxygen available for fetal uptake, especially in clients with severe anemia or sickle cell crisis.**
- Prepare for and assist with intrauterine fetal exchange transfusion as indicated by titers (Kleihauer-Betke test).

Nursing Priority No. 4.

To promote wellness (Teaching/Discharge Considerations):

- Emphasize the normalcy of pregnancy, focus on pregnancy milestones, "countdown to birth." **Avoids or limits perception of "sick role"; promotes sense of hope that modifications or restrictions serve a worthwhile purpose.**
- Discuss implications of preexisting condition and possible impact on pregnancy. **Pregnancy may have no effect or may reduce or exacerbate severity of symptoms of chronic conditions.**
- Provide information about risks of weight reduction during pregnancy and about nourishment needs of client and fetus. **Prenatal calorie restriction and resultant weight loss may result in nutrient deficiency or ketonemia, with negative effects on fetal central nervous system and possible IUGR.**
- Encourage smoking cessation, refer to community program or support group as indicated. **Severe adverse effects of smoking on the fetus may be reduced if mother quits smoking early in pregnancy, and pregnancy outcomes can still be improved if mother stops smoking as late as 32 weeks' gestation.**
- Help client/couple plan restructuring of roles and activities necessitated by complication of pregnancy. **Education, support, and assistance in maintenance of family integrity help foster growth of its individual members and reduce stress that the client may feel from her dependent role.**
- Have client demonstrate new behaviors and therapeutic techniques. **During pregnancy, control of condition may require specific modified or new behaviors.**

Information that appears in brackets has been added by the authors to clarify and enhance the use of nursing diagnoses.

- Recommend client assess uterine tone and contractions for 1 hr, once or twice a day as indicated **to monitor uterine irritability or early indication of premature labor.**
- Encourage close monitoring of blood glucose levels, as appropriate. **Type I or insulin-dependent diabetes mellitus generally need to check blood glucose levels 4 to 12 times/day because insulin needs may increase two to three times above pregravid baseline.**
- Demonstrate technique and specific equipment used when FHR monitoring is done in the home setting.
- Identify danger signals requiring immediate notification of healthcare provider (e.g., PROM, preterm labor, vaginal drainage or bleeding). **Recognizing risk situations encourages prompt evaluation and intervention, which may prevent or limit untoward outcomes.**
- Review availability and use of resources. **Presence or absence of supportive resources can make the difference for the client and family in being able to manage the situation.**
- Refer to community service agencies (e.g., visiting nurse, social service) or resources, such as Sidelines. **Community supports may be needed for ongoing assessment of medical problem, family status, coping behaviors, and financial stressors.** ***Note:*** **Sidelines is a national telephone support group for pregnant women on bedrest.**
- Refer for counseling if family does not sustain positive coping and growth. **May be necessary to promote growth and to prevent family disintegration.**

Documentation Focus

Assessment/Reassessment

- Assessment findings, including weight, signs of pregnancy, safety concerns
- Specific risk factors, comorbidities, and treatment regimen
- Results of screening laboratory tests and diagnostic studies
- Participation in prenatal care
- Cultural beliefs and practices

Planning

- Plan of care, specific interventions, and who is involved in the planning
- Community resources for equipment and supplies
- Specific referrals made
- Teaching plan

Information that appears in brackets has been added by the authors to clarify and enhance the use of nursing diagnoses.

Implementation/Evaluation

- Client/fetal response to treatment and actions performed
- Client's response to teaching provided
- Attainment or progress toward desired outcome(s)
- Modifications to plan of care

Sample Nursing Outcomes & Interventions Classifications (NOC/NIC)

NOC—Prenatal Health Behavior
NIC—High-Risk Pregnancy Care

impaired MEMORY

[Diagnostic Division: Neurosensory]

Definition: Inability to remember or recall bits of information or behavioral skills.

Related Factors

Hypoxia; anemia
Electrolyte imbalance; decrease in cardiac output
Neurological impairment (e.g., positive electroencephalogram [EEG], head trauma, seizure disorders)
Distractions in the environment
[Substance abuse; effects of medications]
[Age]

Defining Characteristics

Subjective

Inability to recall events or factual information

Objective

Inability to recall if a behavior was performed; forgets to perform a behavior at a scheduled time
Inability to learn/retain new skills or information
Inability to perform a previously learned skill
Forgetfulness

Information that appears in brackets has been added by the authors to clarify and enhance the use of nursing diagnoses.

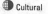

Desired Outcomes/Evaluation Criteria—Client Will:

- Verbalize awareness of memory problems.
- Establish methods to help in remembering essential things when possible.
- Accept limitations of condition and use resources effectively.

Actions/Interventions

Nursing Priority No. 1.

To assess causative factor(s)/degree of impairment:

- Determine physical, biochemical, and environmental factors (e.g., systemic infections; brain injury; pulmonary disease with hypoxia; use of multiple medications; exposure to toxic substances; use or abuse of alcohol or other drugs; traumatic event; removal from known environment) **that may be associated with confusion and loss of memory.**
- Note client's age and potential for depression. **Depressive disorders affecting memory and concentration are particularly prevalent in older adults; however, impairments can occur in depressed persons of any age.**
- Note presence of stressful situation(s) and degree of anxiety. **Can increase client's confusion and disorganization and further interfere with attempts at recall. Stress may also speed up memory decline in person whose cognitive function is already impaired.** (Refer to ND Anxiety for additional interventions as indicated.)
- Collaborate with medical and psychiatric providers in evaluating orientation, attention span, ability to follow directions, send/receive communication, appropriateness of response **to determine presence and/or severity of impairment.**
- Perform or review results of cognitive testing (e.g., Blessed Information-Memory-Concentration [BIMC] test, Mini-Mental State Examination [MMSE]). **A combination of tests may be needed to obtain a complete picture of the client's overall condition and prognosis.**
- Evaluate skill proficiency levels. **Evaluation may include many self-care activities (e.g., daily grooming, steps in preparing a meal, participating in a lifelong hobby, balancing a checkbook, and driving ability) to determine level of independence or needed assistance.**
- Ascertain how client/family view the problem (e.g., practical problems of forgetting and/or role and responsibility impair-

---

Information that appears in brackets has been added by the authors to clarify and enhance the use of nursing diagnoses.

ments related to loss of memory and concentration) **to determine significance and impact of problem.**

Nursing Priority No. 2.

To maximize level of function:

- Assist with treatment of underlying conditions (e.g., electrolyte imbalances, infection, anemia, drug interactions/reaction to medications; alcohol or other drug intoxication; malnutrition, vitamin deficiencies; pain) **where treatment can improve memory processes.**
- Orient/reorient client as needed. Introduce self with each client contact **to meet client's safety and comfort needs.** (Refer to NDs acute/chronic Confusion, for additional interventions.)
- Implement appropriate memory-retraining techniques (e.g., keeping calendars, writing lists, memory cue games, mnemonic devices, using computers).
- Assist with and instruct client and family in associate-learning tasks, such as practice sessions recalling personal information, reminiscing, locating a geographic location (Stimulation Therapy). **Practice may improve performance and integrate new behaviors into the client's coping strategies.**
- Encourage ventilation of feelings of frustration and helplessness. Refocus attention to areas of control and progress **to diminish feelings of powerlessness/hopelessness.**
- Provide for and emphasize importance of pacing learning activities and getting sufficient rest **to avoid fatigue and frustration that may further impair cognitive abilities.**
- Monitor client's behavior and assist in use of stress-management techniques (e.g., music therapy, reading, television, games, socialization) **to reduce boredom and enhance enjoyment of life.**
- Structure teaching methods and interventions to client's level of functioning and/or potential for improvement.
- Determine client's response to and effects of medications prescribed to improve attention, concentration, memory processes, and to lift spirits or modify emotional responses. **Medication for cognitive enhancement can be effective, but benefits need to be weighed against whether quality of life is improved after side effects and cost of drugs are considered.**

Nursing Priority No. 3.

To promote wellness (Teaching/Discharge Considerations):

- Assist client/SO(s) to establish compensation strategies (e.g., menu planning with a shopping list, timely completion of

---

Information that appears in brackets has been added by the authors to clarify and enhance the use of nursing diagnoses.

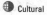

tasks on a daily planner, checklists at the front door to ascertain that lights and stove are off before leaving) **to improve functional lifestyle and safety.** (Refer to NDs acute/chronic Confusion for additional interventions.)

- Refer for follow-up with counselors, rehabilitation programs, job coaches, social or financial support systems **to help deal with persistent or difficult problems.**
- Refer to rehabilitation services **that are matched to the needs, strengths, and capacities of individual and modified as needs change over time.**
- Discuss and encourage safety interventions, as indicated (e.g., assistance with meal preparation, evaluation of driving abilities, cessation of tobacco use or its use only under supervision, removal of guns and other weapons) **to prevent injury to client/others.**
- Assist client to deal with functional limitations (such as loss of driving privileges) and identify resources **to meet individual needs, maximizing independence.**

Documentation Focus

Assessment/Reassessment

- Individual findings, testing results, and perceptions of significance of problem
- Actual impact on lifestyle and independence

Planning

- Plan of care and who is involved in planning process
- Teaching plan

Implementation/Evaluation

- Responses to interventions, teaching, and actions performed
- Attainment or progress toward desired outcome(s)
- Modifications to plan of care

Discharge Planning

- Long-term needs and who is responsible for actions to be taken
- Specific referrals made

Sample Nursing Outcomes & Interventions Classifications (NOC/NIC)

NOC—Memory
NIC—Memory Training

Information that appears in brackets has been added by the authors to clarify and enhance the use of nursing diagnoses.

impaired bed MOBILITY

[Diagnostic Division: Safety]

Definition: Limitation of independent movement from one bed position to another.

Related Factors

Neuromuscular or musculoskeletal impairment
Insufficient muscle strength; physical deconditioning; obesity
Environmental barrier (e.g., bed size or type, equipment, restraints)
Pain; pharmaceutical agent
Insufficient knowledge of mobility strategies
Alteration in cognitive functioning

Defining Characteristics

Objective

Impaired ability to: reposition self in bed, turn from side to side
Impaired ability to move between prone and supine positions, sitting/long sitting and supine positions

Desired Outcomes/Evaluation Criteria—Client/Caregiver Will:

- Verbalize willingness to participate in repositioning program.
- Verbalize understanding of situation and risk factors, individual therapeutic regimen, and safety measures.
- Demonstrate techniques and behaviors that enable safe repositioning.
- Maintain position of function and skin integrity as evidenced by absence of contractures, footdrop, decubitus, and so forth.
- Maintain or increase strength and function of affected and/or compensatory body part.

Actions/Interventions

Nursing Priority No. 1.

To identify causative/contributing factors:

- Determine diagnoses that contribute to immobility (e.g., multiple sclerosis, arthritis, Parkinson's disease,

Information that appears in brackets has been added by the authors to clarify and enhance the use of nursing diagnoses.

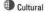

hemi-/para-/tetraplegia, fractures [especially hip joint and long bone fractures], multiple trauma, burns, head injury, depression, dementia).

- Note individual risk factors and current situation, such as surgery, casts, amputation, traction, pain, age, general weakness or debilitation **that can contribute to problems related to bedrest.**
- Determine degree of perceptual or cognitive impairment and/or ability to follow directions. **Impairments related to age; acute or chronic conditions (including severe depression, dementia); trauma; surgery; or medications require alternative interventions or changes in plan of care.**

Nursing Priority No. 2.

To assess functional ability:

- Determine functional level classification 0 to 4. **(The client at level 0 is completely independent; 1 = requires use of equipment or device; 2 = requires help from another person for assistance; 3 = requires help from another person and equipment device; 4 = dependent, does not participate in activity).**
- Note emotional and behavioral responses to problems of immobility. **Can negatively affect self-concept and self-esteem, autonomy, and independence.**
- Note presence of complications related to immobility. **The effects of immobility are rarely confined to one body system and can include decline in cognition, muscle wasting, contractures, pressure sores, constipation, aspiration pneumonia, etc.** (Refer to ND Disuse Syndrome.)

Nursing Priority No. 3.

To promote optimal level of function and prevent complications:

- Assist with treatment of underlying condition(s) **to maximize potential for mobility and optimal function.**
- Ascertain that dependent client is placed in best bed for situation (e.g., correct size, support surface, and mobility functions) **to promote mobility and enhance environmental safety.**
- Change client's position frequently, moving individual parts of the body (e.g., legs, arms, head) using appropriate support and proper body alignment. Encourage periodic changes in head of bed (if not contraindicated by conditions such as an

Information that appears in brackets has been added by the authors to clarify and enhance the use of nursing diagnoses.

acute spinal cord injury), with client in supine and prone positions at intervals **to improve circulation, reduce tightening of muscles and joints, normalize body tone, and more closely simulate body positions an individual would normally use.**

- Turn dependent client frequently, utilizing bed and mattress positioning settings to assist movements; reposition in good body alignment, using appropriate supports.
- Instruct client and caregivers in methods of moving client relative to specific situations (e.g., turning side to side, prone, or sitting) **to provide support for the client's body and to prevent injury to the lifter.**
- Perform and encourage regular skin examination for reddened or excoriated areas. Use a pressure-risk assessment scale (e.g. Braden, Norton) as appropriate. Provide frequent skin care (e.g., cleansing, moisturizing, gentle massage) **to reduce pressure on sensitive areas and prevent development of problems with skin or tissue integrity.** (Refer to NDs impaired Skin Integrity; impaired Tissue Integrity.)
- Provide or assist with daily range-of-motion interventions (active and passive) **to maintain joint mobility, improve circulation, and prevent contractures.**
- Assist with activities of hygiene, feeding, and toileting, as indicated. Assist on and off bedpan and into sitting position (or use cardioposition bed or foot-egress bed) to facilitate elimination.
- Administer medication prior to activity as needed for pain relief **to permit maximal effort and involvement in activity.**
- Observe for change in strength to do more or less self-care **to adjust care as indicated.**
- Provide diversional activities (e.g., television, books, games, music, visiting), as appropriate, **to decrease boredom and potential for depression.**
- Ensure telephone and call bell are within reach **to promote safety and timely response.**
- Provide individually appropriate methods to communicate adequately with client.
- Provide extremity protection (padding, exercises, etc.). (Refer to NDs impaired Skin Integrity; risk for peripheral neurovascular Dysfunction, for additional interventions.)
- Collaborate with rehabilitation team, physical or occupational therapists to create exercise and adaptive program designed specifically for client, identifying assistive devices (e.g., splints, braces, boots) and equipment (e.g., transfer board, sling, trapeze, hydraulic lift, specialty beds).

Information that appears in brackets has been added by the authors to clarify and enhance the use of nursing diagnoses.

- Refer to NDs Activity Intolerance; impaired physical Mobility; impaired wheelchair Mobility; risk for Disuse Syndrome; impaired Transfer Ability; impaired Walking, for additional interventions.

Nursing Priority No. 4.

To promote wellness (Teaching/Discharge Considerations):

- Involve client/SO(s) in determining activity schedule. **Promotes commitment to plan, maximizing outcomes.**
- Encourage continuation of regular exercise regimen **to maintain and enhance gains in strength and muscle control.**
- Obtain, or identify sources for, assistive devices. Demonstrate safe use and proper maintenance.

Documentation Focus

Assessment/Reassessment

- Individual findings, including level of function, ability to participate in specific or desired activities

Planning

- Plan of care and who is involved in the planning

Implementation/Evaluation

- Responses to interventions, teaching, and actions performed
- Attainment or progress toward desired outcome(s)
- Modification to plan of care

Discharge Planning

- Discharge and long-term needs, noting who is responsible for each action to be taken
- Specific referrals made
- Sources for, and maintenance of, assistive devices

Sample Nursing Outcomes & Interventions Classifications (NOC/NIC)

NOC—Body Position: Self-Initiated
NIC—Bed Rest Care

impaired physical MOBILITY

[Diagnostic Division: Safety]

Definition: Limitation in independent, purposeful physical movement of the body or of one or more extremities.

Information that appears in brackets has been added by the authors to clarify and enhance the use of nursing diagnoses.

Related Factors

Activity intolerance; decrease in endurance; physical deconditioning; sedentary lifestyle
Alteration in bone structure integrity; neuromuscular, musculoskeletal, or sensorioperceptual impairment; disuse
Alteration in cognitive functioning; developmental delay
Alteration in metabolism; body mass index above 75th age-appropriate percentile; malnutrition
Anxiety; depression
Cultural belief regarding appropriate activity
Decrease in muscle mass, control or strength; joint stiffness; contractures;
Insufficient environmental support (e.g., phsyical, social)
Insufficient knowledge of value of physical activity
Pain
Pharmaceutical agent
Prescribed movement restrictions; reluctance to initiate movement

Defining Characteristics

Subjective

Discomfort; [reluctance/unwillingness to move]

Objective

Alteration in gait; postural instability
Decrease in fine or gross motor skills; movement-induced tremor
Decrease in range of motion; difficulty turning
Decrease in reaction time; slowed or spastic movement; uncoordinated movement
Engages in substitutions for movement (e.g., attention to other's activities, controlling behavior, focus on pre-illness activity)
Exertional dyspnea

Specify level of independence using a standardized functional scale [such as]

[0—Full self-care
I—Requires use of equipment or device
II—Requires assistance or supervision of another person
III—Requires assistance or supervision of another person and equipment or device
IV—Is dependent and does not participate]

Information that appears in brackets has been added by the authors to clarify and enhance the use of nursing diagnoses.

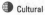

Desired Outcomes/Evaluation Criteria—Client Will:

- Verbalize understanding of situation and individual treatment regimen and safety measures.
- Demonstrate techniques or behaviors that enable resumption of activities.
- Participate in activities of daily living (ADLs) and desired activities.
- Maintain position of function and skin integrity as evidenced by absence of contractures, footdrop, decubitus, and so forth.
- Maintain or increase strength and function of affected and/or compensatory body part.

Actions/Interventions

Nursing Priority No. 1.

To identify causative/contributing factors:

- Determine diagnosis that contributes to immobility (e.g., multiple sclerosis, arthritis, Parkinson's disease, cardiopulmonary disorders, hemi- or paraplegia, depression). **These conditions can cause physiological and psychological problems that can seriously impact physical, social, and economic well-being.**
- Note factors affecting current situation (e.g., surgery, fractures, amputation, tubings [chest tube, Foley catheter, IV tubes, pumps] and potential time involved (e.g., few hours in bed after surgery versus serious trauma requiring long-term bedrest or debilitating disease limiting movement). **Identifies potential impairments and determines types of interventions needed to provide for client's safety.**
- Assess client's developmental level, motor skills, ease and capability of movement, posture, and gait **to determine presence of characteristics of client's unique impairment and to guide choice of interventions.**
- ∞ Note older client's general health status. **While aging, per se, does not cause impaired mobility, several predisposing factors in addition to age-related changes can lead to immobility (e.g., diminished body reserves of musculoskeletal system, chronic diseases, sedentary lifestyle, decreased ability to quickly and adequately correct movements affecting center of gravity).**

Information that appears in brackets has been added by the authors to clarify and enhance the use of nursing diagnoses.

- Assess degree of pain, listening to client's description about manner in which pain limits mobility **to determine if pain management can improve mobility.**
- Ascertain client's perception of activity and exercise needs and impact of current situation. Identify cultural beliefs and expectations affecting recovery or response to long-term limitations. **Helps to determine client's expectations and beliefs related to activity and potential long-term effect of current immobility. Also identifies barriers that may be addressed (e.g., lack of safe place to exercise, focus on pre-illness or disability activity, controlling behavior, depression, cultural expectations, distorted body image).**
- Note decreased motor agility or essential tremor related to age.
- Determine history of falls and relatedness to current situation. **Client may be restricting activity because of weakness or debilitation, actual injury during a fall, or from psychological distress (i.e., fear and anxiety) that can persist after a fall.** (Refer to ND risk for Falls for additional interventions.)
- Assess nutritional status and client's report of energy level. **Deficiencies in nutrients and water, electrolytes, and minerals can negatively affect energy and activity tolerance.**

Nursing Priority No. 2.

To assess functional ability:

- Determine degree of immobility in relation to 0–4 scale, noting muscle strength and tone, joint mobility, cardiovascular status, balance, and endurance. **Identifies strengths and deficits (e.g., ability to ambulate with or without assistive devices, or inability to transfer safely from bed to wheelchair) and may provide information regarding potential for recovery.**
- Determine degree of perceptual or cognitive impairment and ability to follow directions. **Impairments related to age, chronic or acute disease condition, trauma, surgery, or medications require alternative interventions or changes in plan of care.**
- Observe movement when client is unaware of observation **to note any incongruencies with reports of abilities.**
- Note emotional/behavioral responses to problems of immobility. **Feelings of frustration or powerlessness may impede attainment of goals.**
- Determine presence of complications related to immobility. **Effects of immobility are rarely confined to one body sys-**

Information that appears in brackets has been added by the authors to clarify and enhance the use of nursing diagnoses.

tem and can include muscle wasting, contractures, pressure sores, constipation, aspiration pneumonia, thrombotic phenomena, and weakened immune system functioning.(Refer to ND risk for Disuse Syndrome.)

Nursing Priority No. 3.

To promote optimal level of function and prevent complications:

- Assist with treatment of underlying condition causing pain and/or dysfunction **to maximize the potential for mobility and function.**
- Assist or have client reposition self on a regular schedule as dictated by individual situation (including frequent shifting of weight when client is wheelchair bound).
- Instruct in use of siderails, overhead trapeze, roller pads, walker, cane **for position changes, transfers, and ambulation.**
- Support affected body parts or joints using pillows, rolls, foot supports or shoes, gel pads, foam, etc., **to maintain position of function and reduce risk of pressure ulcers.**
- Provide regular skin care to include pressure area management.
- Provide or recommend pressure-reducing mattress, such as egg crate, or pressure-relieving mattress, such as alternating air pressure or water. **Reduces tissue pressure and aids in maximizing cellular perfusion to prevent dermal injury.**
- Encourage adequate intake of fluids and nutritious foods. **Promotes well-being and maximizes energy production.**
- Administer medications prior to activity as needed for pain relief **to permit maximal effort and involvement in activity.**
- Schedule activities with adequate rest periods during the day **to reduce fatigue.**
- Provide client with ample time to perform mobility-related tasks.
- Identify energy-conserving techniques for ADLs, **which limit fatigue, maximizing participation.**
- Encourage participation in self-care; occupational, diversional, or recreational activities. **Enhances self-concept and sense of independence.**
- Discuss discrepancies in movement when client is aware and unaware of observation and methods for dealing with identified problems. **May be necessary when the client is using avoidance or controlling behavior or is not aware of his or her own abilities due to anxiety or fear.**

Information that appears in brackets has been added by the authors to clarify and enhance the use of nursing diagnoses.

- Provide for safety measures as indicated by individual situation, including environmental management and fall prevention.
- Collaborate with physical medicine specialist and occupational or physical therapists in providing range-of-motion exercise (active or passive), isotonic muscle contractions (e.g., flexion of ankles, push-and-pull exercises), assistive devices, and activities (e.g., early ambulation, transfers, stairs) **to develop individual exercise and mobility program, to identify appropriate mobility devices, and to limit or reduce effects and complications of immobility.**
- Refer to NDs Activity Intolerance, risk for Falls, impaired bed Mobility, impaired wheelchair Mobility, impaired Transfer Ability, impaired Sitting, impaired Standing, impaired Walking, or risk for Pressure Ulcer for additional interventions.

Nursing Priority No. 4.

To promote wellness (Teaching/Discharge Considerations):

- Encourage client's/significant other's (SO) involvement in decision making as much as possible. **Enhances commitment to plan, optimizing outcomes.**
- Review safety measures as individually indicated (e.g., use of heating pads, locking wheelchair before transfers, removal or securing of scatter/area rugs).
- Involve client and SO(s) in care, assisting them to learn ways of managing problems of immobility.
- Demonstrate use of standing aids and mobility devices (e.g., walkers, strollers, scooters, braces, prosthetics) and have client/care provider demonstrate knowledge about, and safe use of device. Identify appropriate resources for obtaining and maintaining appliances and equipment. **Promotes independence and enhances safety.**
- Review individual dietary needs. Identify appropriate vitamin or herbal supplements.

Documentation Focus

Assessment/Reassessment

- Individual findings, including level of function, ability to participate in specific or desired activities

Planning

- Plan of care and who is involved in the planning
- Teaching plan

Information that appears in brackets has been added by the authors to clarify and enhance the use of nursing diagnoses.

Implementation/Evaluation

- Responses to interventions, teaching, and actions performed
- Attainment or progress toward desired outcome(s)
- Modifications to plan of care

Discharge Planning

- Discharge and long-term needs, noting who is responsible for each action to be taken
- Specific referrals made
- Sources for, and maintenance of, assistive devices

Sample Nursing Outcomes & Interventions Classifications (NOC/NIC)

NOC—Mobility Level
NIC—Exercise Therapy: [specify]

impaired wheelchair MOBILITY

[Diagnostic Division: Safety]

Definition: Limitation of independent operation of wheelchair within environment.

Related Factors

Neuromuscular or musculoskeletal impairments
Insufficient muscle strength; decrease in endurance; physical deconditioning; obesity
Impaired vision
Pain
Alteration in mood; alteration in cognitive functioning
Insufficient knowledge of wheelchair use
Environmental barrier (e.g., stairs, inclines, uneven surfaces, obstacles, distance)

Defining Characteristics

Impaired ability to operate manual or power wheelchair on even/uneven surface, an incline/decline, or on curbs

NOTE: Specify level of independence using a standardized functional scale. (Refer to ND impaired physical Mobility.)

Information that appears in brackets has been added by the authors to clarify and enhance the use of nursing diagnoses.

Desired Outcomes/Evaluation Criteria—Client Will:

- Move safely within environment, maximizing independence.
- Identify and use resources appropriately.

Caregiver Will:

- Provide safe mobility within environment and community.

Actions/Interventions

Nursing Priority No. 1.

To identify causative/contributing factors:

- Determine diagnosis that contributes to immobility (e.g., amyotrophic lateral sclerosis, spinal cord injury, spastic cerebral palsy, brain injury) and client's functional level and individual abilities.
- Identify factors in environments frequented by the client that contribute to inaccessibility (e.g., uneven floors or surfaces, lack of ramps, steep incline or decline, narrow doorways or spaces).
- Ascertain access to and appropriateness of public and/or private transportation.

Nursing Priority No. 2.

To promote optimal level of function and prevent complications:

- Determine that client's underlying physical, cognitive, and emotional impairment(s) (e.g., brain or spinal cord injury, fractures/other trauma, pain, depression, vision deficits) are treated or being managed **to maximize ability, desire, and motivation to participate in wheelchair activities.**
- Ascertain that wheelchair provides the base mobility to maximize function. **Proper seating and support for people in wheelchairs are critical to their ability to travel, work, learn at school, play, and interact socially. If a family member will be assisting the person using the wheelchair, his or her needs may also need to be considered in the wheelchair selection.**
- Provide for, and instruct client in, safety while in a wheelchair (e.g., adaptive cushions, supports for all body parts, repositioning and transfer assistive devices, and height adjustment).

Information that appears in brackets has been added by the authors to clarify and enhance the use of nursing diagnoses.

- Note evenness of surfaces client would need to negotiate and refer to appropriate sources for modifications. Clear pathways of obstructions.
- Recommend or refer for modifications to home, work, or school and recreational settings frequented by client **to provide safe and suitable environments.**
- Determine need for and capabilities of assistive persons. Provide training and support as indicated.
- Monitor client's use of joystick, sip and puff, sensitive mechanical switches, and so forth, **to provide necessary equipment if condition or capabilities change.**
- Collaborate with physical medicine, physical or occupational therapists in planning activities to improve client's ability to independently operate wheelchair within limits of tolerance and adjustment to various environments. **May require individual instruction and encouragement, strengthening exercises, assistance with various tasks, and close supervision.**
- Monitor client for adverse effects of immobility (e.g., contractures, muscle atrophy, deep venous thrombosis, pressure ulcers). (Refer to NDs Disuse Syndrome; risk for peripheral neurovascular Dysfunction, for additional interventions.)

Nursing Priority No. 3.

To promote wellness (Teaching/Discharge Considerations):

- Identify or refer to medical equipment suppliers **to customize client's wheelchair and accessories (e.g., side guards, head rests, heel loops, brake extensions, tool packs) and electronics suited to client's ability (e.g., sip and puff, head movement, sensitive switches).**
- Encourage client's/significant other's (SO) involvement in decision making as much as possible. **Enhances commitment to plan, optimizing outcomes.**
- Involve client/SO(s) in care, assisting them in managing immobility problems. **Promotes independence.**
- Demonstrate, discuss, and provide information regarding wheelchair safety as individually appropriate, including safe transfers, dealing with uneven surfaces, ramps, and curbs; programming speed on power chairs, etc. Include information and refer for wheelchair preventative maintenance measures (e.g., for wheelchair locks, tires, axles, casters, metal parts, batteries), as indicated. **Wheelchair safety involves people and equipment. This includes not only acquiring the best**

Information that appears in brackets has been added by the authors to clarify and enhance the use of nursing diagnoses.

chair, but also provision for obtaining relief when chair malfunctions.

- Refer to support groups relative to specific medical condition or disability; independence or political action groups. **Provide role modeling, assistance with problem-solving, and social change.**
- Identify community resources **to provide ongoing support.**

Documentation Focus

Assessment/Reassessment

- Individual findings, including level of function, ability to participate in specific or desired activities
- Type of wheelchair and equipment needs

Planning

- Plan of care and who is involved in the planning
- Teaching plan

Implementation/Evaluation

- Responses to interventions, teaching, and actions performed
- Attainment or progress toward desired outcome(s)
- Modifications to plan of care

Discharge Planning

- Discharge and long-term needs, noting who is responsible for each action to be taken
- Specific referrals made
- Sources for, and maintenance of, assistive devices

Sample Nursing Outcomes & Interventions Classifications (NOC/NIC)

NOC—Ambulation: Wheelchair
NIC—Positioning: Wheelchair

impaired MOOD REGULATION

[Diagnostic Division: Ego Integrity]

Definition: A mental state characterized by shifts in mood or affect and which is composed of a constellation of affective, cognitive, somatic, and/or physiological manifestations varying from mild to severe.

Information that appears in brackets has been added by the authors to clarify and enhance the use of nursing diagnoses.

Related Factors

Appetite or weight change; alteration in sleep pattern
Chronic illness; pain; functional impairment
Loneliness; impaired social functioning; social isolation
Recurrent thoughts of death or suicide
Anxiety; hypervigilance; psychosis
Substance misuse

Defining Characteristics

Subjective

Excessive self-awareness, guilt, self-blame
Hopelessness

Objective

Sad affect, withdrawal
Irritability; impaired concentration
Psychomotor agitation, retardation
Changes in verbal behavior; flight of thoughts; dysphoria; disinhibition
Influenced self-esteem

Desired Outcomes/Evaluation Criteria—Client Will:

- Acknowledge reality of mood problems/needs.
- Identify areas of concern.
- Participate in treatment program or therapy regimen.
- Maintain physical health as evidenced by adequate nutrition, weight within normal limits, good sleep habits.

Actions/Interventions

Nursing Priority No. 1.

To assess causative/contributing factors:

- Determine specific reasons for client's mood swings/difficulties. (Refer to related factors and defining characteristics.) **Allows for accurate planning of care for individual.**
- Assess ability to understand current situation. **Mood disturbances are prevalent in many disorders and may affect individual's cognitive functioning and understanding of events.**

Information that appears in brackets has been added by the authors to clarify and enhance the use of nursing diagnoses.

- Review history, evaluate for underlying neurological disorders. Presence of traumatic brain injuries, tumors, stroke, and autism may result in variations of mood and emotional processing deficits.
- Ascertain degree of depression individual is experiencing. **Impaired mood regulation is known to be a factor in vulnerability to depression.**
- Identify behaviors that interfere with person's daily activities. **Awareness of behaviors such as sleep, appetite, concentration, and effect on functioning facilitates identification of treatment options for change.**
- Determine availability and use of resources.

Nursing Priority No. 2.

- Discuss how client perceives the current situation and how it is affecting emotions. **A negative outlook is associated with difficulty in cognitive control and emotional regulation strategies.**
- Determine extent of rumination, reappraisal, and expressive suppression. As the individual goes over and over the negative thoughts, it is more difficult to effect cognitive control and depression can worsen.
- Encourage client to pay attention to emotional states, feelings, identify when they occur, and record in a journal or notebook. **Awareness of one's emotions helps the individual to deal appropriately with them.**
- Clarify meanings of feelings by checking meaning with client and provide feedback. **Validates and ensures accuracy of meaning of the communication.**
- Discuss how negative thinking and rumination intensify depression. **Individual differences can affect the strategies the person uses to recover from a negative mood.**
- Provide information regarding use of electroconvulsive therapy (ECT) as indicated. **It is believed ECT alters brain chemistry and function that relieves severe depression in patients who do not respond to a combination of medication and psychotherapy.**

Nursing Priority No. 3.

To promote wellness (Teaching/Discharge Considerations):

- Involve in cognitive/behavioral, mindful-based or individual psychotherapy. **Having the client identify thinking patterns that result in depression allows the individual to recognize and avoid them, improving the ability to recover.**

Information that appears in brackets has been added by the authors to clarify and enhance the use of nursing diagnoses.

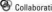

- Discuss the use of and administer medications as indicated. **Antidepressants can be useful in mood disorders and along with psychotherapy can help the client maintain usual activities.**
- Involve in group therapy. **Group discussions promote awareness of others who are experiencing similar difficulties and promotes new ideas for dealing with own concerns.**
- Encourage client to become involved in community activities. **Provides opportunity to develop social skills and interests outside of own concerns.**

Documentation Focus

Assessment/Reassessment

- Individual findings, including client's specific situation, impact on functioning/life
- Description of negative thinking patterns

Planning

- Treatment plan and individual responsibility for activities
- Teaching plan

Implementation/Evaluation

- Client involvement and response to interventions, teaching, and actions performed
- Attainment or progress toward desired outcomes
- Modification to plan of care

Discharge Planning

- Specific referrals made and follow-up plan

Sample Nursing Outcomes & Interventions Classifications (NOC/NIC)

NOC—Mood Equilibrium
NIC—Mood Management

MORAL DISTRESS

[Diagnostic Division: Ego Integrity]

Definition: Response to the inability to carry out one's chosen ethical/moral decision/action.

Information that appears in brackets has been added by the authors to clarify and enhance the use of nursing diagnoses.

Related Factors

Conflict among decision-makers (e.g., family, healthcare providers, insurance payers)
Conflicting information available for moral or ethical decision-making; cultural incongruences
Treatment decision; end-of-life decisions; loss of autonomy
Time constraint for decision-making; physical distance of decision-maker

Defining Characteristics

Subjective

Anguish about acting on one's moral choice (e.g., powerlessness, anxiety, fear)

Desired Outcomes/Evaluation Criteria—Client Will:

- Verbalize understanding of causes for conflict in own situation.
- Be aware of own moral values conflicting with desired/required course of action.
- Identify positive ways or actions necessary to deal with situation.
- Express sense of satisfaction with or acceptance of resolution.

Actions/Interventions

Nursing Priority No. 1.

To identify cause/situation in which moral distress is occurring:

- Determine client's perceptions and specific factors resulting in a sense of distress and all parties involved in situation. **Moral conflict centers around diminishing the harm suffered, with the involved individuals usually struggling with decisions about what "can be done" to prevent, improve, or cure a medical condition or what "ought to be done" in a specific situation, often within financial constraints or scarcity of resources.**
- Note use of sarcasm, avoidance, apathy, crying, or reports of depression or loss of meaning. **Individuals may not understand their feelings of uneasiness/distress or know that the emotional basis for moral distress is anger.**
- Ascertain response of family/significant other (SO)(s) to client's situation or healthcare choices.

Information that appears in brackets has been added by the authors to clarify and enhance the use of nursing diagnoses.

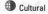

- Identify healthcare goals and expectations. **New treatment options or technology can prolong life or postpone death based on the individual's personal viewpoint, increasing the possibility of conflict with others, including healthcare providers.**
- Ascertain cultural beliefs and values, and degree of importance to client. **Cultural diversity may lead to disparate views or expectations between clients, SO/family members, and healthcare providers. When tensions between conflicting values cannot be resolved, persons experience moral distress.**
- Note attitudes and expressions of dissatisfaction of caregivers/staff. **Client may feel pressure or disapproval if own views are not congruent with expectations of those perceived to be more knowledgeable or in "authority." Furthermore, healthcare providers may themselves feel moral distress in carrying out requested actions/interventions.**
- Determine degree of emotional and physical distress (e.g., fatigue, headaches, forgetfulness, anger, guilt, resentment) individual(s) are experiencing and impact on ability to function. **Moral distress can be very destructive, affecting one's ability to carry out daily tasks or care for self or others, and may lead to a crisis of faith.**
- Assess sleep habits of involved parties. **Evidence suggests that sleep deprivation can harm a person's physical health and emotional well-being, hindering the ability to integrate emotion and cognition to guide moral judgments.**
- Use a moral distress tool, such as the Moral Distress Assessment Questionnaire (MDAQ) **to help measure degree of involvement and identify possible actions to improve situation.**
- Note availability of family/friends for support and encouragement.

Nursing Priority No. 2.

To assist client/involved individuals to develop/effectively use problem-solving skills:

- Encourage involved individuals to recognize and name the experience resulting in moral sensitivity. **Brings concerns out in the open so they can be dealt with.**
- Use skills, such as Active-listening, I-messages, and problem-solving to assist individual(s) **to clarify feelings of anxiety and conflict.**

Information that appears in brackets has been added by the authors to clarify and enhance the use of nursing diagnoses.

- Make time available for support and provide information as desired **to help individuals understand the ethical dilemma that led to moral distress.**
- Provide for privacy when discussing sensitive or personal issues.
- Ascertain coping behaviors client has used successfully in the past that may be helpful in dealing with current situation.
- Provide time for nonjudgmental discussion of philosophic issues/questions about impact of conflict leading to moral questioning of current situation.
- Identify role models (e.g., other individuals who have experienced similar problems in their lives). **Sharing of experiences, identifying options can be helpful to deal with current situation.**
- Involve facility/local ethics committee or ethicist as appropriate **to educate, make recommendations, and facilitate mediation/resolution of issues.**

Nursing Priority No. 3.

To promote wellness (Teaching/Discharge Considerations):

- Engage all parties, as appropriate, in developing plan to address conflict. **Resolving one's moral distress requires making changes or compromises while preserving one's integrity and authenticity.**
- Incorporate identified familial, religious, and cultural factors that have meaning for client.
- Refer to appropriate resources for support and guidance (e.g., pastoral care, counseling, organized support groups, classes), as indicated.
- Assist individuals to recognize that if they follow their moral decisions, they may clash with the legal system. Suggest referral to appropriate resource for legal opinion/options.

Documentation Focus

Assessment/Reassessment

- Individual findings, including nature of moral conflict, individuals involved in conflict.
- Physical and emotional responses to conflict.
- Individual cultural or religious beliefs and values, healthcare goals.
- Responses and involvement of family/SOs.

Planning

- Plan of care and who is involved in planning.
- Teaching plan.

Information that appears in brackets has been added by the authors to clarify and enhance the use of nursing diagnoses.

Implementation/Evaluation

- Responses to interventions, teaching.
- Attainment or progress toward desired outcome(s).
- Modifications to plan of care.

Discharge Planning

- Long-term needs and who is responsible for actions to be taken.
- Available resources.
- Specific referrals made.

Sample Nursing Outcomes & Interventions Classifications (NOC/NIC)

NOC—Decision-Making
NIC—Decision-Making Support

impaired oral MUCOUS MEMBRANE and risk for impaired oral MUCOUS MEMBRANE

[Diagnostic Division: Food/Fluid]

Definition: impaired oral Mucous Membrane: Injury to the lips, soft tissue, buccal cavity, and/or oropharynx.

Definition: risk for impaired oral Mucous Membrane: Vulnerable to Injury to the lips, soft tissue, buccal cavity, and/or oropharynx, which may compromise health.

Related and Risk Factors

Alcohol consumption; smoking
Allergy; stressors
Alteration in cognitive functioning
Autoimmune disease; immunodeficiency; immunosuppression; infection
Autosomal disorder; Syndrome (e.g., Sjorgren's)
Barrier to dental care or oral self-care; insufficient oral hygiene; insufficient knowledge of oral hygiene
Behavior disorder (e.g., attention deficit, oppositional defiant); depression
Chemical injury agent (e.g., burn, capsaicin, methylene chloride, mustard agent)
Chemotherapy; radiation therapy (risk)
Cleft lip or palate; loss of oral support structure
Decrease in hormone level in women

Information that appears in brackets has been added by the authors to clarify and enhance the use of nursing diagnoses.

Decrease in platelets; treatment regimen
Decrease in salivation; dehydration; malnutrition; inadequate nutrition (risk)
Economically disadvantaged (risk)
Mechanical factor (e.g., ill-fitting dentures, orthodontic appliance (risk), braces; endotracheal/nasogastric tube, oral surgery) oral trauma
Mouth breathing; nil per os (NPO) >24 hours
Surgical procedure; trauma (risk)

> **Note:** A risk diagnosis is not evidenced by signs and symptoms, as the problem has not occurred; rather, nursing interventions are directed at prevention.

Defining Characteristics (impaired oral Mucous Membranes)

Subjective

Xerostomia (dry mouth)
Oral pain, discomfort
Bad taste in mouth; decrease in taste sensation; difficulty eating or swallowing
Exposure to pathogen

Objective

Coated tongue; smooth atrophic tongue; geographic tongue
Gingival or mucosal pallor
Stomatitis; hyperemia; macroplasia; vesicles; nodules; papules
White patches or plaques; spongy patches; white, curd-like exudate
Oral lesions or ulcers; fissures; bleeding; cheilitis; desquamation; mucosal denudation
Purulent drainage or exudates; enlarged tonsils
Oral edema
Halitosis
Gingival hyperplasia or recession, pocketing deeper than 4 mm; [carious teeth]
Presence of mass (e.g., hemangiomas)
Difficulty speaking

Desired Outcomes/Evaluation Criteria—Client Will:

- Verbalize understanding of causative **or risk** factors.
- Identify specific interventions to promote healthy oral mucosa.

Information that appears in brackets has been added by the authors to clarify and enhance the use of nursing diagnoses.

• Demonstrate techniques to restore/maintain integrity of oral mucosa.

Actions/Interventions

Nursing Priority No. 1.

To identify causative/contributing factors that or which affecting **or may affect** oral health:

• Perform oral screening or comprehensive assessment upon admission to facility care using tool (e.g., Oral Health Assessment Tool [OHAT] for Long-term Care (or similar tool), as indicated. **Standardized tool is beneficial in evaluating health of entire mouth including lips, tongue, gums and other soft tissues, as well as condition of natural teeth or dentures, and status of oral hygiene.**

• Note presence of systemic or local conditions (e.g., oral infections; dehydration, malnutrition, facial fractures, head or neck cancers or treatment including chemotherapy or, radiation; AIDS, systemic lupus erythematosus [SLE], rheumatoid arthritis, Sjögren syndrome, scleroderma, sarcoidosis, amyloidosis, hypothyroidism, diabetes) **that can affect health of buccal tissues. Note: Oral mucositis is a major complication of chemotherapy and/or radiation therapy.**

• Note presence of illness, disease, or trauma (e.g., gingivitis, periodontal disease; presence of oral ulcerations; bacterial, viral, fungal, or oral infections; gum or palate malformations; facial fractures; generalized debilitating conditions) **that affect health of oral tissues.**

∞ • Note client's age and functional status upon admission to facility care. **The very young, elderly client, or any client with functional deficits (e.g., age-related dependency needs, cognitive or physical impairments, trauma, or complex treatments) may require daily assistance with oral care.**

• Determine if client is resistant to oral care. **Client with behavioral and/or communication difficulties (e.g., dementia, client won't open mouth or is agitated or lethargic, client doesn't understand instructions) may require special equipment, timing of efforts, and/or referral for professional services.**

• Investigate reports of oral pain to determine possible source (e.g., oral lesion, gum disease, tooth abscess, ill-fitting dentures) **to identify needed interventions and reduce risk of complications such as systemic infection.**

Information that appears in brackets has been added by the authors to clarify and enhance the use of nursing diagnoses.

- Obtain history of client's medications **to identify those medications that can impact health of buccal tissues or cause immunosuppression which can impact oral health.**
- Observe for abnormal lesions of mouth, tongue, and cheeks (e.g., white or red patches, ulcers). **White ulcerated spots may be canker sores, especially in children; white curd patches (thrush) are common in infants. Reddened, swollen bleeding gums may indicate infection, poor nutrition, or poor oral hygiene. A red tongue may be related to vitamin deficiencies. Malignant lesions are more common in elderly than younger persons (especially if there is a history of smoking or alcohol use), or in persons who rarely visit a dentist.**
- Observe for chipped, sharp-edged teeth, or malpositioned teeth. Note fit of dentures or other prosthetic devices when used. **Factors that increase the risk of injury to delicate tissues.**
- Note use of tobacco (including smokeless) and alcohol/other drugs (e.g., methamphetamines), **which may predispose gums and mucosa to effects of nutritional deficiencies, infection, cell damage, and cancer.**
- Determine nutrition and fluid intake and reported changes (e.g., avoiding eating, change in taste, chews painstakingly, swallows numerous times for even small bites; insufficient fluid intake/dehydration; unexplained weight loss). **Malnutrition and dehydration are associated with problems with oral mucosa.**
- Determine allergies to food, drugs, other substances **that may result in irritation or disruption of oral mucosa.**
- Review oral hygiene practices, noting frequency and type (e.g., brushing, flossing, water appliances). Inquire about client's professional dental care, regularity and date of last dental examination.
- Evaluate client's ability to provide self-care and availability of necessary equipment or assistance. **Client's age (very young or elderly) impacts client's habits and lifestyle, ability to provide self-care, as well as current health issues (e.g., disease condition or treatment, weakness).**

Nursing Priority No. 2.

To correct identified/developing problems:

- Collaborate in treatment of underlying conditions (e.g., structural defects, infections) **that may correct or limit problem with oral tissues.**

Information that appears in brackets has been added by the authors to clarify and enhance the use of nursing diagnoses.

- Inspect oral cavity and throat routinely for inflammation, sores, lesions, and/or bleeding. **Can help with early identification and management of mucous membrane concerns.**
- Encourage adequate fluids **to prevent dry mouth and dehydration.**
- Encourage use of tart, sour, and citrus foods and drinks; chewing gum; or hard candy **to stimulate saliva.**
- Lubricate lips and provide commercially prepared oral lubricant solution.
- Provide for increased humidity, if indicated, by vaporizer or room humidifier if client is mouth-breather.
- Provide dietary modifications (e.g., food of comfortable texture, temperature, density) **to reduce discomfort and improve intake,** and adequate nutrients and vitamins **to promote healing.**
- Avoid irritating foods and fluids, temperature extremes. Provide soft or pureed diet as required.
- Use lemon/glycerin swabs with caution; **may be irritating if mucosa is injured.**
- Provide or encourage regular oral care (e.g., after meals and at bedtime; and frequently to critically ill client): **Note: Oral care has been determined to be a nursing intervention that decreases colonization of oropharynx and saliva, thereby reducing the incidence of ventilator-associated pneumonia (VAP) in the critically ill client.**

  Use water, or bland rinses or sodium bicarbonate solutions; mucosal coating agents, lubricating agents, topical anesthetics **for oral hydration, or irrigation and treatment of mouth, gums, and mucous membrane surfaces.**

  Avoid mouthwashes containing alcohol **(drying effect)** or hydrogen peroxide **(drying and foul tasting).**

  Use soft-bristle brush or sponge/cotton-tip applicators to cleanse teeth and tongue. **Brushing the teeth is the most effective way to reduce plaque and manage periodontal disease.**

  Floss gently or use Waterpik® **to remove food particles that promote bacterial growth and gum disease.**

  Use foam sticks where indicated **to swab mouth, tongue, and gums when client is intubated or has no teeth.**

  Use lemon/glycerin swabs with caution, following facility policy. **Note: This issue appears to be controversial with some sources stating that glycerin should not be used as it absorbs water and actually dries the oral cavity.**

  Provide or assist with denture care, as needed. **Evidence-based protocol for denture care states that dentures are**

Information that appears in brackets has been added by the authors to clarify and enhance the use of nursing diagnoses.

to be removed and washed at least once daily, removed and rinsed after every meal, and kept in an appropriate solution at night.

- Provide anesthetic lozenges or analgesics such as Stanford solution, viscous lidocaine (Xylocaine), mouthwash containing lidocaine, sucralfate slurry, as indicated **to provide protection and reduce oral discomfort or pain. Note: Pain of mucositis associated with anticancer therapies has been found to be controlled by mouthwashes containing lidocaine to coat the oral cavity.**
- Administer medications, as indicated (e.g., antibiotics, antifungal agents, including antimicrobial mouth rinse or spray) **to treat oral infections or reduce potential for bacterial overgrowth.**
- Change position of endotracheal (ET) tube or airway every 8 hr and as needed when client is on ventilator **to minimize pressure on fragile tissues and improve access to all areas of oral cavity.**
- Suction oral cavity if client cannot swallow secretions. **Note: Saliva contains digestive enzymes that may be erosive to exposed tissues (such as might occur because of heavy drooling following radical neck surgery).**
- Use gentle low-intensity suctioning **to reduce risk of aspiration in intubated clients or those with decreased gag or swallow reflexes.**
- Emphasize avoiding alcohol, smoking, or chewing tobacco especially if periodontal disease present or if client has xerostomia or other oral discomforts, **which may further irritate and damage mucosa.**
- Refer for evaluation of dentures or other prosthetics, structural defects **when impairments are affecting oral health.**

Nursing Priority No. 3.

To promote wellness (Teaching/Discharge Considerations):

- Review current oral hygiene patterns and provide information about oral health as required or desired **to correct deficiencies and encourage proper care.**
- Recommend regular dental checkups and care, and episodic evaluation of oral health prior to certain medical treatments (e.g., chemotherapy, radiation) **to maintain oral health and reduce risks associated with impaired tissues.**
- Instruct parents in oral hygiene techniques and proper dental care for infants/children (e.g., safe use of pacifier, brushing of teeth and gums, avoidance of sweet drinks and candy, recognition and treatment of thrush). **Encourages early initia-**

Information that appears in brackets has been added by the authors to clarify and enhance the use of nursing diagnoses.

tion of good oral health practices and timely intervention for treatable problems. Refer to ND impaired Dentition for additional interventions.

- Discuss special mouth care required during and after illness or trauma or following surgical repair (e.g., cleft lip or palate) **to facilitate healing.**
- Discuss need for and demonstrate use of special "appliances" (e.g., power toothbrushes, dental water jets, flossing instruments, applicators) **to perform own oral care.**
- Discuss and instruct caregiver(s) in special mouth care required during end-of-life care/hospice **to promote optimal comfort in client who has stopped eating or drinking, and who has dry mouth and feeling of thirst.**
- Listen to concerns about appearance and provide accurate information about possible treatments and outcomes. Discuss effect of condition on self-esteem and body image, noting withdrawal from usual social activities or relationships, and/or expressions of powerlessness.
- Review information regarding drug regimen, use of local anesthetics.
- Promote good general health and mental health habits including stress management. **(Altered immune response can affect the oral mucosa.)**
- Provide/refer for nutritional information **to correct deficiencies, reduce gum irritation or disease, prevent dental caries.**
- Recommend avoiding alcohol, smoking, or chewing tobacco **which can contribute to mucosal inflammation and gum disease.**
- Identify community resources (e.g., low-cost dental clinics, smoking cessation resources, cancer information services or support group, meals-on-wheels, food stamps, home-care aide) **to meet individual needs.**

Documentation Focus

Assessment/Reassessment

- Condition of oral mucous membranes, routine oral care habits and interferences
- Availability of oral care equipment and products
- Knowledge of proper oral hygiene and care
- Availability and use of resources

Planning

- Plan of care and who is involved in planning
- Teaching plan

Information that appears in brackets has been added by the authors to clarify and enhance the use of nursing diagnoses.

Implementation/Evaluation

- Responses to interventions, teaching, and actions performed
- Attainment or progress toward desired outcome(s)
- Modifications to plan of care

Discharge Planning

- Long-term needs and who is responsible for actions to be taken
- Specific referrals made, resources for special appliances

Sample Nursing Outcomes & Interventions Classifications (NOC/NIC)

NOC—Oral Hygiene
NIC—Oral Health Restoration

NAUSEA

[Diagnostic Division: Food/Fluid]

Definition: A subjective phenomenon of an unpleasant feeling in the back of the throat and stomach, which may or may not result in vomiting.

Related Factors

Biophysical

Biochemical dysfunction (e.g., uremia, diabetic ketoacidosis); pregnancy
Localized tumors (e.g., acoustic neuroma, brain tumor, bone metastasis); intra-abdominal tumors
Exposure to toxins
Esophageal or pancreatic disease; liver or splenetic capsule stretch
Gastric distention; gastrointestinal irritation
Motion sickness; Ménière's disease; labyrinthitis
Increase in intracranial pressure; meningitis
Treatment regimen

Situational

Noxious taste
Unpleasant visual stimuli; noxious environmental stimuli
Anxiety; fear; psychological disorder

Information that appears in brackets has been added by the authors to clarify and enhance the use of nursing diagnoses.

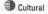

Defining Characteristics

Subjective
Nausea; sour taste

Objective
Aversion toward food
Increase in salivation
Increase in swallowing; gagging sensation

Desired Outcomes/Evaluation Criteria—Client Will:

- Be free of nausea.
- Manage chronic nausea, as evidenced by acceptable level of dietary intake.
- Maintain or regain weight as appropriate.

Actions/Interventions

Nursing Priority No. 1.
To determine causative/contributing factors:

- Assess for presence of conditions of the gastrointestinal (GI) tract (e.g., peptic ulcer disease, bleeding into the stomach; cholecystitis, appendicitis, gastritis, constipation, intestinal blockage, ingestion of "problem" foods; food poisoning; excessive alcohol intake) **that may cause or exacerbate nausea.**
- Note systemic conditions that may result in nausea (e.g., pregnancy, cancer treatment, myocardial infarction, hepatitis, systemic infections, toxins, drug toxicity, presence of neurogenic causes [stimulation of the vestibular system], central nervous system trauma/tumor). **Helps in determining appropriate interventions or need for treatment of underlying condition.**
- Identify situations that client perceives as anxiety inducing, threatening, or distasteful (e.g., "This is nauseating"). **May be able to limit or control exposure to situations or take medication prophylactically.**
- Note psychological factors, including those that are culturally determined (e.g., eating certain foods considered repulsive in one's own culture; seeing or smelling something "gross"; anorexia and bulimia).
- Determine if nausea is potentially self-limiting and/or mild (e.g., first trimester of pregnancy, 24-hr GI viral infection) or

Information that appears in brackets has been added by the authors to clarify and enhance the use of nursing diagnoses.

is severe and prolonged (e.g., advanced cancer with multiple medications accompanied by anorexia, constipation, imbalances of calcium/other blood salts; certain cancer treatments; hyperemesis gravidarum). **Suggests severity of effect on fluid and electrolyte balance and nutritional status.**

- Note client age and developmental level. **Vomiting may occur along with nausea, especially in children (usually part of a short-lived viral infection). Nausea can occur with food intolerances, inner ear problems, pain, or medication reactions in any age client. Nausea in the elderly (in the absence of acute disease condition) may be associated with GI motility dysfunction, or medications, pain, or end-of-life issues. Nausea in a female of childbearing age may indicate pregnancy or hormonal influences associated with menstruation, anorexia, or migraine headaches.**
- Review medication regimen, especially in elderly client on multiple drugs. **Polypharmacy with drug interactions and side effects may cause or exacerbate nausea.**
- Review results of diagnostic studies.

Nursing Priority No. 2.

To promote comfort and enhance intake:

- Administer and monitor response to medications used to treat underlying cause of nausea (e.g., vestibular, bowel obstruction, dysmotility of upper gut, infection, inflammation, toxins) **to determine effectiveness of treatment and to monitor for adverse effects of added medication (e.g., oversedation with risk of aspiration).**
- Select route of medication administration best suited to client's needs (i.e., oral, sublingual, injectable, rectal, transdermal).
- Review pain control regimen. **Converting to long-acting opioids or combination drugs may decrease stimulation of the chemotactic trigger zone, reducing the occurrence of opioid-related nausea.**
- Recommend client try dry foods such as toast, crackers, dry cereal before arising when nausea occurs in the morning or throughout the day, as appropriate.
- Encourage client to begin with ice chips or sips/small amounts of fluids—4 to 8 ounces for adult; 1 ounce or less for child.
- Advise client to drink liquids 30 min before or after meals, instead of with meals.
- Provide diet and snacks of preferred or bland foods (including skinless chicken, rise, toast, pasta, potatoes) and fluids (in-

Information that appears in brackets has been added by the authors to clarify and enhance the use of nursing diagnoses.

cluding caffeine-free nondiet carbonated beverages, clear soup broth, nonacidic fruit juice, gelatin, sherbet, or ices) **to reduce gastric acidity and improve nutrient intake.**

- Avoid milk/dairy products, overly sweet or fried and fatty foods, gas-forming vegetables (e.g., broccoli, cauliflower, cucumbers) **that may increase nausea or be more difficult to digest.**
- Encourage client to eat small meals spaced throughout the day instead of large meals **so stomach does not feel excessively full.**
- Instruct client to eat slowly, chewing food well **to enhance digestion.**
- Recommend client remain seated after meal or with head well elevated above feet if in bed.
- Provide clean, peaceful environment and fresh air with fan or open window. Avoid offending odors, such as cooking smells, smoke, perfumes, mechanical emissions when possible, **as they may stimulate or worsen nausea.**
- Provide frequent oral care (especially after vomiting) **to cleanse mouth and minimize "bad tastes."**
- Encourage deep, slow breathing **to promote relaxation and refocus attention away from nausea.**
- Use distraction with music, chatting with family/friends, watching TV **to refocus attention away from unpleasant sensations.**
- Administer antiemetic on regular schedule before, during, and after administration of antineoplastic agents **to prevent or control side effects of medication.**
- Time chemotherapy doses **for least interference with food intake.**
- Avoid sudden changes in position or excessive motion; move to aisle seat on plane, or front seat or car. Focus on distance, face forward when riding. **The actions may help prevent or limit severity of nausea associated with motion sickness.**
- Investigate use of acupressure point therapy (e.g., elastic band worn around wrist with small, hard bump that presses against acupressure point). **Some individuals with chronic nausea or history of motion sickness report this to be helpful; without sedative effect of medication.**

Nursing Priority No. 3.

To promote wellness (Teaching/Discharge Considerations):

- Review individual factors or triggers causing nausea and ways to avoid problem. **Provides necessary information for client**

Information that appears in brackets has been added by the authors to clarify and enhance the use of nursing diagnoses.

to manage own care. Some individuals develop anticipatory nausea (a conditioned reflex) that recurs each time he or she encounters the situation that triggers the reflex.

- Instruct in proper use, side effects, and adverse reactions of antiemetic medications. **Enhances client safety and effective management of condition.**
- Discuss appropriate use of over-the-counter medications and herbal products (e.g., Dramamine, antacids, antiflatulents, ginger), or the use of THC (Marinol).
- Encourage use of nonpharmacological interventions. **Activities such as self-hypnosis, progressive muscle relaxation, biofeedback, guided imagery, and systemic desensitization promote relaxation, refocus client's attention, increase sense of control, and decrease feelings of helplessness.**
- Advise client to prepare and freeze meals in advance, have someone else cook, or use microwave or oven instead of stove-top cooking **for days when nausea is severe or cooking is impossible.**
- Suggest wearing loose-fitting clothing **to reduce external pressure on abdomen.**
- Recommend recording weight weekly, if appropriate, **to help monitor fluid and nutritional status.**
- Discuss potential complications and possible need for medical follow-up or alternative therapies. **Timely recognition and intervention may limit severity of complications (e.g., dehydration).**
- Review signs of dehydration and emphasize importance of replacing fluids and/or electrolytes (with products such as Gatorade or other electrolyte drinks for adults or Pedialyte for children). **Increases likelihood of preventing potentially serious electrolyte depletion.**
- Review signs (e.g., emesis appears bloody, black, or like coffee grounds; feeling faint) requiring immediate notification of healthcare provider **to prevent serious complications.**

Documentation Focus

Assessment/Reassessment

- Individual findings, including individual factors causing nausea
- Baseline and periodic weight, vital signs
- Specific client preferences for nutritional intake
- Response to medication

Information that appears in brackets has been added by the authors to clarify and enhance the use of nursing diagnoses.

Planning
- Plan of care and who is involved in planning
- Teaching plan

Implementation/Evaluation
- Response to interventions, teaching, and actions performed
- Attainment or progress toward desired outcome(s)
- Modifications to plan of care

Discharge Planning
- Individual long-term needs, noting who is responsible for actions to be taken
- Specific referrals made

Sample Nursing Outcomes & Interventions Classifications (NOC/NIC)

NOC—Nausea & Vomiting Control
NIC—Nausea Management

NONCOMPLIANCE

[Diagnostic Division: Teaching/Learning]

Definition: Behavior of person and/or caregiver that fails to coincide with a health-promoting or therapeutic plan agreed on by the person (and/or family and/or community) and healthcare professional. In the presence of an agreed-upon health-promoting, or therapeutic plan, the person's or caregiver's behavior is fully or partially nonadherent and may lead to clinically ineffective or partially effective outcomes.

NOTE: When the plan of care is reviewed with client/significant other (SO), use of the term *noncompliance* may create a negative response and sense of conflict between healthcare providers and client. Labeling the client noncompliant may also lead to problems with third-party reimbursement. Where possible, use of the ND ineffective Health Management is recommended.

Information that appears in brackets has been added by the authors to clarify and enhance the use of nursing diagnoses.

Related Factors

Healthcare Plan

Lengthy duration or intensity of regimen; complex treatment regimen

Financial barriers; high-cost regimen

Individual

Insufficient knowledge about the regimen; insufficient skills to perform regimen; expectations incongruent with developmental phase

Health beliefs, values, or spiritual values incongruent with plan; cultural incongruence

Insufficient motivation; insufficient social support

Denial; issues of secondary gain

Health System

Insufficient health insurance coverage; insufficient provider reimbursement

Perceived low credibility of provider; difficulty in client-provider relationship; provider discontinuity; insufficient follow-up with provider; ineffective communication or insufficient teaching skills of the provider

Inadequate access or inconvenience of care; low satisfaction with care

Network

Insufficient involvement of members in plan; low social value attributed to plan

Perception that beliefs of significant other differ from plan

Defining Characteristics

Subjective

[Does not believe in efficacy of therapy, unwilling to follow treatment regimen]

Objective

Nonadherence behavior

Failure to progress; exacerbation of symptoms; development-related complication

Failure to meet outcomes; missing of appointments

Information that appears in brackets has been added by the authors to clarify and enhance the use of nursing diagnoses.

Desired Outcomes/Evaluation Criteria—Client Will:

- Verbalize accurate knowledge of condition and understanding of treatment regimen.
- Make choices at level of readiness based on accurate information.
- Verbalize commitment to mutually agreed upon goals and treatment plan.
- Access resources appropriately.
- Demonstrate progress toward health goals.

Actions/Interventions

Nursing Priority No. 1.

To determine reason for alteration/disregard of therapeutic regimen/instructions:

- Determine client's/SO's perception and understanding of the situation (illness, treatment).
- Listen to/active-listen client's complaints/comments. **Helps to identify client's thinking about the treatment regimen (e.g., may be concerned about side effects of medications or success of procedures/transplantation).**
- Note language spoken, read, and understood.
- Be aware of developmental level as well as chronological age of client.
- Assess level of anxiety, locus of control, sense of powerlessness, etc.
- Determine who (e.g., client, SO, other) manages the medication regimen and whether individual knows what the medications are and why they are prescribed.
- Ascertain how client remembers to take medications and how many doses have been missed in the last 72 hr, last week, last 2 weeks, and last month.
- Identify factors that interfere with taking medications or lead to lack of adherence (e.g., depression, active alcohol or other drug use, low literacy, lack of support, lack of belief in treatment efficacy). **Forgetfulness is the most common reason given for not complying with the treatment plan.**
- Note length of illness. **Individuals tend to become passive and dependent in long-term, debilitating illnesses.**
- Clarify value system: cultural and religious values, health and illness beliefs of the client/SO(s).
- Determine social characteristics, demographic and educational factors, as well as personality of the client.

Information that appears in brackets has been added by the authors to clarify and enhance the use of nursing diagnoses.

- Verify psychological meaning of the behavior (e.g., may be denial). Note issues of secondary gain—**family dynamics, school or workplace issues, involvement in legal system may unconsciously affect client's decision making.**
- Assess availability and use of support systems and resources.
- Be aware of nurses'/healthcare providers' attitudes and behaviors toward the client. (Do they have an investment in the client's compliance or recovery? What is the behavior of the client and nurse when client is labeled "noncompliant"?) **Some care providers may be enabling client, whereas others' judgmental attitudes may impede treatment progress.**

Nursing Priority No. 2.

To assist client/SO(s) to develop strategies for dealing effectively with the situation:

- Develop therapeutic nurse-client relationship. **Promotes trust, provides atmosphere in which client/SO(s) can freely express views and concerns. Adherence assessment is most successful when conducted in a positive, nonjudgmental atmosphere.**
- Explore client involvement in or lack of mutual goal setting. **Client will be more likely to follow-through on goals he or she participated in developing.**
- Review treatment strategies. Identify which interventions in the plan of care are most important in meeting therapeutic goals and which are least amenable to compliance. **Sets priorities and encourages problem-solving areas of conflict.**
- Contract with the client for participation in care. **Enhances commitment to follow-through.**
- Encourage client to maintain self-care, providing for assistance when necessary. Accept client's evaluation of own strengths and limitations while working with client to improve abilities.
- Provide for continuity of care in and out of the hospital or care setting, including long-range plans. **Supports trust, facilitates progress toward goals.**
- Provide information and help client to know where and how to find it on own. **Promotes independence and encourages informed decision making.**
- Give information in manageable amounts, using verbal, written, and audiovisual modes at level of client's ability. **Using client's style of learning facilitates learning, enabling client to understand diagnosis and treatment regimen.**

Information that appears in brackets has been added by the authors to clarify and enhance the use of nursing diagnoses.

- Ask client to paraphrase instructions and information heard. **Helps validate client's understanding and reveals misconceptions.**
- Accept the client's choice or point of view, even if it appears to be self-destructive. Avoid confrontation regarding beliefs **to maintain open communication.**
- Establish graduated goals or modified regimen, as necessary (e.g., client with chronic obstructive pulmonary disease who smokes a pack of cigarettes a day may be willing to reduce that amount). **May improve quality of life, encouraging progression to more advanced goals.**

Nursing Priority No. 3.

To promote wellness (Teaching/Discharge Considerations):

- Stress importance of the client's knowledge and understanding of the need for treatment or medication, as well as consequences of actions and choices.
- Develop a system for self-monitoring **to provide a sense of control and enable client to follow own progress and assist with making choices.**
- Suggest using a medication reminder system. **These have been shown to improve client adherence by a significant percentage.**
- Provide support systems **to reinforce negotiated behaviors.** Encourage client to continue positive behaviors, especially if client is beginning to see benefit.
- Refer to counseling, therapy and/or other appropriate resources.
- Refer to NDs ineffective Coping; compromised family Coping; deficient Knowledge [Learning Need (specify)]; Anxiety; ineffective Health Management.

Documentation Focus

Assessment/Reassessment

- Individual findings including deviation from prescribed treatment plan and client's reasons in own words
- Consequences of actions to date

Planning

- Plan of care and who is involved in planning
- Teaching plan

Information that appears in brackets has been added by the authors to clarify and enhance the use of nursing diagnoses.

Implementation/Evaluation

- Response to interventions, teaching, and actions performed
- Attainment or progress toward desired outcome(s)
- Modifications to plan of care

Discharge Planning

- Long-term needs and who is responsible for actions to be taken
- Specific referrals made

Sample Nursing Outcomes & Interventions Classifications (NOC/NIC)

NOC—Compliance Behavior
NIC—Mutual Goal Setting

imbalanced NUTRITION: less than body requirements

[Diagnostic Division: Food/Fluid]

Definition: Intake of nutrients insufficient to meet metabolic needs.

Related Factors

Inability to ingest or digest food; inability to absorb nutrients
Biological factors; psychological disorder
Economically disadvantaged
[Increased metabolic demands (e.g., burns)]

Defining Characteristics

Subjective

Insufficient interest in food; food aversion; alteration in taste sensation; perceived inability to ingest food
Satiety immediately upon ingesting food
Abdominal pain or cramping; sore buccal cavity
Insufficient information; misinformation; misconception

Objective

Body weight 20% or more below ideal weight range; [decreased subcutaneous fat or muscle mass]
Weight loss with adequate food intake
Food intake less than recommended daily allowances

Information that appears in brackets has been added by the authors to clarify and enhance the use of nursing diagnoses.

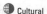

Hyperactive bowel sounds; diarrhea; steatorrhea
Weakness of muscles required for mastication or swallowing; insufficient muscle tone
Pale mucous membranes; capillary fragility
Excessive hair loss [or increased growth of hair on body (lanugo)]; [cessation of menses]
[Abnormal laboratory studies (e.g., decreased albumin, total proteins; iron deficiency; electrolyte imbalances)]

Desired Outcomes/Evaluation Criteria—Client Will:

- Demonstrate progressive weight gain toward goal.
- Display normalization of laboratory values and be free of signs of malnutrition as reflected in Defining Characteristics.
- Verbalize understanding of causative factors when known and necessary interventions.
- Demonstrate behaviors, lifestyle changes to regain and/or maintain appropriate weight.

Actions/Interventions

Nursing Priority No. 1.

To assess causative/contributing factors:

- ∞ Identify client at risk for malnutrition (e.g., institutionalized elderly; client with chronic illness; child or adult living in poverty/low-income area; client with jaw or facial injuries; intestinal surgery, postmalabsorptive or restrictive surgical interventions for weight loss; hypermetabolic states [e.g., burns, hyperthyroidism]; malabsorption syndromes, lactose intolerance; cystic fibrosis; pancreatic disease; prolonged time of restricted intake; prior nutritional deficiencies).
- ∞ Assess pediatric concerns (e.g., changes in nutritional needs related to growth phase; congenital anomalies, including tracheoesophageal fistula, cleft lip/palate; metabolic or malabsorption problems, such as diabetes, phenylketonuria, cerebral palsy; chronic infections).
- Determine client's ability to chew, swallow, and taste food. Evaluate teeth and gums for poor oral health, and note denture fit, as indicated. **All factors that affect ingestion and/or digestion of nutrients.**
- Ascertain understanding of individual nutritional needs **to determine informational needs of client/SO.**
- Determine lifestyle factors that may affect weight. **Socioeconomic resources, amount of money available for**

Information that appears in brackets has been added by the authors to clarify and enhance the use of nursing diagnoses.

purchasing food, proximity of grocery store, and available storage space for food are all factors that may impact food choices and intake.

- Explore specific eating habits, the meaning of food to client (e.g., never eats breakfast, snacks throughout entire day, fasts for weight control, no time to eat properly), and individual food preferences and intolerances/aversions. **Identifies eating practices that may need to be corrected and provides insight into dietary interventions that may appeal to client.**
- Assess drug interactions, disease effects, allergies, use of laxatives, diuretics **that may be affecting appetite, food intake, or absorption.**
- Evaluate impact of cultural, ethnic, or religious desires and influences **that may affect food choices or to identify factors (e.g., dementia, severe depression) that may be interfering with client's appetite and food intake.**
- Determine psychological factors, perform psychological assessment, as indicated, **to assess body image and congruency with reality.**
- Note occurrence of amenorrhea, tooth decay, swollen salivary glands, and report of constant sore throat, **suggesting bulimia and affecting ability to eat.**
- Review usual activities and exercise program noting repetitive activities (e.g., constant pacing) or inappropriate exercise (e.g., prolonged jogging). **May reveal obsessive nature of weight-control measures.**

Nursing Priority No. 2.

To evaluate degree of deficit:

- Assess weight; measure muscle mass, or calculate body fat by means of anthropometric measurements and growth scales **to identify deviations from the norm and to establish baseline parameters.**
- Observe for absence of subcutaneous fat and muscle wasting, loss of hair, fissuring of nails, delayed healing, gum bleeding, swollen abdomen, and so on, **which indicate protein-energy malnutrition.**
- Auscultate bowel sounds. Note characteristics of stool (color, amount, frequency, etc.).
- Assist in nutritional status assessment, using screening tools (e.g., Mini Nutritional Assessment [MNA], the Malnutrition Universal Screening Tool [MUST], or similar tool).
- Review indicated laboratory data (e.g., serum albumin/prealbumin, transferrin, amino acid profile, iron, BUN, nitro-

Information that appears in brackets has been added by the authors to clarify and enhance the use of nursing diagnoses.

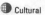

gen balance studies, glucose, liver function, electrolytes, total lymphocyte count, indirect calorimetry).

Nursing Priority No. 3.

To establish a nutritional plan that meets individual needs:

- Note age, body build, strength, activity level, and current condition or treatment needs. **Helps determine nutritional needs.**
- Evaluate total daily food intake. Obtain diary of calorie intake, patterns, and times of eating, **to reveal possible cause of malnutrition and changes that could be made in client's intake.**
- Calculate basal energy expenditure (BEE) using Harris-Benedict (or similar) formula and estimate energy and protein requirements.
- Assist in treating or managing underlying causative factors (e.g., cancer, malabsorption syndrome, impaired cognition, depression, medications that decrease appetite, fad diets, anorexia).
- Collaborate with interdisciplinary team **to set nutritional goals when client has specific dietary needs, malnutrition is profound, or long-term feeding problems exist.**
- Provide diet modifications, as indicated. For example:

  Optimization of client's intake of protein, carbohydrates, fats, calories within eating style and needs

  Several small meals and snacks daily

  Mechanical soft or blenderized tube feedings

  Appetite stimulants (e.g., wine), if indicated

  High-calorie, nutrient-rich dietary supplements, such as meal-replacement shake

  Formula tube feedings; parenteral nutrition infusion
- Administer pharmaceutical agents, as indicated:

  Digestive drugs or enzymes

  Vitamin and mineral (iron) supplements, including chewable multivitamin

  Medications (e.g., antacids, anticholinergics, antiemetics, antidiarrheals)
- Determine whether client prefers or tolerates more calories in a particular meal.
- Use flavoring agents (e.g., lemon and herbs) if salt is restricted **to enhance food satisfaction and stimulate appetite.**
- Encourage use of sugar or honey in beverages if carbohydrates are tolerated well.

Information that appears in brackets has been added by the authors to clarify and enhance the use of nursing diagnoses.

- Encourage client to choose foods or have family member bring foods that seem appealing **to stimulate appetite.**
- Avoid foods that cause intolerances or increase gastric motility (e.g., foods that are gas forming, hot/cold, or spicy; caffeinated beverages; milk products), according to individual needs.
- Limit fiber or bulk, if indicated, **because it may lead to early satiety.**
- Promote pleasant, relaxing environment, including socialization when possible **to enhance intake.**
- Prevent or minimize unpleasant odors or sights. **May have a negative effect on appetite and eating.**
- Assist with or provide oral care before and after meals and at bedtime.
- Encourage use of lozenges and so forth **to stimulate salivation when dryness is a factor.**
- Promote adequate and timely fluid intake. Limit fluids 1 hr prior to meal **to reduce possibility of early satiety.**
- Weigh regularly and graph results **to monitor effectiveness of efforts.**
- Develop individual strategies when problem is mechanical (e.g., wired jaws or paralysis following stroke). Consult occupational therapist **to identify appropriate assistive devices,** or speech therapist **to enhance swallowing ability.** (Refer to ND impaired Swallowing.)
- Refer to structured (behavioral) program of nutrition therapy (e.g., documented time and length of eating period, blenderized food or tube feeding, administered parenteral nutritional therapy) per protocol, **particularly when problem is anorexia nervosa or bulimia.**
- Recommend and support hospitalization **for controlled environment in severe malnutrition or life-threatening situations.**
- Refer to social services or other community resources **for possible assistance with client's limitations in buying and preparing foods.**

Nursing Priority No. 4.

To promote wellness (Teaching/Discharge Considerations):

- Emphasize importance of well-balanced, nutritious intake. Provide information regarding individual nutritional needs and ways to meet these needs within financial constraints.
- Provide positive regard, love, and acknowledgment of "voice within" guiding client with eating disorder.
- Develop consistent, realistic weight goal with client.

Information that appears in brackets has been added by the authors to clarify and enhance the use of nursing diagnoses.

- Weigh at regular intervals and document results **to monitor effectiveness of dietary plan.**
- Consult with dietitian or nutritional support team, as necessary, **for long-term needs.**
- Develop regular exercise and stress reduction program.
- Review drug regimen, side effects, and potential interactions with other medications and over-the-counter drugs.
- Review medical regimen and provide information and assistance, as necessary.
- Assist client to identify and access resources, such as way to obtain nutrient-dense, low-budget foods, Supplemental Nutrition Assistance Program (SNAP), Meals-on-Wheels, community food banks, and/or other appropriate assistance programs.
- Refer for dental hygiene or other professional care, including counseling or psychiatric care, family therapy, as indicated.
- Provide and reinforce client teaching regarding preoperative and postoperative dietary needs when surgery is planned.
- Assist client/SO(s) to learn how to blenderize food and/or perform tube feeding.
- Refer to home health resources **for initiation and supervision of home nutrition therapy when used.**

Documentation Focus

Assessment/Reassessment

- Baseline and subsequent assessment findings to include signs/symptoms as noted in Defining Characteristics and laboratory diagnostic findings
- Caloric intake
- Individual cultural or religious restrictions, personal preferences
- Availability and use of resources
- Personal understanding or perception of problem

Planning

- Plan of care and who is involved in planning
- Teaching plan

Implementation/Evaluation

- Client's responses to interventions, teaching, and actions performed
- Results of periodic weigh-in
- Attainment or progress toward desired outcome(s)
- Modifications to plan of care

Information that appears in brackets has been added by the authors to clarify and enhance the use of nursing diagnoses.

Discharge Planning

- Long-term needs, and who is responsible for actions to be taken
- Specific referrals made

Sample Nursing Outcomes & Interventions Classifications (NOC/NIC)

NOC—Nutritional Status
NIC—Nutrition Management

readiness for enhanced NUTRITION

[Diagnostic Division: Food/Fluid]

Definition: A pattern of nutrient intake that is sufficient for meeting metabolic needs and can be strengthened.

Defining Characteristics

Subjective

Expresses desire to enhance nutrition

Desired Outcomes/Evaluation Criteria—Client Will:

- Demonstrate behaviors to attain or maintain appropriate weight.
- Be free of signs of malnutrition.
- Be able to safely prepare and store foods.

Actions/Interventions

Nursing Priority No. 1.

To determine current nutritional status and eating patterns:

- Review client's knowledge of current nutritional needs and ways client is meeting these needs. **Provides baseline for further teaching and interventions.**
- Assess eating patterns and food and fluid choices in relation to any health risk factors and health goals. **Helps to identify specific strengths and weaknesses that can be addressed.**
- ∞ Verify that age-related and developmental needs are met. **These factors are constantly presented throughout the life span, although differing for each age group. For example, older adults need same nutrients as younger adults, but in**

Information that appears in brackets has been added by the authors to clarify and enhance the use of nursing diagnoses.

smaller amounts, and with attention to certain components, such as calcium, fiber, vitamins, protein, and water. Infants/children require small meals and constant attention to needed nutrients for proper growth and development while dealing with child's food preferences and eating habits.

- Evaluate influence of cultural or religious factors **to determine what client considers to be normal dietary practices, as well as to identify food preferences and restrictions, and eating patterns that can be strengthened and/or altered, if indicated.**
- Assess how client perceives food, food preparation, and the act of eating **to determine client's feelings and emotions regarding food and self-image.**
- Ascertain occurrence of, or potential for, negative feedback from significant other (SO)(s). **May reveal control issues that could impact client's commitment to change.**
- Determine patterns of hunger and satiety. **Helps identify strengths and weaknesses in eating patterns and potential for change (e.g., person predisposed to weight gain may need a different time for a big meal than evening or need to learn what foods reinforce feelings of satisfaction).**
- Assess client's ability to safely store and prepare foods **to determine if health information or resources might be needed.**

Nursing Priority No. 2.

To assist client/SO(s) to develop plan to meet individual needs:

- Determine motivation and expectation for change.
- Assist in obtaining and review results of individual testing (e.g., weight/height, body fat percent, lipids, glucose, complete blood count, total protein) **to determine that client is healthy and/or identify dietary changes that may be helpful in attaining health goals.**
- Encourage client's beneficial eating patterns/habits (e.g., controlling portion size, eating regular meals, reducing high-fat or fast-food intake, following specific dietary program, drinking water and healthy beverages). **Positive feedback promotes continuation of healthy lifestyle habits and new behaviors.**
- Discuss use of nonfood rewards.
- Provide instruction and reinforce information regarding special needs. **Enhances decision-making process and promotes responsibility for meeting own needs.**

Information that appears in brackets has been added by the authors to clarify and enhance the use of nursing diagnoses.

- Encourage reading of food labels and instruct in meaning of labeling, as indicated, **to assist client/SO(s) in making healthful choices.**
- Consult with, or refer to, dietitian, or physician, as indicated. **Client/SO(s) may benefit from advice regarding specific nutrition and dietary issues or may require regular follow-up to determine that needs are being met when a medically prescribed program is to be followed.**
- Develop a system for self-monitoring **to provide a sense of control and enable the client to follow own progress and assist in making choices.**

Nursing Priority No. 3.

To promote optimum wellness:

- Review individual risk factors and provide additional information and response to concerns. **Assists the client with motivation and decision making.**
- Provide bibliotherapy and help client/SO(s) identify and evaluate resources they can access on their own. **When referencing the Internet or nontraditional, unproven resources, the individual must exercise some restraint and determine the reliability of the source/information before acting on it.**
- Encourage variety and moderation in dietary plan **to decrease boredom and encourage client in efforts to make healthy choices about eating and food.**
- Discuss use of nutritional supplements, over-the-counter and herbal products. **Confusion may exist regarding the need for and use of these products in a balanced dietary regimen.**
- Assist client to identify and access community resources when indicated. **May benefit from assistance such as Supplemental Nutrition Assistance Program (SNAP), WIC, budget counseling, Meals-on-Wheels, community food banks, and/or other assistance programs.**

Documentation Focus

Assessment/Reassessment

- Assessment findings, including client perception of needs and desire/expectations for improvement
- Individual cultural or religious restrictions, personal preferences
- Availability and use of resources

Information that appears in brackets has been added by the authors to clarify and enhance the use of nursing diagnoses.

Planning
- Individual goals for enhancement
- Plan for growth and who is involved in planning

Implementation/Evaluation
- Response to activities and learning, and actions performed
- Attainment or progress toward desired outcome(s)
- Modifications to plan

Discharge Planning
- Long-term needs, expectations, and plan of action
- Available resources and specific referrals made

Sample Nursing Outcomes & Interventions Classifications (NOC/NIC)
NOC—Knowledge: Diet
NIC—Nutritional Counseling

OBESITY
[Diagnostic Division: Food/Fluid]

Definition: A condition in which an individual accumulates abnormal or excessive fat for age and gender that exceeds overweight.

Related Factors

Average daily physical activity is less than recommended for gender and age; energy expenditure below energy intake based on standard assessment (e.g., WAVE [weight, activity, variety in diet, excess] assessment)

Consumption of sugar-sweetened beverages; frequent snacking; high frequency of restaurant or fried food; portion sizes larger than recommended

Disordered eating behaviors or perceptions; fear regarding lack of food supply; high disinhibition and restraint eating behavior score

Economically disadvantaged

Formula or mixed-fed infants; overweight in infancy; low dietary calcium intake in children

Information that appears in brackets has been added by the authors to clarify and enhance the use of nursing diagnoses.

Genetic disorder; heritability of interrelated factors (e.g., adipose tissue distribution, energy expenditure, lipid synthesis, lipolysis

Maternal diabetes mellitus, smoking; parental obesity

Defining Characteristics

Objective

ADULT: BMI of >30 kg/m^2

CHILD: <2 years: Term not used with children this age

CHILD: 2–18 years: BMI of >30 kg/m^2 or >95th percentile for age and gender

Desired Outcomes/Evaluation Criteria—Client Will:

- Verbalize a realistic self-concept or body image (congruent mental and physical picture of self).
- Participate in development of, and commit to, a personal weight loss program.
- Demonstrate appropriate changes in lifestyle and behaviors, including eating patterns, food quantity/quality, and exercise program.
- Attain desirable body weight with optimal maintenance of health.

Actions/Interventions

Nursing Priority No. 1.

To identify contributing factors/health status:

- ∞ Obtain weight history, noting if client has weight gain out of character for self or family, is or was obese child, or used to be much more physically active than is now **to identify trends. Note: Obesity is now the most prevalent nutritional disorder among children and adolescents in the United States. Being overweight during older childhood is highly predictive of adult obesity, especially if a parent is also obese.**
- Assess risk and presence of factors or conditions associated with obesity (e.g., familial pattern of obesity; genetic disorders in children [e.g., Prader-Willi syndrome, Laurence-Moon-Biedl syndrome]; hypothyroidism; type 2 diabetes; reproductive dysfunction; menopause; chronic disorders, such as heart disease, kidney disease, chronic pain; food or other

---

Information that appears in brackets has been added by the authors to clarify and enhance the use of nursing diagnoses.

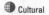

substance addictions; stressful or sedentary lifestyle; depression; use of certain medications such as steroids, birth control pills; physical disabilities or limitations; lack of socioeconomic resources for obtaining or preparing healthy foods) **to determine treatments and interventions that may be indicated in addition to weight management.**

- Ascertain current and previous dieting history. **Client may report normal or excessive intake of food, but calories and intake of certain food groups (e.g., sweets and fats) are often underestimated. Client may report experimentation with numerous types of diets, repeated dieting efforts ("yo-yo" dieting) with varying results, or may never have attempted a weight-management program.**
- Assess client's knowledge of own body weight and nutritional needs, and determine cultural expectations regarding size. **Although nutritional needs are not always understood, being overweight or having large body size may not be viewed negatively by individual, because it is considered within relationship to family eating patterns, peer and cultural influences.**
- Identify familial and cultural influences regarding food. **People of many cultures place high importance on food and food-related events, while some cultures routinely observe fasting days (e.g., Arab, Greek, Irish, Jewish) that may be done for health or religious purposes.**
- Ascertain how client perceives food and the act of eating. **Individual beliefs, values, and types of foods available influence what people eat, avoid, or alter. Client may be eating to satisfy an emotional need rather than physiological hunger, not only because food plays a significant role in socialization but also because food can offer comfort, sense of security, and acceptance.**
- Assess dietary practices by means of diary covering 3–7 days. **Recall of foods and fluids ingested; times, patterns, and place of eating; whether alone or with other(s); and feelings before, during, and after eating can increase client's understanding of eating behavior and serve as the basis for dietary modifications.**
- Identify problems with energy balance. **Few people can accurately estimate the number of calories they should consume in a day for a person their age, height, weight, and physical activity. Eating and physical activity patterns that are focused on consuming fewer calories, making informed food choices, and being physically active can help people attain and maintain a healthy weight.**

Information that appears in brackets has been added by the authors to clarify and enhance the use of nursing diagnoses.

- Collaborate in assessment and interventions for client with disordered eating habits or eating perceptions:

  Obtain comparative body drawing having client draw self on wall with chalk, then standing against it and having actual body outline drawn to note difference between the two. **Determines whether client's view of self-body image is congruent with reality.**

  Ascertain occurrence of negative feedback from SO(s). **May reveal control issues, impact motivation for change.**

  Identify unhelpful eating behaviors (e.g., eating over sink, "gobbling, nibbling, or grazing") and address kinds of activities associated with eating (e.g., watching television or reading, being unmindful of eating or food) **that result in taking in too many calories as well as eliminating the joy of food because of failure to notice flavors or sensation of fullness or satiety.**

  Review daily activity and regular exercise program **for comparative baseline and to identify areas for modification. Note: The 2008 National Health Interview Survey showed that only 33% of American adults participated in leisure-time physical activity on a regular basis.**

- Review laboratory test results (e.g., complete blood count with differential, full lipid panel, fasting glucose, A_1C, and insulin levels; thyroid, leptins; proteins; and eating self-assessment tests or nutritional screening tests such as Mini Nutritional Assessment [MNA]) **that may reveal medical or emotional conditions associated with obesity, and identify problems that may be treated with alterations in diet or medications.**
- Obtain anthropometric measurements **to determine presence and severity of obesity.**
- Calculate body mass index (BMI) **to estimate percentage of body fat. Note: The Centers for Disease Control and Prevention (CDC) have standardized BMI calculations, removing age and sex differences for adults with obesity being defined as 30 and above. Morbid obesity is defined as BMI ≥40. The CDC has recommended that children (over age 2) and adolescents be considered obese if the BMI exceeds the 95th percentiles on growth curves or exceeds 30 kg/m at any age.**
- Refer to ND: Overweight for additional diagnostic studies information.

Information that appears in brackets has been added by the authors to clarify and enhance the use of nursing diagnoses.

Nursing Priority No. 2.

To establish weight-reduction program:

- Collaborate with nutritionist in addressing/implementing client's specific needs (e.g., about foods to incorporate or limit, and how to identify nutrient-dense foods and beverages). **A healthy eating pattern limits intake of sodium, solid fats, added sugars, and refined grains and emphasizes nutrient-dense foods and beverages (e.g., vegetables, fruits, whole grains, fat-free or low-fat milk and milk products), seafood, lean meats and poultry, eggs, beans and peas, and nuts and seeds.**
- Refer to ND: Overweight, Nursing Priority 2 for interventions common to weight loss programs.
- Assist client in using technology to manage food choices/track intake. **Technology offers applications that can assist in monitoring dietary intake and food choices. Some calculate calories, providing immediate feedback, and generating individualized reminders.**
- Engage client and family in structured weight loss programs, as indicated. **Approaches to the treatment of severely obese individuals may include lifestyle modifications, physical activity, very controlled diets, intensive psychiatric interventions, including individual, group, and family therapy.**
- Refer to bariatric physician/surgeon, as indicated. **Evaluation for special measures may be needed (e.g., supervised fasting or bariatric surgery) for obese persons with comorbidities, and for morbidly obese persons with BMI >40.**

Nursing Priority No. 3.

To promote wellness (Teaching/Discharge Considerations):

- **Refer to ND: Overweight for related interventions**

Documentation Focus

Assessment/Reassessment

- Individual findings, including current weight, dietary pattern; perceptions of self, food, and eating; motivation for loss, support or feedback from SO(s)
- Results of laboratory and diagnostic testing

Information that appears in brackets has been added by the authors to clarify and enhance the use of nursing diagnoses.

Planning

- Plan of care, specific interventions, and who is involved in planning
- Teaching plan

Implementation/Evaluation

- Responses to interventions, and actions performed
- Use of available resources, tools to support weight loss program
- Attainment or progress toward desired outcome(s)
- Modifications to plan of care

Discharge Planning

- Long-term needs and who is responsible for actions to be taken
- Specific referrals made

Sample Nursing Outcomes & Interventions Classifications (NOC/NIC)

NOC—Weight Loss Behavior
NIC—Weight Reduction Assistance

OVERWEIGHT and risk for OVERWEIGHT

[Diagnostic Division: Food/Fluid]

Definition: Overweight: A condition in which an individual accumulates abnormal or excessive fat for age and gender.

Definition: risk for Overweight: Vulnerable to abnormal or excessive fat accumulation for age and gender, which may compromise health.

Related and Risk Factors

Average daily physical activity is less than recommended for gender and age; sedentary behavior occurring for >2 hours/day; energy expenditure below energy intake based on standard assessment (e.g., WAVE [weight, activity, variety in diet, excess] assessment)

Consumption of sugar-sweetened beverages; frequent snacking; high frequency of restaurant or fried food; portion sizes larger than recommended

Disordered eating behaviors or perceptions; fear regarding lack of food supply; high disinhibition and restraint eating behavior score

Information that appears in brackets has been added by the authors to clarify and enhance the use of nursing diagnoses.

Economically disadvantaged
Genetic disorder; heritability of interrelated factors (e.g., adipose tissue distribution, energy expenditure, lipid synthesis, lipolysis)
Maternal diabetes mellitus; maternal smoking; parental obesity
Rapid weight gain during infancy, including first week, first 4 months, and first year; solid foods as major food source at <5 months of age
Rapid weight gain during childhood, obesity in childhood; low dietary calcium intake in children; premature pubarche
Shortened sleep time; sleep disorder

Defining Characteristics (Overweight)

Objective

ADULT: BMI >25 kg/m²; Adult: BMI approaching 25 kg/m², (risk)
CHILD <2 years: Weight-for-length >95th percentile; CHILD <2 years: Weight-for-length approaching 95th percentile (risk)
CHILD 2–18 years: BMI >25 kg/m² or >85th but <95th percentile (whichever is smaller); CHILD 2–18 years: BMI 95th percentile, or 25 /kg/m² (whichever is smaller) (risk)

NOTE: A risk diagnosis is not evidenced by signs and symptoms, as the problem has not occurred; rather, nursing interventions are directed at prevention.

Desired Outcomes/Evaluation Criteria—Client Will:

- Verbalize a realistic self-concept or body image (congruent mental and physical picture of self).
- Participate in development of, and commit to, a personal weight loss program.
- Demonstrate appropriate changes in lifestyle and behaviors, including eating patterns, food quantity/quality, and exercise program.
- Attain desirable body weight with optimal maintenance of health.

Actions/Interventions

Nursing Priority No. 1.

To identify contributing **or risk** factors:

Information that appears in brackets has been added by the authors to clarify and enhance the use of nursing diagnoses.

- Obtain weight history, noting if client has weight gain out of character for self or family, is or was an obese child, or used to be much more physically active than is now **to identify trends. Note: Unchecked weight gain can lead to obesity, which is now the most prevalent nutritional disorder among children and adolescents in the United States. (Approximately 21%–24% of American children and adolescents are overweight, and another 16%–18% are obese.)**
- Assess risk and presence of factors or conditions associated with obesity (e.g., familial pattern of obesity; decreased basal metabolic rate or hypothyroidism; type 2 diabetes; reproductive dysfunction; menopause; chronic disorders, such as heart disease, kidney disease, chronic pain; food or other substance addictions; stressful or sedentary lifestyle; depression; use of certain medications such as steroids, birth control pills; physical disabilities or limitations; lack of socioeconomic resources for obtaining or preparing healthy foods) **to determine treatments and interventions that may be indicated in addition to weight management.**
- Assess client's knowledge of own body weight and nutritional needs, and determine cultural expectations regarding size. **Although nutritional needs are not always understood, being overweight or having large body size may not be viewed negatively by an individual, because it is considered in relation to family eating patterns, and peer and cultural influences.**
- Identify familial and cultural influences regarding food. **People of many cultures place a high importance on food and food-related events, while some cultures routinely observe fasting days (e.g., Arab, Greek, Irish, Jewish) that may be done for health or religious purposes.**
- Ascertain how the client perceives food and the act of eating. **The client may be eating to satisfy an emotional need rather than physiological hunger, not only because food plays a significant role in socialization, but also because food can offer comfort, a sense of security, and acceptance.**
- Evaluate the client's routine medications. **Some medications can contribute to weight gain (e.g., cortisol and other glucocorticoids; sulfonylureas, tricyclic antidepressants, monoamine oxidase inhibitors; oral contraceptives; Insulin [in excessive doses]; risperidone; etc.).**
- Assess dietary practices by means of diary covering 3–7 days. **Recall of foods and fluids ingested; times, patterns, and places of eating; whether alone or with other(s); and feelings before, during, and after eating can increase the cli-**

Information that appears in brackets has been added by the authors to clarify and enhance the use of nursing diagnoses.

ent's understanding of eating behaviors and serve as the basis for dietary modifications.**

- Ascertain previous dieting history. **The client may report normal or excessive intake of food, but calories and intake of certain food groups (e.g., sweets and fats) are often underestimated. The client may report experimentation with numerous types of diets, repeated dieting efforts ("yo-yo" dieting) with varying results, or may never have attempted a weight-management program.**
- Collaborate in assessment and interventions for client with disordered eating habits or eating perceptions:

Obtain comparative body drawing having client draw self on wall with chalk, then standing against it and having actual body outline drawn to note difference between the two. **This determines whether the client's view of self-body image is congruent with reality.**

Ascertain occurrence of negative feedback from significant other (SO). **May reveal control issues and may impact motivation for change.**

- Review laboratory test results (e.g., complete blood count with differential, full lipid panel, fasting glucose, A_1C, and insulin levels; thyroid, and leptins; proteins, Mini-Nutritional Assessment) **that may reveal medical conditions associated with obesity, and identify problems that may be treated with alterations in diet or medications.**

Nursing Priority No. 2.

To determine weight loss goals:

- Obtain anthropometric measurements **to determine presence and severity situation**:

Calculate body mass index (BMI) **to estimate the percentage of body fat. Note that the Centers for Disease Control and Prevention (CDC) has standardized BMI calculations, removing age and sex differences for adults, with 25–29.9 kg/m² defining "overweight." The CDC has recommended that children (over age 2) and adolescents be considered overweight if the BMI exceeds the 85th percentile (and is < the 95th percentile) on growth curves or exceeds 25 kg/m² at any age.**

Determine waist circumference, if indicated **Some studies support that waist circumference (WC) is more closely linked to cardiovascular risk factors, than BMI alone, because a high WC can occur in persons with normal or near normal BMIs.**

Information that appears in brackets has been added by the authors to clarify and enhance the use of nursing diagnoses.

- Determine client's motivation for weight loss (e.g., for own satisfaction or self-esteem, to improve health status, or to gain approval from another person). **The client is more likely to succeed and maintain desired weight when change is for self (e.g., acceptance of self "as is," general well-being) rather than to please others.**
- Discuss myths client/SO may have about weight and weight loss **to address misconceptions and possibly enhance motivation for needed behavior changes.**
- Set realistic goals (short and long term) for weight loss. **Reasonable weight loss (1 to 2 lb/week) has been shown to have more lasting effects than rapid weight loss. Note that a loss of 5%–20% of total body weight can reduce many of the health risks associated with obesity in adults.**

Nursing Priority No. 3.

To establish weight-reduction program:

- Obtain commitment or contract for weight loss. **Verbal agreement to goals or written contract formalizes the plan and may enhance efforts and maximize outcomes.**
- Involve SO(s) in the treatment plan as much as possible **to provide ongoing support and increase the likelihood of success.**
- Collaborate with physician and nutritionist **to develop and implement comprehensive weight-loss program that includes food, activity, behavior alteration, and support.**
- Calculate calorie requirements based on physical factors and activity. **While many weight-reduction programs focus on portion size and food components (e.g., low-fat, high-protein, low-glycemic foods), reducing calorie intake is essential for weight loss.**
- Provide information regarding specific nutritional needs. **Depending on client's desires and needs, many weight-management programs are available that focus on particular factors (e.g., low carbohydrates, low fat, low calories). Reducing portion size and following a balanced diet along with increasing exercise is often what is needed to improve health.**
- Discuss modifications to achieve a healthy body weight:

  Eat from each food group (fruits, vegetables, whole grains, lean meats, low-fat dairy, and oils).

  Start with small changes, such as adding one more vegetable/day, and introducing healthier versions of favorite foods.

Information that appears in brackets has been added by the authors to clarify and enhance the use of nursing diagnoses.

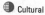

Choose "nutrient-dense" forms of foods that provide substantial amounts of fiber, vitamins, electrolytes, and minerals.

Avoid saturated fats, trans fats, cholesterol, salt (sodium), and added sugars.

Focus on portion sizes. **Calorie-dense foods (high in fat and/or sugar) should be eaten in smaller quantities, whereas high-fiber foods can be eaten in larger quantities.**

Discuss smart snacks (e.g., low-fat yogurt with fruit, nuts, apple slices with peanut butter, low-fat string cheese).

Emphasize the need for adequate fluid intake and taking fluids between meals rather than with meals to provide fluid while leaving more room for food intake at meals **to assist in the digestive process and to quench thirst, which is often mistakenly identified as hunger.**

- Encourage involvement in planned activity program of client's choice and within physical abilities. Refer to formal exercise program, if desired. **Moderately increased physical activity (e.g., 30 to 45 min 3–5 days/week) can support both loss of pounds and maintenance of lower weight. Note: Children should participate in vigorous physical activity throughout adolescence and limit time spent watching television and playing computer games, to facilitate weight control.**
- Recommend weighing only once/week, same time and clothes, and graph on chart. Measure and monitor body fat when possible **to track progress while focusing more on the idea of being health conscious and responsible than on what the scale may reveal.**
- Provide positive reinforcement and encouragement for efforts as well as actual weight loss. **This enhances commitment to the program and enhances the person's sense of self-worth.**
- Refer to bariatric physician/surgeon when indicated. **Evaluation for special measures may be needed (e.g., supervised fasting or bariatric surgery) for obese or morbidly obese persons.** Refer to ND: Obesity for related interventions.

Nursing Priority No. 4.

To promote wellness (Teaching/Discharge Considerations):

- Assist in and encourage periodic evaluation of nutritional status and alteration of dietary plan. **This may be desired or**

Information that appears in brackets has been added by the authors to clarify and enhance the use of nursing diagnoses.

needed for addressing special needs (e.g., diabetes mellitus, age considerations, very low calorie or fasting) and monitoring health status.

- Emphasize the importance of avoiding fad diets **that may be harmful to health and often do not produce long-term positive results.**
- Identify and encourage finding ways to reduce tension when eating. **This promotes relaxation to permit focusing on the act of eating and awareness of satiety.**
- Identify unhelpful eating behaviors (e.g., eating over the sink, "gobbling, nibbling, or grazing") and address kinds of activities associated with eating (e.g., watching television or reading, being unmindful of eating or food) **that result in taking in too many calories as well as eliminating the joy of food because of failure to notice flavors or sensation of fullness or satiety.**
- Review and discuss strategies to deal appropriately with stressful events **to avoid overeating as a means of coping.**
- Discuss importance of an occasional treat by planning for inclusion in diet **to avoid feelings of deprivation arising from self-denial.**
- Advise planning for special occasions (birthday or holidays) by reducing intake before event and/or eating "smart" **to redistribute or reduce calories and allow for participation in food events.**
- Discuss normalcy of ups and downs of weight loss: plateau, set point (at which weight is not being lost), hormonal influences, and so forth. **This prevents discouragement when progress stalls.**
- Encourage buying personal items and clothing **as a reward for weight loss or other accomplishments.**
- Suggest disposing of "fat clothes" **to encourage positive attitude of permanent change and remove "safety valve" of having wardrobe available "just in case" weight is regained.**
- Review prescribed drug regimen (e.g., appetite suppressants, hormone therapy, vitamin and mineral supplements) **for benefits or adverse side effects and drug interactions.**
- Recommend reading labels of nonprescription diet aids if used. **Herbals containing diuretics or ma huang (product similar to ephedrine) may cause adverse side effects in vulnerable persons.**
- Encourage parents and school dieticians to model and offer good nutritional choices (e.g., offer vegetables, fruits, and

---

Information that appears in brackets has been added by the authors to clarify and enhance the use of nursing diagnoses.

lower-fat foods in daily meals and snacks) **to assist child in accepting healthy eating styles. Note: Studies have shown a high correlation between parents and children regarding patterns of food intake and food choices.**

- Refer to community support groups or psychotherapy, as indicated, **to provide role models, address issues of body image or self-worth.**
- Provide contact number for dietitian/nutritionist and/or audiovisual materials, bibliography, reliable Internet sites for resources **to address ongoing nutritional needs and dietary changes.**
- Refer to NDs disturbed Body Image; ineffective Coping, Obesity for additional interventions, as appropriate.

Documentation Focus

Assessment/Reassessment

- Individual findings, including current weight, dietary pattern; perceptions of self, food, and eating; motivation for loss; support or feedback from SO(s)
- Results of laboratory and diagnostic testing
- Results of interval weigh-ins

Planning

- Plan of care, specific interventions, and who is involved in planning
- Teaching plan

Implementation/Evaluation

- Responses to interventions, weekly weight, and actions performed
- Attainment or progress toward desired outcome(s)
- Modifications to plan of care

Discharge Planning

- Long-term needs and who is responsible for actions to be taken
- Specific referrals made

Sample Nursing Outcomes & Interventions Classifications (NOC/NIC)

NOC—Weight Loss Behavior
NIC—Weight Reduction Behavior

Information that appears in brackets has been added by the authors to clarify and enhance the use of nursing diagnoses.

acute PAIN

[Diagnostic Division: Pain/Comfort]

Definition: An unpleasant sensory and emotional experience associated with actual or potential tissue damage, or described in terms of such damage (International Association for the Study of Pain); sudden or slow onset of any intensity from mild to severe with an anticipated or predictable end.

Related Factors

Biological injury agent (e.g., infection, ischemia, neoplasm)
Chemical injury agent (e.g., burn, capsaicin, methylene chloride, mustard agent)
Physical injury agent (e.g. abscess, amputation, burn, cut, heavy lifting, operative procedure, trauma, overtraining)

Defining Characteristics

Subjective

Self-report of intensity using standardized pain scale (e.g., Wong-Baker FACES scale, visual analogue scale, numeric rating scale)
Self-report of pain characteristics using standardized pain instrument (e.g., McGill Pain Questionnaire, Brief Pain Inventory)
Appetite change; hopelessness
Proxy report of pain behavior activity changes (e.g., family member, caregiver)

Objective

Guarding behavior; protective behavior; positioning to ease pain
Facial expression of pain (e.g., eyes lack luster, beaten look, fixed or scattered movement, grimace)
Expressive behavior (e.g., restlessness, crying)
Distraction behavior
Diaphoresis; changes in physiological parameter (e.g., blood pressure, heart rate, respiratory rate, oxygen saturation and end-tidal volume); pupil dilation
Self-focused; narrowed focus (e.g., time perception, thought process, interaction with people and environment)

Information that appears in brackets has been added by the authors to clarify and enhance the use of nursing diagnoses.

Evidence of pain using standard pain behavior checklist for those unable to communicate verbally (e.g., Neonatal Infant Pain Scale, Pain Assessment Checklist for Seniors with Limited Ability to Communicate)

Desired Outcomes/Evaluation Criteria—Client Will:

- Report pain is relieved or controlled.
- Follow prescribed pharmacological regimen.
- Verbalize nonpharmacological methods that provide relief.
- Demonstrate use of relaxation skills and diversional activities, as indicated, for individual situation.
- Verbalize sense of control of response to acute situation and positive outlook for the future.

Actions/Interventions

Nursing Priority No. 1.

To assess etiology/precipitating contributory factors:

- Determine and document presence of possible pathophysiological and psychological causes of pain (e.g., inflammation; tissue trauma, fractures; surgery; infections; heart attack or angina; abdominal conditions [e.g., appendicitis, cholecystitis]; burns; grief; fear, anxiety; depression; and personality disorders). **Acute pain is that which follows an injury, trauma, or procedure such as surgery, or occurs suddenly with the onset of a painful condition (e.g., herniated disk, migraine headache, pancreatitis).**
- ∞ Note client's age and developmental level and current condition (e.g., infant/child, critically ill, ventilated, sedated, or cognitively impaired client) **affecting ability to report pain parameters.**
- Note location of surgical procedures, **as this can influence the amount of postoperative pain experienced; for example, vertical or diagonal incisions are more painful than transverse or S-shaped.**
- Assess for referred pain, as appropriate, **to help determine possibility of underlying condition or organ dysfunction requiring treatment.**
- Note client's attitude toward pain and use of pain medications, including any history of substance abuse.
- Note client's locus of control (internal or external). **Individuals with external locus of control may take little or no responsibility for pain management.**

Information that appears in brackets has been added by the authors to clarify and enhance the use of nursing diagnoses.

Nursing Priority No. 2.

To evaluate client's response to pain:

- Obtain client's/significant other's (SO) assessment of pain to include location, characteristics, onset, duration, frequency, quality, intensity. Identify precipitating or aggravating and relieving factors **in order to fully understand client's pain symptoms.** ***Note:*** **Experts agree that attempts should always be made to obtain self-reports of pain. When that is not possible, credible information can be received from another person who knows the client well (e.g., parent, spouse, caregiver).**
- ∞ Evaluate pain characteristics and intensity. **Use pain rating scale appropriate for age and cognition (e.g., 0 to 10 scale, facial expression or Wong-Baker faces pain scale [pediatric, nonverbal], adolescent pediatric pain tool [APPT], pain assessment scale for seniors with limited ability to communicate [PACSLAC]; behavioral pain scale [BPS]; checklist of nonverbal pain indicators [CNPI], etc.).**
- Perform pain assessment each time pain occurs. Document and investigate changes from previous reports and evaluate results of pain interventions **to demonstrate improvement in status or to identify worsening of underlying condition/developing complications.**
- ∞ Accept client's description of pain. Be aware of the terminology client uses for pain experience (e.g., young child may say "owie" or "hurt"; elderly may say "it aches so bad"). **Pain is a subjective experience and cannot be felt by others. Note: Some elderly clients experience a reduction in perception of pain or have difficulty localizing or describing pain, and pain may be manifested as a change in behavior (e.g., restlessness, loss of appetite, increased confusion or wandering, acting out, change in functional abilities).**
- Note cultural and developmental influences affecting pain response. **Verbal and/or behavioral cues may have no direct relationship to the degree of pain perceived (e.g., client may deny pain even when feeling uncomfortable, or reactions can be stoic or exaggerated, reflecting cultural or familial norms).**
- Observe nonverbal cues and pain behaviors (e.g., how client walks, holds body, sits; facial expression; cool fingertips/toes, which can mean constricted blood vessels) and other objective Defining Characteristics, as noted, especially in persons who cannot communicate verbally. **Observations may not be congruent with verbal reports or may be only indicator present when client is unable to verbalize.**

Information that appears in brackets has been added by the authors to clarify and enhance the use of nursing diagnoses.

- Monitor skin color and temperature and vital signs (e.g., heart rate, blood pressure, respirations), **which are usually altered in acute pain.**
- Ascertain client's knowledge of and expectations about pain management. **Provides baseline for interventions and teaching, provides opportunity to allay common fears and misconceptions.**

Nursing Priority No. 3.

To assist client to explore methods for alleviation/control of pain:

- Collaborate in treatment of underlying condition or disease processes causing pain and proactive management of pain (e.g., epidural analgesia, nerve blockade for postoperative pain).
- Determine client's acceptable level of pain and pain control goals. **One client may not be 100% pain free but may feel that a "3" is a manageable level of discomfort, while another may require medication for pain at the same level, because the experience is subjective.**
- Determine factors in client's lifestyle (e.g., alcohol or other drug use or abuse) **that can affect responses to analgesics and/or choice of interventions for pain management.**
- Note when pain occurs (e.g., only with ambulation, every evening) **to medicate prophylactically, as appropriate.**
- Work with client to prevent pain. Use flow sheet to document pain, therapeutic interventions, response, and length of time before pain recurs. Instruct client to report pain as soon as it begins **as timely intervention is more likely to be successful in alleviating pain.**
- Establish collaborative approach for pain management based on client's understanding about and acceptance of available treatment options. **Pain medications may include pills/liquids or suckers, skin patch, or suppository forms; injections, IV dosing; or patient-controlled analgesia (PCA) or regional analgesia (e.g., epidural and spinal blocking) based on client's symptomatology and mechanism of pain as well as tolerance for pain and various analgesics.**
- Administer analgesics, as indicated, to maximum dosage, as needed, **to maintain "acceptable" level of pain. Notify physician if regimen is inadequate to meet pain control goal. Combinations of medications may be used on prescribed intervals.**
- Demonstrate and monitor use of self-administration/PCA that involves client in plan **to administer own IV pain medication or bolus additional dose when on continual basis drip.**

Information that appears in brackets has been added by the authors to clarify and enhance the use of nursing diagnoses.

- Evaluate and document client's response to analgesia and assist in transitioning or altering drug regimen, based on individual needs and protocols. **Increasing or decreasing dosage, stepped program (switching from injection to oral route, increased time span as pain lessens) helps in self-management of pain.**
- Instruct client in use of transcutaneous electrical stimulation (TENS) unit, when ordered.
- Provide or promote nonpharmacological pain management:

  Quiet environment, calm activities

  Comfort measures (e.g., back rub, change of position, use of heat or cold compresses)

  Use of relaxation exercises (e.g., focused breathing, visualization, guided imagery)

  Diversional or distraction activities, such as television and radio, socialization with others, commercial or individualized tapes (e.g., "white" noise, music, instructional)

  Encourage presence of parent during painful procedures **to comfort child.**

  Identify ways to avoid or minimize pain. **Splinting incision during cough, keeping body in good alignment and using proper body mechanics, and resting between activities can reduce occurrence of muscle tension or spasms, or undue stress on incision.**
- Encourage verbalization of feelings about the pain such as concern about tolerating pain, anxiety, pessimistic thoughts **to evaluate coping abilities and to identify areas of additional concern.**
- Use puppets to demonstrate procedure for child **to enhance understanding and reduce level of anxiety and fear.**

Nursing Priority No. 4.

To promote wellness (Teaching/Discharge Considerations):

- Acknowledge the pain experience and convey acceptance of client's response to pain. **Reduces defensive responses, promotes trust, and enhances cooperation with regimen.**
- Encourage adequate rest periods **to prevent fatigue that can impair ability to manage or cope with pain.**
- Review nonpharmacological ways to lessen pain, including techniques such as Therapeutic Touch (TT), biofeedback, self-hypnosis, and relaxation skills.
- Discuss impact of pain on lifestyle/independence and ways to maximize level of functioning.

Information that appears in brackets has been added by the authors to clarify and enhance the use of nursing diagnoses.

- Provide for individualized physical therapy or exercise program that can be continued by the client after discharge. **Promotes active, rather than passive, role and enhances sense of control.**
- Discuss with SO(s) ways in which they can assist client with pain management. **Family members/SOs may provide assistance by transporting client to prevent walking long distances, or by taking on client's strenuous chores, supporting timely pain control, encouraging eating nutritious meals to enhance wellness, and providing gentle massage to reduce muscle tension.**
- Identify specific signs/symptoms and changes in pain characteristics requiring medical follow-up. **Provides opportunity to modify pain management regimen and allows for timely intervention for developing complications.**

Documentation Focus

Assessment/Reassessment

- Individual assessment findings, including client's description of response to pain, specifics of pain inventory, expectations of pain management, and acceptable level of pain
- Prior medication use; substance abuse

Planning

- Plan of care and who is involved in planning
- Teaching plan

Implementation/Evaluation

- Response to interventions, teaching, and actions performed
- Attainment or progress toward desired outcome(s)
- Modifications to plan of care

Discharge Planning

- Long-term needs, noting who is responsible for actions to be taken
- Specific referrals made

Sample Nursing Outcomes & Interventions Classifications (NOC/NIC)

NOC—Pain Level
NIC—Pain Management

Information that appears in brackets has been added by the authors to clarify and enhance the use of nursing diagnoses.

chronic **PAIN** and chronic **PAIN SYNDROME [CPS]**

[Diagnostic Division: Pain/Discomfort]

Definition: chronic Pain: Unpleasant sensory and emotional experience arising from actual or potential tissue damage or described in terms of such damage (International Association for the Study of Pain); sudden or slow onset of any intensity, from mild to severe, constant or recurring without an anticipated or predictable end and a duration of greater than three (>3) months.

Definition: chronic Pain Syndrome: Recurrent or persistent pain that has lasted at least three months, and that significantly affects daily functioning or well-being.

Author Note: Pain is a signal that something is wrong. Chronic pain may be recurrent and periodically disabling (e.g., migraine headaches, kidney stones, prostatitis) or may be unremitting. It is a complex entity, combining elements from many other NDs, such as risk for Disuse Syndrome; deficient Diversional Activity; disturbed Body Image; compromised family Coping; interrupted Family Processes; Powerlessness; Self-Care Deficit (specify); sexual Dysfunction; Social Isolation]. The nurse is encouraged to refer to other NDs as indicated.

Related Factors (chronic Pain)

Age >50 years; female gender; genetic disorder
Alteration in sleep pattern
Anorexia; emotional distress; fatigue; prolonged increase in cortisol level; whole body vibration
Chronic musculoskeletal condition; muscle injury; damage to the nervous system; imbalance of neurotransmitters, neuromodulators, and receptors; nerve compression; ischemic condition; spinal cord injury; tumor infiltration
Contusion; crush injury; fracture; injury agent; post-trauma related condition (e.g., infection, inflammation)
History of abuse (e.g., physical, psychological, sexual; history of genital mutilation; history of substance abuse
History of overindebtedness
History of static work postures; prolonged computer use (>20 hours/week); repeated handling of heavy loads
Immune disorder (e.g., HIV-associated neuropathy, varicella-zoster virus; impaired metabolic functioning

Information that appears in brackets has been added by the authors to clarify and enhance the use of nursing diagnoses.

Increase in body mass index; malnutrition
Ineffective sexuality pattern; social isolation
Increase in body mass index; malnutrition
Ineffective sexuality pattern; social isolation

Defining Characteristics (chronic Pain)—

Subjective

Self-report of intensity using standardized pain scale (e.g., Wong-Baker FACES scale, visual analogue scale, numeric rating scale);
Self report of pain characteristics using standardized pain instrument (e.g., McGill Pain Questionnaire, Brief Pain Inventory)
Alteration in ability to continue previous activities
Alteration in sleep pattern; anorexia
[Preoccupation with pain]
[Desperately seeks alternative solutions or therapies for relief or control of pain]

chronic Pain Syndrome

Anxiety, fear; stress overload
Constipation
Disturbed sleep pattern, fatigue; insomnia

Objective (chronic pain)

Evidence of pain using standardized pain behavior checklist for those unable to communicate verbally (e.g., Neonatal Infant Pain Scale, Pain Assessment Checklist for Seniors with Limited Ability to Communicate)
Facial expression of pain (e.g., eyes lack luster, beaten look, fixed or scattered movement, grimace); self-focused
Proxy report of pain behavior/activity changes (e.g., family member, caregiver)

chronic Pain Syndrome

Deficient knowledge
Impaired mood regulation; social isolation
Impaired physical mobility
Obesity

Information that appears in brackets has been added by the authors to clarify and enhance the use of nursing diagnoses.

Desired Outcomes/Evaluation Criteria—Client Will:

- Verbalize and demonstrate (nonverbal cues) relief and/or control of pain or discomfort.
- Verbalize recognition of interpersonal and family dynamics and reactions that affect the pain situation.
- Demonstrate and initiate behavioral modifications of lifestyle and appropriate use of therapeutic interventions.
- Verbalize increased sense of control and enhanced enjoyment of life.

Family/SO(s) Will:

- Cooperate in pain management and rehabilitation program. (Refer to ND readiness for enhanced family Coping.)

Actions/Interventions

Nursing Priority No. 1.

To assess etiology/precipitating factors:

- Identify contributing factors (e.g., musculoskeletal trauma with lasting effects, chronic pancreatitis, cancers, osteoporosis, peripheral neuropathies from conditions such as diabetes or AIDS, fibromyalgia, overuse syndromes such as tendonitis, mechanical low back pain, spinal stenosis, amputation, urological disorders, ulcer disease, endometriosis, cardiovascular disease, poor circulation, arthritis, recurrent migraines, bipolar disorders, depression, personality disorders). **These conditions can cause, precipitate, and exacerbate persistent pain.**
- Assist in and/or review diagnostic testing, including physical (e.g., selected tests for identifying and/or monitoring suspected for known disease states; urine or blood toxicology for drug detoxification or therapy; and imaging studies); neurological, psychological evaluation (e.g., Minnesota Multiphasic Personality Inventory [MMPI], pain inventory, psychological interview). **Note: While additional diagnostic studies may be indicated when advanced treatment of the client with chronic pain syndrome (CPS) is initiated, care should be exercised in avoiding duplication of tests. This prevents unnecessary costs, as well as inadvertent reinforcement of client's psychological need for "something to be physically wrong."**

Information that appears in brackets has been added by the authors to clarify and enhance the use of nursing diagnoses.

- Evaluate for presence of/suspected psychological disorders. **Psychological factors may include (and are not limited to) depression, anxiety, somatization, and bipolar personality disorders. Testing may be indicated if organic cause of pain cannot be found, or when psychological factors are known to exist, or pain problems are prolonged and/or life-limiting.**
- Evaluate emotional/psychological components of individual situation. **Many painful conditions cause or exacerbate emotional responses (e.g., depression, withdrawal, agitation, anger) that worsen over time. Individuals with certain psychological syndromes (e.g., major depression, somatization disorder, hypochondriasis) may be prone to develop CPS. Note: Research suggests prevalence of 35% to 50% of people with chronic pain have depression.**
- Determine if client has history of physical or sexual abuse as a child. **A review of the literature shows that abuse in childhood is a strong predictor of depression and physical complaints, both expanded and unexplained, in adulthood.**
- Evaluate client's pattern of coping, and locus of control (internal or external). **Passive and avoidant behavioral patterns or lack of active engagement in self-management activities can contribute to perpetuation of chronic pain. Individuals with external locus of control may take little or no responsibility for pain management.**
- Determine relevant cultural and spirituality factors affecting pain response. **Pain is accepted and expressed in different ways (e.g., moaning aloud or enduring in stoic silence). Some may magnify symptoms to convince others of reality of pain, or believe that suffering in silence helps atone for past wrongdoing. Note: A person with chronic pain who identifies him- or herself as a spiritual being may report the link to divine help as empowering him/her to use strategies for healing.**
- Note gender and age of client. **There may be differences between how women and men perceive and/or respond to pain. Recent studies reveal large numbers of pediatric clients with chronic pain issues affecting academic attendance and function. While the prevalence of chronically painful conditions (e.g., arthritis) and illnesses (e.g., cancers) is common in the elderly, they may be reluctant to report pain.**
- Evaluate current and past analgesic, opioid, other drug use (including alcohol). **Provides clues to options to try or to**

Information that appears in brackets has been added by the authors to clarify and enhance the use of nursing diagnoses.

avoid; identifies need for changes in medication regimen as well as possible need for detoxification program.

Nursing Priority No. 2.

To determine client response to chronic pain situation:

- Evaluate pain behavior, noting past and current pain experience, using pain rating scale or diary, and including functional effects and psychological factors. **Pain behaviors can include the same ones present in acute pain (e.g., crying, grimacing, withdrawal, narrowed focus), but may also include other behaviors (e.g., dramatization of complaints, depression, drug misuse). Pain complaints may be exaggerated because of client's perception that pain reports are not believed or because client believes caregivers are discounting reports of pain.**
- Provide comprehensive assessment of pain problem, noting its duration, who has been consulted, and what therapies (including alternative/complementary) have been used. **The pathophysiology of chronic pain is multifactorial. If the condition causing the persistent pain is physiological and noncurable (e.g., terminal cancer), all diagnostics and treatments may have been exhausted, and pain management becomes the primary goal. If pain is present without a clear etiology or continues unabated, complex rehabilitation techniques may be required.**
- Note lifestyle effects of pain. **Major effects of chronic pain on the client's life can include depressed mood, fatigue, weight loss or gain, sleep disturbances, reduced activity and libido, excessive use of drugs and alcohol, dependent behavior, and disability seemingly out of proportion to impairment.**
- Assess degree of personal maladjustment of the client such as isolationism, anger, irritability, loss of work time or employment, school absenteeism. **Chronic pain reduces client's coping abilities and psychological well-being, often resulting in problems with relationships and life functioning.**
- Determine issues of secondary gain for the client/significant other (SO)(s) (e.g., financial or insurance compensation pending, legal or marital or family concern, school or work issues), **which may be present if there is marked discrepancy between claimed distress and objective findings or there is a lack of cooperation during evaluation and in complying with prescribed treatment.**
- Note codependent components, enabling behaviors of caregivers/family members **that support continuation of the**

Information that appears in brackets has been added by the authors to clarify and enhance the use of nursing diagnoses.

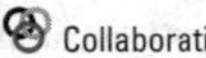

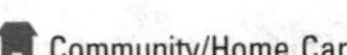

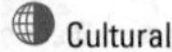

status quo and may interfere with progress in pain management or resolution of situation.**

- Note availability and use of personal and community resources. **Client/SO may need many things (e.g., equipment, financial resources, vocational training, respite services, or placement in rehabilitation facility) in order to manage painful conditions and/or concerns or difficulties associated with condition.**
- Make home visit when indicated, observing such factors as client's safety, equipment, adequate lighting, or family interactions **to note impact of home environment on the client and to determine changes that might be useful in improving client's life (e.g., grab bars in bathrooms and hallways, wider doors, ramps, assistance with activities of daily living [ADLs], housekeeping, yard work).**
- Acknowledge and assess pain matter-of-factly, avoiding undue expressions of concern, as well as expressions of disbelief about client's suffering. **Conveying an attitude of empathic understanding of client's disabling distress can have a beneficial impact on client's perception of health.**

Nursing Priority No. 3.

To assist client to deal with pain:

- Encourage participation in multidisciplinary pain management plan. **Comprehensive team may include physical medicine specialist; physical, occupational, recreational, and vocational therapists; and emotional or behavioral therapists to address complex issues of unresolved pain issues, to set goals for pain relief, and to develop an individualized treatment and evaluation plan.**
- Review client pain management goals and expectations versus reality. **Pain may not be completely resolved but may be significantly lessened to "acceptable level" or managed to the degree that client can participate in desired or needed life activities.**
- Discuss the physiological dynamics of tension and anxiety and how this affects pain.
- Administer or encourage client use of analgesics, as indicated. **Medications may be available in pills, liquids, or suckers to take by mouth, and in injection, skin patch, and suppository forms. Different medications or combinations of drugs may be used to manage persistent pain so that client may find relief and increase level of function. Note: Studies support that people with intense pain can take very high doses of opioids without experiencing side effects.**

Information that appears in brackets has been added by the authors to clarify and enhance the use of nursing diagnoses.

- Provide consistent and sufficient medication for pain relief, tailored to the individual, especially in one who tends to be undermedicated (e.g., elderly, cognitively impaired, person with lifelong pain, those with terminal cancer). **Medications may need to be scheduled around the clock, doses titrated up or down, and dose maximized to optimize pain relief while managing side effects.**
- Recommend or employ nonpharmacological interventions, methods of pain control (e.g., heat or cold applications, progressive muscle relaxation, biofeedback, deep breathing, meditation, visualization or guided imagery, posture correction and muscle strengthening exercises, water therapy, electrical stimulation, massage, acupuncture, Therapeutic Touch [TT]) **to obtain comfort, improve healing, and decrease dependency on analgesics.**
- Address medication misuse with client/SO and refer for appropriate counseling or interventions **when addiction is known or suspected to be interfering with client's well-being. Addicts may misrepresent their pain levels and their activities in order to obtain pain medications or progressively higher doses of medications, and they require specialized evaluation and interventions.**
- Discuss pain management goals and review client expectations versus reality, **because it may be that while pain cannot be completely resolved, it can be significantly reduced or managed to the degree that client can participate in desired or needed life activities, improving quality of life.**
- Assist family in developing a program of coping strategies (e.g., staying active even when modified activities are required, living a healthy lifestyle). **Positive reinforcement, encouraging client to use own control can aid in focusing energies on more productive activities.**
- Encourage limiting attention to pain behaviors, when appropriate (e.g., discussing pain for only a specified time; or acknowledging "I'm sorry your pain returned today, but you need to go to school"; or actively practicing relaxation or coping skills). **Reduces focus on pain, especially if client is highly dependent on pain for secondary gain issues or is addicted to medications.**
- Encourage client to use positive affirmations: "I am healing." "I am relaxed." "I love this life." Have client be aware of internal-external dialogue. Say "cancel" when negative thoughts develop. **Negative thinking can exacerbate feelings of hopelessness, and replacing those thoughts with positive ones can be helpful to pain management.**

Information that appears in brackets has been added by the authors to clarify and enhance the use of nursing diagnoses.

- Encourage right-brain stimulation with activities such as love, laughter, and music. **These actions can release endorphins, enhancing sense of well-being.**
- Encourage use of subliminal tapes **to bypass logical part of the brain by reinforcing: "I am becoming a more relaxed person." "It is all right for me to relax."**
- Use tranquilizers, narcotics, and analgesics sparingly. **These drugs are physically and psychologically addicting and promote sleep disturbances, especially interference with deep rapid eye movement (REM) sleep. Client may need to be detoxified if many medications are currently used.**
- Be alert to changes in pain characteristics **that may indicate a new physical problem or developing complication.**

Nursing Priority No. 4.

To promote wellness (Teaching/Discharge Considerations):

- Provide anticipatory guidance to client with condition in which pain is common and educate about when, where, and how to seek intervention or treatments.
- Assist client and SO(s) to learn how to heal by developing sense of internal control, by being responsible for own treatment, and by obtaining the information and tools to accomplish this.
- Discuss potential for developmental delays in child with chronic pain. Identify current level of function and review appropriate expectations for individual child.
- Instruct client/SO in medication administration, including use of patient-controlled analgesia (PCA) pumps, as indicated. Review safe use of analgesics, including side effects requiring home management (e.g., constipation) or adverse effects requiring medical intervention (e.g., possible drug reactions). **Appropriate instruction in home management increases the accuracy and safety of medication administration.**
- Encourage and assist family member/SO(s) to learn home-care interventions. **Massage and other nonpharmacological pain management techniques benefit the client through reduction of pain level and sense that client is not alone/has support of SO.**
- Incorporate desired folk healthcare practices and beliefs into regimen whenever possible. **Has been shown to increase compliance with pain management treatment plan.**
- Identify and discuss potential hazards of unproved or non-medical therapies or remedies.
- Assist client and SO(s) to learn how to heal **by developing sense of internal control, by being responsible for own**

Information that appears in brackets has been added by the authors to clarify and enhance the use of nursing diagnoses.

treatment, and by obtaining the information and tools to accomplish this.

- Recommend that client and SO(s) take time for themselves. **Provides opportunity to reenergize and refocus on living/tasks at hand.**
- Address client's preferences and wishes for incurable pain or end-of-life pain management via advance directives **in order to assist family/SO in attending to client's needs.**
- Identify community support groups and resources to meet individual needs (e.g., yard care, home maintenance, transportation). **Proper use of resources may reduce negative pattern of "overdoing" heavy activities and then spending several days in bed recuperating.**
- Refer for counseling (e.g., individual, family, marital therapy, parent effectiveness classes) as needed. **Presence of chronic pain affects all relationships and family dynamics.**
- Refer to NDs compromised family Coping, ineffective Coping.

Documentation Focus

Assessment/Reassessment

- Individual findings, including duration of problem, specific contributing factors, previously and currently used interventions
- Perception of pain, effects on lifestyle, and expectations of therapeutic regimen
- Locus of control and cultural beliefs affecting response to pain
- Family's/SO's response to client, and support for change
- Availability and use of resources

Planning

- Plan of care and who is involved in planning
- Teaching plan

Implementation/Evaluation

- Responses to interventions, teaching, and actions performed
- Attainment or progress toward desired outcome(s)
- Modifications to plan of care

Discharge Planning

- Long-term needs and who is responsible for actions to be taken
- Specific referrals made

Information that appears in brackets has been added by the authors to clarify and enhance the use of nursing diagnoses.

Sample Nursing Outcomes & Interventions Classifications (NOC/NIC)

NOC—Pain Control
NIC—Pain Management

labor PAIN

[Diagnostic Division: Pain/Discomfort]

Definition: Sensory and emotional experience that varies from pleasant to unpleasant, associated with labor and childbirth.

Related Factors

Cervical dilation
Fetal expulsion

Defining Characteristics

Subjective

Pain; perineal pressure
Alteration in urinary functioning, sleep pattern
Increase or decrease in appetite; nausea; vomiting

Objective

Uterine contraction
Alteration in blood pressure/heart rate/respiratory rate
Distraction/expressive behavior; protective behavior; positioning to ease pain
Alteration in muscle tension; diaphoresis
Alteration in neuroendocrine functioning
Narrowed focus; self-focused; pupil dilation
Facial expression of pain (e.g., eyes lack luster, beaten look, fixed or scattered movement, grimace)

Desired Outcomes/Evaluation Criteria—Client Will:

- Participate in decision-making for pain management plan to include personal preferences and cultural beliefs.
- Engage in nonpharmacologic measures to reduce discomfort/pain.
- Report pain at manageable level.

Information that appears in brackets has been added by the authors to clarify and enhance the use of nursing diagnoses.

Partner Will:

- Participate in labor process providing client's desired level of support.

Actions/Interventions

Nursing Priority No. 1.

To determine client's individual needs:

- Assess stage of labor, perform vaginal exam noting nature and amount of vaginal show, cervical dilation, effacement, fetal station, and fetal descent. **Choice and timing of medication is affected by degree of dilation and contractile pattern.**
- Note timing of prenatal care and participation in childbirth education classes. **Economic, emotional, and cultural concerns can limit the mother's access or involvement in preparation for labor, increasing her need for information and support.**
- Evaluate degree of discomfort through verbal and nonverbal cues; note cultural influences on pain response. **Attitudes and reactions to pain are individual and based on past experiences, understanding of physiological changes, and familial/cultural expectations.**
- Ascertain presence of a birth plan, individual expectations, and cultural or religious beliefs affecting the labor and delivery process. **Cultural influences may include how the laboring mother views pain management, as well as who attends the mother during the birth process.**
- Determine availability and preparation of support person(s). **Presence of a supportive partner, family/friend, or a doula can provide emotional support and enhance level of comfort.**

Nursing Priority No. 2.

To engage client in nonpharmacologic pain management techniques:

- Provide/encourage use of comfort measures (e.g., back/leg rubs, sacral pressure, back rest, mouth care, repositioning; shower/hot tub use, cool, moist cloths to face and neck, or hot compresses to perineum, abdomen; perineal care, linen changes). **Promotes relaxation and hygiene enhancing feeling of well-being and may reduce the need for analgesia or anesthesia. Position changes can also enhance circulation, reduce muscle tension.**

Information that appears in brackets has been added by the authors to clarify and enhance the use of nursing diagnoses.

- Assess client's desire for physical touch during contractions. **Touch may serve as a distraction, provide supportive reassurance and encouragement, and may aid in maintaining sense of control and reducing pain. Note: Remain respectful of client's preferences regarding touch.**
- Coach use of appropriate breathing/relaxation techniques and abdominal effleurage based on stage of labor. **May block pain impulses within the cerebral cortex through conditioned responses and cutaneous stimulation and gives client a means of coping with and controlling the level of discomfort.**
- Recommend client void every 1–2 hr. **Reduces bladder distention which can increase discomfort and prolong labor.**
- Provide information about available analgesics, usual responses/side effects (client and fetal), and duration of analgesic effect in light of current situation. **Empowers client to make informed choice about means of pain control.**
- Assist with complementary therapies as indicated (e.g., acupressure/acupuncture, moxibustion, hypnosis, reflexology). **Some clients and healthcare providers may prefer a trial of therapies theorized to stimulate/regulate contractions, reduce muscle tension, and mediate perception of pain before pursuing pharmacological interventions.**
- Provide for a quiet environment that is adequately ventilated, dimly lit, and free of unnecessary personnel. **Nondistracting environment provides optimal opportunity for rest and relaxation between contractions.**
- Offer encouragement, provide information about labor progress, and provide positive reinforcement for client's/couple's efforts. **Provides emotional support, which can reduce fear, lower anxiety levels, and help minimize pain.**

Nursing Priority No. 3.

To provide more intensive pain management measures:

- Time and record the frequency, intensity, and duration of uterine contractile pattern per protocol. **Information necessary for choosing appropriate interventions and preventing or limiting undesired side effects of medication.**
- Provide safety measures (e.g., encourage client to move slowly, bed in low position, raise side rails) as indicated post medication administration. **Regional block anesthesia produces vasomotor paralysis, so sudden movement may precipitate hypotension and risk for fall.**
- Administer analgesic, such as butorphanol tartrate (Stadol) or meperidine hydrochloride (Demerol), by IV during contrac-

Information that appears in brackets has been added by the authors to clarify and enhance the use of nursing diagnoses.

tions or deep intramuscular (IM) if indicated during active phase of stage I labor. **IV route provides more rapid and equal absorption of analgesic, and IM route may require up to 45 min to reach adequate plasma levels. Administering IV drug during uterine contraction decreases amount of medication that immediately reaches fetus.**

- Monitor maternal vital signs and fetal heart rate (FHR) variability after drug administration. Note drug's effectiveness and the physiological response. **Narcotics can have a depressant effect on fetus, particularly when administered 2–3 hr before delivery.**
- Assist with epidural or caudal block anesthesia using an indwelling catheter. **Provides relief once active labor is established. Note: Use of ultra–low-dose epidural is being promoted to achieve pain control without negative effect on client's ability to sense contractions and push effectively.**
- Monitor FHR electronically, and note decreased variability or bradycardia. **Decreased FHR variability is a common side effect of many anesthetics/analgesics. These side effects can begin 2–10 min after administration of anesthetic and may last for 5–10 min on occasion.**
- Monitor level of block per protocol. **Migration of decreased sensation from belly button (dermatome T-10) to tip of breastbone (approximately T-6) increases risk of respiratory depression and profound hypotension.**
- Turn client side to side periodically during continuous infusions. **Promotes even distribution of drug to prevent "one-sided" or unilateral block.**
- Inform client of onset of contractions as appropriate. **Client may "sleep" and/or encounter partial amnesia between contractions impairing her ability to recognize contractions as they begin and her ability to initiate pain management techniques.**
- Provide information about type of regional analgesia/anesthesia available at stage II specific to the delivery setting (e.g., local, pudendal block, lumbar epidural reinforcement, spinal block). **Although client is stressed, she still needs to be in control and make informed decisions regarding anesthesia.**

Nursing Priority No. 4.

To support delivery process:

- Note perineal bulging or vaginal show. **Discomfort levels increase as cervix dilates, fetus descends, and small blood vessels rupture.**

Information that appears in brackets has been added by the authors to clarify and enhance the use of nursing diagnoses.

- Assist client in assuming optimal position for bearing down (e.g., squatting or lateral recumbent). **Proper positioning with relaxation of perineal tissue optimizes bearing-down efforts, facilitates labor progress, reducing discomfort.**
- Assist with reinforcement of medication via indwelling lumbar epidural catheter when caput is visible. **Reduces discomfort associated with episiotomy, forceps application if needed, and fetal expulsion.**
- Assist as needed with administration of local anesthetic just before episiotomy, if performed. **Anesthetizes perineum tissue for incision/repair purposes.**

Documentation Focus

Assessment/Reassessment
- Stages of labor, results of vaginal exam, status of fetus/fetal monitoring
- Client's degree of preparation and expectations for labor process
- Choice of support person(s)

Planning
- Specifics of birth plan
- Plan of care and who is involved in planning

Implementation/Evaluation
- Response to actions and interventions performed
- Attainment or progress toward desired outcomes

Discharge Planning
- Postpartal pain management choices

Sample Nursing Outcomes & Interventions Classifications (NOC/NIC)

NOC—Pain Control
NIC—Intrapartal Care

Information that appears in brackets has been added by the authors to clarify and enhance the use of nursing diagnoses.

impaired PARENTING and risk for impaired PARENTING

[Diagnostic Division: Social Interaction]

Definition: impaired Parenting: Inability of the primary caretaker to create, maintain, or regain an environment that promotes the optimum growth and development of the child.

Definition: risk for impaired Parenting: Vulnerable to inability of the primary caretaker to create, maintain, or regain an environment that promotes the optimum growth and development of the child, which may compromise the well-being of the child.

Related and Risk Factors

Infant or Child

Prematurity; multiple births; gender other than desired

Chronic illness; parent-child separation/prolonged separation from parent

Difficult temperament; temperament conflicts with parental expectations

Disabling condition; developmental delay; alteration in perceptual abilities; behavior disorder (e.g., attention deficit, oppositional defiant)

Knowledge

Insufficient knowledge about child development/health maintenance or parenting skills; insufficient response to infant cues

Unrealistic expectations

Low educational level; alteration in cognitive functioning; insufficient cognitive readiness for parenting

Ineffective communication skills

Preference for physical punishment

Physiological

Physical illness

Psychological

Young parental age

Insufficient prenatal care; difficult birthing process; high number of/closely spaced pregnancies

---

Information that appears in brackets has been added by the authors to clarify and enhance the use of nursing diagnoses.

Sleep deprivation/nonrestorative sleep pattern (i.e., due to caregiver responsibilities, parenting practices, sleep partner)
Depression; history of mental illness or substance abuse
Disabling condition

Social

Stressors work difficulty; unemployment; relocation; compromised home environment
Low self-esteem
Insufficient family cohesiveness; conflict between partners; change in family unit; inadequate child-care arrangements
Single parent; father or mother of child not involved/parent-child separation
Insufficient parental role model; insufficient valuing of parenthood/inability to put child's needs before own
Unplanned or unwanted pregnancy/insufficient or late-term prenatal care
Economically disadvantaged; insufficient resources (e.g., financial, social, knowledge); insufficient transportation
Insufficient problem-solving skills; ineffective coping strategies
Insufficient social support; social isolation
History of abuse (e.g., physical. psychological, sexual), or being abusive; legal difficulty

NOTE: A risk diagnosis is not evidenced by signs and symptoms, as the problem has not occurred; rather, nursing interventions are directed at prevention.

Defining Characteristics (impaired Parenting)

Subjective

Parental

Perceived inability to meet child's needs
Speaks negatively about child
Frustration with child; perceived role inadequacy

Objective

Infant or Child

Frequent accidents or illness; failure to thrive
Low academic performance; delay in cognitive development

Information that appears in brackets has been added by the authors to clarify and enhance the use of nursing diagnoses.

Impaired social functioning; behavior disorder (e.g., attention deficit, oppositional defiant)
History of trauma/abuse (e.g., physical, psychological, sexual)
Insufficient attachment behavior; diminished separation anxiety; runaway

Parental

Deficient parental-child interaction; decrease in cuddling
Inadequate child health maintenance; unsafe home environment; inappropriate child care arrangements; inappropriate stimulation (e.g., visual, tactile, auditory)
Inappropriate care-taking skills; inconsistent care/behavior management
Inflexibility in meeting needs of child
Punitive; rejection of child; hostility; history of child abuse (e.g., physical, psychological, sexual); neglects needs of child; abandonment

Desired Outcomes/Evaluation Criteria—Parents Will:

- Verbalize awareness of individual risk factors.
- Verbalize realistic information and expectations of parenting role.
- Verbalize acceptance of the individual situation.
- Demonstrate behavior and lifestyle changes to reduce potential for development of problem or reduce or eliminate effects of risk factors.
- Identify own strengths, individual needs, and methods and resources to meet them.
- Demonstrate appropriate attachment and parenting behaviors.

Actions/Interventions

Nursing Priority No. 1.

To assess causative/contributing **or risk** factors:

- Note family constellation; for example, two-parent, single, extended family, or child living with other relative, such as grandparent. **Helps identify problem areas and strengths to formulate plans to change situation that is currently creating difficulties for the parents.**
- Determine developmental stage of the family (e.g., new baby, adolescent, child leaving or returning home). **These maturational crises bring changes in the family that can be stressful to parents and the family. Provides direction for improving parenting skills and family interactions.**

Information that appears in brackets has been added by the authors to clarify and enhance the use of nursing diagnoses.

- Assess family relationships between individual members and with others.
- Assess parenting skill level, taking into account the individual's intellectual, emotional, and physical strengths and weaknesses. **Parents with significant impairments may need more education and support. Ineffective parenting and unrealistic expectations contribute to problems of abuse and neglect.**
- Observe attachment behaviors between parental figure and child. Determine cultural significance of behaviors. **Failure to bond effectively is thought to affect subsequent parent-child interaction. Behaviors such as eye-to-eye contact, use of en face position, talking to the infant in a high-pitched voice, are indicative of attachment behaviors in American culture but may not be appropriate in another culture.**
- Note presence of factors in the child (e.g., birth defects, hyperactivity) **that may affect attachment and caretaking needs.**
- Identify physical challenges or limitations of the parents (e.g., visual or hearing impairment, quadriplegia, severe depression). **May affect ability to care for child and suggest individual needs for assistance and support.**
- Determine presence and effectiveness of support systems, role models, extended family, and community resources available to the parent(s). **Lack of or ineffective use of support systems increases risk of continued inability to parent effectively.**
- Note absence from home setting or lack of child supervision by parent. **Demands of working long hours, out of town, multiple responsibilities such as working and attending educational classes will affect relationship between parent and child and ability to provide the care and nurturing necessary for children to grow and prosper.**

Nursing Priority No. 2.

To foster development of parenting skills:

- Create an environment in which relationships can be developed and needs of each individual met. **Learning is more effective when individuals feel safe.**
- Make time for listening to concerns of the parent(s).
- Emphasize positive aspects of the situation, maintaining a hopeful attitude toward the parent's capabilities and potential for improving the situation.
- Note staff attitudes toward parent/child and specific problem or disability; for example, needs of disabled parent(s) to be

---

Information that appears in brackets has been added by the authors to clarify and enhance the use of nursing diagnoses.

seen as an individual and to be evaluated apart from a stereotype. **Negative attitudes are detrimental to promoting positive outcomes.**

- Encourage expression of feelings, such as helplessness, anger, frustration. Set limits on unacceptable behaviors. **Individuals who lose control develop feelings of low self-esteem.**
- Acknowledge difficulty of situation and normalcy of feelings. **Enhances feelings of acceptance.**
- ∞ Allow time for parents to express feelings and deal with the "loss." Recognize stages of grieving process when the child is disabled or other than anticipated. **Expectation of a "normal" or desired child (e.g., having a girl instead of boy, child with a prominent birthmark or birth defect such as cleft palate) results in grieving for the loss of that expectation.**
- Encourage attendance at skill classes (e.g., parent effectiveness). **Assists in improving parenting skills by developing communication and problem-solving techniques.**
- Emphasize parenting functions rather than mothering/fathering skills. **By virtue of gender, each person brings something to the parenting role; however, nurturing tasks can be done by both parents.**

Nursing Priority No. 3.

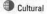

To promote wellness (Teaching/Discharge Considerations):

- Involve all available members of the family in learning.
- Provide information appropriate to the situation, including time management, limit setting, and stress-reduction techniques. **Facilitates satisfactory implementation of plan and new behaviors.**
- Discuss parental beliefs about childrearing, punishment and rewards, teaching. **Identifying these beliefs allows opportunity to provide new information regarding not using spanking and/or yelling and what actions can be substituted for more effective parenting.**
- Develop support systems appropriate to the situation. **Extended family, friends, social worker, home-care services may be needed to help parents cope positively with what is happening.**
- Assist parent to plan time and conserve energy in positive ways. **Enables individual to cope more effectively with difficulties as they arise.**
- Encourage parents to identify positive outlets for meeting their own needs (e.g., going out for dinner, making time for their own interests and each other, dating). **Promotes general**

Information that appears in brackets has been added by the authors to clarify and enhance the use of nursing diagnoses.

well-being, helps parents to be more effective and reduces burnout.

- Refer to appropriate support or therapy groups, as indicated.
- Identify community resources (e.g., childcare services, respite house) **to assist with individual needs, provide respite and support.**
- Report and take necessary actions, as legally and professionally indicated, if child's safety is a concern. **Parents/caregivers who engage in corporal punishment as a technique to ensure desired behavior of child are at increased risk for abusive behavior and possibility of childhood depression.**
- Refer to NDs ineffective Coping; compromised family Coping; risk for Violence [specify]; Self-Esteem [specify]; and interrupted Family Processes, for additional interventions as appropriate.

Documentation Focus

Assessment/Reassessment

- Individual findings, including parenting skill level, deviations from normal parenting expectations, family makeup, and developmental stages
- Availability and use of support systems and community resources

Planning

- Plan of care and who is involved in planning
- Teaching plan

Implementation/Evaluation

- Responses by parent(s)/child to interventions, teaching, and actions performed
- Attainment or progress toward desired outcome(s)
- Modification to plan of care

Discharge Planning

- Long-term needs and who is responsible for actions to be taken
- Specific referrals made

Sample Nursing Outcomes & Interventions Classifications (NOC/NIC)

NOC—Parenting Performance
NIC—Parenting Promotion

Information that appears in brackets has been added by the authors to clarify and enhance the use of nursing diagnoses.

readiness for enhanced **PARENTING**

[Diagnostic Division: Social Interaction]

Definition: A pattern of providing an environment for children or other dependent person(s) to nurture growth and development, which can be strengthened.

Defining Characteristics

Subjective

Expresses desire to enhance parenting
Parent expresses desire to enhance emotional support of children/other dependent person
Children express desire to enhance home environment

Desired Outcomes/Evaluation Criteria—Parents Will:

- Verbalize realistic information and expectations of parenting role.
- Identify own strengths, individual needs, and methods and resources to meet them.
- Participate in activities to enhance parenting skills.
- Demonstrate improved parenting behaviors.

Actions/Interventions

Nursing Priority No. 1.

To determine need/motivation for improvement:

- Ascertain motivation and expectation for change.
- Note family constellation: two parent; single parent; extended family; child living with other relative, such as grandparent; or relationship of dependent person. **Understanding makeup of the family provides information about needs to assist individuals in improving their family connections.**
- Determine developmental stage of the family (e.g., new child, adolescent, child leaving/returning home, retirement). **These maturational crises bring changes in the family, which can provide opportunity for enhancing parenting skills and improving family interactions.**
- Assess family relationships and identify needs of individual members, noting any special concerns that exist, such as birth defects, illness, hyperactivity. **The family is a system, and when members make decisions to improve parenting**

Information that appears in brackets has been added by the authors to clarify and enhance the use of nursing diagnoses.

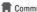

skills, the changes affect all parts of the system. Identifying needs, special situations, and relationships can help in the development of a plan to bring about effective change.

- Assess parenting skill level, taking into account the individual's intellectual, emotional, and physical strengths and weaknesses. **Identifies areas of need for education, skill training, and information on which to base plan for enhancing parenting skills.**
- Observe attachment behaviors between parent(s) and child(ren), recognizing cultural backgrounds that may influence expected behaviors. **Behaviors such as eye-to-eye contact, use of en face position, talking to infant in high-pitched voice, are indicative of attachment behaviors in American culture, but may not be appropriate in another culture. Failure to bond is thought to affect subsequent parent-child interactions.**
- Determine presence and effectiveness of support systems, role models, extended family, and community resources available to the parent(s). **Parents desiring to enhance abilities and improve family life can benefit by role models that help them develop their own style of parenting.**
- Note cultural or religious influences on parenting, expectations of self and child, sense of success or failure. **Expectations may vary with different cultures (e.g., Arab Americans hold children to be sacred, but childrearing is based on negative rather than positive reinforcements and parents are more strict with girls than with boys). These beliefs may interfere with desire to improve parenting skills when there is conflict between the two.**

Nursing Priority No. 2.

To foster improvement of parenting skills:

- Create an environment in which relationships can be strengthened. **A safe environment in which individuals can freely express their thoughts and feelings optimizes learning and positive interactions among family members, thus enhancing relationships.**
- Make time for listening to concerns of the parent(s). **Promotes sense of importance and of being heard and identifies accurate information regarding needs of the family for enhancing relationships.**
- Encourage expression of feelings, such as frustration or anger, while setting limits on unacceptable behaviors. **Identification of feelings promotes understanding of self and enhances connections with others in the family. Unacceptable be-**

Information that appears in brackets has been added by the authors to clarify and enhance the use of nursing diagnoses.

haviors result in diminished self-esteem and can lead to problems in the family relationships.

- Emphasize parenting functions rather than mothering/fathering skills. **By virtue of gender, each person brings something to the parenting role; however, nurturing tasks can be done by both parents, enhancing family relationships.**
- Encourage attendance at skill classes, such as Parent or Family Effectiveness Training. **Assists in developing communication skills of active-listening, I-messages, and problem-solving techniques to improve family relationships and promote a win-win environment.**

Nursing Priority No. 3.

To promote optimal wellness:

- Involve all members of the family in learning. **The family system benefits from all members participating in learning new skills to enhance family relationships.**
- Encourage parents to identify positive outlets for meeting their own needs. **Activities, such as going out for dinner or dating, making time for their own interests and each other, promote general well-being and can enhance family relationships and improve family functioning.**
- Provide information, as indicated, including time management, stress-reduction techniques. **Learning about positive parenting skills, understanding growth and developmental expectations, and discovering ways to reduce stress and anxiety promote the individual's ability to deal with problems that may arise in the course of family relationships.**
- Discuss current "family rules," identifying areas of needed change. **Rules may be imposed by adults, rather than through a democratic process involving all family members, leading to conflict and angry confrontations. Setting positive family rules with all family members participating can promote an effective, functional family.**
- Discuss need for long-term planning and ways in which family can maintain desired positive relationships. **Each stage of life brings its own challenges and understanding, and preparing for each stage enables family members to move through them in positive ways, promoting family unity and resolving inevitable conflicts with win-win solutions.**

Information that appears in brackets has been added by the authors to clarify and enhance the use of nursing diagnoses.

Documentation Focus

Assessment/Reassessment

- Individual findings, including parenting skill level, parenting expectations, family makeup, and developmental stages
- Availability and use of support systems and community resources
- Motivation and expectations for change

Planning

- Plan for enhancement, who is involved in planning
- Teaching plan

Implementation/Evaluation

- Family members' responses to interventions, teaching, and actions performed
- Attainment or progress toward desired outcome(s)
- Modifications to plan

Discharge Planning

- Long-term needs and who is responsible for actions to be taken
- Modification to plan

Sample Nursing Outcomes & Interventions Classifications (NOC/NIC)

NOC—Parenting Performance
NIC—Parent Education: Childrearing Family

disturbed PERSONAL IDENTITY and risk for disturbed PERSONAL IDENTITY

[Diagnostic Division: Ego Integrity]

Definition: disturbed Personal Identity: Inability to maintain an integrated and complete perception of self.

Definition: risk for disturbed Personal Identity: Vulnerable to the inability to maintain an integrated and complete perception of self, which may compromise health.

Information that appears in brackets has been added by the authors to clarify and enhance the use of nursing diagnoses.

Related and Risk Factors

Low self-esteem; dysfunctional family processes
Situational crisis; stages of growth; developmental transition; alteration in social role
Exposure to toxic chemical; pharmaceutical agent
Cultural incongruence; discrimination; perceived prejudice
Manic states; psychiatric disorder; dissociative identity disorder; organic brain disorder
Cult indoctrination

NOTE: A risk diagnosis is not evidenced by signs and symptoms as the problem has not occurred; rather, nursing actions are directed at prevention.

Defining Characteristics (disturbed Personal Identity)

Subjective

Alteration in body image; delusional description of self
Fluctuating feelings about self; feeling of strangeness, emptiness
Confusion about goals, cultural values, or ideological values
Gender confusion
Inability to distinguish between internal and external stimuli

Objective

Inconsistent behavior
Ineffective relationships
Ineffective coping or role performance

Desired Outcomes/Evaluation Criteria—Client Will:

- Acknowledge concern about potential threat to identity.
- Acknowledge perceived or actual threat to personal identity.
- Integrate threat in a healthy, positive manner (e.g., states anxiety is reduced, accepts self in current situation, makes plans for the future).
- Verbalize acceptance of changes that have occurred.
- Use effective coping strategies to deal with situation/stressors.
- State ability to identify and accept self (long-term outcome).

Information that appears in brackets has been added by the authors to clarify and enhance the use of nursing diagnoses.

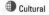

Actions/Interventions

Nursing Priority No. 1.

To assess causative/contributing **or risk** factors:

- Ascertain client's perception of the extent of the threat to self and how client is handling the situation. **Many factors can affect an individual's self-image: illness (chronic or terminal); injuries, changes in body structure (e.g., amputation, spinal cord damage, burns), and client's view of what has happened will affect development of plan of care and interventions to be used.**
- Determine speed of occurrence of threat. **An event that has happened quickly may be more threatening (e.g., a traumatic event resulting in change in body image).**
- Ask client to define own body image. **Body image is the basis of personal identity, and client's perception will affect how changes are viewed, may prevent achievement of ideals and expectations, and have a negative effect.**
- Determine whether issues of gender identity are a concern. **Client may have conflicting feelings about how to deal with realization they are homosexual or transsexual.**
- Note age of client. **An adolescent may struggle with the developmental task of personal or sexual identity, whereas an older person may have more difficulty accepting or dealing with a threat to identity, such as progressive loss of memory.**
- Identify cultural affiliations/discontinuity. **Individuals belonging to subcultures or cults tend to come into conflict with the greater societal views, affecting one's perception of self and perception of reality.**
- Assess availability and use of support systems. Note response of family/significant other (SO)(s). **During stressful situations, support is essential for client to cope with changes that are occurring. Engaging family in choosing supportive interventions will help client and family members deal with situation or illness.**
- Note withdrawn or automatic behavior, regression to earlier developmental stage, general behavioral disorganization, or display of self-mutilation behaviors in adolescent or adult; delayed development, preference for solitary play, unusual display of self-stimulation in child. **Indicators of poor coping skills and need for specific interventions to help client develop sense of self and identity.**

Information that appears in brackets has been added by the authors to clarify and enhance the use of nursing diagnoses.

- Be aware of physical signs of panic state. **Severe anxiety state may progress to panic when concerns seem overwhelming to client.** (Refer to ND Anxiety.)
- Discuss use of alcohol, other drugs. **Individuals often use these substances to avoid painful stressors.**
- Note signs of anxiety. **Use of inadequate coping strategies to deal with changes affecting lifestyle may result in exacerbation of symptoms in anxious person.** (Refer to ND Anxiety [specify level].)
- Determine distortions of reality/symptoms of mental illness. **Requires more in-depth psychological counseling/medication to help client distinguish between self and non-self.**

Nursing Priority No. 2.

To assist client to manage/deal with stressors:

- Make time to listen/active-listen client, encouraging appropriate expression of feelings, including anger and hostility. **Conveys a sense of confidence in client's ability to identify extent of threat, how it is affecting sense of identity, and how to deal with feelings in acceptable way.**
- Discuss client's concerns without confronting unreal ideas. **Irrational beliefs may interfere with ability to manage situation and maintain reality-based perception of self.**
- Provide calm environment. **Helps client to remain calm and able to discuss important issues related to the identity crisis.**
- Use crisis intervention principles as needed **to restore equilibrium when possible.**
- Discuss client's commitment to an identity. **Those who have made a strong commitment to an identity tend to be more comfortable with self and happier than those who have not.**
- Assist client to develop strategies to cope with threat to identity. **Helps reduce anxiety and promotes self-awareness and self-esteem.**
- Engage client in activities to help in identifying self as an individual (e.g., use of mirror for visual feedback, tactile stimulation).
- Provide for simple decisions, concrete tasks, calming activities.
- Allow client to deal with situation in small steps. **May be unable to cope with larger picture when in stress overload.**
- Encourage client to develop and participate in an individualized exercise program (walking is an excellent beginning). **Exercise releases endorphins, thereby reducing stress and anxiety, promoting a sense of well-being.**

Information that appears in brackets has been added by the authors to clarify and enhance the use of nursing diagnoses.

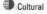

- Provide concrete assistance, as needed (e.g., help with activities of daily living, preparing food).
- Take advantage of opportunities to promote growth. Realize that client will have difficulty learning while in a dissociative state.
- Maintain reality orientation without confronting client's irrational beliefs. **Client may become defensive, blocking opportunity to look at other possibilities.**
- Use humor judiciously, when appropriate. **While humor can lift spirits and provide a moment of levity, it is important to note the mood or receptiveness of the client before using it.**
- Discuss options for dealing with issues of gender identity. **Identification of client's concerns about role dysfunction or conflicting feelings about sexual identity will indicate need for therapies, or possible gender-change surgery.**
- Refer to NDs disturbed Body Image; Self-Esteem [specify]; Spiritual Distress.

Nursing Priority No. 3.

To promote wellness (Teaching/Discharge Considerations):

- Provide accurate information about threat to and potential consequences for individual. **Helps client to make positive decisions for future.**
- Discuss potential changes in lifestyle that may occur with major diagnosis/accident. **Planning for these possibilities can enhance self-confidence and allow client to move forward with life.**
- Refer to appropriate support groups. **Sharing concerns with others in group settings may help client to be realistic regarding concerns about effects of anticipated changes/life challenges.**
- Explore community resources as appropriate. **Additional assistance such as day programs, individual/family counseling, drug/alcohol cessation programs can strengthen client's coping abilities and sense of control.**

Documentation Focus

Assessment/Reassessment

- Findings, noting degree of impairment or possible changes in lifestyle, and future expectations
- Nature of and client's perception of threat or potential threat
- Degree of commitment to own identity

Planning

- Plan of care and who is involved in the planning
- Teaching plan

Information that appears in brackets has been added by the authors to clarify and enhance the use of nursing diagnoses.

Implementation/Evaluation

- Client's response to interventions/teaching and actions performed
- Attainment or progress toward desired outcome(s)
- Modifications to plan of care

Discharge Planning

- Long-term needs and who is responsible for actions to be taken
- Specific referrals made

Sample Nursing Outcomes & Interventions Classifications (NOC/NIC)

NOC—Identity
NIC—Self-Esteem Enhancement

risk for POISONING

[Diagnostic Division: Safety]

Definition: Vulnerable to accidental exposure to, or ingestion of, drugs or dangerous products in sufficient doses that may compromise health.

Risk Factors

Internal

Alteration in cognitive functioning
Emotional disturbance
Inadequate precautions against poisoning; inadequate knowledge of poisoning prevention
Inadequate knowledge of pharmacological agents; [narrow therapeutic margin of safety of specific pharmaceutical agents (e.g., therapeutic versus toxic level, half-life, method of uptake and degradation in body, adequacy of organ function)]
Occupational setting without adequate safeguards
Reduced vision
[Cultural or religious beliefs or practices]

External

Access to dangerous product
Access to pharmaceutical agent; access to large supply of pharmaceutical agents in house

Information that appears in brackets has been added by the authors to clarify and enhance the use of nursing diagnoses.

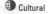

Access to illicit drugs potentially contaminated by poisonous additives
[Use of multiple herbal supplements or megadosing]

NOTE: A risk diagnosis is not evidenced by signs and symptoms, as the problem has not occurred; rather, nursing interventions are directed at prevention.

Desired Outcomes/Evaluation Criteria—Client/Caregiver Will:

- Verbalize understanding of dangers of poisoning.
- Identify hazards that could lead to accidental poisoning.
- Correct external hazards as identified.
- Demonstrate necessary actions/lifestyle changes to promote safe environment.

Refer to NDs Contamination; risk for Contamination, for additional interventions related to poisoning associated with environmental contaminants.

Actions/Interventions

Nursing Priority No. 1.

To assess causative/contributing factors:

- Identify internal and external risk factors in client's environment, including presence of infants, young children, or frail elderly **(who are at risk for accidental poisoning)** and teenagers or young adults **(who are at risk for medication experimentation);** confused or chronically ill person on multiple medications; person with potential for suicidal action; person who partakes in illicit drug use/dealing (e.g., marijuana, cocaine, heroin); person who manufactures drugs in home (e.g., methamphetamines).
- Note client's age, gender, socioeconomic status, developmental stage, decision-making ability, level of cognition and competence. **Affects client's ability to protect self/others and influences choice of interventions/teaching.**
- Determine client's allergies to medications and foods **in order to avoid exposure to substances causing potentially lethal reaction.**
- Assess mood, coping abilities, personality styles (e.g., temperament, impulsive behavior, level of self-esteem) **that may result in carelessness/increased risk taking without consideration of consequences.**

Information that appears in brackets has been added by the authors to clarify and enhance the use of nursing diagnoses.

- Assess client's knowledge of safe use of drugs/herbal supplements, safety hazards in the environment, and ability to respond to potential threat. **People may believe "if a little is good, a lot is better," placing them at risk for overdose, adverse drug effects, or interactions. Knowledge and use also affect the client's storage (e.g., may not use labeled bottles) and/or taking of medications that look alike (potentiating risk of overdose or adverse drug interactions). The elderly may unintentionally take the wrong medication at the wrong time or "double up," forgetting that they already took their daily dose of a prescription medicine.**
- Evaluate for alcohol/other drug use/abuse (e.g., cocaine, methamphetamine, lysergic acid diethylamide [LSD], methadone). **These substances have potential for adverse reactions, cumulative affects with other substances, and risk for intentional and accidental overdose.**
- Identify environmental hazards:

  Storage of household chemicals (e.g., oven, toilet bowl, or drain cleaners; dishwasher products; bleach; hydrogen peroxide; fluoride preparations; essential oils; furniture polish; lighter fluid; lamp oil; kerosene; paints; turpentine; rust remover; lubricant oils; bug sprays or powders; fertilizers). **These are all readily available toxins in various forms that are often improperly stored.**

  Review client's home, employment, or work environment **for exposure to chemicals, including vapors and fumes.**

  Refer to ND risk for Contamination for environmental issues.

- Review results of laboratory tests and toxicology screening, as indicated.

Nursing Priority No. 2.

To assist in correcting factors that can lead to accidental poisoning:

- Discuss medication safety with client/SO(s) **to prevent accidental poisoning:**

  Stress importance of supervising infant, child, frail elderly, or individuals with cognitive limitations.

  Keep medicines and vitamins out of sight or reach of children or cognitively impaired persons.

  Use child-resistant or tamper-resistant caps and lock medication cabinets.

  Recap medication containers immediately after obtaining current dosage. Do not leave open container out.

  Code medicines for the visually impaired.

Information that appears in brackets has been added by the authors to clarify and enhance the use of nursing diagnoses.

- Administer children's medications as drugs, not candy.
- Prevent duplication or possible overdose:

  Keep updated list of all medications (prescription, over the counter [OTC], herbals, supplements) and review with healthcare providers when medications are changed, new ones added, or new healthcare providers are consulted.

  Keep prescription medication in original bottle with label. Do not mix with other medication/place in unmarked containers.

  Have responsible SO(s)/home health nurse supervise medication regimen/prepare medications for the cognitively or visually impaired or obtain prefilled medication box from pharmacy.

  Take prescription medications, as prescribed on label.

  Do not adjust medication dosage.

  Retain and read safety information that accompanies prescriptions about expected effects, minor side effects, reportable or adverse affects that require medical intervention, and how to manage forgotten dose.

- Prevent taking medications that interact with one another or OTCs, herbals, or other supplements in an undesired or dangerous manner:

  Keep list of and reveal medication allergies, including type of reaction, to healthcare providers/pharmacist.

  Wear medical alert bracelet or necklace, as appropriate.

  Do not take outdated or expired medications. Do not save partial prescriptions to use another time.

  Encourage discarding outdated or unused drug safely (disposing in hazardous waste collection areas, not down drain or toilet).

  Do not take medications prescribed for another person.

  Coordinate care when multiple healthcare providers are involved to limit number of prescriptions and dosage levels.

Nursing Priority No. 3.

To promote wellness (Teaching/Discharge Considerations):

- Discuss general poison prevention measures:
- Encourage parent/caregiver to place safety stickers on dangerous products (drugs and chemicals) **to warn children of harmful contents.**
- Teach children about hazards of poisonous substances and to "ask first" before eating or drinking anything.
- Review drug side effects, potential interactions, and possibilities of misuse or overdosing (as with vitamin megadosing, etc.).

Information that appears in brackets has been added by the authors to clarify and enhance the use of nursing diagnoses.

- Discuss issues regarding drug use in home (e.g., alcohol, marijuana, heroin) **to provide opportunity to address potential for client's/SO's accidental overdose or accidental ingestion by children when drugs or drug paraphernalia are in the home.**
- Refer substance abuser to detoxification programs, inpatient/outpatient rehabilitation, counseling, support groups, psychotherapy.
- Provide list of emergency numbers (i.e., local or national poison control numbers, physician's office) to be placed by telephone **for use if poisoning occurs.**
- Encourage client to obtain regular screening tests at prescribed intervals (e.g., prothrombin time/international normalized ratio [INR] for Coumadin; drug levels for Dilantin, digoxin; liver function studies when lipid-lowering agents [statins] are prescribed; or renal and thyroid function and serum glucose levels for antimanics [lithium] use) **to ascertain that circulating blood levels are within therapeutic range and absence of adverse effects.**
- Encourage participation in community awareness and education programs (e.g., CPR and First Aid class, home and workplace safety, hazardous materials disposal, access to emergency medical personnel) **to assist individuals to identify and correct risk factors in environment and be prepared for emergency situation.**
- Discuss vitamins (especially those containing iron) that can be poisonous or lethal to children.
- Review common analgesic safety (e.g., acetaminophen is an ingredient in many OTC medications, and unintentional overdose can occur).
- Discuss use of ipecac syrup in home. **The use of ipecac is controversial, as it may delay appropriate medical treatment (e.g., reduce the effectiveness of activated charcoal or oral antidotes) or be used inappropriately with adverse effects. Therefore, use in the home without direct advice from poison control professionals is not recommended.**
- Refer substance abuser to detoxification programs, inpatient/outpatient rehabilitation, counseling, support groups, and psychotherapy as appropriate.
- Encourage emergency measures, awareness, and education (e.g., CPR/First Aid class, community safety programs, ways to access emergency medical personnel) **to assist individuals to identify and correct risk factors in environment and be prepared for emergency situation.**

Information that appears in brackets has been added by the authors to clarify and enhance the use of nursing diagnoses.

Documentation Focus

Assessment/Reassessment

- Identified risk factors noting internal and external concerns
- Drug allergies or sensitivities
- Current medications prescribed or available to individual, use of OTC medications, herbals or supplements, illicit drug use

Planning

- Plan of care and who is involved in the planning
- Teaching plan

Implementation/Evaluation

- Response to interventions, teaching, and actions performed
- Attainment or progress toward desired outcome(s)
- Modification to plan of care

Discharge Planning

- Long-term needs and who is responsible for actions to be taken
- Specific referrals made

Sample Nursing Outcomes & Interventions Classifications (NOC/NIC)

NOC—Knowledge: Medication
NIC—Medication Management

risk for perioperative POSITIONING INJURY

[Diagnostic Division: Safety]

Definition: Vulnerable to inadvertent anatomical and physical changes as a result of posture or equipment used during an invasive/surgical procedure, which may compromise health.

Risk Factors

Disorientation; sensory/perceptual disturbances from anesthesia
Immobilization; muscle weakness; [preexisting musculoskeletal conditions]
Obesity; emaciation; edema

Information that appears in brackets has been added by the authors to clarify and enhance the use of nursing diagnoses.

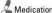

NOTE: A risk diagnosis is not evidenced by signs and symptoms, as the problem has not occurred; rather, nursing interventions are directed at prevention.

Desired Outcomes/Evaluation Criteria—Client Will:

- Be free of injury related to perioperative disorientation or altered consciousness.
- Be free of untoward skin and tissue injury or changes lasting beyond 24 to 48 hours postprocedure.

Actions/Interventions

Nursing Priority No. 1.

To identify individual risk factors/needs:

- Review client's history, noting age, weight and height, nutritional status, physical limitations or preexisting conditions (e.g., elderly person with arthritis; extremes of weight; diabetes or other conditions affecting peripheral vascular health; nutrition and hydration impairments). **Affects choice of perioperative positioning and affects skin and tissue integrity during surgery.**
- Evaluate and document client's preoperative reports of neurological, sensory, or motor deficits **for comparative baseline of perioperative and postoperative sensations.**
- Note anticipated length of procedure and customary position **to increase awareness of potential postoperative complications (e.g., supine position may cause low back pain and skin pressure at heels, elbows, and sacrum; lateral chest position can cause shoulder and neck pain, or eye and ear injury on the client's downside).**
- Evaluate environmental conditions/safety issues surrounding the sedated client (e.g., client alone in holding area, side rails up on bed and cart, use of tourniquets and arm boards, need for local injections) **that predispose client to potential tissue injury.**
- Assess the individual's responses to preoperative sedation/medication, noting level of sedation and/or adverse effects (e.g., drop in blood pressure) and report to surgeon, as indicated. **Hypotension is a common factor associated with nerve ischemia.**

Information that appears in brackets has been added by the authors to clarify and enhance the use of nursing diagnoses.

Nursing Priority No. 2.

To position client to provide protection for anatomical structures and to prevent client injury:

- Stabilize and lock cart or bed in place; support client's body and limbs; use adequate number of personnel during transfer **to prevent client fall or shear and friction injuries.**
- Place safety strap strategically to secure client for specific procedure **to prevent unintended movement.**
- Protect body from contact with metal parts of the operating table, **which could produce burns or electric shock injury.**
- Prevent pooling of prep and irrigating solutions, and body fluids. **Pooling of liquids in areas of high pressure under client increases risk of pressure ulcer development and presents electrical hazard.**
- Maintain body alignment as much as possible using pillows, padding, and safety straps **to reduce potential for neurovascular complications associated with compression, overstretching, or ischemia of nerve(s).**
- Ascertain that eyelids are closed and secured **to prevent corneal abrasions.**
- Apply and periodically reposition padding of pressure points and bony prominences (e.g., arms, elbows, sacrum, ankles, heels) and neurovascular pressure points (e.g., breasts, knees) **to maintain position of safety, especially when repositioning client and/or table attachments.**
- Check peripheral pulses and skin color and temperature periodically **to monitor circulation.**
- Reposition slowly at transfer and in bed (especially halothane-anesthetized client) **to prevent severe drop in blood pressure, dizziness, or unsafe transfer.**
- Protect airway and facilitate respiratory effort following extubation.
- Determine specific position reflecting procedure guidelines (e.g., head of bed elevated following spinal anesthesia, **to prevent headache;** turn to unoperated side following pneumonectomy) **to facilitate maximal respiratory effort.**

Nursing Priority No. 3.

To promote wellness (Teaching/Discharge Considerations):

- Maintain equipment in good working order **to identify potential hazards in the surgical suite and implement corrections as appropriate.**

Information that appears in brackets has been added by the authors to clarify and enhance the use of nursing diagnoses.

- Provide perioperative teaching relative to client safety issues, including not crossing legs during procedures performed under local or light anesthesia, postoperative needs and limitations, and signs/symptoms requiring medical evaluation **to reduce incidence of preventable complications.**
- Inform client and postoperative caregivers of expected/transient reactions (such as low backache, localized numbness, and reddening or skin indentations, all of which should disappear in 24 hr).
- Assist with therapies and perform routine nursing actions, including skin care measures, application of elastic stockings, early mobilization **to enhance circulation and promote skin and tissue integrity.**
- Encourage and assist with frequent range-of-motion exercises, especially when joint stiffness occurs.
- Refer to appropriate resources, as needed.

Documentation Focus

Assessment/Reassessment

- Findings, including individual risk factors for problems in the perioperative setting or need to modify routine activities or positions
- Periodic evaluation of monitoring activities

Planning

- Plan of care and who is involved in planning
- Teaching plan

Implementation/Evaluation

- Response to interventions and actions performed
- Attainment or progress toward desired outcome(s)
- Modifications to plan of care

Discharge Planning

- Long-term needs and who is responsible for actions to be taken

Sample Nursing Outcomes & Interventions Classifications (NOC/NIC)

NOC—Risk Control
NIC—Positioning: Intraoperative

Information that appears in brackets has been added by the authors to clarify and enhance the use of nursing diagnoses.

POST-TRAUMA SYNDROME and risk for POST-TRAUMA SYNDROME

[Diagnostic Division: Ego Integrity]

Definition: Post-Trauma Syndrome: Sustained maladaptive response to a traumatic, overwhelming event.

Definition: risk for Post-Trauma Syndrome: Vulnerable to sustained maladaptive response to a traumatic, overwhelming event, which may compromise health.

Related Factors (Post-Trauma Syndrome)

Exposure to disaster (natural or man-made); destruction of one's home
Event outside the range of usual human experience; exposure to event involving multiple deaths;
Exposure to war; history of being a prisoner of war
History of abuse (e.g., physical, psychological, sexual); history of criminal victimization; history of torture; witnessing mutilation or violent death
Self-injurious behavior;
Serious accident (e.g., industrial, motor vehicle); serious injury to loved one
Serious threat to self or loved one

Risk Factors

Diminished ego strength; environment not conducive to needs; insufficient social support
Displacement from home
Duration of traumatic event; perceives event as traumatic; survival role
Exaggerated sense of responsibility
Human service occupations (e.g., police, fire, rescue, corrections, emergency room, mental health)

NOTE: A risk diagnosis is not evidenced by signs and symptoms, as the problem has not occurred; rather, nursing interventions are directed at prevention.

Information that appears in brackets has been added by the authors to clarify and enhance the use of nursing diagnoses.

Defining Characteristics (Post-Trauma Syndrome)

Subjective

Intrusive thoughts or dreams; nightmares; flashbacks; [excessive verbalization of the traumatic event]

Heart palpitations; headache; [loss of interest in usual activities, loss of feeling of intimacy or sexuality]

Hopelessness; shame; guilt; [verbalization of survival guilt or guilt about behavior required for survival]

Anxiety; fear; grieving; depression; horror

Reports feeling numb

Gastrointestinal irritation; [change in appetite]

Alteration in concentration

[Change in sleep; fatigue]

Objective

Alteration in mood; [poor impulse control or explosiveness]; panic attacks

Hypervigilance; exaggerated startle response; irritability; neurosensory irritability

Anger; rage; aggression

Avoidance behaviors; denial; repression; alienation;

History of detachment; dissociative amnesia

Substance abuse; compulsive behavior

Enuresis

[Difficulty with interpersonal relationships; dependence on others; work or school failure]

NOTE:
[Stages:
ACUTE: Begins within 6 months and does not last longer than 6 months
CHRONIC: Lasts more than 6 months
DELAYED ONSET: **Period of latency of 6 months or more before onset of symptoms]**

Desired Outcomes/Evaluation Criteria—Client Will:

- Express own feelings or reactions, avoiding projection.
- Verbalize a positive self-image.
- Report absence of severe anxiety; or reduced anxiety or fear when memories occur.
- Demonstrate ability to deal with emotional reactions in an individually appropriate manner.

Information that appears in brackets has been added by the authors to clarify and enhance the use of nursing diagnoses.

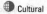

- Demonstrate appropriate changes in behavior and lifestyle (e.g., share experiences with others, seek or get support from significant others [SO(s)] as needed, change in job or residence).
- Report relief or absence of physical manifestations (pain, nightmares or flashbacks, fatigue) associated with event.

Actions/Interventions

Nursing Priority No. 1.

To assess causative **or risk** factor(s) and individual reaction:

Acute

- Identify client who survived or witnessed traumatic event (e.g., airplane or motor vehicle crash, mass shooting, fire destroying home and lands, robbery at gunpoint, other violent act) **to recognize individual at high risk for post-trauma syndrome.**
- Note occupation (e.g., police, fire, rescue, emergency department staff; corrections officer; mental health worker; disaster responders; soldier or support personnel in combat zone; as well as family members). **These occupations carry a high risk for constantly being involved in traumatic events and the potential for exacerbation of stress response and block to recovery.**
- Assess client's knowledge of and anxiety related to potential for work-related trauma (e.g., shooting in line of duty or viewing body of murdered child); and number, duration, and intensity of recurring situations (e.g., emergency medical technician [EMT] personnel exposed to numerous on-the-job traumatic incidents; rescuers searching for victims of natural or man-made disasters).
- Observe for and elicit information about physical or psychological injury and note associated stress-related symptoms (e.g., "numbness," headache, tightness in chest, nausea, pounding heart). **Anxiety is viewed as a normal reaction to a realistic danger or threat, and noting these factors can identify the severity of the anxiety the client is experiencing in the circumstances. In post-traumatic stress disorder (PTSD), this anxiety reaction is changed or damaged.**
- Identify psychological responses: anger, shock, acute anxiety, confusion, denial. Note laughter, crying, calm or agitated or excited (hysterical) behavior, expressions of disbelief, guilt or self-blame, labile emotions. **Indicators of severe response to trauma that client has experienced and need for specific interventions.**
- Assess client's knowledge of and anxiety related to the situation. Note ongoing threat to self (e.g., contact with perpetra-

---

Information that appears in brackets has been added by the authors to clarify and enhance the use of nursing diagnoses.

tor and/or associates). **Client may be aware but speak as though the incident is related to someone else. Flashbacks may occur with the individual reliving the incident/event.**

- Identify social aspects of trauma or incident (e.g., disfigurement, chronic conditions or permanent disabilities, loss of home or community) **that affect ability to return to normal involvement in activities and work.**
- Ascertain ethnic background and cultural or religious perceptions and beliefs about the occurrence. **Individual's view of how he or she is coping is influenced by cultural background, religious beliefs, and family influence. Client (or significant others) may believe occurrence is retribution from God or result of some indiscretion on client's part.**
- Determine degree of disorganization (e.g., task-oriented activity is not goal directed, organized, or effective; individual is overwhelmed by emotion most of the time). **Presence of persistent problems may interfere with ability to manage daily living, work, and relationships with others.**
- Identify how client's past experiences may affect current situation. **Individual who has had previous experiences with traumatic events may be more susceptible to PTSD and ineffective coping abilities.**
- Listen for comments of guilt, humiliation, shame, or taking on responsibility (e.g., "I should have been more careful/gone back to get her"; "Don't call me a hero, I couldn't save my partner"; "My kids are the same age as the ones that died").
- Evaluate for life factors or stressors currently or recently occurring, such as displacement from home due to catastrophic event (e.g., fire, flood, violent storm) happening to individual whose child is dying with cancer or who suffered abuse as a child. **This individual is at greater risk for developing traumatic symptoms (acute added to delayed-onset reactions).**
- Determine disruptions in relationships (e.g., family, friends, coworkers, SOs). **Support persons may not know how to deal with client/situation (e.g., may be oversolicitous or withdraw).**
- Note withdrawn behavior, use of denial, and use of chemical substances or impulsive behaviors (e.g., chain smoking, overeating), **which are indicators of severity of anxiety and client's coping responses.**
- Be aware of signs of increasing anxiety (e.g., silence, stuttering, inability to sit still). **Increasing anxiety may indicate risk for violence.**
- Note verbal and nonverbal expressions of guilt or self-blame when client has survived trauma in which others died. Vali-

Information that appears in brackets has been added by the authors to clarify and enhance the use of nursing diagnoses.

date congruency of observations with verbalizations. **Sense of own responsibility (blame) and guilt about not having done something to prevent incident or not having been "good enough" to deserve survival are strong beliefs, especially in individuals who are influenced by background, religious, and cultural factors.**

- Identify client's general health and coping mechanisms. **Resolution of the post-trauma response is largely dependent on the coping skills the client has developed throughout own life and is able to bring to bear on current situation.**
- Assess signs and stage of grieving for self and others.
- Identify development of phobic reactions to ordinary articles (e.g., knives); situations (e.g., walking in groups of people, strangers ringing doorbell). **These may trigger feelings from original trauma and need to be dealt with sensitively, accepting reality of feelings and stressing ability of client to deal with them.**

Chronic (In addition to previous assessment)

- Evaluate continued somatic complaints (e.g., gastric irritation, anorexia, insomnia, muscle tension, headache). Investigate reports of new or changes in symptoms.
- Note manifestations of chronic pain or pain symptoms in excess of degree of physical injury. **Psychological responses may magnify or exacerbate physical symptoms, indicating need for interventions to help client deal with pain.**
- Be aware of signs of severe or prolonged depression. Note presence of flashbacks, intrusive memories, nightmares; panic attacks; poor impulse control; problems with memory or concentration, thoughts, and perceptions; conflict, aggression, or rage. **Symptoms are not uncommon following a trauma of such magnitude, although client may feel that he or she is "going crazy."**
- Assess degree of dysfunctional coping (e.g., use or abuse of alcohol or other drugs; suicidal or homicidal ideation) and consequences. **Individuals display different levels of dysfunctional behavior in response to stress, and often the choice of chemical substances or substance abuse is a way of deadening psychic pain.**

Nursing Priority No. 2.

To assist client to deal with situation **or risk** that exists:

Acute

- Provide a calm, safe environment. **Promotes sense of trust and safety in which client can deal with disruption of life.**

Information that appears in brackets has been added by the authors to clarify and enhance the use of nursing diagnoses.

- Listen as client recounts incident or concerns—possibly repeatedly. (If client does not want to talk, accept silence.) **Provides psychological support.**
- Evaluate client's perceptions of events and personal significance (e.g., police officer—who is also a parent—investigating death of a child).
- Provide emotional and physical presence **to strengthen client's coping abilities.**
- Listen to and investigate physical complaints, and take note of lack of physical complaints when injury may have occurred. **Emotional reactions may limit client's ability to recognize or verbalize physical injury.**
- Identify supportive persons for the individual (e.g., loved ones, counselor, spiritual advisor or pastor).
- Provide environment in which client can talk freely about feelings and fears (including concerns about relationship with and response of SO) and trauma experiences and sensations (e.g., loss of control, "near-death experience").
- Be aware of and assist client to use ego strengths in a positive way by acknowledging ability to handle what is happening. **Enhances self-concept, supports self-esteem, and reduces sense of helplessness.**
- Help child express feelings about event using techniques appropriate to developmental level (e.g., play for young child, stories or puppets for preschooler, peer group for adolescent). **Children are more likely to express in play what they may not be able to verbalize directly. Adolescents may benefit from groups that help them gain knowledge, support, and a decreased sense of isolation.**
- Allow client to work through own kind of adjustment. If the client is withdrawn or unwilling to talk, do not force the issue.
- Listen for expressions of fear of crowds and/or people.
- Administer anti-anxiety, sedative, or hypnotic medications with caution.
- Assist in dealing with practical concerns and effects of the incident, such as documentation for police report, court appearances, altered relationships with SO(s), employment problems. **In the period immediately following the traumatic incident, thinking becomes difficult, and assistance with practical matters will help manage necessary activities for the person to move through this time.**

Chronic

- Continue listening to expressions of concern. **May have recurring thoughts, thus necessitating the need to continue talking about the incident.**

Information that appears in brackets has been added by the authors to clarify and enhance the use of nursing diagnoses.

- Permit free expression of feelings (may continue from the crisis phase). Avoid rushing client through expressions of feelings too quickly and refrain from providing reassurance inappropriately. **Client may believe pain and/or anguish is misunderstood and may be depressed. Statements such as "You don't understand" or "You weren't there" are a defense, a way of pushing others away.**
- Encourage client to talk out experience when ready, expressing feelings of fear, anger, loss, or grief. (Refer to NDs, Grieving, complicated Grieving.)
- Ascertain and monitor sleep pattern of children as well as adults. **Sleep disturbances and/or nightmares may develop, delaying resolution and/or impairing coping abilities.**
- Encourage client to become aware of and accept own feelings and reactions as being normal reactions in an abnormal situation.
- Acknowledge reality of loss of self that existed before the incident. Help client to move toward a state of acceptance as to the potential for growth that still exists within client. **Recognition that individual can never go back to being the person he or she was before the incident allows progress toward life as a different person.**
- Continue to allow client to progress at own pace.
- Give "permission" to express and deal with anger at the assailant or situation in acceptable ways.
- Avoid prompting discussion of issues that cannot be resolved. Keep discussion on practical and emotional level rather than intellectualizing the experience, **which allows client to deal with reality while taking time to work out feelings.**
- Provide for sensitive, trained counselors/therapists and engage in therapies, such as psychotherapy, Implosive Therapy (flooding), hypnosis, relaxation, Rolfing, memory work, cognitive restructuring, Eye Movement Desensitization and Reprocessing (EMDR), physical and occupational therapies.
- Administer psychotropic medications, as indicated.

Nursing Priority No. 3.

To promote wellness (Teaching/Discharge Considerations):

- Educate high-risk persons and families about signs/symptoms of post-trauma response, especially if it is likely to occur in their occupation/life.
- Encourage client to identify and monitor feelings on an ongoing basis, and/or while therapy is occurring.
- Identify and discuss client's strengths (e.g., very supportive family, usually copes well with stress) as well as vulnerabil-

---

Information that appears in brackets has been added by the authors to clarify and enhance the use of nursing diagnoses.

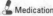

ities (e.g., client tends toward alcohol or other drugs for coping, client has witnessed a murder). **Knowing one's strengths and weaknesses helps client know what actions to take to cope with and prevent anxiety from becoming overwhelming.**

- Provide information about what reactions client may expect during each phase. Let client know these are common reactions. Be sure to phrase in neutral terms of "You may or you may not . . . ." **Helps reduce fear of the unknown.**
- Assist client to identify factors that may have created a vulnerable situation and that he or she may have power to change **to protect self in the future.**
- Avoid making value judgments.
- Discuss lifestyle changes client is contemplating and how they may contribute to recovery. **Helps client evaluate appropriateness of plans and identify shortcomings (e.g., moving away from effective support group).**
- Encourage learning stress-management techniques, such as deep breathing, meditation, relaxation, exercise. **Reduces stress, enhancing coping skills, and helping to resolve situation.**
- Discuss recognition of, and ways to manage, "anniversary reactions," reinforcing normalcy of recurrence of thoughts and feelings at this time.
- Discuss drug regimen, potential side effects of prescribed medications, and necessity of prompt reporting of untoward effects.
- Recommend participation in debriefing sessions that may be provided following major events. **Dealing with the stressor promptly may facilitate recovery from event or prevent exacerbation, although issues about best timing of debriefing continue to be debated.**
- Explain that post-traumatic symptoms can emerge months or sometimes years after a traumatic experience and that help and support can be obtained when needed or desired if client begins to experience intrusive memories or other symptoms.
- Identify employment, community resource groups (e.g., Assistance Support and Self Help in Surviving Trauma [ASSIST], employee peer-assistance programs, Red Cross or other survivor support services, Compassionate Friends). **Provides opportunity for ongoing support to deal with recurrent stressors.**
- Encourage psychiatric consultation, especially if client is unable to maintain control, is violent, is inconsolable, or does not seem to be making an adjustment.

Information that appears in brackets has been added by the authors to clarify and enhance the use of nursing diagnoses.

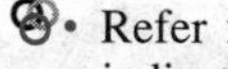

- Refer for long-term individual/family/marital counseling, if indicated.
- Refer to NDs Powerlessness; ineffective Coping; Grieving; complicated Grieving.

Documentation Focus

Assessment/Reassessment

- Identified risk factors noting internal and external concerns
- Client's perception of event and personal significance
- Individual findings, noting current dysfunction and behavioral and emotional responses to the incident
- Specifics of traumatic event
- Reactions of family/SO(s)
- Availability and use of resources

Planning

- Plan of care and who is involved in the planning
- Teaching plan

Implementation/Evaluation

- Responses to interventions, teaching, and actions performed
- Emotional changes
- Attainment or progress toward desired outcome(s)
- Modifications to plan of care

Discharge Planning

- Long-term needs and who is responsible for actions to be taken
- Specific referrals made

Sample Nursing Outcomes & Interventions Classifications (NOC/NIC)

NOC—Comfort Status: Psychospiritual
NIC—Crisis Intervention
NIC—Support System Enhancement

Information that appears in brackets has been added by the authors to clarify and enhance the use of nursing diagnoses.

POWERLESSNESS and risk for POWERLESSNESS

[Diagnostic Division: Ego Integrity]

Definition: Powerlessness: The lived experience of lack of control over a situation, including a perception that one's own actions do not significantly affect an outcome.

Definition: risk for Powerlessness: Vulnerable to the lived experience of lack of control over a situation, including a perception that one's actions do not significantly affect an outcome, which may compromise health.

Related Factors (Powerlessness)

Dysfunctional institutional environment
Insufficient interpersonal interactions
Complex treatment regimen

Risk Factors

Anxiety; ineffective coping strategies; low self-esteem
Caregiver role
Economically disadvantaged
Illness; progressive illness; unpredictability of illness trajectory; pain
Insufficient knowledge to manage a situation
Insufficient social support; social marginalization; stigmatization

NOTE: A risk diagnosis is not evidenced by signs and symptoms, as the problem has not occurred; rather, nursing interventions are directed at prevention.

Defining Characteristics (Powerlessness)

Subjective

Alienation; shame
Depression
Doubt about inability to perform previous activities; insufficient sense of control

Objective

Dependency
Inadequate participation in care

Information that appears in brackets has been added by the authors to clarify and enhance the use of nursing diagnoses.

Desired Outcomes/Evaluation Criteria—Client Will:

- Express sense of control over the present situation and future outcome.
- Make choices related to and be involved in care.
- Verbalize positive self-appraisal in current situation.
- Identify areas over which individual has control.
- Acknowledge reality that some areas are beyond individual's control.

Actions/Interventions

Nursing Priority No. 1.

To assess causative/contributing **or risk** factors:

- Identify situational circumstances (e.g., unfamiliar environment, immobility, diagnosis of terminal or chronic illness, lack of support system, lack of knowledge about situation).
- Determine client's perception and knowledge of condition and treatment plan.
- Ascertain client's response to treatment regimen. Does client see reason(s) and understand regimen is in the client's best interest, or is client compliant and helpless?
- Identify client's locus of control: internal (expressions of responsibility for self and ability to control outcomes—"I didn't quit smoking") or external (expressions of lack of control over self and environment—"Nothing ever works out"; "What bad luck to get lung cancer"). **Locus of control is a term used in reference to an individual's sense of mastery or control over events. Those with internal locus of control tend to be more optimistic about their ability to deal with adversity even in the face of current difficulties. Individuals with external locus of control may attribute feelings of powerlessness to an external source perceiving it as beyond his or her control.**
- Note cultural factors or religious beliefs that may contribute to how client is handling the situation. **One's values and beliefs may dictate gender roles. influence client's belief in ability to manage situation, participate in decision making, and direct own life.**
- Assess degree of mastery client has exhibited in life. **Passive individual may have more difficulty being assertive and standing up for rights.**

Information that appears in brackets has been added by the authors to clarify and enhance the use of nursing diagnoses.

- Determine if there has been a change in relationships with significant other (SO)(s). **Conflict in the family, loss of a family member, or divorce can contribute to feelings of powerlessness and lack of ability to manage situation.**
- Note availability and use of resources. **Client who has few options for assistance or who is not knowledgeable about how to use resources needs to be given information and assistance to know how and where to seek help.**
- Investigate caregiver practices to determine if they support client control and responsibility.

Nursing Priority No. 2.

To assess degree of powerlessness experienced by client:

- Listen to statements client makes: "They don't care"; "It won't make any difference"; "Are you kidding?" **Indicators of sense of powerlessness and hopelessness and need for specific interventions to provide sense of control over what is happening.**
- Note expressions that indicate "giving up," such as "It won't do any good." **May indicate suicidal intent, indicating need for immediate evaluation and interventions.**
- Note behavioral responses (verbal and nonverbal) including expressions of fear, interest or apathy, agitation, withdrawal.
- Note lack of communication, flat affect, and lack of eye contact. **May indicate more severe state of mind, such as psychotic episode and need for immediate evaluation and treatment.**
- Identify the use of manipulative behavior and reactions of client and caregivers. **Manipulation is used for management of powerlessness because of distrust of others, fear of intimacy, search for approval, and validation of sexuality.**

Nursing Priority No. 3.

To assist client to clarify needs relative to ability to meet them:

- Show concern for client as a person.
- Make time to listen to client's perceptions and concerns and encourage questions.
- Accept expressions of feelings, including anger and hopelessness.
- Avoid arguing or using logic with hopeless client. **Client will not believe it can make a difference.**

Information that appears in brackets has been added by the authors to clarify and enhance the use of nursing diagnoses.

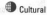

- Deal with manipulative behavior by being straightforward and honest with your communication and letting client know that this is a better way to get needs met. **Steps can be taken to recognize the behaviors and feelings and begin to change them.**
- Express hope for the client. **(There is always hope of something.)**
- Identify strengths and assets, and past coping strategies that were successful. **Helps client to recognize own ability to deal with difficult situation.**
- Assist client to identify what he or she can do for self. Identify things the client can and cannot control. **Accomplishing something can provide a sense of control and helps client understand that there are things he or she can manage. Accepting that some things cannot be controlled helps client to stop wasting efforts and refocus energy.**

Nursing Priority No. 4.

To promote independence:

- Use client's locus of control to develop individual plan of care (e.g., for client with internal control, encourage client to take control of own care; for those with external control, begin with small tasks and add, as tolerated).
- Develop contract with client specifying goals agreed on. **Enhances commitment to plan, optimizing outcomes.**
- Treat expressed decisions and desires with respect. Avoid critical parenting behaviors and communications. **Comments that are heard as critical or condescending will block communication and growth.**
- Provide client opportunities to control as many events as energy and restrictions of care permit.
- Discuss needs openly with client and set up agreed-on routines for meeting identified needs. **Minimizes use of manipulation.**
- Minimize rules and limit continuous observation to the degree that safety permits **to provide sense of control for the client.**
- Support client efforts to develop realistic steps to put plan into action, reach goals, and maintain expectations.
- Provide positive reinforcement for desired behaviors.
- Direct client's thoughts beyond present state to future when appropriate. **Focusing on possibilities in small steps can**

Information that appears in brackets has been added by the authors to clarify and enhance the use of nursing diagnoses.

help the client see that there can be hope in small things each day.

- Schedule frequent brief visits **to check on client, deal with client needs, and let client know someone is available.**
- Involve SO(s) in client care as appropriate. **Personal involvement by supportive family members can help client see the possibilities for resolving problems related to feelings of powerlessness.**

Nursing Priority No. 5.

To promote wellness (Teaching/Discharge Considerations):

- Encourage client to think productively and positively and to take responsibility for choosing own thoughts and reactions. **Can enhance feelings of power and sense of positive self-esteem.**
- Instruct in and encourage use of anxiety and stress-reduction techniques.
- Provide accurate verbal and written information about what is happening and discuss with client/SO(s). Repeat as often as necessary.
- Assist client to set realistic goals for the future. **Provides opportunity for client to decide what direction is desired and to gain confidence from completion of each goal.**
- Assist client to learn and use assertive communication skills. **Use of I-messages, active-listening, and problem-solving encourages client to be more in control of own life.**
- Refer to occupational therapist or vocational counselor, as indicated. **Facilitates return to a productive role in whatever capacity possible for the individual.**
- Encourage client to think productively and positively and take responsibility for choosing own thoughts. **Negative thinking can result in feelings of powerlessness, and learning to use positive thinking can reverse this pattern, promoting feelings of control and self-worth.**
- Model problem-solving process with client/SO(s). **Outcome is more likely to be accepted when arrived at by all parties involved, and participating in win-win solutions promotes sense of self-worth.**
- Suggest periodic review of own needs and goals.
- Refer to support groups for chronic conditions or disability (e.g., National Multiple Sclerosis Society, Easter Seals, Alzheimer's Association, Al-Anon) or counseling or therapy, as appropriate.

Information that appears in brackets has been added by the authors to clarify and enhance the use of nursing diagnoses.

Documentation Focus

Assessment/Reassessment

- Individual findings, noting degree of powerlessness, locus of control, individual's perception of the situation
- Specific cultural or religious factors
- Availability and use of support system and resources

Planning

- Plan of care and who is involved in the planning
- Teaching plan

Implementation/Evaluation

- Responses to interventions, teaching, and actions performed
- Specific goals and expectations
- Attainment or progress toward desired outcome(s)
- Modifications to plan of care

Discharge Planning

- Long-term needs and who is responsible for actions to be taken
- Specific referrals made

Sample Nursing Outcomes & Interventions Classifications (NOC/NIC)

NOC—Personal Autonomy
NIC—Self-Responsibility Facilitation

readiness for enhanced POWER

[Diagnostic Division: Ego Integrity]

Definition: A pattern of participating knowingly in change for well-being, which can be strengthened.

Defining Characteristics

Subjective

Expresses desire to enhance: power; knowledge for participation in change; awareness of possible changes; identification of choices that can be made for change

---

Information that appears in brackets has been added by the authors to clarify and enhance the use of nursing diagnoses.

Expresses desire to enhance: independence with actions for change; involvement in change; participation in choices for daily living and health

> **NOTE:** Even though power (a response) and empowerment (an intervention approach) are different concepts, the literature related to both concepts supports the defining characteristics of this diagnosis.

Desired Outcomes/Evaluation Criteria—Client Will:

- Verbalize knowledge of what changes he or she wants to make.
- Express awareness of own ability to be in charge of changes to be made.
- Participate in classes or group activities to learn new skills.
- State readiness to take power over own life.

Actions/Interventions

Nursing Priority No. 1.

To determine need/motivation for improvement:

- Determine current situation and circumstances that client is experiencing, leading to desire to improve life.
- Ascertain motivation and expectations for change.
- Identify emotional climate in which client and relationships live and work. **The emotional climate has a great impact between people. When a power differential exists in relationships, the atmosphere is largely determined by the person or people who have the power.**
- Identify client's locus of control: internal (expressions of responsibility for self and ability to control outcomes) or external (expressions of lack of control over self and environment). **Understanding locus of control can help client work toward positive, internal control as he or she develops ability to freely recognize and choose own actions.**
- Determine cultural factors/religious beliefs influencing client's self-view.
- Assess degree of mastery client has exhibited in his or her life. **Helps client understand how he or she has functioned in the past and what is needed to improve.**

Information that appears in brackets has been added by the authors to clarify and enhance the use of nursing diagnoses.

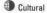

- Note presence of family/significant other (SO)(s) that can, or do, act as support systems for client.
- Determine whether client knows and/or uses assertiveness skills.

Nursing Priority No. 2.

To assist client to clarify needs relative to ability to improve feelings of power:

- Discuss needs and how client is meeting them at this time.
- Listen/active-listen client's perceptions and beliefs about how power can be gained in his or her life.
- Identify strengths, assets, and past coping strategies that were successful and can be built on **to enhance feelings of control.**
- Discuss the importance of assuming personal responsibility for life and relationships. **This skill requires one to be open to new ideas and experiences and different values and beliefs and to be inquisitive.**
- Identify things client can and cannot control. **Avoids wasting time on things that are not in the control of the client.**
- Treat expressed desires and decisions with respect. Avoid critical parenting expressions.

Nursing Priority No. 3.

To promote optimum wellness, enhancing power (Teaching/Discharge Considerations):

- Assist client to set realistic goals for the future.
- Provide accurate verbal and written information about what is happening and discuss with client. **Reinforces learning and promotes self-paced review.**
- Assist client to learn and use assertive communication skills. **These techniques require practice, but as the client becomes more proficient, he or she will help client to develop more effective relationships.**
- Use I-messages instead of You-messages. **I-messages acknowledge ownership of what is said, while You-messages suggest that the other person is wrong or bad, fostering resentment and resistance instead of understanding and cooperation.**
- Discuss importance of client paying attention to nonverbal communication. **Messages are often confusing or misinterpreted when verbal and nonverbal communications are not congruent.**

Information that appears in brackets has been added by the authors to clarify and enhance the use of nursing diagnoses.

- Help client learn to problem-solve differences. **Promotes win-win solutions.**
- Instruct and encourage use of stress-reduction techniques.
- Refer to support groups or classes, as indicated (e.g., assertiveness training, effectiveness for women, "Be your best").

Documentation Focus

Assessment/Reassessment

- Individual findings, noting determination to improve sense of power, locus of control
- Motivation and expectations for change

Planning

- Plan of care, specific interventions, and who is involved in planning
- Teaching plan

Implementation/Evaluation

- Client's responses to interventions, teaching, and actions performed
- Attainment or progress toward desired outcome(s)
- Modifications to plan of care

Discharge Planning

- Long-term needs and who is responsible for actions to be taken
- Specific referrals made

Sample Nursing Outcomes & Interventions Classifications (NOC/NIC)

NOC—Personal Autonomy
NIC—Self-Modification Assistance

risk for PRESSURE ULCER

[Diagnostic Division: Safety]

Definition: Vulnerable to localized injury to the skin and/or underlying tissue usually over a bony prominence as a result of pressure, or pressure in combination with shear [National Pressure Ulcer Advisory Panel (NPUAP, 2007)].

Information that appears in brackets has been added by the authors to clarify and enhance the use of nursing diagnoses.

Risk Factors

ADULT: Braden scale score of <18; CHILD: Braden scale score of ≤16; American Society of Anesthesiologists (ASA) Physical Status classification score ≥2; low score on Risk Assessment Pressure Sore (RAPS) scale; New York Heart Association (NYHA) Functional Classification ≥2

Alteration in cognitive functioning

Alteration in sensation; decrease in mobility; extended period of immobility on hard surface (e.g., surgical procedure ≥2 hours)

Anemia; decrease in tissue oxygenation or perfusion; impaired circulation; lymphopenia

Cardiovascular disease; history of cerebral vascular accident

Dehydration; dry or scaly skin; skin moisture; edema

Elevated skin temperature by 1–2°C; hyperthermia

Extremes of age or weight

Female gender

Hip fracture; history of trauma; physical immobilization

History of pressure ulcer

Inadequate nutrition; reduced triceps skin fold thickness; decrease in serum albumin

Incontinence

Insufficient caregiver knowledge of pressure ulcer prevention

Non blanchable erythema; pressure over bony prominence

Pharmaceutical agents (e.g., vasopressors, antidepressant, norepinephrine)

Self-care deficit

Shearing forces; friction

Use of linen with insufficient moisture wicking property

Smoking

NOTE: A risk diagnosis is not evidenced by signs and symptoms, as the problem has not occurred; rather, nursing interventions are directed at prevention.

Desired Outcomes/Evaluation Criteria—Client Will:

- Display and maintain healthy skin in risk areas (e.g., bony prominences, skin folds) during time in care facility.
- Participate in prevention measures and treatment program.
- Verbalize understanding of risk factors and when to contact healthcare provider.

Information that appears in brackets has been added by the authors to clarify and enhance the use of nursing diagnoses.

- Demonstrate behaviors or lifestyle changes to improve circulation (e.g., engage in regular exercise, cessation of smoking, weight reduction, disease management).

Client/Caregiver Will:

- Participate in prevention measures.

Actions/Interventions

Nursing Priority No. 1.

To assess risk and contributing factors:

- Identify presence of underlying condition that increases risk of pressure ulcer. **Skin integrity problems can be the result of (1) disease processes that affect circulation and perfusion of tissues (e.g., arteriosclerosis, venous insufficiency, hypertension, obesity, diabetes, malignant neoplasms); (2) medications (e.g., vasopressors, antidepressants, anticoagulants, corticosteroids, immunosuppressives, antineoplastics) that adversely affect or impair healing; (3) burns or radiation (can break down internal tissues as well as skin); and (4) nutrition and hydration (e.g., malnutrition deprives the body of protein and calories required for cell growth and repair, and dehydration impairs transport of oxygen and nutrients).**
- Evaluate client's risk for developing pressure ulcer upon admission to care, using Braden (or similar scale per facility policy) risk scale as listed above. **Using susceptibility factors of sensory perception, skin moisture, activity, mobility, nutritional status, friction, and shear potential, the client's risk can be quickly determined.**
- Determine client's age and developmental factors affecting skin/tissue health. **Infant's skin is predisposed to a dry, flaky, and impaired skin barrier. Studies have shown that similar to adult patients, acutely ill infants and children are at risk for pressure ulcers. In older adults, reduced epidermal regeneration, fewer sweat glands, less subcutaneous fat, elastin, and collagen, cause skin to become thinner, drier, and less responsive to pain sensations.**
- Note skin color discoloration (e.g., nonblanchable erythema, persistent red, blue, or purple hues) in pressure areas **suggestive of impaired tissue health. Note: It may be necessary in a darker skinned individual to focus more on other evidence of pressure ulcer development, such as bogginess, induration, coolness, or increased warmth as well as signs of skin discoloration.**

Information that appears in brackets has been added by the authors to clarify and enhance the use of nursing diagnoses.

- Ascertain current medication regimen. **Individual may be on medications which affect wound healing (e.g., vasopressors, anticoagulants, immunosuppressives, antineoplastics) that can adversely affect the skin).**
- Review laboratory results (e.g., hemoglobin/hematocrit [Hb/Hct], blood glucose, blood and/or wound culture and sensitivities for infectious agents [viral, bacterial, fungal], albumin, prealbumin, transferrin, protein) **to evaluate for potential risk factors or ability to heal. Note: Albumin <3.5 correlates to decreased wound healing and increased incidence of pressure ulcers.**

Nursing Priority No. 2.

To maintain optimal skin/tissue integrity:

- Monitor for incontinence, changing diapers, padding, and bedding as needed. **Maintains skin that is clean, dry, and free of contaminants which can cause/exacerbate skin/tissue breakdown.**
- Develop regularly timed repositioning schedule for client with mobility and sensation impairments; encourage or assist with periodic weight shifts for client in chair **to reduce stress on pressure points and to promote circulation to tissues.**
- Use proper turning and transfer techniques and sufficient personnel when repositioning client. **Avoids movements that cause friction or shearing (e.g., pulling client with parallel force, dragging movements).**
- Use appropriate padding or pressure-reducing devices (e.g., egg crate, gel pads, heel rolls, or foam boots) or pressure-relieving devices (e.g., air or water mattress) when indicated **to reduce pressure on sensitive areas and enhance circulation.**
- Participate in practices that prevent medical device–related pressure ulcers:

  Choose the correct size of medical device(s) (e.g., ET tube, anti-embolism stocking splints, other tubings) to fit the individual

  Remove or move the device daily to assess skin

  Avoid placement of device(s) over sites of prior, or existing pressure ulceration

  Protect skin with cushioning in high risk areas (e.g., nasal bridge, ears, sacrum, heels, occipital area of head in infants/small children)

  Educate other care providers about client's devices and prevention of skin breakdown interventions

Information that appears in brackets has been added by the authors to clarify and enhance the use of nursing diagnoses.

- Provide optimum nutrition (including adequate protein, lipids, calories, trace minerals, and multivitamins [e.g., A, C, D, E]) **to promote skin and tissue health, and to maintain general good health.** Refer to nutritionist as indicated.
- Provide adequate hydration (e.g., oral, tube feeding, IV, ambient room humidity) **to reduce and replenish transepidermal water loss.**

Nursing Priority No. 3.

To promote wellness (Teaching/Discharge Considerations):

- Encourage regular inspection and monitoring of skin for changes or failure to heal. **Early detection and reporting to healthcare providers promotes timely evaluation and intervention.**
- Encourage good nutrition, adequate hydration, early and ongoing mobility, and range of motion and strengthening exercises **to enhance circulation and promote health of skin and other organs.**
- Discuss proper and safe use of equipment or appliances (e.g., heating pad, ostomy appliances, padding straps of braces).
- Encourage abstinence from smoking, **which causes vasoconstriction, impairing circulation.**

Documentation Focus

Assessment/Reassessment

- Individual findings, including specific risk factors, condition of skin, ability to manage/direct own care

Planning

- Plan of care and who is involved in planning
- Teaching plan

Implementation/Evaluation

- Responses to interventions, teaching, and actions performed
- Attainment or progress toward desired outcome(s)
- Modifications to plan of care

Discharge Planning

- Long-term needs and who is responsible for actions to be taken
- Specific referrals made

Information that appears in brackets has been added by the authors to clarify and enhance the use of nursing diagnoses.

Sample Nursing Outcomes & Interventions Classifications (NOC/NIC)

NOC—Risk Control
NIC—Pressure Ulcer Prevention

ineffective PROTECTION

[Diagnostic Division: Safety]

Definition: Decrease in the ability to guard self from internal or external threats such as illness or injury.

Related Factors

Extremes of age
Inadequate nutrition
Substance abuse
Abnormal blood profile [e.g., leukopenia, thrombocytopenia, anemia]
Pharmaceutical agent [e.g., antineoplastic, corticosteroid, immune, thrombolytic]
Treatment regimen
Cancer; immune disorder (e.g., HIV-associated neuropathy, varicella-zoster virus)

Defining Characteristics

Subjective

Neurosensory impairment
Chilling
Itching
Insomnia; fatigue; weakness
Anorexia

Objective

Deficient immunity
Impaired healing; alteration in clotting
Maladaptive stress response
Alteration in perspiration
Dyspnea; coughing
Restlessness; immobility
Disorientation
Pressure ulcer

Information that appears in brackets has been added by the authors to clarify and enhance the use of nursing diagnoses.

NOTE: The purpose of this diagnosis seems to combine multiple NDs under a single heading for ease of planning care when a number of variables may be present. Outcomes/evaluation criteria and interventions are specifically tied to individual related factors that are present, such as:

Extremes of age: Concerns may include body temperature or thermoregulation; memory or sensory-perceptual alterations, as well as impaired mobility, risk for falls, sedentary lifestyle, self-care deficits; risk for trauma, suffocation, or poisoning; problems with skin or tissue integrity; and fluid volume imbalances.

Inadequate nutrition: Brings up issues of nutrition, unstable blood glucose; infection, delayed surgical recovery; swallowing difficulties; impaired skin or tissue integrity; trauma, problems with coping, and family processes.

Substance abuse: May be situational or chronic, with problems ranging from impaired respiration, decreased cardiac output, impaired liver function, and fluid volume deficits, to nutritional concerns, infection, trauma, risk for violence, and coping or family process difficulties.

Abnormal blood profile: Suggests possibility of fluid volume imbalances, decreased tissue perfusion, problems with oxygenation, activity intolerance, or risk for infection or injury.

Pharmaceutical agents and treatment-related side effects or concerns: Would include ineffective tissue perfusion, activity intolerance; cardiovascular, respiratory, and elimination concerns; risk for infection, fluid volume imbalances, impaired skin or tissue integrity, impaired liver function; pain, nutritional problems, fatigue or sleep difficulties; ineffective health management; and emotional responses (e.g., anxiety, sorrow, grieving, coping difficulties).

It is suggested that the user refer to specific NDs based on identified related factors and individual concerns for this client to find appropriate outcomes and interventions, as well as for Documentation Focus.

Sample Nursing Outcomes & Interventions Classifications (NOC/NIC)

NOC/NICs also depend on the specifics of the client's situation such as:

NOC—Symptom Control

NIC—Bleeding Precautions; Infection Protection; Postanesthesia Care

---

Information that appears in brackets has been added by the authors to clarify and enhance the use of nursing diagnoses.

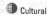

RAPE-TRAUMA SYNDROME

[Diagnostic Division: Ego Integrity]

Definition: Sustained maladaptive response to a forced, violent, sexual penetration against the victim's will and consent. [Rape is not a sexual crime, but a crime of violence, and it is identified as sexual assault. Although attacks are most often directed toward women, men also may be victims.]

Related Factors

Rape [actual or attempted forced sexual penetration]

Defining Characteristics

Subjective

Embarrassment; humiliation; shame; guilt; self-blame
Helplessness; powerlessness
Shock; fear; anxiety; anger; thoughts of revenge
Nightmares; alteration in sleep pattern
Change in relationship(s); sexual dysfunction

Objective

Physical trauma; muscle tension or spasm
Confusion; disorganization; impaired decision-making
Agitation; hyperalertness; aggression
Mood swings; perceived vulnerability; dependency; low self-esteem; depression
Substance abuse; history of suicide attempts
Denial; phobias; paranoia; dissociative identity disorder

Desired Outcomes/Evaluation Criteria—Client Will:

- Deal appropriately with emotional reactions as evidenced by behavior and expression of feelings.
- Report absence of physical complications, pain, and discomfort.
- Verbalize a positive self-image.
- Verbalize recognition that incident was not of own doing.
- Identify behaviors or situations within own control that may enhance sense of safety, reduce risk of recurrence.
- Deal with practical aspects (e.g., court appearances).

Information that appears in brackets has been added by the authors to clarify and enhance the use of nursing diagnoses.

- Demonstrate appropriate changes in lifestyle (e.g., change in job, residence) as necessary and seek or obtain support from significant other (SO)(s) as needed.
- Interact with individuals and groups in desired and acceptable manner.

Actions/Interventions

Nursing Priority No. 1.

To assess trauma and individual reaction, noting length of time since occurrence of event:

- Observe for and elicit information about physical injury and assess stress-related symptoms, such as numbness, headache, tightness in chest, nausea, and pounding heart.
- Identify psychological responses: anger, shock, acute anxiety, confusion, denial. Note laughter, crying, calm or agitated state, excited (hysterical) behavior, expressions of disbelief, and/or self-blame.
- Note signs of increasing anxiety (e.g., silence, stuttering, inability to sit still). **Indicates need for immediate interventions to prevent panic reaction.**
- Determine degree of disorganization. **(May need help to manage activities of daily living and other aspects of life.)**
- Identify whether incident has reactivated preexisting or coexisting situations (physical/psychological). **Can affect how the client views the current trauma and exacerbate preexisting problems.**
- Ascertain cultural values or religious beliefs that may affect how client views incident, self, and expectations of SO/family reaction.
- Determine sexual orientation of the survivor. **Heterosexual men/boys may believe that they are now gay and need to be assured that is not true.**
- Determine disruptions in relationships with men and with others (e.g., family, friends, coworkers, SO[s]). **Many women find that they react to men in general in a different way, seeing them as reminders of the assault. Male survivors may withdraw entirely from sexual relations.**
- Identify development of phobic reactions to ordinary articles (e.g., knives, buildings) and situations (e.g., walking in groups of people, strangers ringing doorbell).
- Note degree of intrusive repetitive thoughts, sleep disturbances.

Information that appears in brackets has been added by the authors to clarify and enhance the use of nursing diagnoses.

- Assess degree of dysfunctional coping (e.g., use of alcohol, other drugs, suicidal/homicidal ideation, marked change in sexual behavior).

Nursing Priority No. 2.

To assist client to deal with situation that exists:

- Explore own feelings (nurse/caregiver) regarding rape or incest issue prior to interacting with the client. **Need to recognize own biases to prevent imposing them on the client.**

Acute Phase

- Stay with the client, do not leave child unattended. **Provides reassurance and sense of safety.**
- Involve rape response team where available. Provide same-sex examiner when appropriate.
- Evaluate infant, child, or adolescent as dictated by age, sex, and developmental level. **Age of the victim is an important consideration in deciding plan of care and appropriate interventions.** ***Note:*** **While underreported, it is believed that 1 in 10 men are sexually assaulted and 1 in 6 boys will be sexually assaulted or abused before the age of 18.**
- Assist with documentation of incident for police or child protective services reports, maintain sequencing and collection of evidence (chain of evidence), label each specimen, and store and package properly. **Protecting evidence is important to the judicial process when offender goes to trial.**
- Provide environment in which client can talk freely about feelings and fears, including concerns about relationship with and response of SO(s), pregnancy, sexually transmitted infections.
- Provide psychological support by listening and remaining with client. If client does not want to talk, accept silence. **May indicate Silent Reaction.**
- Listen to and investigate physical complaints. Assist with medical treatments, as indicated. **Emotional reactions may limit client's ability to recognize physical injury.**
- Assist with practical realities (e.g., safe temporary housing, money, or other needs).
- Determine client's ego strengths and assist client to use them in a positive way by acknowledging client's ability to handle what is happening.
- Identify support persons for this individual. **The client's partner can be important to her or his recovery by being pa-**

Information that appears in brackets has been added by the authors to clarify and enhance the use of nursing diagnoses.

tient and comforting. When partners talk through the incident, the relationship can be strengthened.

Postacute Phase

- Allow the client to work through own kind of adjustment (may be withdrawn or unwilling to talk); do not force the issue, but be available, if needed.
- Listen for expressions of fear of crowds, men, being alone in home, and so forth. **May reveal developing phobias.**
- Discuss specific concerns and fears. Identify appropriate actions (e.g., diagnostic testing for pregnancy, sexually transmitted infections) and provide information, as indicated.
- Include written instructions that are concise and clear regarding medical treatments, crisis support services, and so forth. **Reinforces teaching, provides opportunity to deal with information at own pace.**

Long-Term Phase

- Continue listening to expressions of concern. May need to continue to talk about the assault. Note persistence of somatic complaints (e.g., nausea, anorexia, insomnia, muscle tension, headache).
- Permit free expression of feelings (may continue from the crisis phase). Refrain from rushing client through expressions of feelings and avoid reassuring inappropriately. **Client may believe pain and/or anguish is misunderstood, and depression may limit responses.**
- Acknowledge reality of loss of self that existed before the incident. Assist client to move toward an acceptance of the potential for growth that exists within individual.
- Continue to allow client to progress at own pace.
- Give "permission" to express/deal with anger at the perpetrator and situation in acceptable ways. Set limits on destructive behaviors. **Facilitates resolution of feelings without diminishing self-concept.**
- Keep discussion on practical and emotional level rather than intellectualizing the experience, **which allows client to avoid dealing with feelings.**
- Assist in dealing with ongoing concerns about and effects of the incident, such as court appearance, pregnancy, sexually transmitted infection, and relationship with SO(s).
- Provide for sensitive, trained counselors, considering individual needs. (**Male or female counselors may be best determined on an individual basis as counselor's gender may be an issue for some clients, affecting ability to disclose.**)

Information that appears in brackets has been added by the authors to clarify and enhance the use of nursing diagnoses.

Nursing Priority No. 3.

To promote wellness (Teaching/Discharge Considerations):

- Provide information about what reactions client may expect during each phase. Let client know these are common reactions and phrase in neutral terms of "You may or may not . . . ." (Be aware that although male rape perpetrators are usually heterosexual, the male victim may be concerned about his own sexuality and may exhibit a homophobic response.)
- Assist client to identify factors that may have created a vulnerable situation and that she or he may have power to change **to protect self in the future.**
- Avoid making value judgments.
- Discuss lifestyle changes client is contemplating and how they will contribute to recovery. **Helps client evaluate appropriateness of plans and make decisions that will be helpful to eventual recovery.**
- Encourage psychiatric consultation if client is violent, inconsolable, or does not seem to be making an adjustment. **Participation in a group may be helpful.**
- Refer to family/marital counseling, as indicated.
- Refer to NDs Powerlessness; ineffective Coping; Grieving; complicated Grieving; Anxiety; Fear.

Documentation Focus

Assessment/Reassessment

- Individual findings, including nature of incident, individual reactions and fears, degree of trauma (physical and emotional), effects on lifestyle
- Cultural or religious factors
- Reactions of family/SO(s)
- Samples gathered for evidence, disposition, and storage (chain of evidence)

Planning

- Plan of action and who is involved in planning
- Teaching plan

Implementation/Evaluation

- Responses to interventions, teaching, and actions performed
- Attainment or progress toward desired outcome(s)
- Modifications to plan of care

Information that appears in brackets has been added by the authors to clarify and enhance the use of nursing diagnoses.

Discharge Planning

- Long-term needs and who is responsible for actions to be taken
- Specific referrals made

Sample Nursing Outcomes & Interventions Classifications (NOC/NIC)

NOC—Abuse Recovery: Sexual
NIC—Rape-Trauma Treatment

risk for adverse REACTION TO IODINATED CONTRAST MEDIA

[Diagnostic Division: Safety]

Definition: Vulnerable to noxious or unintended reaction associated with the use of iodinated contrast media that can occur within seven days after contrast agent injection, which may compromise health.

Risk Factors

Anxiety
Chronic illness
Concurrent use of pharmaceutical agents (e.g., beta-blockers, interleukin-2, metformin, nephrotoxins)
Contrast media precipitates adverse event (e.g., iodine concentration, viscosity, high osmolality, iron toxicity)
Dehydration
Extremes of age, generalized debilitation
Fragile veins (e.g., chemotherapy or radiation in limb to be injected; indwelling line in place for more than 24 hours; axillary lymph node dissection in limb to be injected; distal intravenous access site)
History of allergies, or previous adverse effect from iodinated contrast media [ICM]
Unconsciousness

NOTE: A risk diagnosis is not evidenced by signs and symptoms, as the problem has not occurred; the nursing interventions are directed at prevention.

Information that appears in brackets has been added by the authors to clarify and enhance the use of nursing diagnoses.

Desired Outcomes/Evaluation Criteria–Client Will:

- Experience no adverse reaction from ICM.
- Verbalize understanding of individual risks and responsibilities to avoid exposure.
- Recognize need for/seek assistance to limit allergic response/complications.

Actions/Interventions

Nursing Priority No. 1.

To identify causative/precipitating factors related to risk:

- Identify the client at risk for adverse reaction prior to procedures. **A history of allergies, asthma, diabetes, renal insufficiency, including solitary kidney with elevated creatinine, thyroid dysfunction, hypertension, heart failure, current or recent use of nephrotoxic medications, or reaction to previous ICM administration places individual at increased risk.**
- Ascertain type of reaction client experienced when there is a history of past reaction. **There are two types of reactions, idiosyncratic and nonidiosyncratic, both of which could change decisions about using ICM for diagnostic purposes.**

Nursing Priority No. 2.

To assist client/caregiver to reduce or correct individual risk factors:

- Administer infusions using "6 rights" system (right client, right medication, right route, right dose, right time, and right documentation) **to prevent client from receiving improper contrast agent or dosage.**
- Perform imaging tests that do not require contrast media where possible **when client is at high risk for reaction.**
- Administer IV fluids as appropriate **to reduce incidence of contrast medium-induced nephropathy.**
- Administer medications (e.g., prednisone [Deltasone] or Benadryl) before, during, and after injection or procedures **to reduce risk or severity of reaction.**
- Observe IV injection site frequently **to ascertain that no extravasation of contrast solution is occurring.**
- Halt infusion immediately if client reports site discomfort or redness or swelling is noted **to prevent tissue damage from contrast agent.**

Information that appears in brackets has been added by the authors to clarify and enhance the use of nursing diagnoses.

- Monitor results of lab studies (e.g., creatinine clearance) **to ascertain status of kidney function.**

Nursing Priority No. 3.

To promote wellness (Teaching/Discharge Criteria):

- Instruct client regarding signs and symptoms that should be reported to physician after a procedure. **Any delayed signs of reaction should be reported to physician immediately for timely intervention.**
- Instruct client/care provider about puncture sites and to report redness, soreness, or pain **to reduce risk of complications associated with extravasation.**
- Encourage client to use Medic Alert bracelet **to alert health-care providers of history of prior reaction to contrast media.**

Documentation Focus

Assessment/Reassessment

- Individual risk factors identified
- Client concerns or difficulty making and following through with plans

Planning

- Plan of care and who is involved in planning
- Teaching plan

Implementation/Evaluation

- Response to interventions, teaching, and actions performed
- Attainment or progress toward outcomes

Discharge Planning

- Referrals to other resources
- Long-term need and who is responsible for actions

Sample Nursing Outcomes & Interventions Classifications (NOC/NIC)

NOC—Allergic Response: Systemic
NIC—Allergy Management

Information that appears in brackets has been added by the authors to clarify and enhance the use of nursing diagnoses.

ineffective **RELATIONSHIP** and risk for ineffective **RELATIONSHIP**

[Diagnostic Division: Ego Integrity]

Definition: ineffective Relationship: A pattern of mutual partnership that is insufficient to provide for each other's needs.

Definition: risk for ineffective Relationship: Vulnerable to developing a pattern that is insufficient for providing a mutual partnership to provide for each other's needs.

Related and Risk Factors

Stressors; developmental crisis
Substance abuse
Unrealistic expectations
Ineffective communication skills
History of domestic violence
Alteration in cognitive functioning in one partner
Incarceration of one partner

NOTE: A risk diagnosis is not evidenced by signs and symptoms, as the problem has not occurred; rather, nursing interventions are directed at prevention.

Defining Characteristics (ineffective Relationship)

Subjective

Dissatisfaction with complementary relation between partners
Dissatisfaction with physical or emotional need fulfillment between partners
Dissatisfaction with information or idea sharing between partners

Objective

Unsatisfactory communication with partner
Insufficient balance in autonomy or collaboration between partners
Insufficient mutual respect between partners
Insufficient mutual support in daily activities between partners
Inadequate understanding of partner's compromised functioning (e.g., physical, social, psychological)
Delay in meeting of developmental goals appropriate for family life-cycle stage
Partner not identified as support person

Information that appears in brackets has been added by the authors to clarify and enhance the use of nursing diagnoses.

Desired Outcomes/Evaluation Criteria—Client Will:

- Verbalize a desire to develop realistic plan to improve relationship with partner.
- Acknowledge worth and value of partner as a key person.
- Seek information regarding physical and emotional needs of partner.
- Express a desire to improve communication skills, or engage in effective communication skills for both partners.
- Participate in marital therapy sessions to learn ways to develop a satisfactory relationship.

Actions/Interventions

Nursing Priority No. 1.

To assess current situation and determine needs:

- ∞ Determine makeup of family, length of relationship, financial situation—parents/children, older/younger, other members of household. **Stressors of family relationships within a household, difficulties with childrearing, older adult needing care, and financial difficulties can strain the relationship between partners.**
- Discuss individual's perception of own and other's needs and how partner sees own needs. **Identifies misperceptions and areas of disagreement.**
- Determine each person's self-image and locus of control. **View of self as a positive or negative individual who is in control or controlled by others influences behavior and how partners react to each other.**
- Assess emotional intelligence skills of each individual. **This is the ability to recognize and control one's own emotions and recognize the emotions of the other.**
- Investigate cultural factors that may be affecting relationship and contributing to conflict. **Roles from family of origin for each person may promote conflict when beliefs clash and neither is willing to change or even discuss their thinking.**
- Determine style of communication and understanding of nonverbal cues used by partners. **Poor communication is unclear and indirect, leading to conflict, ineffective problem-solving, and poor emotional bonding in families with problems.**
- Determine how partners deal with conflict. **Many individuals try to avoid conflict instead of working to resolve it.**

Information that appears in brackets has been added by the authors to clarify and enhance the use of nursing diagnoses.

- Determine how family as a whole functions. **Situational dynamics can create conflict as individuals take sides in disagreements, escalating the situation.**
- Ascertain ways in which family members deal with conflict. **Conflict is inevitable in relationships, and partners need to identify whether how they deal with it is effective or ineffective.**
- Identify concerns about sexual aspects of relationship from both partners' viewpoints. **Intimacy is an important part of a relationship, and if both individuals are avoiding that activity, they will need to discuss specific ways to resolve these problems.**
- Note medical problems that may be affecting sexual relationship. **Conditions, such as hysterectomy, prostatitis, breast cancer, erectile dysfunction may cause partners to withdraw from one another.**

Nursing Priority No. 2.

To assist partners to resolve existing conflict, **or improve relationship**:

- Maintain positive attitude toward partners and family members. **Safe environment allows individuals to speak freely, knowing they will not be judged for comments and opinions.**
- Discuss surface symptoms of dysfunctional relationships and the fact that these are not the problems that need to be dealt with. **Individuals are often not aware of underlying emotions that are influencing their behavior and continue to focus on surface issues.**
- Explore each partner's emotional needs. **Unconscious desires to gain acceptance, recognition, sense of being cared about or valued are often motivators for relationships.**
- Discuss and clarify nonverbal communication. **Partners need to be aware of and ask about the meaning of body language, tone of voice, and subtle movements that convey positive or negative messages.**
- Assist partners/family to learn effective conflict resolution skills such as the win-win method. **Resolving to listen to each other's needs and agree on a mutually acceptable solution provides new ways to resolve problems and enhances relationship.**
- Provide information about Active-listening techniques. **Avoids giving advice and encourages other person to find own solution, enhancing self-esteem.**

Information that appears in brackets has been added by the authors to clarify and enhance the use of nursing diagnoses.

- Have partners identify thoughts and feelings when starting a discussion with each other.
- Recommend individuals verify what they believe the other has said. **Allows speaker to correct misperception and respond more effectively.**
- Have partners role-play a specific conflict that is a frequent issue. **Practicing how to defuse arguments and repair hurt feelings helps to identify other's feelings and use new skills for resolution.**
- Encourage partners to maintain a calm demeanor. **Staying focused enables individuals to think more rationally and come to a desired solution.**
- Have each person verify what he or she heard the other person say. **Provides opportunity for the speaker to correct or acknowledge what was said.**
- Discuss sexual concerns and provide opportunity for questions. **Conflict in the relationship inevitability affects these concerns, and providing information and discussing them can enhance intimacy.**
- Promote non-blameful self-disclosure when having a discussion. **Not placing blame results in a more considerate and respectful resolution.**

Nursing Priority No. 3.

To promote optimal functioning of couple/family (Teaching/Discharge Considerations):

- Help family members learn skill of Active-listening. **Avoids giving advice and allows others to find their own solution, enhancing self-esteem.**
- Have partners acknowledge beliefs they have become aware of during therapy.
- Encourage use of relaxation, mindfulness techniques. **Helps individuals to ease anxiety and learn to relate to each other in a calm manner.**
- Discuss the appropriate use of humor and laughter in daily lives. **Helps to break the tension and lighten difficult moments.**
- Recommend books, Web sites to provide additional information.
- Refer to support groups, classes as indicated. **Parenting, assertiveness, financial assistance will help partners learn new skills as needed.**
- Include all family members in discussions, as indicated. **Promotes involvement, provides opportunities for communication and clarification of family dynamics and enhances commitment to achieving goals.**

Information that appears in brackets has been added by the authors to clarify and enhance the use of nursing diagnoses.

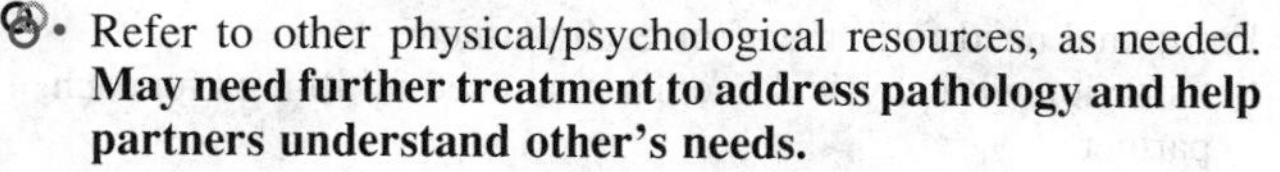

- Refer to other physical/psychological resources, as needed. **May need further treatment to address pathology and help partners understand other's needs.**

Documentation Focus

Assessment/Reassessment
- Individual's perception of situation and self
- Partner's views and expectations
- How partners communicate and deal with conflict

Planning
- Plan of care and who is involved in planning
- Teaching plan

Implementation/Evaluation
- Response of partners to plan, interventions, and actions performed
- Attainment or progress toward desired outcomes

Discharge Planning
- Long-range plan and who is responsible for actions to be taken
- Referrals made

Sample Nursing Outcomes & Interventions Classifications (NOC/NIC)

NOC—Role Performance
NIC—Conflict Mediation

readiness for enhanced RELATIONSHIP

[Diagnostic Division: Ego Integrity]

Definition: A pattern of mutual partnership to provide for each other's needs, which can be strengthened.

Defining Characteristics

Subjective

Expresses desire to enhance:

Communication between partners
Satisfaction with information/idea sharing between partners

Information that appears in brackets has been added by the authors to clarify and enhance the use of nursing diagnoses.

Emotional need fulfillment for each partner
Satisfaction with physical or emotional need fulfillment for each partner
Satisfaction with complementary relation between partners
Mutual respect between partners
Autonomy or collaboration between partners
Understanding of partner's functional deficit (e.g., physical, social, psychological)

Desired Outcomes/Evaluation Criteria—Client Will (Include Specific Time Frames):

- Verbalize a desire to learn more effective communication skills.
- Verbalize understanding of current relationship with partner.
- Seek information to improve emotional and physical needs of both partners.
- Talk with partner about circumstances that can be improved.
- Develop realistic plans to strengthen relationship.

Actions/Interventions

Nursing Priority No. 1.

To assess current situation and determine needs:

- Determine makeup of family (e.g., includes couple only, parents and children, older and younger members). **Life changes, such as developmental, situational, health-illness, can affect relationship between partners and require readjustment and thinking of ways to enhance situation.**
- Discuss client's perception of needs and how partner sees desire to improve relationship.
- Identify use of effective communication skills. **May need to improve understanding of words partners use in discussion of sensitive subjects.**
- Help client identify thoughts and feelings when starting a discussion with partner. **A system of thinking (referred to as a paradigm) forms the basis for how we look at and experience life and determines how we perceive our world, forms the basis for our reality, and exists below our level of consciousness.**
- Ask partners how they deal with conflict.
- Ascertain client's view of sexual aspects of relationship. **Changes that occur with aging or medical conditions, such as a hysterectomy or erectile dysfunction, can affect the relationship and need specific interventions to resolve.**

Information that appears in brackets has been added by the authors to clarify and enhance the use of nursing diagnoses.

- Identify cultural factors relating to individual's view of role in relationship.
- Discuss how family as a whole functions. **Interrelationships with members of the family, personal and family history, and situational dynamics can improve the functioning of the whole family.**

Nursing Priority No. 2.

To assist the client to enhance existing situation:

- Maintain positive attitude toward client. **Promotes safe relationship in which client can feel free to speak openly and plan for a positive future.**
- Have couple discuss paradigms that they have become aware of in own thinking that interfere with relationship.
- Determine how each person views himself or herself as a positive or negative person. **One's self-image influences behavior and how one relates to others. When emotional needs are met, individuals relate to others in positive ways, while unmet needs result in low self-image and insecurity.**
- Discuss the skills of emotional intelligence that are important for maintaining positive relationships. **This is the ability to recognize and effectively control our own emotions and to recognize the emotions of others.**
- Help couple to recognize that surface symptoms of dysfunctional relationships are not the problems that need to be dealt with. **Underlying emotions influence our behaviors, and individuals often are not aware of them and continue to deal with the superficial conflicts.**
- Explore individual's emotional needs. **Relationships are often motivated by unconscious desires to gain acceptance, recognition, sense of being cared about or valued.**
- Note client's awareness of nonverbal communications. **Body language, tone of voice, a roll of the eyes, or subtle movements convey strong messages, positive or negative, that need to be discussed and clarified.**
- Discuss effective conflict-resolution skills.
- Encourage client to remain calm and focused regardless of circumstances. **Maintaining a calm demeanor helps individual to be able to think more clearly and be more rational in dealing with situation.**
- Recommend cross-checking or verifying what listener believes speaker said. **Clarifies communication and allows speaker to respond or correct perception of listener as needed.**
- Help partners to learn win-win method of conflict resolution.

Information that appears in brackets has been added by the authors to clarify and enhance the use of nursing diagnoses.

- Role-play ways to defuse arguments and repair injured feelings. **Provides a realistic situation where each person can identify own and partner's view and practice new ways of interacting.**
- Provide open environment for partners to discuss sexual concerns and questions.
- Discuss nonblameful self-disclosure when having a dialogue. **Partners take turns talking about own needs and feelings without blaming the other, resulting in being able to find a solution in a climate of mutual consideration and respect.**

Nursing Priority No. 3.

To promote optimal functioning (Teaching/Discharge Considerations):

- Provide information for partners, using bibliotherapy and appropriate Web sites.
- Encourage couple to use humor and playfulness in their relationship. **Sharing laughter and enjoying life helps weather difficult times.**
- Discuss the importance of being an empathic, understanding, and nonjudgmental listener when either partner has a problem.
- Help individuals to learn to use the skill of Active-listening. **This avoids giving advice and helps other person to find own solution, enhancing self-esteem.**
- Refer to support groups, classes on assertiveness, parenting, as indicated by individual needs.
- Include family members in discussions as needed.
- Refer for care as indicated by psychological or physical concerns of either individual.

Documentation Focus

Assessment/Reassessment

- Baseline information, individuals' perception of situation and self
- Reasons for desire to improve relationship
- Motivation and expectations for change

Planning

- Plan of care and who is involved in planning
- Teaching plan

Implementation/Evaluation

- Response of partners to plan, interventions, and actions performed
- Attainment or progress toward desired outcomes(s)

Information that appears in brackets has been added by the authors to clarify and enhance the use of nursing diagnoses.

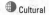

Discharge Planning

- Long-range plan and who is responsible for actions to be taken

Sample Nursing Outcomes & Interventions Classifications (NOC/NIC)

NOC—Social Interaction Skills
NIC—Role Enhancement

impaired RELIGIOSITY and risk for impaired RELIGIOSITY

[Diagnostic Division: Ego Integrity]

Definition: impaired Religiosity: Impaired ability to exercise reliance on beliefs and/or participate in rituals of a particular faith tradition.

Definition: risk for impaired Religiosity: Vulnerable to an impaired ability to exercise reliance on beliefs and/or participate in rituals of a particular faith tradition, which may compromise health.

NOTE: NANDA recognizes that the term "religiosity" may be culture specific; however, the term is useful in the United States and is well supported in the U.S. literature.

Related and Risk Factors

Developmental and Situational

Aging; end-stage life crisis
Life transition (actual and risk)

Environmental (risk)

Insufficient transportation
Barrier to practicing religion

Physical

Illness; pain

Psychological

Ineffective coping strategies; insufficient or ineffective social support

Information that appears in brackets has been added by the authors to clarify and enhance the use of nursing diagnoses.

Anxiety; fear of death
Depression (risk)
Personal crisis; insecurity
History of religious manipulation

Sociocultural
Cultural or environmental barrier to practicing religion
Insufficient social integration or sociocultural interaction

Spiritual
Spiritual crises; suffering

> **NOTE:** A risk diagnosis is not evidenced by signs and symptoms, as the problem has not occurred; rather, nursing interventions are directed at prevention.

Defining Characteristics (impaired Religiosity)

Subjective
Distress about separation from faith community
Desire to reconnect with previous belief pattern or customs
Questioning of religious belief patterns or customs
Difficulty adhering to prescribed religious beliefs and rituals (e.g., ceremonies, regulations, clothing, prayer, services, holiday observances)

Desired Outcomes/Evaluation Criteria—Client Will:

- Express understanding of relation of situation/health status to thoughts and feelings of concern about ability to participate in desired religious activities.
- Seek solutions to individual factors that may interfere with reliance on religious beliefs/participation in religious rituals.
- Express ability to once again participate in beliefs and rituals of desired religion.
- Discuss beliefs and values about spiritual or religious issues.
- Attend religious or worship services of choice as desired.
- Verbalize concerns about end-of-life issues and fear of death.

Information that appears in brackets has been added by the authors to clarify and enhance the use of nursing diagnoses.

Actions/Interventions

Nursing Priority No. 1.

To assess causative/contributing **or risk** factors:

- Ascertain current situation (e.g., illness, hospitalization, prognosis of death, depression, lack of support systems, financial concerns). **Identifies problems client is dealing with in the moment that may be affecting desire to be involved with religious activities.**
- Note client's/significant other's (SO) reports and expressions of anger, alienation from God, sense of guilt or retribution. **Perception of guilt may cause spiritual crisis and suffering, resulting in rejection of religious symbols.**
- Determine sense of futility, feelings of hopelessness, lack of motivation to help self. **Indicators that client may see no, or only limited, options, alternatives, or personal choices.**
- Assess extent of depression client may be experiencing. **Some studies suggest that a focus on religion may protect against depression.**
- Note recent changes in behavior (e.g., withdrawal from others or religious activities; dependence on alcohol or medications). **Lack of connectedness with self/others impairs ability to trust others or feel worthy of trust from others or God.**
- Determine client's usual religious or spiritual beliefs, past or current involvement in specific church activities. **Helps in directing discussions and potential interventions that client may find helpful,**
- Note quality of relationships with SO(s) and friends. **Individual may withdraw from others in reaction to stress of illness, pain, and suffering. Other people may be encouraging client to rely on religious beliefs at a time when individual is questioning own beliefs in the current situation.**
- Identify cultural values and expectations regarding religious beliefs or practices. **Individuals grow up in a family that instills a value system within them. As the person grows up, ideas, values, and expectations may change or be strengthened by new information, different questioning, and alternative viewpoints, which may affect current situation.**
- Ascertain substance use or abuse. **Individuals may turn to use of various substances during times of distress, and this can affect the ability to deal with problems in a positive manner.**

Information that appears in brackets has been added by the authors to clarify and enhance the use of nursing diagnoses.

- Note socioeconomic status of individual/family. **The poor may have high levels of personal religiosity yet may participate less in organized religion because they feel stigmatized by their situation (e.g., single mothers, those receiving public assistance, or those engaging in a lifestyle that conflicts with church norms).**

Nursing Priority No. 2.

To assist client/SO(s) to deal with feelings/situation:

- Use therapeutic communication skills of reflection and Active-listening. **Communicates acceptance and enables client to find own solutions to concerns.**
- Encourage expression of feelings about illness, condition, death. **As people age, they become more concerned about their own mortality, and others often see them as in poor health and as spiritual and religious. If they have been diagnosed with a long-term chronic or terminal illness, they may be feeling more angry and rejecting of God than seeking his help,**
- Have client identify and prioritize current or immediate needs. **Dealing with current needs is easier than trying to predict the future.**
- Provide time for nonjudgmental discussion of individual's spiritual beliefs and fears about impact of current illness and/or treatment regimen. **Helps clarify thoughts and promote ability to deal with stresses of what is happening.**
- Review with client past difficulties in life and coping skills that were used at those times.
- Suggest use of journaling and reminiscence. **Promotes life review and can assist in clarifying values and ideas, recognizing and resolving feelings or situation.**
- Discuss differences between grief and guilt and help client to identify and deal with each. Point out consequences of actions based on guilt.
- Encourage client to identify individuals (e.g., spiritual advisor, parish nurse) who can provide needed support.
- Review client's religious affiliation, associated rituals, and beliefs. **Helps client examine what has been important in the past.**
- Provide opportunity for nonjudgmental discussion of philosophical issues related to religious belief patterns and customs. **Open communication can assist client to check reality of perceptions and identify personal options and willingness to resume desired activities.**

Information that appears in brackets has been added by the authors to clarify and enhance the use of nursing diagnoses.

- Discuss desire to continue or reconnect with previous belief patterns, customs, and current barriers. **As client begins to think about current feelings of alienation from previous religious connections, these discussions can help to clarify and allow client to think about how these beliefs can be regained.**
- Identify ways to strengthen spiritual or religious expression. **There are multiple options for enhancing participation in faith community (e.g., joining prayer or study group, volunteering time to community projects, singing in the choir, reading spiritual writings).**
- Involve client in refining healthcare goals and therapeutic regimen, as appropriate. **Identifies role illness is playing in current concerns about ability to participate or appropriateness of participating in desired religious activities.**

Nursing Priority No. 3.

To promote spiritual wellness (Teaching/Discharge Considerations):

- Have client identify support systems available.
- Help client learn relaxation techniques, meditation, guided imagery, and mindfulness/living in the moment and enjoying it.
- Take the lead from the client in initiating participation in religious activities, prayer, other activities. **Client may be vulnerable in current situation and must be allowed to decide own participation in these actions.**
- Provide privacy for meditation, prayer, or performance of rituals, as appropriate.
- Explore alternatives or modifications of ritual based on setting and individual needs and limitations. **Individual may not be able to go to a church or temple, so providing another setting—chapel in the facility or quiet room with appropriate religious artifacts or material—can provide the setting desired.**
- Assist client to identify spiritual resources that could be helpful (e.g., contacting spiritual advisor who has qualifications and experience in dealing with specific problems individual is concerned about). **Provides answers to spiritual questions, assists in the journey of self-discovery, and can help client learn to accept and forgive self.**

Documentation Focus

Assessment/Reassessment

- Individual findings, including risk factors or nature of spiritual conflict, effects of participation in treatment regimen

Information that appears in brackets has been added by the authors to clarify and enhance the use of nursing diagnoses.

- Physical and emotional responses to conflict
- Availability and use of resources

Planning
- Plan of care and who is involved in planning
- Teaching plan

Implementation/Evaluation
- Responses to interventions, teaching, and actions performed
- Attainment or progress toward desired outcome(s)
- Modifications to plan of care

Discharge Planning
- Long-term needs and who is responsible for actions to be taken
- Available resources, specific referrals made

Sample Nursing Outcomes & Interventions Classifications (NOC/NIC)

NOC—Spiritual Health
NIC—Spiritual Support

readiness for enhanced RELIGIOSITY

[Diagnostic Division: Ego Integrity]

Definition: A pattern of reliance on religious beliefs and/or participation in rituals of a particular faith tradition, which can be strengthened.

Defining Characteristics

Subjective

Expresses desire to enhance belief patterns or religious customs used in the past

Expresses desire to enhance participation in religious experiences or practices (e.g., ceremonies, regulations, clothing, prayer, services, holiday observances)

Expresses desire to enhance religious options, use of religious materials

Expresses desire to enhance connection with a religious leader

Expresses desire to enhance forgiveness

Information that appears in brackets has been added by the authors to clarify and enhance the use of nursing diagnoses.

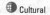

Desired Outcomes/Evaluation Criteria—Client Will:

- Acknowledge need to strengthen religious affiliations and continue or resume previously comforting rituals.
- Verbalize willingness to seek help to enhance desired religious beliefs.
- Become involved in spiritually based programs of own choice.
- Recognize the difference between belief patterns and customs that are helpful and those that may be harmful.

Actions/Interventions

Nursing Priority No. 1.

To determine spiritual state/motivation for growth:

- Determine client's current thinking about desire to learn more about religious beliefs and actions.
- Ascertain religious beliefs of family of origin and climate in which client grew up. **Early religious training deeply affects children and is carried on into adulthood. Conflict between family's beliefs and client's current learning may need to be addressed.**
- Discuss client's spiritual commitment, beliefs, and values. **Enables examination of these issues and helps client learn more about self and what he or she desires/believes.**
- Explore how spirituality and religious practices have affected client's life.
- Ascertain motivation and expectations for change.

Nursing Priority No. 2.

To assist client to integrate values and beliefs to strengthen sense of wholeness and achieve optimum balance in daily living:

- Establish nurse-client relationship in which dialogue can occur. **Client can feel safe to say anything and know it will be accepted.**
- Identify barriers and beliefs that might hinder growth and/or self-discovery. **Previous practices and beliefs may need to be considered and accepted or discarded in new search for religious beliefs.**
- Discuss cultural beliefs of family of origin and how they have influenced client's religious practices. **As client expands options for learning new or other religious beliefs and prac-**

Information that appears in brackets has been added by the authors to clarify and enhance the use of nursing diagnoses.

tices, these influences will provide information for comparing and contrasting new information.

- Explore connection of desire to strengthen belief patterns and customs to daily life. **Becoming aware of how these issues affect the individual's daily life can enhance ability to incorporate them into everything he or she does.**
- Identify ways in which individual can develop a sense of harmony with self and others.

Nursing Priority No. 3.

To enhance optimum spiritual wellness:

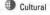

- Encourage client to seek out and experience different religious beliefs, services, and ceremonies. **Trying out different religions will give client more information to contrast and compare what will fit his or her belief system.**
- Provide bibliotherapy or reading materials pertaining to spiritual issues client is interested in learning about.
- Help client learn about stress-reducing activities (e.g., meditation, relaxation exercises, mindfulness). **Promotes general well-being and sense of control over self and ability to choose religious activities desired. Mindfulness is a method of being in the moment.**
- Encourage participation in religious activities, worship or religious services, reading religious materials or reviewing multimedia sources, study groups, volunteering in choir, or undertaking other needed duties.
- Refer to community resources (e.g., parish nurse, religion classes, other support groups).

Documentation Focus

Assessment/Reassessment

- Assessment findings, including client's religious beliefs and practices, perception of need
- Motivation and expectations for growth or enhancement

Planning

- Plan for growth and who is involved in planning

Implementation/Evaluation

- Response to activities, learning, and actions performed
- Attainment or progress toward desired outcome(s)
- Modifications to plan

Information that appears in brackets has been added by the authors to clarify and enhance the use of nursing diagnoses.

Discharge Planning

- Long-term needs/expectations and plan of action
- Specific referrals made

Sample Nursing Outcomes & Interventions Classifications (NOC/NIC)

NOC—Spiritual Health
NIC—Spiritual Growth Facilitation

RELOCATION STRESS SYNDROME and risk for RELOCATION STRESS SYNDROME

[Diagnostic Division: Ego Integrity]

Definition: Relocation Stress Syndrome: Physiological and/or psychosocial disturbance following transfer from one environment to another.

Definition: risk for Relocation Stress Syndrome: At risk for physiological and/or psychosocial disturbance following transfer from one environment to another.

Related and Risk Factors

Move from one environment to another; significant environmental change (risk)
Compromised health status (risk); deficient mental competence (risk)
History of loss; powerlessness;
Insufficient support system; insufficient predeparture counseling; unpredictability of experience
Social Isolation; language barrier
Impaired psychosocial functioning; ineffective coping strategies
[Increased confusion, cognitive impairment]

NOTE: A risk diagnosis is not evidenced by signs and symptoms, as the problem has not occurred; rather, nursing interventions are directed at prevention.

Defining Characteristics (Relocation Stress Syndrome)

Subjective

Anxiety (e.g., separation); anger
Insecurity; worry; fear

Information that appears in brackets has been added by the authors to clarify and enhance the use of nursing diagnoses.

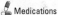

Loneliness; depression
Unwillingness to move; concern about relocation
Alteration in sleep pattern

Objective

Increase in verbalization of needs
Pessimism; frustration
Increase in physical symptoms or illness
Withdrawal; aloneness; alienation
Loss of identity or self-worth; low self-esteem; dependency
Increased confusion or cognitive impairment

Desired Outcomes/Evaluation Criteria—Client Will:

- Verbalize understanding of reason(s) for change.
- Demonstrate appropriate range of feelings and reduced fear.
- Participate in routine and special or social events as able.
- Verbalize acceptance of situation.
- Experience no catastrophic event.

Actions/Interventions

Nursing Priority No. 1.

To assess causative/contributing **or risk** factors:

- Determine situation or cause for relocation (e.g., planned move for new job; deployment or returning from military duty; loss of home or community due to natural or man-made disaster such as fire, earthquake, flood, war or act of terror; older adult unable to care for self, caregiver burnout; change in marital or health status). **Influences needs and choice of interventions.**
- Determine physical and emotional health status. **Stress associated with a move, even if desired, can cause or exacerbate health problems.**
- ∞ Note client's age, developmental level, role in family. **Age and position in life cycle make a difference in the impact of issues involved in relocating. For example, a child can be traumatized by transfer to new school/loss of peers; elderly persons may be affected by loss of long-term home, neighborhood setting, and support persons.**
- Ascertain if client participated in the decision to relocate and perceptions about change(s) and expectations for the future. **Decision may have been made without client's input or**

Information that appears in brackets has been added by the authors to clarify and enhance the use of nursing diagnoses.

understanding of event or consequences, which can impact adjustment.

- Note whether relocation will be temporary (e.g., extended care for rehabilitation therapies, moving in with family while house is being repaired after fire) or long term or permanent (e.g., move from home of many years; placement in retirement center or long-term care facility). **Client may be willing to relocate on temporary basis, seeing it as step to health and independence, but may view long-term placement as unbearable loss.**
- Identify cultural and/or religious concerns or conflicts **that may affect client's coping or impact social interactions and expectations. For example. client's cultural norm may be that elders are cared for by family—not placed in a facility—causing client to feel abandoned; or individual may be required to defer to family decision maker and feel powerless in determining own destiny.**
- Note ethnic ties and primary language spoken and read. Obtain interpreter where appropriate. **Affects client, significant other (SO)(s), and healthcare providers who must try to reduce the client's feelings of alienation, while communicating with client of another primary language, or client who is displaced from cultural attachments.**
- Monitor behavior, noting presence of anxiety, suspiciousness or paranoia, irritability, defensiveness. Compare with SO's/staff's description of customary responses. **Move may temporarily exacerbate mental deterioration (cognitive inaccessibility) and impair communication (social inaccessibility).**
- Determine involvement of family/SO(s). Note availability and use of support systems and resources.
- Identify issues of safety that may be involved **such as difficulty adjusting to new environment (e.g., navigating streets or choosing correct bus; locating dining hall or bathroom in facility), concerns of elopement or running away.**

Nursing Priority No. 2.

To assist client to deal with situation/changes **or to prevent/minimize adverse response to change:**

- Collaborate in treatment of underlying conditions (e.g., chronic confusional states, brain injury, post-trauma rehabilitation) and physical stress symptoms **that are potentially exacerbating relocation stress or that may affect the length of time that relocation is required.**

Information that appears in brackets has been added by the authors to clarify and enhance the use of nursing diagnoses.

- Anticipate and address feelings of distress and grieving in family/caregivers when placing loved one in a different environment (e.g., nursing home, foster care). **Support and referrals may be needed to help SOs in practical issues and adjustment.**
- Begin relocation planning with client and SO(s) as early as possible. Provide support and advocate for client who is unable to participate in decisions. **Having a well-organized plan for move with support and advocacy may reduce anxiety.**
- Allow as much time as possible for move preparation and provide information and support in planning.
- ∞ Discuss relocation or move with child, providing information aimed at level of understanding and interest. **Child lacks ability to put problem into perspective, so minor mishap may seem catastrophic, and child is more vulnerable to stress because he or she has less control over environment than most adults.**
- ∞ Avoid moving adolescent in middle of school year when possible. **Adolescent is vulnerable to emotional, social, and cognitive dysfunction because of the great importance of peer group and loss of friends and social standing caused by relocation.**
- Support self-responsibility and coping strategies **to foster sense of control and self-worth.**
- Suggest contact with someone (friend, family, business associate) who has been to or lived in new area where move is being planned **to absorb some of his or her experience and knowledge.**
- Encourage free expression of feelings about reason for relocation, including venting of anger; grief; loss of personal space, belongings, or friends; financial strains; powerlessness; and so forth. Acknowledge reality of situation and maintain hopeful attitude regarding move/change. Refer to NDs relating to client's particular situation (e.g., Grieving; ineffective Coping) for additional interventions.
- Identify strengths and successful coping behaviors the individual has used previously. **Incorporating these into problem-solving builds on past successes.**
- Encourage client to maintain contact with friends (e.g., telephone, e-mail, video or audio tapes, arranged visits) **to reduce sense of isolation.**
- Orient to surroundings and schedules. Introduce to neighbors, staff members, roommate, or residents. Provide clear, honest information about actions and events.

Information that appears in brackets has been added by the authors to clarify and enhance the use of nursing diagnoses.

- Encourage individual/family to personalize area with pictures, own belongings, as possible and appropriate. **Enhances sense of belonging and creates personal space.**
- Determine client's usual schedule of activities and incorporate into routine as possible. **Reinforces sense of importance of individual.**
- Take practical steps to alleviate stress for child. Encourage parents to walk with child to school or rehearse boarding the school bus, visit new classroom, contact friends child left behind, drive past places of interest to child, find a safe play place, unpack child's favorite toys, invite neighborhood children to a get-acquainted party, and so forth. **Helps child to maintain ties and develop new ones, thus reducing sense of loss and shifting focus to the future.**
- Introduce planned diversional activities, such as movies, meals with new acquaintances, art therapy, music, religious activities. **Involvement increases opportunity to interact with others, decreasing isolation.**
- Place client with dementia in private facility room, if appropriate, and include SO(s)/family in care activities, mealtimes, especially early in transition stage. **Keeping client secluded may be needed under some circumstances (e.g., advanced Alzheimer's disease with fear or aggressive reactions) to decrease the client's stress reactions to new environment.**
- Encourage hugging and use of touch unless client prefers to abstain from hugging, is paranoid, or agitated at the moment. **Human connection reaffirms acceptance of individual.**
- Deal with aggressive behavior by imposing calm, firm limits. Control environment and protect others from client's disruptive behavior. **Promotes safety for client and others.**
- Remain composed, place in a quiet environment, providing time out, as indicated, **to prevent escalation into panic state and violent behavior.**
- Refer to professionals (e.g., social worker, financial resources, mental healthcare provider, minister/spiritual advisor) if serious difficulties develop (e.g., depression, alcohol or other drug abuse, deteriorating behavior of child) **to assist client with special needs and/or persistent problems with adaptation.**

Nursing Priority No. 3.

To promote wellness (Teaching/Discharge Considerations):

- Involve client in formulating goals and plan of care when possible. **Supports independence and commitment to achieving outcomes.**

Information that appears in brackets has been added by the authors to clarify and enhance the use of nursing diagnoses.

- Encourage communication between client/family/SO **to provide mutual support and problem-solving opportunities.**
- Discuss benefits of adequate nutrition, rest, and exercise **to maintain physical well-being.**
- Involve in anxiety- and stress-reduction activities (e.g., meditation, progressive muscle relaxation, group socialization), as able, **to enhance psychological well-being and coping abilities.**
- Encourage participation in activities, hobbies, and personal interactions as appropriate. **Promotes creative endeavors, stimulating the mind.**
- Provide client with information and list of organizations or community services (e.g., Welcome Wagon, senior citizens or teen clubs, churches, singles' groups, sports leagues) **to provide contacts for client to develop new relationships and learn more about the new setting.**
- Discuss safety issues regarding new environment (e.g., how to navigate streets or choose correct bus; locate dining hall or bathroom in facility), concerns of elopement or running away.
- Anticipate variety of emotions and reactions. **May vary from insomnia and loss of appetite to becoming involved with alcohol or other drugs or exacerbation of health problems, onset of serious illness, or behavioral problems. Awareness provides opportunity for timely intervention.**

Documentation Focus

Assessment/Reassessment

- Assessment findings, individual's perception of the situation and changes, sense of loss, specific behaviors
- Cultural or religious concerns
- Safety issues

Planning

- Note plan of care, who is involved in planning, and who is responsible for proposed actions
- Teaching plan

Implementation/Evaluation

- Response to interventions (especially time out or seclusion), teaching, and actions performed
- Sentinel events
- Attainment or progress toward desired outcome(s)
- Modifications to plan of care

Information that appears in brackets has been added by the authors to clarify and enhance the use of nursing diagnoses.

 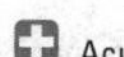  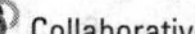  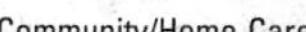 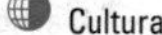

Discharge Planning

- Long-term needs and who is responsible for actions to be taken
- Specific referrals made

Sample Nursing Outcomes & Interventions Classifications (NOC/NIC)

NOC—Psychosocial Adjustment: Life Change
NIC—Relocation Stress Reduction

risk for ineffective RENAL PERFUSION

[Diagnostic Division: Circulatory]

Definition: Vulnerable to a decrease in blood circulation to the kidney, which may compromise health.

Risk Factors

Alteration in metabolism; diabetes mellitus
Renal disease (e.g., polycystic kidney, renal artery stenosis, failure); bilateral cortical necrosis; exposure to nephrotoxin; glomerulonephritis; interstitial nephritis; polynephritis
Burns; infection; systemic inflammatory response syndrome (SIRS)
Cardiac surgery; vascular embolism; vasculitis
Abdominal compartment syndrome
Extremes of age; female gender
Hypertension; malignant hypertension; hypovolemia; hypoxemia
Malignancy
Smoking; substance abuse
Trauma; treatment regimen

NOTE: A risk diagnosis is not evidenced by signs and symptoms, as the problem has not occurred; rather, nursing interventions are directed at prevention.

Desired Outcomes/Evaluation Criteria—Client Will:

- Demonstrate adequate renal perfusion as evidenced by urine output appropriate for individual, balanced intake and output, absence of edema formation or inappropriate weight gain.

Information that appears in brackets has been added by the authors to clarify and enhance the use of nursing diagnoses.

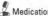

- Verbalize understanding of condition, therapy regimen, side effects of medication, and when to contact healthcare provider.
- Engage in behaviors/lifestyle changes to improve circulation (e.g., smoking cessation, diabetic glucose control, medication management).

Actions/Interventions

Nursing Priority No. 1.

To assess causative/contributing factors:

- Determine history or presence of severe hypotension and hypoxemia or shock (may be cardiogenic, hypovolemia, obstructive, or septic shock), blunt or penetrating trauma, surgery with excess bleeding or fluid loss, prolonged dehydration, poorly controlled diabetes, and so forth—**conditions associated with decreased systemic circulation and kidney ischemia.**
- Note history or presence of abrupt onset or severe hypertension, persistent hypertension (>160/100) over time, or hypertension resistant to appropriately dosed antihypertensive therapy, **any of which places client at high risk for kidney damage associated with renovascular hypertension.**
- Assess hydration status. **Dehydration reduces glomerular filtration rate.**
- Ascultate for bruit over each renal artery in abdomen at midclavicular line, **suggesting renal artery stenosis, which is associated with renal insufficiency.**
- Determine usual voiding pattern and investigate reported deviations, such as low output or need for diuretics, **which may indicate problems with kidney perfusion.**
- Note urine color—pale (dilute) or dark (concentrated)—and measure specific gravity, as indicated, **to evaluate hydration status and kidney's ability to concentrate the urine.**
- Monitor fluid intake, urine output, and weight on a regular schedule **to provide noninvasive assessment of cardiovascular and renal function.**
- Monitor for edema. **May be present with increased fluid retention due to impaired renal function related to decreased renal perfusion.**
- Note mentation and behavior. **Adverse changes may be the consequence of fluid shifts, accumulation of toxins,**

Information that appears in brackets has been added by the authors to clarify and enhance the use of nursing diagnoses.

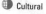

acid-based and/or electrolyte imbalances when kidney dysfunction is occurring.

- Review medication regimen, observing for certain antimicrobials, antivirals, chemotherapy agents, analgesics, immunosuppressives, herbals, and diagnostic agents. Monitor peak and trough blood levels when client receiving nephrotoxic agents such as aminoglycosides (e.g.,Vancomycin), **known for potential side or toxic effects that may substantially alter kidney perfusion.**
- Discuss client's history of and current alcohol and illicit substance use/abuse. **Most street drugs, including heroin, cocaine, and ecstasy can cause high blood pressure, a risk factor for impaired renal function. Alcohol (when used heavily), cocaine, heroin, and amphetamines also can cause kidney damage.**
- Review laboratory studies (e.g., complete blood count, blood urea nitrogen/creatinine levels, protein, specific gravity, 24-hr creatinine clearance, glucose, electrolytes) **to evaluate kidney function.**
- Review diagnostic studies, as indicated, including Doppler ultrasonography, computed tomography, renogram, IV pyelogram; contrast or magnetic resonance angiography, **to evaluate kidney size, perfusion, and function.**

Nursing Priority No. 2.

To reduce or correct individual risk factors:

- Collaborate in treatment of underlying conditions (e.g., angioplasty with stent placement, surgical revascularization procedures, fluids, electrolytes, nutrients, antibiotics, thrombolytics, oxygen) **to improve tissue perfusion/organ function.**
- Administer medications (e.g., vasoactive medications, including antihypertensive agents, insulin) as indicated **to treat underlying condition and improve renal blood flow and function.**
- Exercise caution when administering nephrotoxic agents, particularly when dehydration is present, **to reduce risk for acute or chronic renal failure.**
- Provide for fluid and diet restrictions as indicated, while providing adequate calories and hydration **to meet the body's needs without overtaxing kidney function.**
- Refer to NDs deficient or excess Fluid Volume, impaired urinary Elimination for additional interventions.

Information that appears in brackets has been added by the authors to clarify and enhance the use of nursing diagnoses.

Nursing Priority No. 3.

To promote wellness (Teaching/Discharge Considerations):

- Discuss individual risk factors (e.g., family history, obesity, age, smoking, hypertension, diabetes, clotting disorders) and potential outcomes of atherosclerosis such as systemic and peripheral vascular disease. **Information necessary for client to make informed choices about remedial risk factors and consider lifestyle changes to prevent onset of complications or manage symptoms when condition present.**
- Identify necessary changes in lifestyle and assist client to incorporate disease management into activities of daily living. **Promotes independence; enhances self-concept regarding ability to deal with change and manage own needs.**
- Emphasize need to manage blood pressure when client is hypertensive. Instruct about individual's antihypertensive medications (e.g., angiotensin-converting enzyme inhibitors, diuretics, beta-adrenergic blockers), and necessity for taking them as prescribed and with physician follow-up **to reduce cardiovascular complications and slow progression of renal dysfunction.**
- Instruct in home blood pressure monitoring; advise purchase of appropriate equipment; refer to community resources as indicated. **Facilitates management of hypertension, which is a major risk factor for damage to blood vessels and organ function.**
- Encourage client to quit smoking, join Smoke-out or other smoking-cessation programs. **Smoking causes vasoconstriction, compromising renal perfusion.**
- Review specific fluid and dietary requirements with client/significant other (SO) (e.g., reduction of cholesterol, carbohydrates, or sodium) as indicated by individual situation **to promote circulatory health and kidney function.**
- Establish regular exercise program **to enhance circulation and promote general well-being.**
- Encourage regular medical and laboratory follow-up **to provide monitoring and earlier intervention for underlying conditions and to evaluate effectiveness of therapeutic interventions.**
- Refer to specific support groups, counseling as appropriate **to assist with problem-solving, provide role model, enhance coping ability.**

Information that appears in brackets has been added by the authors to clarify and enhance the use of nursing diagnoses.

Documentation Focus

Assessment/Reassessment

- Individual physical findings; identified risk factors
- Baseline kidney function
- Input and output and weight as indicated

Planning

- Plan of care and who is involved in planning
- Teaching plan

Implementation/Evaluation

- Response to interventions, teaching, and actions performed
- Attainment or progress toward desired outcome(s)
- Modifications to plan of care

Discharge Planning

- Long-term needs and who is responsible for actions to be taken
- Available resources, specific referrals made

Sample Nursing Outcomes & Interventions Classifications (NOC/NIC)

NOC—Kidney Function
NIC—Fluid/Electrolyte Management

impaired RESILIENCE and risk for impaired RESILIENCE

[Diagnostic Division: Ego Integrity]

Definition: impaired Resilience: Decreased ability to sustain a pattern of positive responses to an adverse situation or crisis.

Definition: risk for impaired Resilience: Vulnerable to decreased ability to sustain a pattern of positive responses to an adverse situation or crisis, which may compromise health.

Related Factors

Community violence; exposure to violence
Demographics that increase changes of maladjustment; ethnic minority status
Economically disadvantaged; perceived vulnerability

Information that appears in brackets has been added by the authors to clarify and enhance the use of nursing diagnoses.

Female gender; large family size
Inconsistent parenting; parental mental illness; psychological disorder
Low intellectual ability; low maternal educational level
Insufficient impulse control; substance abuse

Risk Factors

Chronicity of existing crisis
Multiple coexisting adverse situations
New crisis (e.g., unplanned pregnancy, loss of housing, death of family member)

NOTE: A risk diagnosis is not evidenced by signs and symptoms, as the problem has not occurred; rather, nursing interventions are directed at prevention.

Defining Characteristics (impaired Resilience)

Subjective

Depression; guilt; shame
Impaired health status
Renewed elevation of distress
Decreased interest in academic or vocational activities

Objective

Ineffective coping skills; social isolation; low self-esteem

Desired Outcomes/Evaluation Criteria—Client Will:

- Acknowledge reality of current situation or crisis.
- Express positive feelings about self and situation.
- Seek appropriate resources to change circumstances that affect adaptation and resilience.
- Be involved in programs to address problems presenting in life (e.g., substance abuse, low self-esteem, poverty).

Actions/Interventions

Nursing Priority No. 1.

To assess causative/contributing factors **or potential stressors/challenges:**

Information that appears in brackets has been added by the authors to clarify and enhance the use of nursing diagnoses.

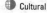

- Determine individuals, family, children involved and ages and current circumstances. **Understanding the family makeup provides information that will guide choice of interventions.**
- Note underlying stressors, health concerns, debilitating conditions, mental health or behavioral issues such as unemployment, poverty, diabetes, obesity, chronic obstructive pulmonary disease, Alzheimer's disease, parental mental illness.
- Assess functional capacity and how it affects client's ability to manage daily needs.
- Identify locus of control. **Individuals with external locus of control are less likely to feel in control or to rely on their own abilities or judgment to manage a situation.**
- Determine client's education level, family dynamics, and parenting styles, if relevant. **Drug use, violence, and poor impulse control affect individual's ability to develop resilience in adverse situations or crisis. Individual may see self as a victim rather than a survivor.**
- Evaluate client's ability to verbalize and understand current situation and impact of new crisis. **Informed choice cannot be made without a good understanding of reality of situation.**
- Note communication patterns within the family. **Skills learned within the family can determine whether the individual develops low self-esteem or positive feelings about self.**
- Identify maladaptive coping skills used by individual and in the family. **Focusing on negative in situations impairs one's ability to adjust positively and learn attributes of resiliency.**
- Note parental status including age and maturity. **Young parents may lack ability to deal with family responsibilities, financial concerns, factors associated with low socioeconomic status.**
- Ascertain stability of relationship, presence of separation or divorce. **Family members are vulnerable to break-up of the family unit and may see it as causing long-term harm.**
- Determine availability and use of resources, family, support groups, financial aid.
- Note cultural factors and religious beliefs that may affect interpretation of, or response to, situation. **Helps determine individual needs and possible options.**

Nursing Priority No. 2.

To assist client to improve skills to deal with adverse situations or crises.

Information that appears in brackets has been added by the authors to clarify and enhance the use of nursing diagnoses.

- Encourage free expressions of feelings, including feelings of anger and hostility, setting limits on unacceptable behavior. **Unacceptable behavior leads to feelings of shame and guilt if not controlled.**
- Listen to client's concerns and acknowledge difficulty of adversity and making changes in situation. **Being listened to provides opportunity for client to feel valued, capable, and like a survivor rather than a victim.**
- Help client assume responsibility for own life, look at situation as a challenge rather than an obstacle, and refrain from viewing crisis as insurmountable. **People learn and develop resilience as they deal with adversities of life.**
- Provide information at client's level of comprehension, being honest in explanations. **Provides data to assist in decision-making process.**
- Have client paraphrase information provided during teaching session to **ensure understanding and to provide opportunity to correct misunderstandings.**
- Promote parents' involvement in developing a positive mind-set for fostering resilience in their children. **Parents are concerned that their children grow up to be competent adults. They can learn the parenting skills that promote optimal growth and resilience in their children for the problems they will face as grown-ups.**
- Facilitate communication skills between client and family. **Sometimes, individuals who find themselves in difficult situations withdraw because they do not know what to do or say.**
- Focus on strengths of the individual as the problems are being assessed and diagnosed. **Improving the future for the client is based on developing the capacity to deal successfully with the obstacles he or she meets in life.**
- Teach client/parents to practice empathy with family members.
- Discuss individual issues, such as obesity, substance use, poor impulse control, violent behavior; provide information about the risks and help client/parent understand how they can help family members develop habits that will promote physical and mental well-being.

Nursing Priority No. 3.

To promote wellness (Teaching/Discharge Considerations):

- Reinforce that client is responsible for self, for choices made, and actions taken. **The road to resilience is developed by**

Information that appears in brackets has been added by the authors to clarify and enhance the use of nursing diagnoses.

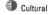

the individual accepting that change is a part of living and then beginning to live life more fully.

- Encourage an attitude of realistic hope. **Client can accept that change is a part of living and, while some plans cannot be obtained because of crisis or new circumstances, new goals can be developed and life can move forward.**
- Provide anticipatory guidance relevant to current situation and long-term expectations.
- Provide or identify learning opportunities specific to individual needs. **Activities such as assertiveness, regular exercise, parenting classes can enhance knowledge and help develop a resilient mind-set.**
- Discuss use of the problem-solving method to set mutually agreed-on goals. **As family accepts solutions that are acceptable to each member, their self-esteem is enhanced, and individuals are more apt to follow through on decisions.**
- Provide anticipatory guidance relevant to current situation and long-term expectations. **Client may have many issues to resolve, and planning ahead can help individuals make changes, have hope for the future, and have a sense of control over their lives.**
- Encourage client/parents to take time for themselves. **Provides opportunity for personal growth; respite allows individuals to pursue own interests and return to tasks of life/parenting with renewed vigor.**
- Determine need or desire for religious or spiritual counselor and make arrangements for visit. **Providing client an opportunity to discuss concerns about what has happened helps to build resilience to face future stressors.**
- Refer to community resources as appropriate, such as social services, financial, domestic violence/elder abuse program, family therapy, divorce counseling, special needs support services.

Documentation Focus

Assessment/Reassessment

- Findings, including specifics of individual situations, parental concerns, perceptions, expectations
- Locus of control and cultural beliefs

Planning

- Plan of care and who is involved in the planning
- Teaching plan

Information that appears in brackets has been added by the authors to clarify and enhance the use of nursing diagnoses.

Implementation/Evaluation

- Response to interventions, teaching, and actions performed
- Attainment or progress toward desired outcome(s)
- Modifications to plan of care

Discharge Planning

- Long-term needs and who is responsible for actions to be taken
- Specific referrals made

Sample Nursing Outcomes & Interventions Classifications (NOC/NIC)

NOC—Personal Resiliency
NIC—Resiliency Promotion

readiness for enhanced RESILIENCE

[Diagnostic Division: Ego Integrity]

Definition: A pattern of positive responses to an adverse situation or crisis, which can be strengthened.

Defining Characteristics

Subjective

Expresses desire to enhance: communication skills, relationships with others
Expresses desire to enhance use of: coping skills, conflict management strategies
Expresses desire to enhance: resilience, self-esteem
Expresses desire to enhance: involvement in activities, own responsibility for action, sense of control
Expresses desire to enhance: goal-setting, progress toward goal
Expresses desire to enhance: support system, available resources, use of resources
Expresses desire to enhance: environmental safety

Objective

Demonstrates positive outlook
Exposure to crisis

Information that appears in brackets has been added by the authors to clarify and enhance the use of nursing diagnoses.

Desired Outcomes/Evaluation Criteria—Client Will:

- Describe current situation accurately.
- Identify positive responses currently being used.
- Verbalize feelings congruent with behavior.
- Express desire to strengthen ability to deal with current situation or crisis.

Actions/Interventions

Nursing Priority No. 1.

To determine needs and desires for improvement:

- Evaluate client's perception and ability to provide a realistic view of the situation. **Provides information about how client views the situation and specific expectations to aid in formulating plan of care.**
- Determine client's coping abilities in current situation and expectations for change. **Motivation to improve and high expectations can encourage client to make changes that will improve his or her life. However, unrealistic expectations may hamper efforts.**
- Note client's verbal expressions indicating belief that he or she owns the responsibility for how to deal with adverse situation. **When client has internal locus of control, he or she accepts that life has its adversities and one needs to deal with them.**
- Discuss religious and cultural beliefs held by the individual.
- Identify support systems available to client.

Nursing Priority No. 2.

To assist client to enhance resilience to adverse situation:

- Active-listen and identify client's concerns about situation. **Reflecting client's statements helps to clarify what he or she is thinking and promotes accurate interpretation of reality.**
- Determine previous methods of dealing with adversity. **Helps client to remember successful skills used in the past, and see what might be helpful in current situation.**
- Discuss desire to improve ability to handle adverse situations that arise throughout life. **Willingness to be open to change requires a curiosity, listening to others' ideas and beliefs, looking at new ways to do things.**
- Discuss concept of what can be changed versus what cannot be changed.

Information that appears in brackets has been added by the authors to clarify and enhance the use of nursing diagnoses.

- Determine how client is dealing with activities of daily living. **While client may have some transient problems with sleeping or managing daily affairs, most people have the ability to function in a healthy manner over time.**
- Help client to learn how to empathize with others. **Understanding own emotions as well as feelings of others enhances one's resiliency during stressful times.**

Nursing Priority No. 3.

To promote optimum growth and resiliency:

- Provide factual information and anticipatory guidance relevant to current situation and long-term expectations. **Planning ahead allows for problem-solving and review of options in a relaxed atmosphere, reinforcing sense of control and hope for the future.**
- Review factors that might impact individual's response to stress.
- Encourage client to maintain or establish good relationships with family and friends.
- Help client avoid seeing situation as insurmountable. **While one cannot change the fact of the circumstances, how individual interprets and responds is within one's control.**
- Recommend setting realistic goals and doing something regularly, even if it is small.
- Encourage client to maintain a hopeful outlook, nurture a positive view of self, and take care of self. **Keeping a long-term perspective and paying attention to own needs help maintain and build resilience.**
- Refer to classes and/or reading materials as appropriate.

Documentation Focus

Assessment/Reassessment

- Baseline information, including client's perception of situation, view of own ability to be resilient, and support systems available
- Ways of dealing with previous life problems
- Motivation and expectations for change
- Cultural or religious influences

Planning

- Plan of care and who is involved in planning
- Educational plan

Information that appears in brackets has been added by the authors to clarify and enhance the use of nursing diagnoses.

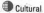

Implementation/Evaluation

- Responses to interventions, teaching, and actions performed
- Attainment or progress toward desired outcomes(s)
- Modifications to plan

Discharge Planning

- Long-term needs and who is responsible for actions to be taken
- Specific referrals made

Sample Nursing Outcomes & Interventions Classifications (NOC/NIC)

NOC—Personal Resiliency
NIC—Resiliency Promotion

parental ROLE CONFLICT

[Diagnostic Division: Social Interaction]

Definition: Parental experience of role confusion and conflict in response to crisis.

Related Factors

Parent-child separation
Intimidation by invasive modalities (e.g., intubation); by restrictive modalities (e.g., isolation)
Home care of a child with special needs
Living in nontraditional setting (e.g., foster, group, or institutional care)
Change in marital status; [conflicts of the role of single parent]
Interruptions in family life due to home-care regimen (e.g., treatments, caregivers, lack of respite)

Defining Characteristics

Subjective

Perceived inadequacy to provide for child's needs (e.g., physical, emotional)
Concern about change in parental role; concern about family (e.g., functioning, communication, health)
Perceived loss of control over decisions relating to child
Guilt; frustration; anxiety; fear

Information that appears in brackets has been added by the authors to clarify and enhance the use of nursing diagnoses.

Objective

Disruption in caregiver routines
Reluctance to participate in usual caregiver activities

Desired Outcomes/Evaluation Criteria—Parent(s) Will:

- Verbalize understanding of situation and expected parent's/child's role.
- Express feelings about child's illness or situation and effect on family life.
- Demonstrate appropriate behaviors in regard to parenting role.
- Assume caretaking activities as appropriate.
- Handle family disruptions effectively.

Actions/Interventions

Nursing Priority No. 1.

To assess causative/contributory factors:

- Assess individual situation and parent's perception of/concern about what is happening and expectations of self as caregiver.
- Note parental status, including age and maturity, stability of relationship, single parent, other responsibilities. **For example, increasing numbers of elderly individuals are providing full-time care for young grandchildren whose parents are unavailable or unable to provide care.**
- Ascertain parent's understanding of child's developmental stage and expectations for the future **to identify misconceptions and strengths.**
- Note coping skills currently being used by each individual as well as how problems have been dealt with in the past. **Provides basis for comparison and reference for client's coping abilities.**
- Determine use of substances (e.g., alcohol, other drugs, including prescription medications). **May interfere with individual's ability to cope and problem-solve.**
- Assess availability and use of resources, including extended family, support groups, and financial.
- Perform testing, such as Parent-Child Relationship Inventory, for further evaluation as indicated.

Nursing Priority No. 2.

To assist parents to deal with current crisis:

Information that appears in brackets has been added by the authors to clarify and enhance the use of nursing diagnoses.

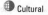

- Encourage free verbal expression of feelings (including negative feelings of anger and hostility), setting limits on inappropriate behavior.
- Acknowledge difficulty of situation and normalcy of feeling overwhelmed and helpless. Encourage contact with parents who experienced similar situation with child and had positive outcome.
- Provide information, including technical information when appropriate, **to meet individual needs and correct misconceptions.**
- Promote parental involvement in decision making and care as much as possible/desired. **Enhances sense of control.**
- Encourage interaction/facilitate communication between parent(s) and children.
- Promote use of assertiveness, relaxation skills **to help individuals deal with situation/crisis.**
- Assist parent(s) to learn proper administration of medications and treatments, as indicated.
- Provide for, or encourage use of, respite care, parental time off **to enhance emotional well-being.**
- Help single parent distinguish between parent love and partner love. **Love is constant, but attention can be given to one or the other, as appropriate.**

Nursing Priority No. 3.

To promote wellness (Teaching/Discharge Considerations):

- Provide anticipatory guidance **to encourage making plans for future needs.**
- Encourage parents to set realistic and mutually agreed-on goals.
- Discuss attachment behaviors such as breastfeeding on cue, cosleeping, baby-wearing (carrying baby around on chest/back), and playing. **Dealing with ill child/home-care pressures can strain the bond between parent and child. Activities such as these encourage secure relationships.**
- Provide and identify learning opportunities specific to needs (e.g., parenting classes, healthcare equipment use/troubleshooting).
- Refer to community resources, as appropriate (e.g., visiting nurse, respite care, social services, psychiatric care or family therapy, well-baby clinics, special needs support services).
- Refer to ND impaired Parenting for additional interventions.

Information that appears in brackets has been added by the authors to clarify and enhance the use of nursing diagnoses.

Documentation Focus

Assessment/Reassessment

- Findings, including specifics of individual situation/parental concerns, perceptions, expectations

Planning

- Plan of care and who is involved in the planning
- Teaching plan

Implementation/Evaluation

- Parent's responses to interventions, teaching, and actions performed
- Attainment or progress toward desired outcome(s)
- Modifications to plan of care

Discharge Planning

- Long-term needs and who is responsible for each action to be taken
- Specific referrals made

Sample Nursing Outcomes & Interventions Classifications (NOC/NIC)

NOC—Parenting Performance
NIC—Parenting Promotion

ineffective ROLE PERFORMANCE

[Diagnostic Division: Social Interaction]

Definition: A pattern of behavior and self-expression that does not match the environmental context, norms, and expectations.

NOTE: There is a typology of roles (e.g., sociopersonal [friendship, family, marital, parenting, community]; home management; intimacy [sexuality, relationship building]; leisure, exercise, or recreation; self-management; socialization [developmental transitions], community contributor; and religious) that can help to understand ineffective Role Performance.

Information that appears in brackets has been added by the authors to clarify and enhance the use of nursing diagnoses.

Related Factors

Knowledge

Insufficient role model
Insufficient role preparation (e.g., role transition, skill rehearsal, validation)
Low educational level
Unrealistic role expectations

Physiological

Alteration in body image; neurological deficit; physical illness; low self-esteem
Mental health issue (e.g., depression, psychosis, personality disorder, substance abuse)
Fatigue; pain

Social

Insufficient role socialization
Young age; developmental level inappropriate for role expectation
Insufficient resources (e.g., financial, social, knowledge); economically disadvantaged
Stressors; conflict; high demands of job schedule
[Family conflict]; domestic violence
Insufficient support system; insufficient rewards
Inappropriate linkage with the healthcare system

Defining Characteristics

Subjective

Alteration in role perception; change in self-/other's perception of role
Change in usual pattern of responsibility or in capacity to resume role
Insufficient opportunity for role enactment
Role dissatisfaction; role denial
Discrimination; powerlessness

Objective

Insufficient knowledge of role requirements
Ineffective adaptation to change; inappropriate developmental expectations
Insufficient confidence, motivation, self-management, or skills
Ineffective coping strategies; ineffective role performance
Inadequate external support for role enactment

Information that appears in brackets has been added by the authors to clarify and enhance the use of nursing diagnoses.

Role strain, conflict, confusion, or ambivalence; [failure to assume role]
Uncertainty; anxiety; depression; pessimism
Domestic violence; harassment; system conflict

Desired Outcomes/Evaluation Criteria—Client Will:

- Verbalize understanding of role expectations and obligations.
- Verbalize realistic perception and acceptance of self in changed role.
- Talk with family/significant other (SO)(s) about situation and changes that have occurred and limitations imposed.
- Develop realistic plans for adapting to new role or role changes.

Actions/Interventions

Nursing Priority No. 1.

To assess causative/contributing factors:

- Identify type of role dysfunction: for example, developmental (adolescent to adult); situational (husband to father, gender identity); transitions from health to illness.
- Determine client role in family constellation.
- Identify how client sees self as a man or woman in usual lifestyle or role functioning.
- Ascertain client's view of sexual functioning (e.g., loss of childbearing ability following hysterectomy).
- Identify cultural factors relating to individual's sexual roles. **Cultures define male and female roles differently (e.g., Muslim culture demands that the woman adopt a subservient role, whereas the man is seen as the powerful one in the relationship).**
- Determine client's perceptions or concerns about current situation. **May believe current role is more appropriate for the opposite sex (e.g., passive role of the patient may be somewhat less threatening for women).**
- Interview SO(s) regarding their perceptions and expectations. **Influences client's view of self.**

Nursing Priority No. 2.

To assist client to deal with existing situation:

- Discuss perceptions and significance of the situation as seen by client.
- Maintain positive attitude toward the client.

Information that appears in brackets has been added by the authors to clarify and enhance the use of nursing diagnoses.

- Provide opportunities for client to exercise control over as many decisions as possible. **Enhances self-concept and promotes commitment to goals.**
- Offer realistic assessment of situation while communicating sense of hope.
- Discuss and assist client/SO(s) to develop strategies for dealing with changes in role related to past transitions, cultural expectations, and value or belief challenges. **Helps those involved deal with differences between individuals (e.g., adolescent task of separation in which parents clash with child's choices; individual's decision to change religious affiliation).**
- Acknowledge reality of situation related to role change and help client express feelings of anger, sadness, and grief. Encourage celebration of positive aspects of change and expressions of feelings.
- Provide open environment for client to discuss concerns about sexuality. **Embarrassment can block discussion of sensitive subject.** (Refer to NDs Sexual Dysfunction; ineffective Sexuality Pattern.)
- Identify role model for client. Educate about role expectations using written and audiovisual materials.
- Use the techniques of role rehearsal to help client develop new skills **to cope with changes.**

Nursing Priority No. 3.

To promote wellness (Teaching/Discharge Considerations):

- Make information available for client to learn about role expectations or demands that may occur. **Provides opportunity to be proactive in dealing with changes.**
- Accept client in changed role. Encourage and give positive feedback for changes and goals achieved. **Provides reinforcement and facilitates continuation of efforts.**
- Refer to support groups, employment counselors, parent effectiveness classes, counseling/psychotherapy, as indicated by individual need(s). **Provides ongoing support to sustain progress.**
- Refer to NDs Self-Esteem [specify]; impaired, risk for impaired, or readiness for enhanced Parenting.

Documentation Focus

Assessment/Reassessment

- Individual findings, including specifics of predisposing crises or situation, perception of role change
- Expectations of SO(s)

Information that appears in brackets has been added by the authors to clarify and enhance the use of nursing diagnoses.

Planning
- Plan of care and who is involved in planning
- Teaching plan

Implementation/Evaluation
- Responses to interventions, teaching, and actions performed
- Attainment or progress toward desired outcome(s)
- Modifications to plan of care

Discharge Planning
- Long-term needs and who is responsible for actions to be taken
- Specific referrals made

Sample Nursing Outcomes & Interventions Classifications (NOC/NIC)

NOC—Role Performance
NIC—Role Enhancement

caregiver ROLE STRAIN and risk for caregiver ROLE STRAIN

[Diagnostic Division: Social Interaction]

Definition: caregiver Role Strain: Difficulty in performing family/significant other caregiver role.

Definition: risk for caregiver Role Strain: Vulnerable to difficulty in performing the family/significant other caregiver role, which may compromise health.

Related Factors (caregiver Role Strain)—

Care Receiver Health Status
Alteration in cognitive functioning
Chronic illness; illness severity; increase in care needs; unpredictability of illness trajectory; unstable health condition
Codependency; dependency; substance abuse
Problematic behavior; psychiatric disorder

Caregiver Health Status
Alteration in cognitive functioning; physical conditions
Codependency; substance abuse
Ineffective coping strategies; insufficient fulfillment of others' or self-expectations; unrealistic care receiver expectations

Information that appears in brackets has been added by the authors to clarify and enhance the use of nursing diagnoses.

Caregiver–Care Receiver Relationship

Abusive or violent relationship; pattern of ineffective relationships

Care receiver's condition inhibits conversation; unrealistic care receiver expectations

Caregiving Activities

Around-the-clock care responsibilities; change in nature or complexity of care activities

Duration of caregiving; unpredictability of care situation

Excessive caregiving activities; recent discharge home with significant care needs;

Family Processes

Pattern of ineffective family coping or family dysfunction

Resources

Caregiver is not developmentally ready for caregiver role; insufficient time

Difficulty accessing assistance, support, or community resources; insufficient knowledge about community resources; insufficient community services (e.g., respite, recreation, social support); insufficient transportation

Financial crisis (e.g., debt, insufficient finances)

Insufficient emotional resilience, social support, time, or energy

Insufficient physical environment or equipment for providing care

Socioeconomic

Alienation or social isolation

Competing role commitments

Insufficient recreation

Risk Factors (risk for caregiver Role Strain)

Illness severity of the care receiver; alteration in cognitive functioning in care receiver; psychological disorder in care receiver; care receiver exhibits bizarre or deviant behavior

Care receiver discharged home with significant needs; prematurity; congenital disorder; developmental delay

Unpredictable illness trajectory; instability in care receiver's health

Substance abuse; codependency

Extended duration of caregiving required; inexperience with caregiving; caregiving task complexity; excessive caregiving activities

---

Information that appears in brackets has been added by the authors to clarify and enhance the use of nursing diagnoses.

Caregiver health impairment; psychological disorder in caregiver
Partner is caregiver, female
Caregiver is not developmentally ready for caregiver role [e.g., a young adult needing to provide care for middle-aged parent]; developmental delay of caregiver
Stressors; caregiver's competing role commitments
Inadequate physical environment for providing care
Family or caregiver isolation
Insufficient caregiver respite or recreation
Ineffective family adaptation; pattern of family dysfunction prior to the caregiving situation
Ineffective caregiver coping pattern
Pattern of ineffective relationship between caregiver and care receiver
Exposure to violence; presence of abuse (e.g., physical, psychological, sexual)

NOTE: A risk diagnosis is not evidenced by signs and symptoms, as the problem has not occurred; rather, nursing interventions are directed at prevention.

Defining Characteristics (caregiver Role Strain)

Subjective

Caregiving Activities

Apprehensiveness about: future ability to provide care or well-being of care receiver if unable to provide care; apprehensiveness about future health or institutionalization of care receiver; to provide care

Caregiver Health Status—Physiological

Fatigue; gastrointestinal distress; headache, rash, weight change
Hypertension; cardiovascular disease; diabetes

Caregiver Health Status—Emotional

Alteration in sleep pattern
Anger, emotional vacillation; depression; frustration, impatience; nervousness
Insufficient time to meet personal needs; stressors

Caregiver Health Status—Socioeconomic

Change in leisure activities; low work productivity; refuses career advancement

---

Information that appears in brackets has been added by the authors to clarify and enhance the use of nursing diagnoses.

Caregiver-Care Receiver Relationship
Difficulty watching care receiver with illness
Grieving changes or uncertainty in relationship with care receiver

Family Processes—Caregiving Activities
Concern about family members; family conflict

Objective

Caregiving Activities
Difficulty performing or completing required tasks
Dysfunctional change in caregiving activities
Preoccupation with care routine

Caregiver Health Status—Physiological
Cardiovascular disease; diabetes mellitus
Hypertension; weight change; rash

Caregiver Health Status—Emotional
Anger, emotional vacillation; depression; frustration, impatience; nervousness
Ineffective coping strategies
Somatization

Caregiver Health Status—Socioeconomic
Low work productivity, refusal of career advancement; social isolation

Family Processes
Family conflict

> **NOTE:** The presence of this problem may encompass other numerous problems/high-risk concerns, such as deficient Diversional Activity; Insomnia; Fatigue; Anxiety; ineffective Coping; compromised family Coping; disabled family Coping; Decisional Conflict [specify]; ineffective Denial; Grieving; Hopelessness; Powerlessness; Spiritual Distress; ineffective Health Maintenance; impaired Home Maintenance; ineffective Sexuality Pattern; readiness for enhanced family Coping; interrupted Family Processes; and Social Isolation. Careful attention to data gathering will identify and clarify the client's specific needs, which can then be coordinated under this single diagnostic label.

Information that appears in brackets has been added by the authors to clarify and enhance the use of nursing diagnoses.

Desired Outcomes/Evaluation Criteria—Caregiver Will:

- Identify resources within self to deal with situation.
- Provide opportunity for care receiver to deal with situation in own way.
- Express more realistic understanding and expectations of the care receiver.
- Demonstrate behavior or lifestyle changes to cope with or resolve problematic factors.
- Report improved general well-being, ability to deal with situation.

Actions/Interventions

Nursing Priority No. 1.

To assess factors affecting current situation or degree of impaired function:

- Inquire about and observe physical condition of care receiver and surroundings, as appropriate. **Important to determine factors that may indicate problems that can interfere with ability for caregiving.**
- Assess caregiver's current state of health, and functioning (e.g., caregiver has multiple medical issues; is unable to get enough sleep, has poor nutritional intake, personal appearance and demeanor are indicating stress). **Provides basis for determining needs that indicate caregiver is having difficulty dealing with role.**
- Determine use of prescription/over-the-counter drugs or alcohol to deal with situation.
- Identify safety issues concerning caregiver and care receiver.
- Assess current actions of caregiver and how they are viewed by the care receiver (e.g., caregiver may be trying to be helpful, but is not perceived as helpful; may be too protective or may have unrealistic expectations of care receiver). **May lead to misunderstanding and conflict.**
- Note choice and frequency of social involvement and recreational activities.
- Determine use and effectiveness of resources and support systems. **People are often not aware of available resources, or may need help in using them to the best advantage.**

Nursing Priority No. 2.

To identify the causative, contributing, **or risk** factors relating to the impairment:

Information that appears in brackets has been added by the authors to clarify and enhance the use of nursing diagnoses.

- Note presence of high-risk situations (e.g., elderly client with total care dependence on spouse; or caregiver with several small children with one child requiring extensive assistance due to physical condition or developmental delays). **Such situations result in added stress (e.g., imposing unwanted role reversal, or placing excessive demands on parenting skills).**
- Determine current knowledge of the situation, noting misconceptions and lack of information. **May interfere with caregiver/care receiver response to illness/condition.**
- Identify relationship of caregiver to care receiver (e.g., spouse/lover, parent/child, sibling, friend). **Close relationships may make it more difficult to manage guilt, loneliness, anger, and resentment.**
- Determine quality of couple's relationship/presence of intimacy issues. **Disease/condition, caregiving activities, and possible change in role responsibilities may strain relationship adding to sense of loss and unmet needs.**
- Ascertain proximity of caregiver to care receiver. **Caregiver could be living in the home of care receiver (e.g., spouse or parent of disabled child) or be an adult child stopping by to check on elderly parent each day, providing support, food preparation/shopping, and assistance in emergencies. Either situation can be taxing.**
- Note care receiver's physical and mental condition, as well as the complexity of required therapeutic regimen. **Caregiving activities can be complex, requiring hands-on care, problem-solving skills, clinical judgment, and organizational and communication skills that can tax the caregiver.**
- Determine caregiver's level of involvement in/preparedness for the responsibilities of caring for the client and anticipated length of care.
- Ascertain caregiver's physical and emotional health and developmental level, as well as additional responsibilities of caregiver (e.g., job, raising family). **Provides clues to potential stressors and possible supportive interventions.**
- Use assessment tool, such as Burden Interview, when appropriate, **to further determine caregiver's coping abilities.**
- Identify individual cultural factors and impact on caregiver. **Helps clarify expectations of caregiver/receiver, family, and community.**
- Note codependency needs and enabling behaviors of caregiver. **These behaviors can interfere with competent caregiving and contribute to caregiver burnout.**
- Determine availability/use of support systems and resources.

Information that appears in brackets has been added by the authors to clarify and enhance the use of nursing diagnoses.

Nursing Priority No. 3.

To assist caregiver in identifying feelings and in beginning to deal with problems (caregiver Role Strain):

- Establish a therapeutic relationship, conveying empathy and unconditional positive regard. **A compassionate approach, blending the nurse's expertise in healthcare with the caregiver's firsthand knowledge of the care receiver can provide encouragement, especially in a long-term difficult situation.**
- Acknowledge difficulty of the situation for the caregiver/ family. **Research shows that the two greatest predictors of caregiver strain are poor health and the feeling that there is no choice but to take on additional responsibilities.**
- Discuss caregiver's view of and concerns about situation, including quality of couple's relationship/presence of intimacy issues. **Important to identify issues so planning and solutions can be developed.**
- Encourage caregiver to acknowledge and express feelings. Discuss normalcy of the reactions without using false reassurance.
- Discuss caregiver's and family members' life goals, perceptions, and expectations of self **to clarify unrealistic thinking and identify potential areas of flexibility or compromise.**
- Discuss caregiver's perception of impact of and ability to handle role changes necessitated by situation. **People initially do not realize changes that will be encountered as situation develops, and it helps to identify and plan for changes before they arise.**

Nursing Priority No. 4.

To enhance caregiver's ability to deal with current **or future** situation:

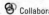

- Identify strengths of caregiver and care receiver. **Bringing these to the individual's awareness promotes positive thinking and helps with problem-solving to deal more effectively with circumstances.**
- Discuss strategies to coordinate caregiving tasks and other responsibilities (e.g., employment, care of children/ dependents, or housekeeping activities).
- Facilitate family conference, as appropriate, **to share information and develop plan for involvement in care activities.**
- Identify classes and/or needed specialists (e.g., first aid/CPR classes, enterostomal specialist, physical therapist).

Information that appears in brackets has been added by the authors to clarify and enhance the use of nursing diagnoses.

- Determine need for, and sources of, additional resources (e.g., financial, legal, respite care, social, and spiritual).
- Provide information or demonstrate techniques for dealing with acting out, violent, or disoriented behavior. **Presence of dementia necessitates learning these techniques or skills to enhance safety of caregiver and receiver.**
- Identify equipment needs or adaptive aids and resources **to enhance the independence and safety of the care receiver.**
- Provide contact person/case manager **to partner with care provider(s) in coordinating care, providing physical/social support, and assisting with problem-solving, as needed/desired.**

Nursing Priority No. 5.

To promote wellness (Teaching/Discharge Considerations):

- Emphasize importance of self-nurturing (e.g., pursuing self-development interests, personal needs, hobbies, and social activities) **to improve/maintain quality of life for caregiver.**
- Advocate for/assist caregiver to plan for and implement changes that may be necessary (e.g., home care providers, adult day care, placement in long-term care facility, hospice care).
- Support caregiver in setting practical goals for self (and care receiver) that are realistic for care receiver's condition/prognosis and caregiver's own abilities.
- Review signs of burnout (e.g., emotional/physical exhaustion; changes in appetite and sleep; and withdrawal from friends, family, life interests).
- Discuss/demonstrate stress management techniques (e.g., accepting own feelings/frustrations and limitations, talking with trusted friend, taking a break from situation) and importance of self-nurturing (e.g., eating and sleeping regularly and pursuing self-development interests, personal needs, hobbies, social activities, spiritual enrichment). **May provide care provider with options to look after self.**
- Encourage involvement in caregiver/other specific support group(s).
- Refer to classes/other therapies, as indicated.
- Identify available 12-step program, when indicated, **to provide tools to deal with enabling/codependent behaviors that impair level of function.**
- Refer to counseling or psychotherapy, as needed.

Information that appears in brackets has been added by the authors to clarify and enhance the use of nursing diagnoses.

- Provide bibliotherapy of appropriate references and Web sites for self-paced learning and updated information, and contact with other caregivers. **Further information can help individuals understand what is happening and manage more effectively.**

Documentation Focus

Assessment/Reassessment

- Assessment findings, functional level or degree of impairment, caregiver's understanding and perception of situation
- Identified risk factors and caregiver perceptions of situation
- Reactions of care receiver and family
- Involvement of family members and others

Planning

- Plan of care and individual responsibility for specific activities
- Needed resources, including type and source of assistive devices and durable equipment
- Teaching plan

Implementation/Evaluation

- Caregiver/receiver response to interventions, teaching, and actions performed
- Identification of inner resources, behavior, and lifestyle changes to be made
- Attainment or progress toward desired outcome(s)
- Modifications to plan of care

Discharge Planning

- Plan for continuation and follow-through of needed changes
- Referrals for assistance and reevaluation

Sample Nursing Outcomes & Interventions Classifications (NOC/NIC)

NOC—Caregiver Role Endurance
NOC—Caregiver Stressors
NIC—Caregiver Support

Information that appears in brackets has been added by the authors to clarify and enhance the use of nursing diagnoses.

bathing, dressing, feeding, toileting SELF-CARE DEFICIT

[Diagnostic Division: Hygiene]

Definition: Impaired ability to perform or complete bathing, dressing, feeding, or toileting activities for self [on a temporary, permanent, or progressing basis].

NOTE: Self-care also may be expanded to include the practices used by the client to promote health, the individual responsibility for self, a way of thinking. Refer to NDs impaired Home Maintenance; ineffective Health Maintenance.

Related Factors

Alteration in cognitive functioning; perceptual impairment
Weakness; fatigue; decrease in motivation; anxiety
Neuromuscular or musculoskeletal impairment
Environmental barrier; [mechanical restrictions such as cast, splint, traction, ventilator]
Pain; discomfort
Inability to perceive body part or spatial relationship [bathing]
Impaired mobility or transfer ability [toileting]

Defining Characteristics

bathing Self-Care Deficit

Impaired ability to: access bathroom [tub], gather bathing supplies, access water, regulate bath water, wash or dry body

dressing Self-Care Deficit

Impaired ability to: choose clothing, gather clothing, pick up clothing, put clothing on upper or lower body, fasten clothing
Impaired ability to: put on/remove various items of clothing (e.g., shirt, socks, shoes)
Impaired ability to: use zipper or assistive device, maintain appearance

feeding Self-Care Deficit

Impaired ability to: prepare food, open containers
Impaired ability to: handle utensils, get food onto utensil, bring food to the mouth, use assistive device, pick up cup

---

Information that appears in brackets has been added by the authors to clarify and enhance the use of nursing diagnoses.

Impaired ability to: manipulate food in mouth, chew food, swallow food or swallow sufficient amount of food, self-feed a complete meal in an acceptable manner

toileting Self-Care Deficit

Impaired ability to: reach toilet, manipulate clothing for toileting, sit on or rise from toilet, complete toilet hygiene, flush toilet

Desired Outcomes/Evaluation Criteria—Client Will:

- Identify individual areas of weakness or needs.
- Verbalize knowledge of healthcare practices.
- Demonstrate techniques and lifestyle changes to meet self-care needs.
- Perform self-care activities within level of own ability.
- Identify personal and community resources that can provide assistance.

Actions/Interventions

Nursing Priority No. 1.

To identify causative/contributing factors:

- Determine age and developmental issues **affecting ability of individual to participate in own care.**
- Note concomitant medical problems or existing conditions that may be factors for care (e.g., recent trauma or surgery, heart disease, renal failure, spinal cord injury, cerebral vascular accident, multiple sclerosis, malnutrition, pain, Alzheimer's disease).
- Review medication regimen **for possible effects on alertness/mentation, energy level, balance, perception.**
- Note other etiological factors present, including language barriers, speech impairment, visual acuity or hearing problem, emotional stability. (Refer to NDs impaired verbal Communication; risk for Unilateral Neglect; [disturbed Sensory Perception specify], for related interventions.)
- Assess barriers to participation in regimen **that can limit use of resources or choice of options (e.g., lack of information, insufficient time for discussion, psychological or intimate family problems that may be difficult to share, fear of appearing stupid or ignorant, social or economic limitations, work or home environment problems).**

Nursing Priority No. 2.

To assess degree of disability:

- Identify degree of individual impairment and functional level according to scale (as listed in ND impaired physical Mobility).

Information that appears in brackets has been added by the authors to clarify and enhance the use of nursing diagnoses.

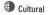

- Assess memory and intellectual functioning. Note developmental level to which client has regressed or progressed.
- Determine individual strengths and skills of the client.
- Note whether deficit is temporary or permanent, should decrease or increase with time.

Nursing Priority No. 3.

To assist in correcting/dealing with situation:

- Collaborate in treatment of underlying conditions **to enhance client's capabilities, maximize rehabilitation potential.**
- Provide accurate and relevant information regarding current and future needs **so that client can incorporate into self-care plans while minimizing problems (e.g., heightened anxiety, depression, resistance) often associated with change.**
- Perform or assist with meeting client's needs (e.g., personal care assistance is part of nursing care and should not be neglected while self-care independence is promoted and integrated).
- Promote client's/significant other's (SO's) participation in problem identification and desired goals and decision making. **Enhances commitment to plan, optimizing outcomes, and supporting recovery and/or health promotion.**
- Develop plan of care appropriate to individual situation, scheduling activities to conform to client's usual or desired schedule.
- Active-listen client's/SO(s)' concerns. **Exhibits regard for client's values and beliefs, clarifies barriers to participation in self-care, provides opportunity to work on problem-solving solutions and to provide encouragement and support.**
- Practice and promote short-term goal setting and achievement **to recognize that today's success is as important as any long-term goal, accepting ability to do one thing at a time and conceptualization of self-care in a broader sense.**
- Provide for communication among those who are involved in caring for or assisting the client. **Enhances coordination and continuity of care.**
- Instruct in or review appropriate skills necessary for self-care, using terms understandable to client (e.g., child, adult, cognitively impaired person) and with sensitivity to developmental needs for practice, repetition, or reluctance. **Individualized teaching best affords reinforcement of learning. Sensitivity to special needs attaches value to the client's needs.**

Information that appears in brackets has been added by the authors to clarify and enhance the use of nursing diagnoses.

- Establish remotivation or resocialization programs when indicated.
- Establish "contractual" partnership with client/SO(s), if appropriate, **for motivation or behavioral modification.**
- Refer to and assist with rehabilitation program **to enhance client's capabilities and promote independence.**
- Provide privacy and equipment within easy reach during personal care activities.
- Allow sufficient time for client to accomplish tasks to fullest extent of ability. Avoid unnecessary conversation or interruptions.
- Assist with necessary adaptations to accomplish activities of daily living. Begin with familiar, easily accomplished tasks **to encourage client and build on successes.**
- Collaborate with rehabilitation professionals to identify and obtain assistive devices, mobility aids, and home modification as necessary (e.g., adequate lighting, visual aids; bedside commode; raised toilet seat and grab bars for bathroom; modified clothing; modified eating utensils).
- Identify energy-saving behaviors (e.g., sitting instead of standing when possible). (Refer to NDs Activity Intolerance; Fatigue, for additional interventions.)
- Implement bowel or bladder training program, as indicated. (Refer to NDs Constipation; bowel Incontinence; impaired urinary Elimination, for appropriate interventions.)
- Encourage food and fluid choices reflecting individual likes and abilities that meet nutritional needs. Provide assistive devices or alternate feeding methods, as appropriate. (Refer to ND impaired Swallowing for related interventions.)
- Assist with medication regimen as necessary, encouraging timely use of medications (e.g., taking diuretics in morning when client is more awake and able to manage toileting, use of pain relievers prior to activity to facilitate movement, postponing intake of medications that cause sedation until self-care activities completed).
- Make home visit, as indicated **to assess environmental and discharge needs.**

Nursing Priority No. 4.

To meet specific self-care needs:

Bathing deficit

- Ask client/SO for input on bathing habits or cultural bathing preferences. **Creates opportunities for client to (1) keep long-standing routines (e.g., bathing at bedtime to im-**

Information that appears in brackets has been added by the authors to clarify and enhance the use of nursing diagnoses.

prove sleep) and (2) exercise control over situation. This enhances self-esteem, while respecting personal and cultural preferences.

- Bathe or assist client in bathing, providing for any or all hygiene needs as indicated. **Type (e.g., bed bath, towel bath, tub bath, shower) and purpose (e.g., cleansing, removing odor, or simply soothing agitation) of bath is determined by individual need.**
- Obtain hygiene supplies (e.g., soap, toothpaste, toothbrush, mouthwash, lotion, shampoo, razor, towels) for specific activity to be performed and place in client's easy reach **to provide visual cues and facilitate completion of activity.**
- Ascertain that all safety equipment is in place and properly installed (e.g., grab bars, antislip strips, shower chair, hydraulic lift) and that client/caregiver(s) can safely operate equipment.
- Instruct client to request assistance when needed and place call device within easy reach, or stay with client as dictated by safety needs.
- ∞ Provide for adequate warmth (e.g., covering client during bed bath or warming bathroom). **Certain individuals (especially infants, the elderly, and very thin or debilitated persons) are prone to hypothermia and can experience evaporative cooling during and after bathing.**
- Determine that client can perceive water temperature, adjust water temperature safely, or that water is correct temperature for client's bath or shower **to prevent chilling or burns. This step requires that client is cognitively and physically able to perceive hot and cold and to adjust faucets safely.**
- Assist client in and out of shower or tub as indicated.
- Provide for or assist with grooming activities (e.g., shaving, hair care, cleaning and clipping nails, makeup) on a routine, consistent basis. Encourage participation, guiding client's hand through tasks, as indicated. **Experiencing the normal process of a task through established routine and guided practice facilitates optimal relearning.**

Dressing deficit

- Ascertain that appropriate clothing is available. **Clothing may need to be modified for client's particular medical condition or physical limitations.**
- Assist client in choosing clothing or lay out clothing as indicated.
- Dress client or assist with dressing, as indicated. **Client may need assistance in putting on or taking off items of clothing**

Information that appears in brackets has been added by the authors to clarify and enhance the use of nursing diagnoses.

(e.g., shoes and socks, or over-the-head shirt) or may require partial or complete assistance with fasteners (e.g., buttons, snaps, zippers, shoelaces).

- Allow sufficient time for dressing and undressing.
- Use adaptive clothing as indicated (e.g., clothing with front closure, wide sleeves and pant legs, Velcro or zipper closures). **These may be helpful for client with limited arm or leg movement or impaired fine motor skills or cognitively impaired person who desires to dress self but cannot do so with regular clothing fasteners.**
- Teach client to dress affected side first, then unaffected side (when client has paralysis or injury to one side of body).

Feeding deficit

- Assess client's need and ability to prepare food as indicated (including shopping, cooking, cutting food, opening containers, etc.).
- Encourage food and fluid choices reflecting individual likes and abilities and that meet nutritional needs **to maximize food intake.**
- Ascertain that client can swallow safely, checking gag and swallow reflexes, as indicated. (Refer to ND impaired Swallowing for related interventions.)
- Provide food and fluid of appropriate consistency **to facilitate swallowing.** Cut food into bite-size pieces **to prevent overfilling mouth and reduce risk of choking.**
- Assist client to handle utensils or in guiding utensils to mouth. **May require specialized equipment (e.g., rocker knife, plate guard, built-up handles) to increase independence or assistance with movement of arms and hands.**
- Assist client with small cup, glass, or bottle for liquids, using straw or adaptive lids as indicated **to enhance fluid intake while reducing spills.**
- Allow client time for intake of sufficient food **for feeling satisfied or completing a meal.**
- Assist client with social graces when eating with others; provide privacy when manners might be offensive to others or client could be embarrassed.
- Collaborate with nutritionist, speech-language pathologist, occupational therapist, or physician **for special diets or feeding methods necessary to provide adequate nutrition.**
- Feed client, allowing adequate time for chewing and swallowing, **when client is not able to obtain nutrition by self-feeding.** Avoid providing fluids until client has swallowed food and mouth is clear. **Prevents "washing down" foods, reducing risk of choking.**

Information that appears in brackets has been added by the authors to clarify and enhance the use of nursing diagnoses.

Toileting deficit

- Provide mobility assistance to bathroom or commode or place on bedpan or offer urinal, as indicated.
- Direct or accompany cognitively impaired client to bathroom, as needed.
- Observe for behaviors such as pacing, fidgeting, holding crotch **that may be indicative of need for prompt toileting.**
- Provide privacy **to enhance self-esteem and improve ability to urinate or defecate.**
- Assist with manipulation of clothing, if needed, **to decrease incidence of functional incontinence caused by difficulty removing clothing/underwear.**
- Observe need for and assist in obtaining modified clothing or fasteners **to assist client in manipulation of clothing, fostering independence in self-toileting.**
- Provide or assist with use of assistive equipment (e.g., raised toilet seat, support rails, spill-proof urinals, fracture pans, bedside commode) **to promote independence and safety in sitting down or arising from toilet or for aiding elimination when client is unable to go to bathroom.**
- Keep toilet paper or wipes and hand-washing items within client's easy reach.
- Implement bowel or bladder training/retraining programs as indicated.

Nursing Priority No. 5.

To promote wellness (Teaching/Discharge Considerations):

- Assist the client to become aware of rights and responsibilities in health and healthcare and to assess own health strengths—physical, emotional, and intellectual.
- Support client in making health-related decisions and assist in developing self-care practices and goals that promote health.
- Provide for ongoing evaluation of self-care program, identifying progress and needed changes.
- Review and modify program periodically to accommodate changes in client's abilities. **Assists client to adhere to plan of care to fullest extent.**
- Encourage keeping a journal of progress and practicing of independent living skills **to foster self-care and self-determination.**
- Review safety concerns. Modify activities or environment **to reduce risk of injury and promote successful community functioning.**

Information that appears in brackets has been added by the authors to clarify and enhance the use of nursing diagnoses.

- Refer to home care provider, social services, physical or occupational therapy, rehabilitation, and counseling resources, as indicated.
- Identify additional community resources (e.g., senior services, Meals-on-Wheels).
- Review instructions from other members of healthcare team and provide written copy. **Provides clarification, reinforcement; allows periodic review by client/caregivers.**
- Give family information about respite or other care options. **Allows them free time away from the care situation to renew themselves.** (Refer to ND caregiver Role Strain for additional interventions.)
- Assist and support family with alternative placements as necessary. **Enhances likelihood of finding individually appropriate situation to meet client's needs.**
- Be available for discussion of feelings about situation (e.g., grieving, anger). **Provides opportunity for client/family to get feelings out in the open and begin to problem-solve solutions as indicated.**
- Refer to NDs risk for Falls; risk for Injury; ineffective Coping; compromised family Coping; risk for Disuse Syndrome; situational low Self-Esteem; impaired physical Mobility; Powerlessness, as appropriate.

Documentation Focus

Assessment/Reassessment

- Individual findings, functional level, and specifics of limitation(s)
- Needed resources and adaptive devices
- Availability and use of community resources
- Who is involved in care or provides assistance

Planning

- Plan of care and who is involved in planning
- Teaching plan

Implementation/Evaluation

- Response to interventions, teaching, and actions performed
- Attainment or progress toward desired outcome(s)
- Modifications of plan of care

Discharge Planning

- Long-term needs and who is responsible for actions to be taken

---

Information that appears in brackets has been added by the authors to clarify and enhance the use of nursing diagnoses.

- Type of and source for assistive devices
- Specific referrals made

Sample Nursing Outcomes & Interventions Classifications (NOC/NIC)

Bathing Deficit
NOC—Self-Care: Bathing
NIC—Self-Care Assistance: Bathing/Hygiene

Dressing Deficit
NOC—Self-Care: Dressing
NIC—Self-Care Assistance: Dressing/Grooming

Feeding Deficit
NOC—Self-Care: Eating
NIC—Self-Care Assistance: Feeding

Toileting Deficit
NOC—Self-Care: Toileting
NIC—Self-Care Assistance: Toileting

readiness for enhanced SELF-CARE

[Diagnostic Division: Teaching/Learning]

Definition: A pattern of performing activities for oneself to meet health-related goals, which can be strengthened.

Defining Characteristics

Subjective

Expresses desire to enhance independence with life, health, personal development, or well-being
Expresses desire to enhance self-care, knowledge for strategies for self-care

[NOTE: Based on the definition and defining characteristics of this ND, the focus appears to be broader than simply meeting routine basic activities of daily living and addresses independence in maintaining overall health, personal development, and general well-being.]

Information that appears in brackets has been added by the authors to clarify and enhance the use of nursing diagnoses.

Desired Outcomes/Evaluation Criteria—Client Will:

- Maintain responsibility for planning and achieving self-care goals and general well-being.
- Demonstrate proactive management of chronic conditions, potential complications or changes in capabilities.
- Identify and use resources appropriately.
- Remain free of preventable complications.

Actions/Interventions

Nursing Priority No. 1.

To determine current self-care status and motivation for growth:

- Determine individual strengths and skills of the client. **Establishes comparative baseline for potential growth and/or modifications in current strategies.** ***Note:*** **Assessment might include use of an instrument to evaluate client's current functional status, in addition to client's self-report.**
- Ascertain motivation and expectations for change.
- Note availability and use of resources, supportive person(s), assistive devices **to ascertain that client has means for sharing common concerns, needs, and wishes as well as has access to social support and approval (e.g., support group participants, family members, professionals).**
- ∞ Determine age and developmental issues, presence of medical conditions **that could impact potential for growth or interrupt client's ability to meet own needs.**
- Assess for potential barriers to enhanced participation in self-care (e.g., lack of information, insufficient time for discussion, sudden or progressive change in health status, catastrophic events).

Nursing Priority No. 2.

To assist client's/significant other's (SO's) plan to meet individual needs:

- Discuss client's understanding of current situation **to determine areas that can be clarified or strengthened.**
- Provide accurate and relevant information regarding current and future needs **so that client can incorporate into self-care plans, while minimizing problems associated with change.**
- Review coping skills (e.g., assertiveness, interpersonal relations, decision making, problem-solving, stigma management, time management) **that are useful in managing a wide range of stressful conditions.** Encourage client to ask for assistance, as needed or desired.

Information that appears in brackets has been added by the authors to clarify and enhance the use of nursing diagnoses.

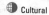

- Promote client's/SO's participation in problem identification and decision making. **Optimizes outcomes and supports health promotion.**
- Active-listen client's/SO's concerns **to exhibit regard for client's values and beliefs, to support positive responses, and to address questions or concerns.**
- Encourage communication among those who are involved in the client's health promotion. **Periodic review allows for clarification of issues, reinforcement of successful interventions, and possibility for early intervention (where needed) to manage chronic conditions.**

Nursing Priority No. 3.

To promote optimum functioning (Teaching/Discharge Considerations):

- Assist client to set realistic goals for the future.
- Support client in making health-related decisions and pursuit of self-care practices that promote health **to foster self-esteem and support positive self-concept.**
- Identify reliable reference sources regarding individual needs and strategies for self-care. **Reinforces learning and promotes self-paced review.**
- Provide for ongoing evaluation of self-care program **to identify progress and needed changes for continuation of health, adaptation in management of limiting conditions.**
- Review safety concerns and modification of medical therapies or activities and environment, as needed, **to prevent injury and enhance successful functioning.**
- Refer to home care provider, social services, physical or occupational therapy, rehabilitation, and counseling resources, as indicated or requested, **for education, assistance, adaptive devices, and modifications that may be desired.**
- Identify additional community resources (e.g., senior services, handicap transportation van for appointments, accessible and safe locations for social or sports activities, Meals-on-Wheels).

Documentation Focus

Assessment/Reassessment

- Individual findings including strengths, health status, and any limitation(s)
- Availability and use of community resources, support person(s), assistive devices
- Motivation and expectations for change

Information that appears in brackets has been added by the authors to clarify and enhance the use of nursing diagnoses.

Planning
- Plan of care, specific interventions, and who is involved in planning
- Teaching plan

Implementation/Evaluation
- Client's responses to interventions, teaching, and actions performed
- Attainment or progress toward desired outcome(s)
- Modifications to plan

Discharge Planning
- Long-term needs and who is responsible for actions to be taken
- Type of and source for assistive devices
- Specific referrals made

Sample Nursing Outcomes & Interventions Classifications (NOC/NIC)
NOC—Self-Care Status
NIC—Self-Modification Assistance

readiness for enhanced SELF-CONCEPT

[Diagnostic Division: Ego Integrity]

Definition: A pattern of perceptions or ideas about the self, which can be strengthened.

Defining Characteristics

Subjective
Expresses desire to enhance self-concept, role performance
Acceptance of strengths, limitations
Confidence in abilities
Satisfaction with thoughts about self, sense of worth
Satisfaction with body image, personal identity

Objective
Actions congruent with verbal expressions

Information that appears in brackets has been added by the authors to clarify and enhance the use of nursing diagnoses.

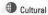

Desired Outcomes/Evaluation Criteria—Client Will:

- Verbalize understanding of own sense of self-concept.
- Participate in programs and activities to enhance self-esteem.
- Demonstrate behaviors and lifestyle changes to promote positive self-esteem.
- Participate in family, group, or community activities to enhance self-concept.

Actions/Interventions

Nursing Priority No. 1.

To assess current situation and desire for improvement:

- Determine current status of individual's belief about self. **Self-concept consists of the physical self (body image), the personal self (identity), and self-esteem. Information about client's current thinking about self provides a beginning for making changes to improve self.**
- Determine availability and quality of family/SO(s) support. **Presence of supportive people who reflect positive attitudes regarding the individual promotes a positive sense of self.**
- Identify family dynamics—present and past. **Self-esteem begins in early childhood and is influenced by perceptions of how the individual is viewed by significant others (SOs). Provides information about family functioning that will help to develop plan of care for enhancing client's self-concept.**
- Note willingness to seek assistance and motivation for change. **Individuals who have a sense of their own self-image and are willing to look at themselves realistically will be able to progress in the desire to improve.**
- Determine client's concept of self in relation to cultural or religious ideals and beliefs. **Cultural characteristics are learned in the family of origin and shape how the individual views self.**
- Observe nonverbal behaviors and note congruence with verbal expressions. Discuss cultural meanings of nonverbal communication. **Incongruencies between verbal and nonverbal communication require clarification. Interpretation of nonverbal expressions is culturally determined and needs to be clarified to avoid misinterpretation.**

Information that appears in brackets has been added by the authors to clarify and enhance the use of nursing diagnoses.

Nursing Priority No. 2.

To facilitate personal growth:

- Develop therapeutic relationship. Be attentive, maintain open communication, use skills of Active-listening and I-messages. **Promotes trusting situation in which client is free to be open and honest with self and others.**
- Validate client's communication, provide encouragement for efforts.
- Accept client's perceptions or view of current status. **Provides opportunity for client to develop realistic plan for improving self-concept, while feeling safe in existing view of self.**
- Be aware that people are not programmed to be rational. **Individuals must seek information, choosing to learn, and to think rather than merely to accept or react in order to have respect for self, facts, and honesty and to develop positive self-esteem.**
- Discuss client perception of self, confronting misconceptions and identifying negative self-talk. Address distortions in thinking, such as self-referencing (beliefs that others are focusing on individual's weaknesses or limitations); filtering (focusing on negative and ignoring positive); catastrophizing (expecting the worst outcomes). **Addressing these issues openly allows client to identify things that may negatively affect self-esteem and provides opportunity for change.**
- Have client list current and past successes and strengths. **Emphasizes fact that client is and has been successful in many actions taken.**
- Use positive I-messages rather than praise. **Praise is a form of external control, coming from outside sources, whereas I-messages allow the client to develop internal sense of self-esteem.**
- Discuss what behavior does for client (positive intention). Ask what options are available to the client/SO(s). **Encourages thinking about what inner motivations are and what actions can be taken to enhance self-esteem.**
- Give reinforcement for progress noted. **Positive words of encouragement support development of effective coping behaviors.**
- Encourage client to progress at own rate. **Adaptation to a change in self-concept depends on its significance to the individual and disruption to lifestyle.**
- Involve in activities or exercise program of choice, promote socialization. **Enhances sense of well-being and can help to energize client.**

Information that appears in brackets has been added by the authors to clarify and enhance the use of nursing diagnoses.

Nursing Priority No. 3.

To promote optimum sense of self-worth and happiness:

- Assist client to identify goals that are personally achievable. Provide positive feedback for verbal and behavioral indications of improved self-view. **Increases likelihood of success and commitment to change.**
- Refer to vocational or employment counselor, educational resources, as appropriate. **Assists with improving development of social or vocational skills.**
- Encourage participation in classes, activities, or hobbies that client enjoys or would like to experience. **Provides opportunity for learning new information and skills that can enhance feelings of success, improving self-esteem.**
- Reinforce that current decision to improve self-concept is ongoing. **Continued work and support are necessary to sustain behavior changes and personal growth.**
- Discuss ways to develop optimism. **Optimism is a key ingredient in happiness and can be learned.**
- Suggest assertiveness training classes. **Enhances ability to interact with others and develop more effective relationships, enhancing one's self-concept.**
- Emphasize importance of grooming and personal hygiene and assist in developing skills to improve appearance and dress for success as needed. **Looking one's best improves sense of self-esteem, and presenting a positive appearance enhances how others see one.**

Documentation Focus

Assessment/Reassessment

- Individual findings, including evaluations of self and others, current and past successes
- Interactions with others, lifestyle
- Motivation for and willingness to change

Planning

- Plan of care and who is involved in planning
- Educational plan

Implementation/Evaluation

- Responses to interventions, teaching, and actions performed
- Attainment or progress toward desired outcome(s)
- Modifications to plan of care

Information that appears in brackets has been added by the authors to clarify and enhance the use of nursing diagnoses.

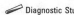

Discharge Planning

- Long-term needs and who is responsible for actions to be taken
- Specific referrals made

Sample Nursing Outcomes & Interventions Classifications (NOC/NIC)

NOC—Self-Esteem
NIC—Self-Modification Assistance

chronic low SELF-ESTEEM and risk for chronic low SELF-ESTEEM

[Diagnostic Division: Ego Integrity]

Definition: chronic low Self-Esteem: Long-standing negative self-evaluation/feelings about self or self-capabilities.

Definition: risk for chronic low Self-Esteem: Vulnerable to long-standing negative self-evaluating/feelings about self or self-capabilities, which may compromise health.

Related and Risk Factors

Repeated negative reinforcement, failures
Receiving insufficient affection, approval from others
Inadequate belonging; insufficient group membership
Inadequate respect from others
Cultural or spiritual incongruencies
Exposure to traumatic situation
Ineffective coping with loss
Psychiatric disorder

NOTE: A risk diagnosis is not evidenced by signs and symptoms, as the problem has not occurred; rather, nursing interventions are directed at prevention.

Defining Characteristics (chronic low Self-Esteem)

Subjective

Shame; guilt
Underestimation of ability to deal with situation
Rejection of positive feedback

Information that appears in brackets has been added by the authors to clarify and enhance the use of nursing diagnoses.

Objective

Hesitant to try new experiences
Repeatedly unsuccessful in life events
Exaggerates negative feedback about self
Overly conforming; dependent on others' opinions
Poor eye contact
Nonassertive or indecisive behavior; passivity
Excessive seeking of reassurance

Desired Outcomes/Evaluation Criteria—Client Will:

- Verbalize understanding of negative evaluation of self and reasons for this problem.
- Participate in treatment program to promote change in self-evaluation.
- Demonstrate behaviors and lifestyle changes to promote positive self-image.
- Verbalize increased sense of self-worth in relation to current situation.
- Participate in family, group, or community activities to enhance change.

Actions/Interventions

Nursing Priority No. 1.

To assess causative/contributing **or risk** factors:

- ∞ Note age and developmental level of client and circumstances surrounding current situation. **Younger people may not have learned skills to deal with negative occurrences and/or rejection from others.**
- Elicit client's perceptions of current situation.
- Determine factors of low self-esteem related to current situation (e.g., family crises, physical disfigurement, social isolation). **Current crises may exacerbate long-standing feelings and perception of self-evaluation as not being worthwhile.**
- Assess content of negative self-talk. Note client's perceptions of how others view him or her. **Constant repetition of negative words and thoughts reinforces idea that individual is worthless and belief that others view him or her in a negative manner.**
- Observe nonverbal behavior (e.g., nervous movements, lack of eye contact) and how it relates to verbal statements. **Incongruence between verbal and nonverbal needs to be**

Information that appears in brackets has been added by the authors to clarify and enhance the use of nursing diagnoses.

clarified to be sure perceived meaning of communication is accurate.

- Determine availability and quality of family/significant other (SO) support. **The development of a positive sense of self depends on how the person relates to members of the family, as they are growing up and in the current situation.**
- Identify family dynamics—present and past—and cultural influences. **Family may engage in "put-downs" or "teasing" in ways that give client the message that he or she is worthless.**
- Be alert to client's concept of self in relation to cultural/religious ideal(s). **Composition and structure of nuclear family influences individual's sense of who he or she is in relation to others in the family and in society.**
- Note nonverbal behavior (e.g., nervous movements, lack of eye contact). **Incongruencies between verbal/nonverbal communication require clarification.**
- Determine degree of participation and cooperation with therapeutic regimen. **Maintaining therapeutic regimen requires ongoing evaluation to determine efficacy or need for change.**

Nursing Priority No. 2.

To promote client sense of self-esteem in dealing with current situation **or changes in life:**

- Develop therapeutic relationship. Be attentive, validate client's communication, provide encouragement for efforts, maintain open communication, use skills of Active-listening and I-messages. **Promotes trusting situation in which client is free to be open and honest with self and therapist.**
- Address presenting medical/safety issues. **Client's self-esteem may be affected by physical changes of current medical conditions. Changes in body (e.g., weight loss or gain, amputation) will affect how client sees self as a person. Attitude may contribute to depression and lack of attention to personal safety requiring evaluation and assistance.**
- Accept client's perceptions or view of situation. Avoid threatening existing self-esteem.
- Be aware that people are not programmed to be rational. **To have respect for self, facts, honesty, and to develop positive self-esteem, one must seek information, choosing to learn, and to think, rather than merely accepting/reacting.**
- Discuss client perceptions of self related to what is happening; confront misconceptions and negative self-talk. Address distortions in thinking, such as self-referencing (belief that others are focusing on individual's weaknesses/limitations), filtering

---

Information that appears in brackets has been added by the authors to clarify and enhance the use of nursing diagnoses.

(focusing on negative and ignoring positive), catastrophizing (expecting the worst outcomes). **Addressing these issues openly provides opportunity for change.**

- Emphasize need to avoid comparing self with others. Encourage client to focus on aspects of self that can be valued.
- Have client review past successes and strengths. **May help client see that he or she can develop an internal locus of control (a belief that one's successes and failures are the result of one's efforts).**
- Use positive I-messages rather than praise. **Praise may be heard as manipulative and insincere and be rejected. Use of positive I-messages communicates a feeling that is genuine and allows client to feel good about himself or herself, developing internal sense of self-esteem.**
- Discuss what a given behavior does for client (positive intention). What options are available to the client/SO(s)? **Helping client begin to look at what actions might be taken to achieve the same rewards in a more positive way can provide a realistic and accurate self-appraisal, enhancing sense of competence and self-worth.**
- Assist client to deal with sense of powerlessness. (Refer to ND Powerlessness.)
- Set limits on aggressive or problem behaviors such as acting out, suicide preoccupation, or rumination. Put self in client's place (empathy not sympathy). **These negative behaviors diminish sense of self-concept.**
- Give reinforcement for progress noted. **Positive words of encouragement promote continuation of efforts, supporting development of coping behaviors.**
- Encourage client to progress at own rate. **Adaptation to a change in self-concept depends on its significance to individual, disruption to lifestyle, and length of illness/debilitation.**
- Assist client to recognize and cope with events, alterations, and sense of loss of control by incorporating changes accurately into self-concept.
- Involve in activities or exercise program, promote socialization. **Enhances sense of well-being/can help energize client.**

Nursing Priority No. 3.

To promote wellness (Teaching/Discharge Considerations):

- Discuss inaccuracies in self-perception with client/SO(s).
- Model behaviors being taught, involving client in goal setting and decision making. **Facilitates client's developing trust in own unique strengths.**

Information that appears in brackets has been added by the authors to clarify and enhance the use of nursing diagnoses.

- Prepare client for events/changes that are expected, when possible **to provide opportunity for client to prepare self, or reduce negative reactions associated with the unknown.**
- Provide structure in daily routine/care activities.
- Emphasize importance of grooming and personal hygiene. Assist in developing skills as indicated (e.g., makeup classes, dressing for success). **People feel better about themselves when they present a positive outer appearance.**
- Assist client to identify goals that are personally achievable. **Increases likelihood of success and commitment to change.**
- Provide positive feedback for verbal and behavioral indications of improved self-view.
- Refer to vocational or employment counselor, educational resources, as appropriate. **Assists with development of social or vocational skills, enhancing sense of self-concept and inner locus of control.**
- Encourage participation in class, activities, or hobbies that client enjoys or would like to experience. **Meaningful accomplishment, assuming self-responsibility, and participating in new activities engenders one's sense of competence and self-worth.**
- Reinforce that this therapy is a brief encounter in overall life of the client/SO(s), with continued work and ongoing support being necessary **to sustain behavior changes and personal growth.**
- Refer to classes (e.g., assertiveness training, positive self-image, communication skills) **to assist with learning new skills to promote self-esteem.**
- Refer to counseling, therapy, mental health, or special-needs support groups, as indicated.

Documentation Focus

Assessment/Reassessment

- Individual findings, including early memories of negative evaluations (self and others), subsequent or precipitating failure events
- Effects on interactions with others, lifestyle
- Specific medical and safety issues
- Motivation for and willingness to change

Planning

- Plan of care and who is involved in planning
- Teaching plan

Information that appears in brackets has been added by the authors to clarify and enhance the use of nursing diagnoses.

Implementation/Evaluation

- Responses to interventions, teaching, and actions performed
- Attainment or progress toward desired outcome(s)
- Modifications to plan of care

Discharge Planning

- Long-term needs and who is responsible for actions to be taken
- Specific referrals made

Sample Nursing Outcomes & Interventions Classifications (NOC/NIC)

NOC—Self-Esteem
NIC—Self-Esteem Enhancement

situational low SELF-ESTEEM and risk for situational low SELF-ESTEEM

[Diagnostic Division: Ego Integrity]

Definition: situational low Self-Esteem: Development of a negative perception of self-worth in response to a current situation.

Definition: risk for situational low Self-Esteem: Vulnerable to developing a negative perception of self-worth in response to a current situation, which may compromise health.

Related Factors (situational low Self-Esteem)

Developmental transition
Functional impairment; alteration in body image
History of loss
Alteration in social role
Pattern of failure; history of rejection; inadequate recognition
Behavior inconsistent with values

Risk Factors

Alteration in body image; physical illness
Alteration in social role; history of abandonment
Behavior inconsistent with values; unrealistic self-expectations
Decrease in control over environment

Information that appears in brackets has been added by the authors to clarify and enhance the use of nursing diagnoses.

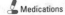

Developmental transition; functional impairment
History neglect or rejection; history of abuse (e.g., physical, psychological, sexual)
Inadequate recognition; pattern of failure; pattern of helplessness

> **NOTE:** A risk diagnosis is not evidenced by signs and symptoms, as the problem has not occurred; rather, nursing interventions are directed at prevention.

Defining Characteristics (situational low Self-Esteem)

Subjective

Helplessness; purposelessness
Underestimates ability to deal with situation

Objective

Situational challenge to self-worth
Self-negating verbalizations
Indecisive or nonassertive behavior

Desired Outcomes/Evaluation Criteria—Client Will:

- Acknowledge factors that lead to possibility of feelings of low self-esteem.
- Verbalize understanding of individual factors that precipitated current situation.
- Identify feelings and underlying dynamics for negative perception of self.
- Demonstrate self-confidence by setting realistic goals and actively participating in life situation.
- Express positive self-appraisal.

Actions/Interventions

Nursing Priority No. 1.

To assess causative/contributing **or risk** factors:

- Determine individual situation (e.g., family crisis, termination of a relationship, loss of employment, physical disfigurement) related to low self-esteem in the present circumstances.
- Identify client's basic sense of self-esteem and image client has of self: existential, physical, psychological. **Each aspect**

Information that appears in brackets has been added by the authors to clarify and enhance the use of nursing diagnoses.

plays a role in the client's ability to deal with current situation/crisis.

- Assess degree of threat and perception of client in regard to crisis. **One individual views a serious situation as manageable, while another individual may be overly concerned about a minor problem.**
- Ascertain sense of control client has (or perceives self to have) over self and situation. Note client's locus of control (internal or external). **Important in determining whether the client believes he or she has control over the situation or whether one is at the mercy of fate or luck.**
- Determine client's awareness of own responsibility for dealing with situation, personal growth, and so forth. **When client is aware of and accepts own responsibility, may indicate internal locus of control.**
- Verify client's concept of self in relation to cultural/religious ideals. **Cultural and religious influences during the individual's life affect beliefs about self, measure of worth, and ability to deal with current situation or crisis.**
- Review past coping skills in relation to current episode.
- Assess negative attitudes and/or self-talk. **An individual who is feeling unimportant, incompetent, and not in control often is unconsciously saying negative things to himself or herself that contribute to a loss of self-esteem and an attitude of despair.**
- Note nonverbal body language. **Incongruencies between verbal and nonverbal communication require clarification.**
- Assess for self-destructive or suicidal behavior. (Refer to ND risk for Suicide, as appropriate.)
- Identify previous adaptations to illness or disruptive events in life. **May be predictive of current outcome.**
- Assess family/significant other (SO) dynamics and support of client.
- Note availability and use of resources.

Nursing Priority No. 2.

To assist client to deal with loss/change and recapture **or maintain** sense of positive self-esteem:

- Assist with treatment of underlying condition when possible. **For example, cognitive restructuring and improved concentration in mild brain injury often result in restoration of positive self-esteem.**
- Encourage expression of feelings, anxieties. **Facilitates grieving the loss.**

Information that appears in brackets has been added by the authors to clarify and enhance the use of nursing diagnoses.

- Active-listen client's concerns and negative verbalizations without judgment. **Conveys a message of acceptance and confidence in client's ability to deal with whatever occurs.**
- Identify individual strengths and assets and aspects of self that remain intact and can be valued. Reinforce positive traits, abilities, self-view.
- Help client identify own responsibility and control or lack of control in situation. **When able to acknowledge what is out of his or her control, client can focus attention on area of own responsibility.**
- Assist client to problem-solve situation, developing plan of action and setting goals to achieve desired outcome. **Enhances commitment to plan, optimizing outcomes.**
- Convey confidence in client's ability to cope with current situation. **Validation helps client accept own ability to deal with what is happening.**
- Mobilize support systems. **Support systems can provide role modeling and the help needed to engender hope and enhance self-esteem.**
- Provide opportunity for client to practice alternative coping strategies, including progressive socialization opportunities.
- Encourage use of visualization, guided imagery, and relaxation **to promote positive sense of self and coping ability.**
- Provide feedback of client's self-negating remarks or behavior, using I-messages, **to allow the client to experience a different view.**
- Encourage involvement in decisions about care when possible.
- Give reinforcement for progress noted. **Positive words of encouragement promote continuation of efforts, supporting development of coping behaviors.**

Nursing Priority No. 3.

To promote wellness (Teaching/Discharge Considerations):

- Encourage client to set long-range goals for achieving necessary lifestyle changes. **Supports view that this is an ongoing process.**
- Support independence in activities of daily living or mastery of therapeutic regimen. **Confident individual is more secure and positive in self-appraisal.**
- Promote attendance in therapy or support group, as indicated.
- Involve extended family/SO(s) in treatment plan. **Increases likelihood they will provide appropriate support to client.**

Information that appears in brackets has been added by the authors to clarify and enhance the use of nursing diagnoses.

- Provide information to assist client in making desired changes. **Appropriate books, DVDs, or other resources allow client to learn at own pace.**
- Suggest participation in group or community activities (e.g., assertiveness classes, volunteer work, support groups).

Documentation Focus

Assessment/Reassessment

- Individual findings, noting precipitating crisis, client's perceptions, effects on desired lifestyle/interaction with others
- Underlying dynamics and duration of current situation
- Past history of self-esteem issues
- Cultural values or religious beliefs, locus of control
- Family support, availability and use of resources

Planning

- Plan of care and who is involved in planning
- Teaching plan

Implementation/Evaluation

- Responses to interventions, teaching, actions performed, and changes that may be indicated
- Attainment or progress toward desired outcome(s)
- Modifications to plan of care

Discharge Planning

- Long-term needs and goals and who is responsible for actions to be taken
- Specific referrals made

Sample Nursing Outcomes & Interventions Classifications (NOC/NIC)

NOC—Self-Esteem
NIC—Self-Esteem Enhancement

Information that appears in brackets has been added by the authors to clarify and enhance the use of nursing diagnoses.

SELF-MUTILATION and risk for SELF-MUTILATION

[Diagnostic Division: Safety]

Definition: Self-Mutilation: Deliberate self-injurious behavior causing tissue damage with the intent of causing nonfatal injury to attain relief of tension.

Definition: risk for Self-Mutilation: Vulnerable to deliberate self-injurious behavior causing tissue damage with the intent of causing nonfatal injury to attain relief of tension.

Related and Risk Factors

Absence of family confidant; disturbance in interpersonal relationships

Adolescence; ineffective communication between parent and adolescent; eating disorder

Alteration in body image; impaired or low self-esteem

Autism; childhood illness or surgery; developmental delay

Borderline personality or character disorder; depersonalization; dissociation; psychotic disorder; emotional disorder; labile behavior (risk)

Family divorce; family history of substance abuse or self-destructive behavior; violence between parental figures

Feeling threatened with loss of significant relationship; loss of significant relationship(s) (risk)

History of childhood abuse (e.g., physical, psychological, sexual)

History of self-directed violence; irresistible urge for self-directed violence or to cut self

Impulsiveness; ineffective coping strategies; inability to express tension verbally; mounting tension that is intolerable; requires rapid stress reduction

Incarceration

Isolation from peers; peers who self-mutilate

Living in nontraditional setting (e.g., foster, group, or institutional care)

Negative feeling (e.g., depression, rejection, self-hatred, separation anxiety, guilt, depersonalization); perfectionism

Loss of control over problem-solving (risk); pattern of inability to plan solutions or to see long-term consequences; history of manipulation to obtain nurturing relationship with others

Sexual identity crisis

Substance abuse

Information that appears in brackets has been added by the authors to clarify and enhance the use of nursing diagnoses.

> **NOTE:** A risk diagnosis is not evidenced by signs and symptoms, as the problem has not occurred; rather, nursing interventions are directed at prevention.

Defining Characteristics (Self-Mutilation)

Subjective

Self-inflicted burn
Ingestion or inhalation of harmful substance

Objective

Cuts or scratches on body
Picking at wound
Biting; abrading
Insertion of object into body orifice
Hitting
Severing or constricting a body part

Desired Outcomes/Evaluation Criteria—Client Will:

- Verbalize understanding of reasons for wanting to cut or harm self, or occurrence of behavior.
- Identify precipitating factors or awareness of arousal state that occurs prior to incident.
- Express increased self-concept or self-esteem.
- Demonstrate self-control as evidenced by lessened (or absence of) episodes of self-injury.
- Engage in use of alternative methods for managing feelings and individuality.
- Seek help when feeling anxious and having thoughts of harming self.

Actions/Interventions

Nursing Priority No. 1.

To assess causative/contributing **or risk** factors:

- Determine underlying dynamics of individual situation as listed in Related/Risk Factors. Note presence of inflexible, maladaptive personality traits (e.g., impulsive, unpredictable, inappropriate behaviors, intense anger, lack of control of anger) **reflecting personality or character disorder, mental illness (e.g., bipolar disorder).**

Information that appears in brackets has been added by the authors to clarify and enhance the use of nursing diagnoses.

- Evaluate history of mental illness (e.g., borderline personality, identity disorder, bipolar disorder).
- Identify previous episodes of self-mutilation behavior. **Some body piercing (e.g., ears) is generally accepted as decorative; piercing of multiple sites often is an attempt to establish individuality, addressing issues of separation and belonging, but is not considered self-injury behavior.**
- Note beliefs, cultural and religious practices that may be involved in choice of behavior. **Growing up in a family that did not allow feelings to be expressed, individuals learn that feelings are bad or wrong. Family dynamics may come out of religious or cultural expectations that believe in strict punishment for transgressions.**
- Note use or abuse of addicting substances. **Client may be trying to resist impulse to self-injure by turning to drugs.**
- Review laboratory findings (e.g., blood alcohol, polydrug screen, glucose, and electrolyte levels). **Drug use may affect self-injury behavior.**
- Note degree of impairment in social and occupational functioning. **May dictate treatment setting (e.g., specific outpatient program, short-stay inpatient).**

Nursing Priority No. 2.

To structure environment to maintain client safety:

- Assist client to identify feelings leading up to desire for self-mutilation. **Early recognition of recurring feelings provides opportunity to seek and learn other ways of coping.**
- Provide external controls/limit setting. **May decrease the opportunity to self-mutilate.**
- Include client in development of plan of care. **Commitment to plan increases likelihood of adherence.**
- Encourage appropriate expression of feelings. **Identifies feelings and promotes understanding of what leads to development of tension.**
- Keep client in continuous staff view and provide special observation checks during inpatient therapy **to promote safety.**
- Structure inpatient milieu to maintain positive, clear, open communication among staff and clients, with an understanding that "secrets are not tolerated" and failure to maintain openness will be confronted.
- Develop schedule of alternative, healthy, success-oriented activities, including involvement in such groups as Self-Harm

Information that appears in brackets has been added by the authors to clarify and enhance the use of nursing diagnoses.

Support Group, Cutters Awareness & Support Group (or similar program) based on individual needs; self-esteem activities including positive affirmations, connecting with friends and like-minded peers, and exercise.

- Note feelings of healthcare providers and family, such as frustration, anger, defensiveness, need to rescue. **Client may be manipulative, evoking defensiveness and conflict. These feelings need to be identified, recognized, and dealt with openly with staff/family and client.**
- Provide care for client's wounds when self-mutilation occurs in a matter-of-fact manner **that conveys empathy and concern.** Refrain from offering sympathy or additional attention **that could provide reinforcement for maladaptive behavior and may encourage its repetition.**

Nursing Priority No. 3.

To promote movement toward positive behaviors:

- Discuss with client/family normalcy of adolescent task of separation and ways of achieving.
- Assist client to learn assertive behavior. Include the use of effective communication skills, focusing on developing self-esteem by replacing negative self-talk with positive comments.
- Involve client in developing goals for stopping behavior. **Enhances commitment, optimizing outcomes.**
- Develop a contract between client and counselor **to enable the client to stay physically safe, such as "I will not cut or harm myself for the next 24 hours."** Renew contract on a regular basis and have both parties sign and date each contract.
- Provide avenues of communication **for times when client needs to talk to avoid cutting or damaging self.**
- Use interventions that help the client to reclaim power in own life (e.g., experiential and cognitive).
- Involve client/family in group therapies as appropriate.

Nursing Priority No. 4.

To promote wellness (Teaching/Discharge Considerations):

- Discuss commitment to safety and ways in which client will deal with precursors to undesired behavior. **Provides opportunity for client to assume responsibility for self.**
- Mobilize support systems.
- Promote the use of healthy behaviors, identifying consequences and outcomes of current actions.

Information that appears in brackets has been added by the authors to clarify and enhance the use of nursing diagnoses.

- Discuss living arrangements when client is discharged/relocated. **May need assistance with transition to changes required to avoid recurrence of self-mutilating behaviors.**
- Involve family/significant other (SO) in planning for discharge and in group therapies, as appropriate. **Promotes coordination and continuation of plan, commitment to goals.**
- Discuss information about the role neurotransmitters play in predisposing an individual to beginning this behavior. **It is believed that problems in the serotonin system may make the person more aggressive and impulsive, especially when combined with an environment where he or she learned that feelings are bad or wrong, leading client to turn aggression on self.**
- Provide information and discuss the use of medication, as appropriate. **Antidepressant medications may be useful, but they need to be weighed against the potential for overdosing.**
- Refer to NDs Anxiety; impaired Social Interaction; Self-Esteem [specify].

Documentation Focus

Assessment/Reassessment

- Individual findings, including risk factors present, underlying dynamics, prior episodes
- Cultural or religious practices
- Laboratory test results
- Substance use or abuse

Planning

- Plan of care and who is involved in planning
- Teaching plan

Implementation/Evaluation

- Response to interventions, teaching, and actions performed
- Attainment or progress toward desired outcome(s)
- Modifications to plan of care

Discharge Planning

- Long-term needs and who is responsible for actions to be taken
- Community resources, referrals made

Information that appears in brackets has been added by the authors to clarify and enhance the use of nursing diagnoses.

Sample Nursing Outcomes & Interventions Classifications (NOC/NIC)

NOC—Self-Mutilation Restraint
NIC—Behavior Management: Self-Harm

SELF-NEGLECT

[Diagnostic Division: Hygiene]

Definition: A constellation of culturally framed behaviors involving one or more self-care activities in which there is a failure to maintain a socially accepted standard of health and well-being (Gibbons, Lauder, & Ludwick, 2006).

Related Factors

Stressor; psychiatric/psychotic disorder
Frontal lobe dysfunction; deficient executive function; alteration in cognitive functioning; Capgras syndrome
Functional impairment; learning disability
Lifestyle choice; substance abuse; malingering
Inability to maintain control; fear of institutionalization

Defining Characteristics

Objective

Insufficient personal or environmental hygiene
Nonadherence to health activity

Desired Outcomes/Evaluation Criteria—Client Will:

- Acknowledge difficulty maintaining hygiene practices.
- Demonstrate ability to manage lifestyle changes and medication regimen.
- Perform activities of daily living within level of own ability.

Caregiver Will:

- Assist individual with personal and environmental hygiene as needed.
- Identify and assist client with medical, dental, and other healthcare appointments as indicated.

Information that appears in brackets has been added by the authors to clarify and enhance the use of nursing diagnoses.

Actions/Interventions

Nursing Priority No. 1.

To identify causative or precipitating factors:

- Determine existing health problems, age, developmental level, and cognitive psychological factors, including presence of delusions affecting ability to care for own needs. **A wide variety of impairments can cause a person to neglect hygiene needs, particularly aging, homelessness, and dementia.**
- Use an appropriate screening instrument, such as the Elder Assessment Instrument (EAI). **Neglect and elder abuse is underreported, and the use of a good tool can help identify presence.**
- Identify other problems that may interfere with ability to care for self. **Visual or hearing impairment, language barrier, emotional instability or lability can create difficulties for individual to manage daily tasks.**
- Note recent life events or changes in circumstances. **Losses such as of a loved one, financial security, or physical independence can trigger or exacerbate self-neglect behaviors.**
- Review circumstances of client illness, possible monetary rewards, sympathy or attention from family. **On occasion self-neglect may be malingering as an attempt to gain something from others or relinquish unwanted responsibilities.**
- Perform mental status examination. **Mental illness (e.g., psychosis, depression, dementia) can affect individual's ability or desire to maintain self-care activities or care for home surroundings.**
- Review studies evaluating frontal lobe dysfunction and possibility of Diogenes syndrome. **These clients present with severe self-neglect and may have coexisting medical and psychiatric conditions.**
- Assess economic factors and living arrangements. **May live alone or with family members who are not helpful or may be homeless; may have little or no financial resources, resulting in inability to achieve or lack of concern about personal well-being.**
- Determine availability and use of resources. **Depending on disability of client, agencies can work together to develop a plan to meet needs, noting whether individual is availing self of help.**
- Interview significant other (SO)/family members to determine level of involvement and support. **Client may be exhibiting**

Information that appears in brackets has been added by the authors to clarify and enhance the use of nursing diagnoses.

acting-out/paranoid behaviors, stressing caregivers, who may not realize that cognitive impairment prevents individual from exercising self-control.

Nursing Priority No. 2.

To determine degree of impairment:

- Perform head-to-toe assessment inspecting scalp and skin, noting personal hygiene, body odor, rashes, bruising, skin tears, lesions, burns, presence of vermin; inspecting oral cavity for gum disease, inflammation, lesions, loose or broken teeth, fit of dentures. **Identifies specific needs and may reveal signs of trauma or abuse.**
- Perform nutritional assessment as indicated. **Neglecting oneself often includes not eating meals regularly or not eating nutritionally balanced foods, especially when alcoholism or drug abuse is present.**
- Review medication regimen. **In addition to neglecting self-care activities, client will likely not pay attention to taking prescriptions as ordered, resulting in exacerbation of medical problem. Some psychotropic medications may cause individual to "feel different" or not in control of self, resulting in reluctance to take drug.**
- Determine client's willingness to change situation.

Nursing Priority No. 3.

To assist in correcting/dealing with situation:

- Develop multidisciplinary team specific to individual needs, such as case manager, physician, dietitian, physical or occupational therapist, rehabilitation specialist. **To develop a plan appropriate to the individual situation, making use of client's capabilities and maximizing potential.**
- Establish therapeutic relationship with client and with family, if available and willing to be involved.
- Identify specific priorities and goals of client/SOs. **Helps client to look at possibilities for dealing with difficult situation of no longer being able to maintain lifestyle and moving on to a new way of managing.**
- Promote client's/SO's participation in problem identification and decision making.
- Evaluate need for safety, balancing client's need for autonomy. **The ethical challenge of providing individual safety within the current laws for client's right to refuse care in face of self-neglect and self-destructive behaviors, which can impact others as well as the client, is difficult to manage.**

Information that appears in brackets has been added by the authors to clarify and enhance the use of nursing diagnoses.

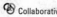

- Perform home assessment **to determine safety issues, cleanliness, compulsive hoarding, neglected property concerns.**
- Demonstrate or review skills necessary for caring for self, using terms appropriate to client's level of understanding.
- Plan time for listening to client's/SO's concerns. **Provides opportunity to determine whether plan is being followed and identify the barriers to participation.**
- Refer to NDs Self-Care Deficit [specify]; ineffective Health Maintenance; impaired Home Maintenance; [disturbed Sensory Perception], for additional interventions as appropriate.

Nursing Priority No. 4.

To promote wellness (Discharge/Evaluation Criteria):

- Establish remotivation or resocialization program when indicated. **Depending on where the client is residing, isolation may become a problem as individual withdraws from contact with others.**
- Assist with setting up medication regimen as indicated.
- Discuss dietary needs and client's ability to provide nutritious meals. **May require support such as food assistance, community pantry, elder meal program, Meals-on-Wheels.**
- Provide for ongoing evaluation of self-care program. **Helps to identify whether client is managing effectively or whether cognitive functioning is deteriorating and a new plan needs to be developed.**
- Evaluate for appropriateness of providing a companion animal. **Taking responsibility for another life and sharing unconditional love can provide purpose and motivation for client to take more interest in own situation.**
- Refer to support services such as home care, day-care program, social services, food assistance, community clinic, physical/occupational therapy, senior services, as indicated.
- Investigate alternative placements as indicated.
- Discuss need for respite for family members. **Care of cognitively impaired member can be wearing, and time away allows for renewing oneself and enhancing ability to cope with continued care responsibilities.**
- Refer for counseling as indicated. **Accurate mental health diagnoses may reveal the need for appropriate services, psychiatric, social services, home care.**

Documentation Focus

Assessment/Reassessment

- Individual findings, functional level and limitations, mental status

Information that appears in brackets has been added by the authors to clarify and enhance the use of nursing diagnoses.

- Personal safety issues
- Needed resources, possible need for placement

Planning

- Plan of care and who is involved in planning
- Teaching plan

Implementation/Evaluation

- Response to interventions, teaching, and actions performed
- Attainment or progress toward desired outcomes
- Modifications of plan of care

Discharge Planning

- Long-term needs and who is responsible for actions to be taken
- Type of assistance and resources needed
- Specific referrals made

Sample Nursing Outcomes & Interventions Classifications (NOC/NIC)

NOC—Self-Care Status
NIC—Self-Responsibility Facilitation

[disturbed SENSORY PERCEPTION: Specify visual, auditory, kinesthetic, gustatory, tactile, olfactory]

[Diagnostic Division: Neurosensory]

Definition: Change in the amount or patterning of incoming stimuli accompanied by a diminished, exaggerated, distorted, or impaired response to such stimuli.

Related Factors

Insufficient environmental stimuli (therapeutically restricted environments [e.g., isolation, intensive care, bedrest, traction, confining illnesses, incubator]; socially restricted environment [e.g., institutionalization, homebound, aging, chronic or terminal illness, infant deprivation]; stigmatized [e.g., mental illness, developmentally delayed, disabled])

Excessive environmental stimuli

Altered sensory reception, transmission, or integration

Biochemical imbalances (e.g., elevated blood urea nitrogen, ammonia; hypoxia); electrolyte imbalance; [drugs (e.g., stimulants or depressants, mind-altering drugs)]

Psychological stress; [sleep deprivation]

Information that appears in brackets has been added by the authors to clarify and enhance the use of nursing diagnoses.

Defining Characteristics

Subjective

[Reported] change in sensory acuity (e.g., photosensitivity, hypoesthesias or hyperesthesias, diminished or altered sense of taste, inability to tell position of body parts [proprioception])

Sensory distortions

Objective

[Measured] change in sensory acuity

Change in usual response to stimuli

Change in behavior pattern; restlessness; irritability

Change in problem-solving abilities; poor concentration

Disorientation; hallucinations; [illusions]

Impaired communication

Motor incoordination, altered sense of balance/falls (e.g., Ménière's syndrome)

Desired Outcomes/Evaluation Criteria—Client Will:

- Regain or maintain usual level of cognition.
- Recognize and correct or compensate for sensory impairments.
- Verbalize awareness of sensory needs and presence of overload and/or deprivation.
- Identify and modify external factors that contribute to alterations in sensory or perceptual abilities.
- Use resources effectively and appropriately.
- Be free of injury.

Actions/Interventions

Nursing Priority No. 1.

To assess causative/contributing factors and degree of impairment:

- Identify client with condition that can affect sensing, interpreting, and communicating stimuli. **Specific clinical concerns (e.g., neurological disease or trauma, intensive care unit confinement, surgery, pain, biochemical imbalances, psychosis, substance abuse, toxemia) have the potential for altering one or more of the senses, with resultant change in the reception, sensitivity, or interpretation of sensory input.**

Information that appears in brackets has been added by the authors to clarify and enhance the use of nursing diagnoses.

- Note age and developmental stage. **Problems with sensory perception may be known to client/caregiver (e.g., child wearing hearing aid, elderly adult with known macular degeneration), where compensatory interventions are in place. Screening or evaluation may be required if sensory impairments are suspected but not obvious.**
- Review results of sensory and motor neurological testing and laboratory studies (e.g., cognitive testing or laboratory values, such as electrolytes, chemical profile, arterial blood gases, serum drug levels) **to note presence or possible cause of changes in response to sensory stimuli.**
- Evaluate medication regimen and determine possible use or misuse of drugs (prescription, over-the-counter [OTC], illicit) **to identify effects, side effects, or drug interactions that may cause or exacerbate sensory or perceptual problems.**
- Assess ability to speak, hear, interpret, and respond to simple commands **to obtain an overview of client's mental and cognitive status and ability to interpret stimuli.**
- Evaluate sensory awareness: stimulus of hot and cold, dull or sharp; smell, taste, visual acuity, and hearing; gait, mobility; location and function of body parts.
- Determine response to painful stimuli **to note whether response is appropriate to stimulus and is immediate or delayed.**
- Observe for behavioral responses (e.g., illusions, hallucinations, delusions, withdrawal, hostility, crying, inappropriate affect, confusion or disorientation) **that may indicate mental or emotional problems or chemical toxicity (as might occur with digoxin or other drug overdose or reaction) or be associated with brain or neurological trauma or infection.**
- Note inattention to body parts, segments of environment; lack of recognition of familiar objects or persons. **Loss of comprehension of auditory, visual, or other sensations may be indicative of unilateral neglect or inability to recognize and respond to environmental cues.**
- Ascertain client's/significant other's (SO's) perception of problem/changes in activities of daily living. **Client may or may not be aware of changes (e.g., diabetic with neuropathy may not realize he or she has lost discrimination for pain in feet; or parents may notice child's problem with coordination or difficulty with words).** Listen to and respect client's expressions of deprivation and take these into consideration in planning care.
- Refer to additional NDs Anxiety; acute/chronic Confusion; Unilateral Neglect, as appropriate and based on findings.

Information that appears in brackets has been added by the authors to clarify and enhance the use of nursing diagnoses.

Nursing Priority No. 2.

To promote normalization of response to stimuli:

- Address client by name and have personnel wear name tags and reintroduce self, as needed, **to preserve client's sense of identity and orientation.**
- Reorient to person, place, time, and events, as necessary **to reduce confusion and provide sense of normalcy to client's daily life.**
- Explain procedures and activities, expected sensations, and outcomes.
- Provide means of communication, as indicated by client's current situation.
- Encourage use of listening devices (e.g., hearing aid, audiovisual amplifier, closed-caption TV, signing interpreter) **to assist in managing auditory impairment.**
- Interpret stimuli and offer feedback **to assist client to separate reality from fantasy or altered perception.**
- Avoid isolation of client, physically or emotionally, **to prevent sensory deprivation and limit confusion.**
- Promote a stable environment with continuity of care by same personnel as much as possible.
- Eliminate extraneous noise and stimuli, including nonessential equipment, alarms or audible monitor signals when possible.
- Provide undisturbed rest and sleep periods.
- Speak to visually impaired or unresponsive client during care **to provide auditory stimulation and prevent startle reflex.**
- Provide tactile stimulation as care is given. **Touching is an important part of caring and a deep psychological need communicating presence and connection with another human being.**
- Provide sensory stimulation, including familiar smells and sounds, tactile stimulation with a variety of objects, changing of light intensity, and other cues (e.g., clocks, calendars).
- Encourage SO(s) to bring in familiar objects, talk to, and touch the client frequently.
- Minimize discussion of negatives (e.g., client and personnel problems) within client's hearing. **Client may misinterpret and believe references are to himself or herself.**
- Provide diversional activities, as able (e.g., TV, radio, conversation, large-print or talking books). (Refer to ND deficient Diversional Activity.)
- Promote meaningful socialization. (Refer to ND Social Isolation.)

Information that appears in brackets has been added by the authors to clarify and enhance the use of nursing diagnoses.

- Collaborate with other health team members in providing rehabilitative therapies and stimulating modalities (e.g., music therapy, sensory training, remotivation therapy) **to achieve maximal gains in function and psychosocial well-being.**
- Identify and encourage use of resources and prosthetic devices (e.g., hearing aids, computerized visual aid, glasses with a level plumbline for balance). **Useful for augmenting senses.**

Nursing Priority No. 3.

To prevent injury/complications:

- Record perceptual deficit on chart **so that caregivers are aware.**
- Place call bell or other communication device within reach and be sure client knows where it is and how to use it.
- Provide safety measures, as needed (e.g., siderails, bed in low position, adequate lighting; assistance with walking; use of vision or hearing devices).
- Review basic and specific safety information (e.g., "I am on your right side"; "This water is hot"; "Swallow now"; "Stand up"; "You cannot drive").
- Position doors and furniture so they are out of travel path for client with impaired vision or strategically place items or grab bars **to aid in maintaining balance.**
- Ambulate with assistance and devices **to enhance balance.**
- Describe where affected areas of body are when moving client.
- Limit and carefully monitor use of sedation, especially in the elderly **who are more sensitive to side effects and drug interactions affecting sensory perception and interpretation.**
- Monitor use of heating pads or ice packs; use thermometer to measure temperature of bath water **to protect from thermal injury.**
- Refer to NDs risk for Thermal Injury; risk for Trauma; risk for Falls.

Nursing Priority No. 4.

To promote wellness (Teaching/Discharge Considerations):

- Review ways to prevent or limit exposure to conditions affecting sensory functions (e.g., how exposure to loud noise and toxins can impair hearing; early childhood screening for speech and language disorders; vaccines to prevent measles, mumps, meningitis, **once known to be major causes of hearing loss).**

Information that appears in brackets has been added by the authors to clarify and enhance the use of nursing diagnoses.

- Assist client/SO(s) to learn effective ways of coping with and managing sensory disturbances, anticipating safety needs according to client's sensory deficits and developmental level.
- Identify alternative ways of dealing with perceptual deficits (e.g., vision and hearing aids; augmentative communication devices; computer technologies; specific deficit-compensation techniques).
- Provide explanations of and plan care with client, involving SO(s) as much as possible. **Enhances commitment to and continuation of plan, optimizing outcomes.**
- Review home safety measures pertinent to deficits.
- Discuss drug regimen, noting possible toxic side effects of both prescription and over-the-counter drugs. **Prompt recognition of side effects allows for timely intervention/change in drug regimen.**
- Demonstrate use and care of sensory prosthetic devices (e.g., assistive vision or listening devices, etc.).
- Identify resources and community programs for acquiring and maintaining assistive devices.
- Refer to appropriate helping resources, such as Society for the Blind, Self-Help for the Hard of Hearing (SHHH), or local support groups, screening programs, as indicated.
- Refer to additional NDs Anxiety; acute/chronic Confusion; Unilateral Neglect, as appropriate.

Documentation Focus

Assessment/Reassessment

- Individual findings, noting specific deficit and associated symptoms, perceptions of client/SO(s)
- Assistive device needs

Planning

- Plan of care, including who is involved in planning
- Teaching plan

Implementation/Evaluation

- Responses to interventions, teaching, and actions performed
- Attainment or progress toward desired outcome(s)
- Modifications to plan of care

Discharge Planning

- Long-term needs and who is responsible for actions to be taken
- Available resources; specific referrals made

Information that appears in brackets has been added by the authors to clarify and enhance the use of nursing diagnoses.

Sample Nursing Outcomes & Interventions Classifications (NOC/NIC)

Auditory

NOC—Sensory Function: Hearing
NIC—Communication Enhancement: Hearing Deficit

Visual

NOC—Sensory Function: Vision
NIC—Communication Enhancement: Visual Deficit

Gustatory/Olfactory

NOC—Sensory Function: Taste & Smell
NIC—Nutrition Management

Kinesthetic

NOC—Sensory Function: Proprioception
NIC—Body Mechanics Promotion

Tactile

NOC—Sensory Function: Cutaneous
NIC—Peripheral Sensation Management

SEXUAL DYSFUNCTION

[Diagnostic Division: Sexuality]

Definition: A state in which an individual experiences a change in sexual function during the sexual response phases of desire, excitation, and/or orgasm, which is viewed as unsatisfying, unrewarding, or inadequate.

Related Factors

Inadequate role model; absence of significant other (SO)
Absence of privacy
Misinformation or insufficient knowledge about sexual function
Vulnerability
Presence of abuse (e.g., physical, psychological, sexual); psychosocial abuse (e.g., controlling, manipulation, verbal abuse)
Alteration in body function or structure (due to pregnancy, surgery, medication, anomaly, disease, trauma, radiation, etc.)
Value conflict

Information that appears in brackets has been added by the authors to clarify and enhance the use of nursing diagnoses.

Defining Characteristics

Subjective

Change in sexual role
Perceived sexual limitation
Alteration in sexual activity, excitation, or satisfaction; decrease in sexual desire
Undesired change in sexual function
Seeks confirmation of desirability
Change in self-interest/interest toward others

Desired Outcomes/Evaluation Criteria—Client Will:

- Verbalize understanding of sexual anatomy and function and alterations that may affect function.
- Verbalize understanding of individual reasons for sexual problems.
- Identify stressors in lifestyle that may contribute to the dysfunction.
- Identify satisfying and acceptable sexual practices and alternative ways of dealing with sexual expression.
- Discuss concerns about body image, sex role, desirability as a sexual partner with partner/SO.

Actions/Interventions

Nursing Priority No. 1.

To assess causative/contributing factors:

- Do a complete history and physical, including a sexual history, which would include usual pattern of functioning and level of desire. Note vocabulary used by the individual to maximize communication/understanding.
- Have client describe problem in own words.
- Determine importance of sex to individual/partner and client's motivation for change. **Interpersonal problems (marital and relationship), lack of trust or open communication between partners can contribute to client's concern.**
- Be alert to comments of client, **as sexual concerns are often disguised as humor, sarcasm, and/or offhand remarks.**
- Assess knowledge of client/SO regarding sexual anatomy and function and effects of current situation or condition. **Individuals are often ignorant of anatomy of sexual system and**

Information that appears in brackets has been added by the authors to clarify and enhance the use of nursing diagnoses.

how it works, impacting client's understanding of situation and expectations.

- Determine preexisting problems that may be factors in current situation (e.g., marital or job stress, role conflicts).
- Identify current stress factors in individual situation. **These factors may be producing enough anxiety to cause depression or other psychological reaction(s) leading to physiological symptoms.**
- Discuss cultural values, religious beliefs, or conflicts present. **Client may have anxiety and guilt as a result of family beliefs about sex and genital area of the body because of how sexuality was communicated to the client as he or she was growing up.**
- Determine pathophysiology, illness, surgery, or trauma involved and impact on (perception of) individual/SO. **The client may be more concerned about these issues when the sexual parts of the body are involved (e.g., mastectomy, hysterectomy, prostatectomy).**
- Review medication regimen and drug use (prescriptions, over the counter, illegal, alcohol) and cigarette use. **Antihypertensives may cause erectile dysfunction; monoamine oxidase inhibitors and tricyclics can cause erection or ejaculation problems and anorgasmia in women; narcotics and alcohol can produce impotence and inhibit orgasm; smoking creates vasoconstriction and may be a factor in erectile dysfunction.**
- Observe behavior and stage of grieving when related to body changes or loss of a body part (e.g., pregnancy, obesity, amputation, mastectomy).
- Discuss client's view of body, concern about penis size, failure with performance.
- Assist with diagnostic studies to determine cause of erectile dysfunction. **More than half of the cases have a physical cause such as diabetes, vascular problems.** Monitor penile tumescence during REM sleep **to assist in determining physical ability.**
- Explore with client the meaning of client's behavior. **(Masturbation, for instance, may have many meanings or purposes, such as for relief of anxiety, sexual deprivation, pleasure, a nonverbal expression of need to talk, way of alienating.)** (*Note:* Nurse needs to be aware of and be in control of own feelings and response to client expressions or self-revelation.)
- Avoid making value judgments, **as they do not help the client to cope with the situation.**

Information that appears in brackets has been added by the authors to clarify and enhance the use of nursing diagnoses.

Nursing Priority No. 2.

To assist client/SO to deal with individual situation:

- Establish therapeutic nurse-client relationship **to promote treatment and facilitate sharing of sensitive information and feelings.**
- Assist with treatment of underlying medical conditions, including changes in medication regimen, weight management, and cessation of smoking.
- Provide factual information about individual condition involved. **Promotes informed decision making.**
- Determine what client wants to know **to tailor information to client needs.** *Note:* Information affecting client safety or consequences of actions may need to be reviewed and reinforced.
- Encourage and accept expressions of concern, anger, grief, fear. **Client needs to talk about these feelings to begin resolution.**
- Assist client to be aware of and deal with stages of grieving for loss or change.
- Encourage client to share thoughts and concerns with partner and to clarify values and impact of condition on relationship.
- Provide for or identify ways to obtain privacy **to allow for sexual expression for individual and/or between partners without embarrassment and/or objections of others.**
- Assist client/SO to problem-solve alternative ways of sexual expression. **When client is unable to perform in usual manner, there are many ways the couple can learn to satisfy sexual needs.**
- Provide information about availability of corrective measures such as medication (e.g., papaverine or sildenafil [Viagra] for erectile dysfunction) or reconstructive surgery (e.g., penile/breast implants) when indicated.
- Refer to appropriate resources, as needed (e.g., healthcare coworker with greater comfort level and/or knowledgeable clinical nurse specialist or professional sex therapist, family counseling).

Nursing Priority No. 3.

To promote wellness (Teaching/Discharge Considerations):

- Provide sex education, explanation of normal sexual functioning when necessary.
- Provide written material appropriate to individual needs (include list of books related to client's concerns) **for reinforcement at client's leisure and readiness to deal with sensitive materials.**

Information that appears in brackets has been added by the authors to clarify and enhance the use of nursing diagnoses.

- Encourage ongoing dialogue and take advantage of teachable moments that occur. **Nurse needs to become comfortable with talking about sexual issue so he or she can recognize these moments and be willing to discuss the client's concerns.**
- Demonstrate and assist client to learn relaxation and/or visualization techniques.
- Encourage client to engage in regular self-examination, as indicated (e.g., breast/testicular examinations).
- Identify community resources for further assistance (e.g., Reach for Recovery, CanSurmount, Ostomy Association, family or sex therapist).
- Refer for further professional assistance concerning relationship difficulties, low sexual desire, and other sexual concerns (e.g., premature ejaculation, vaginismus, painful intercourse).
- Identify resources for assistive devices or sexual "aids."

Documentation Focus

Assessment/Reassessment

- Individual findings including nature of dysfunction, predisposing factors, perceived effect on sexuality and relationships
- Cultural or religious factors, conflicts
- Response of SO
- Motivation for change

Planning

- Plan of care and who is involved in planning
- Teaching plan

Implementation/Evaluation

- Response to interventions, teaching, and actions performed
- Attainment or progress toward desired outcome(s)
- Modifications to plan of care

Discharge Planning

- Long-term needs, referrals made, and who is responsible for actions to be taken
- Community resources, specific referrals made

Sample Nursing Outcomes & Interventions Classifications (NOC/NIC)

NOC—Sexual Functioning
NIC—Sexual Counseling

Information that appears in brackets has been added by the authors to clarify and enhance the use of nursing diagnoses.

ineffective SEXUALITY PATTERN

[Diagnostic Division: Sexuality]

Definition: Expressions of concern regarding own sexuality.

Related Factors

Insufficient knowledge or skill deficit about alternatives related to sexuality
Absence of privacy
Impaired relationship with a significant other (SO); absence of SO
Inadequate role model
Conflict about sexual orientation or variant preference
Fear of pregnancy or sexually transmitted infection

Defining Characteristics

Subjective

Alteration in relationship with SO
Alteration in/difficulty with sexual activity or behavior
Change in sexual role
Value conflict

Desired Outcomes/Evaluation Criteria—Client Will:

- Verbalize understanding of sexual anatomy and function.
- Verbalize knowledge and understanding of sexual limitations, difficulties, or changes that have occurred.
- Verbalize acceptance of self in current (altered) condition.
- Demonstrate improved communication and relationship skills.
- Identify individually appropriate method of contraception.

Actions/Interventions

Nursing Priority No. 1.

To assess causative/contributing factors:

- Obtain complete physical and sexual history, as indicated, including perception of normal function. **Sexuality is multifaceted, beginning with one's body, biological sex, and**

Information that appears in brackets has been added by the authors to clarify and enhance the use of nursing diagnoses.

gender (biological, social, and legal status as girls or boys, women or men).

- Note use of vocabulary (assessing basic knowledge) and comments or concerns about sexual identity. **Components of sexual identity include one's gender identity (how one feels about his or her gender) as well as one's sexual orientation (straight, lesbian, gay, bisexual, transgendered).**
- Determine importance of sex and a description of the problem in the client's own words. Be alert to comments of client/SO (e.g., discounting overt or covert sexual expressions such as "He's just a dirty old man"). **Sexual concerns are often disguised as sarcasm, humor, or in offhand remarks.**
- Elicit impact of perceived problem on SO/family. **One's values about life, love, and the people in one's life are also components of one's sexuality.**
- Note cultural values or religious beliefs and conflicts that may exist. **Individuals are enculturated as they grow up and, depending on particular family views and taboos, may harbor feelings of shame and guilt about their sexual feelings.**
- Assess stress factors in client's environment that might cause anxiety or psychological reactions (e.g., power issues involving SO, adult children, aging, employment, loss of prowess).
- Explore knowledge of effects of altered body function/limitations precipitated by illness (e.g., multiple sclerosis, arthritis, mutilating cancer surgery) or medical treatment of alternative sexual responses and expressions (e.g., undescended testicle in young male, gender change or reassignment procedure).
- Review history of substance use (prescription medications, over-the-counter drugs, alcohol, illicit drugs). **May be used by client to handle underlying feelings or anxiety.**
- Explore issues and fears associated with sex (pregnancy, sexually transmitted, trust and control issues, inflexible beliefs, preference confusion, altered performance).
- Determine client's interpretation of the altered sexual activity or behavior (e.g., a way of controlling, relief of anxiety, pleasure, lack of partner). **These behaviors (when related to body changes, including pregnancy, weight loss or gain, or loss of body part) may reflect a stage of grieving.**
- Assess life cycle issues, such as adolescence, young adulthood, menopause, aging. **All people are sexual beings from birth to death. Each transition has its own concerns and needs specific education to help the client deal with it in a healthy manner.**

Information that appears in brackets has been added by the authors to clarify and enhance the use of nursing diagnoses.

Nursing Priority No. 2.

To assist client/SO to deal with individual situation:

- Provide atmosphere in which discussion of sexual problems is encouraged and permitted. **Sense of trust or comfort enhances ability to discuss sensitive matters.**
- Avoid value judgments—**they do not help the client cope with the situation.**
- Provide information about individual situation, determining client needs and desires.
- Encourage discussion of individual situation, with opportunity for expression of feelings without judgment. **Sexuality also includes feelings, attitudes, relationships, self-image, ideals, and behaviors, and influences how one experiences the world.** (*Note:* Nurse needs to be aware of and in control of own feelings and responses to the client's expressions and/or concerns.)
- Provide specific information and suggestions about interventions directed toward the identified problems.
- Identify alternative forms of sexual expression that might be acceptable to both partners. **When illness or trauma (e.g., rheumatoid arthritis, paraplegia, long-term chronic condition) interferes with usual sexual expression, there are many different methods that can be used to obtain sexual satisfaction.**
- Discuss ways to manage individual devices or appliances (e.g., ostomy bag, breast prostheses, urinary collection device) **when change in body image or medical condition is involved.**
- Provide anticipatory guidance about losses that are to be expected (e.g., loss of known self when transsexual surgery is planned).
- Introduce client to individuals who have successfully managed a similar problem. **Provides positive role model and support for problem-solving.**

Nursing Priority No. 3.

To promote wellness (Teaching/Discharge Considerations):

- Provide factual information about problem(s), as identified by the client.
- Engage in ongoing dialogue with the client and SO(s), as situation permits.
- Discuss methods, effectiveness and side effects of contraceptives, if indicated. **Assists individual/couple to make an informed decision on a method that meets own values or religious beliefs.**

Information that appears in brackets has been added by the authors to clarify and enhance the use of nursing diagnoses.

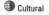

- Refer to community resources (e.g., Planned Parenthood; gender identity clinic; social services; Parents, Families and Friends of Lesbians and Gays), as indicated.
- Refer for intensive individual or group psychotherapy, which may be combined with couple or family and/or sex therapy, as appropriate.
- Refer to NDs Sexual Dysfunction; disturbed Body Image; Self-Esteem [specify].

Documentation Focus

Assessment/Reassessment

- Individual findings, including nature of concern, perceived difficulties, limitations or changes, specific needs and desires
- Cultural or religious beliefs, conflicts
- Response of SO(s)

Planning

- Plan of care and who is involved in the planning
- Teaching plan

Implementation/Evaluation

- Response to interventions, teaching, and actions performed
- Attainment or progress toward desired outcome(s)
- Modifications to plan of care

Discharge Planning

- Long-term needs, teaching, and referrals made, and who is responsible for actions to be taken
- Community resources, specific referrals made

Sample Nursing Outcomes & Interventions Classifications (NOC/NIC)

NOC—Sexual Identity
NIC—Sexual Counseling

risk for SHOCK

[Diagnostic Division: Circulation]

Definition: Vulnerable to an inadequate blood flow to the body's tissues that may lead to life-threatening cellular dysfunction, which may compromise health.

Information that appears in brackets has been added by the authors to clarify and enhance the use of nursing diagnoses.

Risk Factors

Hypotension
Hypovolemia
Hypoxemia, hypoxia
Infection, sepsis; systemic inflammatory response syndrome (SIRS)

NOTE: A risk diagnosis is not evidenced by signs and symptoms, as the problem has not occurred; rather, nursing interventions are directed at prevention.

Desired Outcomes/Evaluation Criteria—Client Will:

- Display hemodynamic stability as evidenced by vital signs within normal range for client; prompt capillary refill; adequate urinary output with normal specific gravity; usual level of mentation.
- Be afebrile and free of other signs of infection, achieve timely wound healing.
- Verbalize understanding of disease process, risk factors, and treatment plan.

Actions/Interventions

Nursing Priority No. 1.

To assess causative/contributing factors:

- Note possible medical diagnoses or disease processes that can result in one or more types of shock, such as major trauma with heavy internal or external bleeding; heart failure; head or spinal cord injury; allergic reactions; pregnancy-related complications; intra-abdomimal infections, open wounds, or other conditions associated with sepsis.
- Assess for history or presence of conditions leading to hypovolemic shock, such as trauma, surgery, inadequate clotting, anticoagulant therapy; gastrointestinal or other organ hemorrhage; prolonged vomiting and diarrhea; diabetes insipidus; misuse of diuretics. **These conditions deplete the body's circulating blood volume and ability to maintain organ perfusion and function.**
- Assess for conditions associated with *cardiogenic shock,* including myocardial infarction, cardiac arrest, lethal ventricular dysrhythmias, severe valvular dysfunction, cardiomyopathies, malignant hypertension. **These conditions directly impair the heart muscle and ability to pump.**

Information that appears in brackets has been added by the authors to clarify and enhance the use of nursing diagnoses.

- Assess for conditions associated with *obstructive shock,* including pulmonary embolus, aortic stenosis, cardiac tamponade, tension pneumothorax. **In these conditions, the heart itself may be healthy but cannot pump because of conditions outside the heart that prevent normal filling or adequate outflow.**
- Assess for conditions associated with *distributive shock—neural induced,* including pain, anesthesia, spinal cord or head injury; or *chemical induced,* including peritonitis, sepsis, burns, anaphylaxis, hyperglycemia. **These situations result in loss of sympathetic tone, blood vessel dilation, pooling of venous blood and increased capillary permeability with shifting of fluids.**
- Monitor for persistent or heavy fluid loss, including wounds, drains, vomiting, gastrointestinal tube, chest tube. Check all secretions and excretions for occult blood. Refer to NDs risk for Bleeding; risk for imbalanced Fluid Volume (for additional interventions).
- Inspect skin, noting presence of traumatic or surgical wounds, erythema, edema, tenderness, petechiae; rashes or hives **for evidence of hemorrhage, localized infections, or hypersensitivity reaction.**
- Investigate reports of increased or sudden pain in wounds or body parts, **which could indicate ischemia or infection.**
- Be aware of invasive devices such as urinary and intravascular cathethers, endotrachial tube, implanted prosthetic devices **that potentiate risk for localized and systemic infections.**
- Assess vital signs and tissue and organ perfusion **for changes associated with shock states:**

Heart rate and rhythm—noting progressive changes in heart rate **(reflecting an attempt to increase cardiac output)** and development of dysrhythmias, **suggesting electrolyte imbalances, hypoxia.**

Respirations—noting rapid, shallow breathing, use of accessory muscles **(in an attempt to increase vital capacity and compensate for metabolic acidosis associated with poor tissue perfusion and anaerobic metabolism),** which can progress to respiratory failure.

Blood pressure—noting hypotension, postural hypotension, and narrowed pulse pressure. **May indicate hypovolemia and/or failure of cardiac pumping or compensatory mechanisms.**

Pulses and neck veins—noting rapid, weak, thready peripheral pulses; congested or flat neck veins. **Signs associated with changes in circulating volume, cardiac ouput, and**

Information that appears in brackets has been added by the authors to clarify and enhance the use of nursing diagnoses.

progressive changes in vascular tone and/or capillary permeability.**

Temperature—higher than 100.4°F (38°C) or lower than 96.8°F (36°C) may indicate infectious process. **Temperature changes in presence of elevated heart and respiratory rate, along with mildly elevated white blood cell (WBC) count in absence of documented infection, is suggestive of systemic inflammatory response syndrome (SIRS).**

State of consciousness and mentation—noting anxiety, restlessness, confusion, lethargy, or unresponsiveness. **Can occur because of changes in oxygenation, acid-base imbalances, and toxins associated with hypoperfusion.**

Skin color and moisture—noting overall flushing or pallor; bluish lips and fingernails, slow capillary refill; or cool, clammy skin.

Urine output—noting substantially decreased ouput. **One of the most sensitive indicators of change in circulating volume or poor perfusion.**

Urine characteristics—noting color and odor **suggestive of infection source.**

Bowel sounds—noting diminished or absent bowel sounds; other changes in gastrointestinal function such as vomiting; or change in color, amount, or frequency of stools, **reflecting hypoperfusion of gastrointestinal tract.**

- Measure invasive hemodynamic parameters when available—central venous pressure (CVP), mean arterial pressure (MAP), cardiac output (CO)—**to determine if intravascular fluid deficit or cardiac dysfunction exists.**
- Obtain specimens of wounds, drains, central lines, blood for culture and sensitivity.
- Review laboratory data such as complete blood count with WBCs and differential; platelet numbers and function; other coagulation factors; tests for cardiac, renal, and hepatic function; pulse oximetry/arterial blood gas; serum lactate, blood urine cultures **to identify potential sources of shock and degree of organ involvement.**
- Review diagnostic studies such as x-rays, electrocardiogram, echocardiogram, angiography with ejection fraction; computed tomography or magnetic resonance imaging scans, ultrasound **to determine presence of injuries or disorders that could cause or lead to shock conditions.**

Nursing Priority No. 2.

To prevent/correct potential causes of shock:

Information that appears in brackets has been added by the authors to clarify and enhance the use of nursing diagnoses.

- Collaborate in prompt treatment of underlying conditions such as trauma, heart failure, infections, and prepare for/assist with medical and surgical interventions **to maximize systemic circulation and tissue and organ perfusion.**
- Administer oxygen by appropriate route (e.g., nasal prongs, mask, ventilator) **to maximize oxygenation of tissues.**
- Administer fluids, electrolytes, colloids, blood or blood products, as indicated, **to rapidly restore or sustain circulating volume, electrolyte balance, and prevent shock state.**
- Administer medications as indicated (e.g., vasoactive drugs, cardiac glycosides, thrombolytics, anticoagulants, antimicrobials, analgesics).
- Provide client care with infection prevention interventions, such as diligent attention to hand hygiene, aseptic wound care or dressing changes, isolation precautions, early intervention in potential infectious condition.
- Provide nutrition by best means—oral, enteral, or parenteral feeding. Refer to nutritionist or dietitian **to provide foods rich in nutrients, vitamins, and minerals needed to promote healing and support immune system health.**
- Refer to NDs ineffective peripheral Tissue Perfusion; risk for decreased cardiac Tissue Perfusion; risk for ineffective cerebral Tissue Perfusion; risk for ineffective Gastrointestinal Perfusion; risk for ineffective Renal Perfusion, for additional interventions and rationales.

Nursing Priority No. 3.

Promote wellness (Teaching/Discharge Considerations):

- Instruct client/SO in ways to prevent and/or manage underlying conditions that cause shock, including heart disease, injuries, dehydration, infection.
- Identify reportable signs and symptoms, including unrelieved pain, unresolved bleeding, excessive fluid loss, persistent fever and chills, change in skin color accompanied by chest pain **for timely evaluation and intervention.**
- Emphasize need for recognition of substances that cause hypersensitivity or allergic reactions (e.g., insects, medicines, foods, latex) **to reduce risk of anaphylactic shock state.**
- Teach client purpose, dosage, schedule, precautions, and potential side effects of medications given to treat underlying conditions. **Enhances compliance with drug regimen, reducing individual risk.**
- Instruct in wound and skin care as indicated **to prevent infection and promote healing.**

Information that appears in brackets has been added by the authors to clarify and enhance the use of nursing diagnoses.

- Teach client/caregivers importance of good hand hygiene, clean environment, and avoiding crowds when ill, especially if client is immunocompromised.
- Reinforce importance of immunization against infections such as influenza and pneumonia, especially in client with chronic conditions.
- Encourage consumption of healthy diet, participation in regular exercise, and adequate rest **for healing and immune system support.**
- Recommend that client at risk for hypersensitivity reactions wear medical alert bracelet, maintain readily accessible emergency medication (e.g., Benadryl and/or EpiPen).

Documentation Focus

Assessment/Reassessment

- Individual risk factors such as blood loss, presence of infection
- Assessment findings, including respiratory rate, character of breath sounds; heart rate and rhythm; temperature; frequency, amount, and appearance of secretions; presence of cyanosis; and mentation level
- Results of laboratory tests and diagnostic studies

Planning

- Plan of care, specific interventions, and who is involved in the planning
- Teaching plan

Implementation/Evaluation

- Client's responses to treatment, teaching, and actions performed
- Attainment or progress toward desired outcome(s)
- Modifications to plan of care

Discharge Planning

- Long-term needs, identifying who is responsible for actions to be taken
- Community resources for equipment and supplies postdischarge
- Specific referrals made

Sample Nursing Outcomes & Interventions Classifications (NOC/NIC)

NOC—Circulation Status
NIC—Shock Management

Information that appears in brackets has been added by the authors to clarify and enhance the use of nursing diagnoses.

impaired SITTING

[Diagnostic Division: Safety]

Definition: Limitation of ability to independently and purposefully attain and/or maintain a rest position that is supported by the buttocks and thighs in which the torso is upright.

Related Factors

Alteration in cognitive functioning; psychological disorder
Impaired metabolic functioning; malnutrition; sarcopenia
Insufficient endurance
Neurological disorder
Orthopedic surgery
Pain
Prescribed posture; self-imposed relief posture

Defining Characteristics

Objective

Impaired ability to attain or maintain a balanced position of the torso; impaired ability to stress torso with body weight
Impaired ability to adjust position of one or both lower limbs on uneven surface
Impaired ability to flex or move both hips or knees
Insufficient muscle strength

Desired Outcomes/Evaluation Criteria—Client Will:

- Verbalize understanding of individual treatment regimen and safety measures.
- Attain and maintain sitting position that enables activities.
- Participate in activities of daily living (ADLs) and desired activities and prevent complications.

Actions/Interventions

Nursing Priority No. 1.

To identify causative/contributing factors:

- Determine diagnosis that contributes to sitting balance problems (e.g., MS, arthritis, Parkinson's disease, cardiopulmonary disorders, back pain conditions with client use of com-

Information that appears in brackets has been added by the authors to clarify and enhance the use of nursing diagnoses.

pensatory positions to reduce pain; traumatic brain injury, spinal cord injury with hemi-/paraplegia; lower-limb injuries or amputations; psychiatric conditions including severe depression, dementias). **These conditions can cause postural impairments, muscular weakness, and inadequate range of motion. Sensory deficits may also be involved (e.g., impaired proprioception, and/or visual processing, cognitive impairments).**

- Note factors affecting current situation (e.g., surgery, fractures, amputation, tubings [chest tube, indwelling catheter, IVs, pumps] and potential time involved [e.g., few hours in bed after surgery versus serious trauma requiring long-term bedrest or debilitating disease or pain limiting movement]). **Identifies potential impairments and determines type of interventions needed to provide for client's safety.**
- ∞ Note older client's general health status. **Several aging-related changes can lead to immobility (e.g., sarcopenia with diminished endurance and core strength; impaired vision; and loss of balance; and decreased ability to quickly and adequately correct movements affecting center of gravity). Thus, falls are a major risk and source of morbidity and mortality.**
- Assess nutritional and hydration status and client's report of energy level. **Deficiencies in nutrients and water, electrolytes, and minerals can negatively affect energy and activity tolerance. Note: Research supports that obese individuals show lower sitting functional reach abilities when compared to normal and overweight subject.**

Nursing Priority No. 2.

To assess functional ability:

- Determine functional status in relation to 0 to 4 scale, noting muscle strength and tone, joint mobility, cardiovascular status, balance, and endurance. **Identifies strengths and deficits (e.g., inability to sit upright, or reach forward, or transfer safely from bed to wheelchair) and may provide information regarding potential for recovery.**
- Determine degree of perceptual or cognitive impairment and ability to follow directions. **Impairments related to age, chronic or acute disease condition, trauma, surgery, or medications require alternative interventions or changes in plan of care.**
- Refer to physician, physical therapy specialists, for special testing, as indicated. **May include many different functional**

Information that appears in brackets has been added by the authors to clarify and enhance the use of nursing diagnoses.

tests to determine potential for improvement and direction for therapies.

Nursing Priority No. 3.

To promote optimal level of function and prevent complications:

- Assist with treatment of underlying condition(s) **to maximize potential for optimal function.**
- Encourage client's participation in self-care activities, and in physical or occupational therapies. **Improves body strength and function. enhances self-concept and sense of independence. Note: Sitting balance affects activities of daily living (ADLs) including feeding, dressing, bathing, transfers, and mobility.**
- Support trunk and extremities when in seated position, using pillows or rolls, braces, shoes, gel pads, and so forth, **to maintain upright position and optimal internal organ function, and to reduce risk of pressure ulcers.**
- Demonstrate and assist with use of assistive devices (e.g., side rails, overhead trapeze, roller pads, safety belt, hydraulic lifts, or chairs) **for position changes and safe transfers.**
- Avoid routinely doing for client those activities that client can do for self. **Caregivers can contribute to deficits by being overprotective or helping too much.**
- Provide for safety measures as indicated by individual situation, including environmental management and fall prevention. (Refer to ND risk for Falls.)
- Note changes in ability to do more or less self-care (e.g., hygiene, feeding, toileting, therapies) **to promote psychological and physical benefits of self-care and to adjust level of assistance as indicated.**
- Collaborate with physical medicine specialist and occupational or physical therapists in providing range-of-motion exercise (active or passive), isotonic muscle contractions (e.g., sitting reach, push, and pull exercises), assistive devices, and activities.
- Administer pain medications before activity as needed **to promote maximal effort and involvement in activity.**
- Collaborate with nutritionist in providing nutritious foods and needed feeding assistance, maximizing client's abilities in ingesting and swallowing (upright position) **to optimize available energy for activities.**
- Refer to NDs Activity Intolerance, impaired bed Mobility, impaired wheelchair Mobility, impaired Transfer Ability, im-

---

Information that appears in brackets has been added by the authors to clarify and enhance the use of nursing diagnoses.

paired Standing, and impaired Walking for additional interventions.

Nursing Priority No. 4.

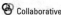

To promote wellness (Teaching/Discharge Considerations):

- Encourage client's/significant other's (SO's) involvement in decision making as much as possible. **Enhances commitment to plan, optimizing outcomes.**
- Demonstrate use of mobility devices (e.g., walkers, strollers, scooters, braces, prosthetics) and have client/care provider demonstrate knowledge about and safe use of device. Identify appropriate resources for obtaining and maintaining appliances or equipment. **Safe use of mobility aids promotes client's independence and enhances quality of life and safety for client and caregiver.**
- Discuss ways that client can exercise safely. **Options may be limited, but attending regular rehab sessions may provide best opportunity for improvement in function, including self-care, social independence, and recreation.**
- Involve client and SO(s) in care, assisting them to learn ways of managing problems of immobility and imbalanced sitting, especially when impairment is expected to be long term. Refer to support and community services as indicated **to provide care, supervision, companionship, respite services, nutritional and ADL assistance, adaptive devices or changes to living environment, financial assistance, and so forth.**

Documentation Focus

Assessment/Reassessment

- Individual findings, including level of function and ability to participate in specific or desired activities

Planning

- Plan of care and who is involved in the planning
- Teaching plan

Implementation/Evaluation

- Responses to interventions, teaching, and actions performed
- Attainment or progress toward desired outcome(s)
- Modifications to plan of care

Discharge Planning

- Discharge and long-term needs, noting who is responsible for each action to be taken

---

Information that appears in brackets has been added by the authors to clarify and enhance the use of nursing diagnoses.

- Specific referrals made
- Sources of and maintenance for assistive devices

Sample Nursing Outcomes & Interventions Classifications (NOC/NIC)

NOC—Body Mechanics Performance
NIC—Body Mechanics Promotion

impaired SKIN INTEGRITY and risk for impaired SKIN INTEGRITY

[Diagnostic Division: Safety]

Definition: impaired Skin Integrity: Altered epidermis and/or dermis.

Definition: risk for impaired Skin Integrity: Vulnerable to alteration in epidermis and/or dermis, which may compromise health.

Related and Risk Factors

External

Hyperthermia; hypothermia
Chemical injury agent (e.g., burn, capsaicin, methylene chloride, mustard agent); radiation therapy; pharmaceutical agent
Humidity; moisture; [excretions or secretions]
Mechanical factor (e.g., shearing forces, pressure, physical immobility [restraint]); [trauma: injury, surgery]
Extremes of age

Internal

Alteration in metabolism; inadequate nutrition [e.g., obesity, emaciation]; alteration in fluid volume [including presence of edema]
Pressure over bony prominence; alteration in skin turgor
Impaired circulation; alteration in sensation (resulting from spinal cord injury, diabetes mellitus, etc.); alteration in pigmentation
Immunodeficiency
Psychogenic factor [e.g., obsessive compulsive disorder] (risk)

NOTE: A risk diagnosis is not evidenced by signs and symptoms as the problem has not occurred; rather, nursing interventions are directed at prevention.

Information that appears in brackets has been added by the authors to clarify and enhance the use of nursing diagnoses.

NOTE: Risk should be determined by use of a standardized risk assessment tool (e.g., Braden, Norton [or similar] Scale).

Defining Characteristics (impaired Skin Integrity)

Subjective

[Reports of itching, pain, numbness of affected or surrounding area]

Objective

Alteration in skin integrity [i.e., disruption of skin surface (epidermis), destruction of skin layers (dermis)]
Foreign matter piercing skin
[Invasion of body structures]

Desired Outcomes/Evaluation Criteria—Client Will:

- Identify individual risk factors.
- Display timely healing of skin lesions, wounds, or pressure sores without complication.
- Participate in prevention measures and treatment program.

Actions/Interventions

Nursing Priority No. 1.

To assess causative/contributing **or risk** factors:

- Identify underlying condition or pathology involved. **Skin integrity problems can be the result of (1) disease processes that affect circulation and perfusion of tissues (e.g., arteriosclerosis, venous insufficiency, hypertension, obesity, diabetes, malignant neoplasms); (2) medications (e.g., anticoagulants, corticosteroids, immunosuppressives, antineoplastics) that adversely affect or impair healing; (3) burns or radiation (can break down internal tissues as well as skin); and (4) nutrition and hydration (e.g., malnutrition deprives the body of protein and calories required for cell growth and repair, and dehydration impairs transport of oxygen and nutrients). Disruption in skin integrity can be intentional (e.g., surgical incision) or unintentional (e.g., accidental trauma, drug effect, allergic reaction) and closed (e.g., contusion, abrasion, rash) or open (e.g., laceration, skin tears, penetrating wound, ulcerations).**

Information that appears in brackets has been added by the authors to clarify and enhance the use of nursing diagnoses.

- Determine client's age and developmental factors or ability to care for self. **Newborn/infant's skin is thin and provides ineffective thermal regulation, and nails are thin. Babies and children are prone to skin rashes associated with viral, bacterial, and fungal infections and allergic reactions. In adolescence, hormones stimulate hair growth and sebaceous gland activity. In adults, it takes longer to replenish epidermis cells, resulting in increased risk of skin cancers and infection. In older adults, there is decreased epidermal regeneration, fewer sweat glands, less subcutaneous fat, elastin, and collagen, causing skin to become thinner, drier, and less responsive to pain sensations.**
- Assess skin, noting moisture, color, and elasticity.
- Review with client/significant other (SO) history of past skin problems (e.g., allergic reactions, rashes, easy bruising or skin tears) **that may indicate particular vulnerability.**
- Evaluate client's skin care practices and hygiene issues. **Individual's skin may be oily, dry and scaly, or sensitive and is affected by bathing frequency (or lack of bathing), temperature of water, types of soap and other cleansing agents. Incontinence (urinary or bowel) and ineffective hygiene can result in serious skin impairment and discomfort.**
- Determine nutritional status and potential for delayed healing or tissue injury exacerbated by malnutrition (e.g., pressure points on emaciated and/or elderly client).
- Review medication and therapy regimen (e.g., steroid use, chemotherapy, radiation).
- Evaluate client with impaired cognition, developmental delay, need for or use of restraints, long-term immobility **to identify risk for injury and safety requirements.**
- Note presence of compromised mobility, sensation, vision, hearing, or speech **that may impact client's self-care as relates to skin care (e.g., diabetic with impaired vision probably cannot satisfactorily examine own feet).**
- Assess blood supply (e.g., capillary return time, color, and warmth) and sensation of skin surfaces and affected area on a regular basis **to provide comparative baseline and opportunity for timely intervention when problems are noted.**
- Calculate ankle-brachial index (ABI) **to evaluate actual/potential for impairment of circulation to lower extremities.** ***Note:*** **Result less than 0.9 indicates need for close monitoring or more aggressive intervention (e.g., tighter blood glucose and weight control in diabetic client).**
- Review laboratory results pertinent to causative factors (e.g., studies such as hemoglobin/hematocrit, blood glucose, infec-

Information that appears in brackets has been added by the authors to clarify and enhance the use of nursing diagnoses.

tious agents [viral, bacterial, fungal], albumin and protein). (*Note:* **Albumin less than 3.5 correlates to decreased wound healing and increased frequency of pressure ulcers.**)

- Obtain specimen from draining wounds when appropriate for culture and sensitivities or Gram stain **to determine appropriate therapy.**

Nursing Priority No. 2.

To assess extent of involvement/injury: (impaired Skin Integrity)

- Obtain a complete history of current skin condition(s) (especially in children where recurrent rash or lesions are common), including age at onset, date of first episode, duration, original site, characteristics of lesions, and any changes that have occurred. **Common skin manifestations of sensitivity or allergies are hives, eczema, and contact dermatitis. Contagious rashes include measles, rubella, roseola, chicken pox, and scarlet fever. Bacterial, viral, and fungal infections can also cause skin problems (e.g., impetigo, cellulitis, cold sores, shingles, athlete's foot, *candidiasis* diaper rashes).**
- Perform routine skin inspections describing observed changes. Note skin color, texture, and turgor. Assess areas of least pigmentation for color changes (e.g., sclera, conjunctiva, nailbeds, buccal mucosa, tongue, palms, and soles of feet).
- Palpate skin lesions for size, shape, consistency, texture, temperature, and hydration.
- Determine degree and depth of injury or damage to integumentary system (i.e., involves epidermis, dermis, and/or underlying tissues).
- Measure length, width, depth of ulcer or wound. Note extent of tunneling or undermining, if present.
- Inspect surrounding skin for erythema, induration, maceration.
- Photograph lesion(s)/burns, as appropriate, **to document status and provide visual baseline for future comparisons.**
- Note odors emitted from the skin, lesion, or wound.
- Classify ulcer using tool such as Wagner Ulcer Classification System. **Provides consistent terminology for documentation.**

Nursing Priority No. 3.

To determine impact of condition: (impaired Skin Integrity)

- Determine if wound is acute (e.g., injury from surgery or trauma) or chronic (e.g., venous or arterial insufficiency),

---

Information that appears in brackets has been added by the authors to clarify and enhance the use of nursing diagnoses.

which affects healing time and the client's emotional and physical responses.

- Determine client's level of discomfort (e.g., can vary widely from minor itching or aching, to deep pain with burns, or excoriation associated with drainage) **to clarify intervention needs and priorities.**
- Ascertain attitudes of individual/SO(s) about condition (e.g., cultural values, stigma). Note misconceptions. **Identifies areas to be addressed in teaching plan and potential referral needs.**
- Determine impact on life (e.g., work, leisure, increased caregiver requirements).
- Obtain psychological assessment of client's emotional status, as indicated, noting potential for sexual problems arising from presence of condition.
- Note presence of compromised vision, hearing, or speech. **Touch is a particularly important avenue of communication for this population, and when skin is compromised, communication may be affected.**

Nursing Priority No. 4.

To assist client with correcting/minimizing condition **or maintain skin integrity at optimal level**:

- Perform routine skin inspections, assessing color, temperature, surface changes, texture, and contours. Evaluate color changes in areas of least pigmentation (e.g., sclera, conjunctiva, nailbeds, buccal mucosa, tongue, palms, soles of feet). Report potential problem areas (e.g., reddened/blanched areas or rashes) promptly. **Systematic inspection can identify developing problems and promotes early intervention, thus reducing likelihood of progression to skin breakdown.**
- Handle client gently (particularly infant, young child, elderly). **Epidermis of infants and very young children is thin and lacks subcutaneous depth that will develop with age. Skin of the older client is also thin, less elastic, and prone to injury, such as bruising and skin tears.**
- Inspect skin surfaces and pressure points routinely, especially in mobility-impaired client.
- Observe for reddened or blanched areas or skin rashes, and institute treatment immediately. **Reduces likelihood of progression to skin breakdown.**
- Maintain and instruct in good skin hygiene (e.g., shower instead of bath, washing thoroughly, using mild nondetergent soap, drying gently and lubricating with lotion or emollient,

---

Information that appears in brackets has been added by the authors to clarify and enhance the use of nursing diagnoses.

as indicated) **to reduce risk of dermal trauma, improve circulation, and promote comfort.**

- Develop regularly timed repositioning schedule for client with mobility and sensation impairments, using turn sheet, as needed; encourage or assist with periodic weight shifts for client in chair **to reduce stress on pressure points and to promote circulation to tissues.**
- Provide adequate clothing or covers; protect from drafts **to prevent vasoconstriction.**
- Keep bedclothes dry and wrinkle free; use nonirritating linens.
- Use appropriate padding or pressure reducing devices (e.g., egg crate, gel pads, heel rolls or foam boots) or pressure-relieving devices (e.g., air or water mattress), when indicated, **to reduce pressure on sensitive areas and enhance circulation to compromised tissues.**
- Use paper tape or a nonadherent dressing on frail skin and remove it gently or use stockinette, gauze wrap, or any other similar type of wrap instead of tape to secure dressings and drains.
- Avoid use of latex products **when client has known or suspected sensitivity.** (Refer to ND Latex Allergy Response.)
- Apply hot and cold applications judiciously **to reduce risk of dermal injury in persons with circulatory and neurosensory impairments.**
- Encourage early ambulation or mobilization. **Promotes circulation and reduces risks associated with immobility.**
- Provide for safety measures during ambulation and other therapies that might cause dermal injury (e.g., use of properly fitting hose and footwear, safe use of heating pads or lamps, restraints).
- Provide preventive skin care to incontinent client. Change continence pads/briefs or diapers frequently; cleanse perineal skin daily; and after each incontinence episode, apply skin protectant ointment **to minimize contact with irritants (urine, stool, excessive moisture).**
- Avoid or limit use of plastic material (e.g., plastic-backed linen savers). Remove wet and wrinkled linens promptly. **Moisture potentiates skin breakdown.**
- Provide optimum nutrition, including vitamins (e.g., A, C, D, E) and protein, **to provide a positive nitrogen balance to aid in skin and tissue healing and to maintain general good health.**
- Keep surgical area clean and dry, carefully dress wounds, support incision (e.g., use of Steri-Strips, splinting when cough-

---

Information that appears in brackets has been added by the authors to clarify and enhance the use of nursing diagnoses.

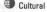

ing), prevent infection, manage incontinence, and stimulate circulation to surrounding areas **to assist body's natural process of repair.**

- Assist with débridement or enzymatic therapy, as indicated (e.g., burns, severe pressure sores), **to remove nonviable, contaminated, or infected tissue.**
- Use appropriate barrier dressings, wound coverings, drainage appliances, vacuum-assisted closure device (wound vac), and skin-protective agents for open, draining wounds and stomas **to protect the wound and/or surrounding tissues.**
- Apply appropriate dressing (e.g., adhesive or nonadhesive film, hydrofiber or gel, acrylics, hydropolymers) **for wound healing and to best meet needs of client and caregiver or care setting.**
- Maintain appropriate moisture environment for particular wound (e.g., expose lesion or ulcer to air and light **if excess moisture is impeding healing** or use occlusive dressings **to maintain a moist environment for autolytic débridement of wound**), as indicated.
- Periodically remeasure and photograph wound and observe for complications (e.g., infection, dehiscence) **to monitor progress of wound healing.**
- Monitor periodic laboratory studies relative to general well-being and status of specific problem.
- Consult with wound or stoma specialist, as indicated, **to assist with developing plan of care for problematic or potentially serious wounds.**

Nursing Priority No. 5.

To promote wellness (Teaching/Discharge Considerations):

- Review importance of health, intact skin, as well as measures to maintain proper skin functioning.
- Assist the client/SO(s) in understanding and following medical regimen and developing a program of preventive care and daily maintenance. **Enhances commitment to plan, optimizing outcomes.**
- Encourage continuation of regular exercise program (active or assistive) **to enhance circulation.**
- Recommend elevation of lower extremities when sitting **to enhance venous return and reduce edema formation.**
- Encourage abstinence from smoking, **which causes vasoconstriction.**
- Suggest use of ice, colloidal bath, lotions **to decrease irritable itching.**

Information that appears in brackets has been added by the authors to clarify and enhance the use of nursing diagnoses.

- Recommend keeping nails short or wearing gloves **to reduce risk of dermal injury when severe itching is present.**
- Discuss importance of avoiding exposure to sunlight in specific conditions (e.g., systemic lupus, tetracycline or psychotropic drug use, radiation therapy) as well as potential for development of skin cancer.
- Review measures to avoid spread of communicable disease or reinfection.
- Emphasize importance of proper fit of clothing and shoes, use of specially lined shock-absorbing socks or pressure-reducing insoles for shoes **in presence of reduced sensation/circulation.**
- Identify safety factors for use of equipment or appliances (e.g., heating pad, ostomy appliances, padding straps of braces).
- Encourage client to verbalize feelings and discuss how or if condition affects self-concept or self-esteem. (Refer to NDs disturbed Body Image; situational low Self-Esteem.)
- Assist client to work through stages of grief and feelings associated with individual condition.
- Lend psychological support and acceptance of client, using touch, facial expressions, and tone of voice.
- Assist client to learn stress-reduction and engage in alternate therapy techniques **to control feelings of helplessness and deal with situation.**
- Refer to dietitian or certified diabetes educator, as appropriate, **to enhance healing, reduce risk of recurrence of diabetic ulcers.**

Documentation Focus

Assessment/Reassessment

- Individual findings, including individual risk factors
- Characteristics of lesion(s) or condition, ulcer classification
- Causative and contributing factors
- Impact of condition on personal image and lifestyle

Planning

- Plan of care and who is involved in planning
- Teaching plan

Implementation/Evaluation

- Responses to interventions, teaching, and actions performed
- Attainment or progress toward desired outcome(s)
- Modifications to plan of care

Information that appears in brackets has been added by the authors to clarify and enhance the use of nursing diagnoses.

Discharge Planning

- Long-term needs and who is responsible for actions to be taken
- Specific referrals made

Sample Nursing Outcomes & Interventions Classifications (NOC/NIC)

NOC—Risk Control
NOC—Tissue Integrity: Skin & Mucous Membranes
NIC—Skin Surveillance

readiness for enhanced SLEEP

[Diagnostic Division: Activity/Rest]

Definition: A pattern of natural, periodic suspension of relative consciousness to provide rest and sustain a desired lifestyle, which can be strengthened.

Defining Characteristics

Subjective

Expresses desire to enhance sleep

Desired Outcomes/Evaluation Criteria—Client Will:

- Identify individually appropriate interventions to promote sleep.
- Adjust lifestyle to accommodate routines that promote sleep.
- Verbalize feeling rested after sleep.

Actions/Interventions

Nursing Priority No. 1.

To determine motivation for continued growth:

- Listen to client's reports of sleep quantity and quality. Determine client's/significant other's (SO's) perception of adequate sleep. **Reveals client's experience and expectations. Provides opportunity to address misconceptions or unrealistic expectations and plan for interventions.**
- Observe and/or obtain feedback from client/SO(s) regarding usual bedtime, desired rituals and routines, number of hours

Information that appears in brackets has been added by the authors to clarify and enhance the use of nursing diagnoses.

of sleep, time of arising, and environmental needs **to determine usual sleep pattern and provide comparative baseline for improvements.**

- Ascertain motivation and expectation for change.
- Note client report of potential for alteration of habitual sleep time (e.g., change of work pattern, rotating shifts) or change in normal bedtime (e.g., hospitalization). **Helps identify circumstances that are known to interrupt sleep patterns and that could disrupt the person's biological rhythms.**

Nursing Priority No. 2.

To assist client to enhance sleep/rest:

- Review client's usual bedtime rituals, routines, and sleep environment needs. **Provides information on client's management of the situation and identifies areas that might be modified when the need arises.**
- Implement effective age-appropriate bedtime rituals for infant/child (e.g., soothing bath, rocking, story reading, cuddling, favorite blanket or toy). **Rituals can enhance ability to fall asleep, reinforce that bed is a place to sleep, and promote sense of security for child.**
- Provide quiet environment and comfort measures (e.g., back rub, washing hands and face, cleaning and straightening sheets). **Promotes relaxation and readiness for sleep.**
- Arrange care **to provide for uninterrupted periods for rest.** Explain necessity of disturbances for monitoring vital signs and/or other care when client is hospitalized. Do as much care as possible without waking client during night. **Allows for longer periods of uninterrupted sleep, especially during night.**
- Discuss dietary matters, such as limiting intake of chocolate and caffeine or alcoholic beverages (especially prior to bedtime), **which are substances known to impair falling or staying asleep. *Note:* Use of alcohol at bedtime may help individual initially fall asleep, but ensuing sleep is then fragmented.**
- Limit fluid intake in evening if nocturia or bedwetting is a problem **to reduce need for nighttime elimination.**
- Recommend appropriate changes to usual bedtime rituals. Explore use of warm bath, comfortable room temperature, use of soothing music, favorite calming TV show. **Nonpharmaceutical aids can enhance falling asleep.**
- Assist client in use of necessary equipment, instructing as necessary. **Client may use oxygen or continuous positive**

Information that appears in brackets has been added by the authors to clarify and enhance the use of nursing diagnoses.

airway pressure (CPAP) system to improve sleep/rest if hypoxia or sleep apnea is diagnosed.

- Investigate use of sleep mask, darkening shades or curtains, earplugs, low-level background ("white") noise. **Aids in blocking out light and disturbing noise.**
- Recommend continuing same schedule for sleep throughout week—including days off. **Maintaining same sleep-wake pattern helps sustain biological rhythms.**

Nursing Priority No. 3.

To promote optimum sleep and wellness:

- Assure client that occasional sleeplessness should not threaten health. **Knowledge that occasional insomnia is universal and usually not harmful may promote relaxation and relief from worry.**
- Encourage regular exercise during the day **to aid in stress control and release of energy. *Note:* Exercise at bedtime may stimulate rather than relax client and actually interfere with sleep.**
- Address sleep management techniques that may be useful during stressful conditions or lifestyle changes (e.g., pregnancy, new baby, menopause, medical procedures, new job, moving, change in relationship, grief).
- Advise using barbiturates and/or other sleeping medications sparingly. **These medications, while useful for promoting sleep in the short term, can interfere with REM sleep.**

Documentation Focus

Assessment/Reassessment

- Assessment findings, including specifics of current and past sleep pattern, and effects on lifestyle and level of functioning
- Medications, interventions, and previous therapies used
- Motivation and expectations for change

Planning

- Plan of care and who is involved in planning
- Teaching plan

Implementation/Evaluation

- Client's response to interventions, teaching, and actions performed
- Attainment or progress toward desired outcome(s)
- Modifications to plan of care

Information that appears in brackets has been added by the authors to clarify and enhance the use of nursing diagnoses.

Discharge Planning

- Long-term needs and who is responsible for actions to be taken
- Specific referrals made

Sample Nursing Outcomes & Interventions Classifications (NOC/NIC)

NOC—Sleep
NIC—Sleep Enhancement

SLEEP DEPRIVATION

[Diagnostic Division: Activity/Rest]

Definition: Prolonged periods of time without sleep (sustained natural, periodic suspension of relative consciousness).

Related Factors

Overstimulating environment; environmental barrier; treatment regimen
Average daily physical activity is less than recommended for gender and age; sustained circadian asynchrony; age-related sleep stage shifts
Sustained inadequate sleep hygiene; nonrestorative sleep pattern (i.e., due to caregiver responsibilities, parenting practices, sleep partner)
Prolonged discomfort (e.g., physical, psychological); conditions with periodic limb movement (e.g., restless leg syndrome, nocturnal myoclonus); sleep-related enuresis/painful erections
Nightmares; sleepwalking; sleep terror
Sleep apnea
Sundowner's syndrome; dementia
Idiopathic central nervous system hypersomnolence; narcolepsy; familial sleep paralysis

Defining Characteristics

Subjective

Decrease in functional ability
Malaise; lethargy; fatigue

Information that appears in brackets has been added by the authors to clarify and enhance the use of nursing diagnoses.

Anxiety
Perceptual disorders; heightened sensitivity to pain

Objective

Restlessness; irritability
Alteration in concentration; decrease in reaction time
Drowsiness; listlessness; apathy
Fleeting nystagmus; hand tremors
Confusion; transient paranoia; agitation; combativeness; hallucinations

Desired Outcomes/Evaluation Criteria—Client Will:

- Identify individually appropriate interventions to promote sleep.
- Verbalize understanding of sleep disorder.
- Adjust lifestyle to accommodate chronobiological rhythms.
- Report improvement in sleep and rest pattern.

Family Will:

- Deal appropriately with parasomnias.

Actions/Interventions

Nursing Priority No. 1.

To assess causative/contributing factors:

- ∞ Note client's age and developmental stage. **The average adult requires 7 to 8 hr sleep; teenagers about 9 hr, infants about 16 hr. Pregnant women and new mothers, while needing more sleep, are usually sleep deprived; adolescents and young adults do not get enough sleep, have irregular sleep patterns, and are at risk for problem sleepiness; menopausal women often report interrupted sleep because of hot flashes or hormonal influences; elderly persons sleep fewer hours, report less restful sleep and need for more sleep.**
- Determine presence of physical or psychological stressors, including night-shift working hours or rotating shifts, pain, current or recent illness, death of a spouse.
- Note medical diagnoses that affect sleep (e.g., dementia, encephalitis, brain injury, narcolepsy, depression, asthma, nocturnal myoclonus [jerking of legs causing repeated awakening]).

Information that appears in brackets has been added by the authors to clarify and enhance the use of nursing diagnoses.

- Review results of studies that may be done to assess for sleep-induced respiratory disorders or obstructive sleep apnea.
- Evaluate for use of medications and/or other drugs affecting sleep. **Diet pills or other stimulants, sedatives, antidepressants, antihypertensives, diuretics, narcotics, agents with anticholinergic effects, and need for medications requiring nighttime dosing can inhibit getting to sleep or remaining asleep.**
- Note environmental factors affecting sleep (e.g., unfamiliar or uncomfortable sleep environment, excessive noise and light, uncomfortable temperature, roommate actions [e.g., snoring, watching TV late at night]).
- Determine presence of parasomnias: nightmares, terrors, or somnambulism (e.g., sitting, sleepwalking, or other complex behavior during sleep).
- Note reports of terror, brief periods of paralysis, sense of body being disconnected from the brain. **Occurrence of sleep paralysis (although not widely recognized in the United States, has been well documented elsewhere) may result in feelings of fear and reluctance to go to sleep.**

Nursing Priority No. 2.

To assess degree of impairment:

- Determine client's usual sleep pattern and expectations. **Provides comparative baseline.**
- Ascertain duration of current problem and effect on life and functional ability.
- Listen to client's/significant other's (SO's) subjective reports of client's sleep quality and family concerns.
- Observe for physical signs of fatigue (e.g., frequent yawning, restlessness, irritability; inability to tolerate stress; disorientation; problems with concentration or memory; behavioral, learning, or social problems).
- Determine interventions client has tried in the past. **Helps identify appropriate options.**
- Distinguish client's beneficial bedtime habits from detrimental ones (e.g., drinking late-evening milk versus drinking late-evening coffee).
- Instruct client and/or bed partner to keep a sleep-wake log **to document symptoms and identify factors that are interfering with sleep.**
- Do a chronological chart **to determine peak performance rhythms.**

Information that appears in brackets has been added by the authors to clarify and enhance the use of nursing diagnoses.

Nursing Priority No. 3.

To assist client to establish optimal sleep pattern:

- Review medications being taken and their effect on sleep, suggesting modifications in regimen, **if medications are found to be interfering.**
- Encourage client to restrict late afternoon or evening intake of caffeine, alcohol, and other stimulating substances and to avoid eating large evening or late-night meals. **These factors are known to disrupt sleep patterns.**
- Recommend light bedtime snack (protein, simple carbohydrate, and low fat) for individuals who feel hungry 15 to 30 min before retiring. **Sense of fullness and satiety promotes sleep and reduces likelihood of gastric upset.**
- Promote adequate physical exercise activity during day. **Enhances expenditure of energy and release of tension so that client feels ready for sleep or rest.**
- Suggest abstaining from daytime naps **because they may impair ability to sleep at night.**
- Investigate anxious feelings **to help determine basis and appropriate anxiety-reduction techniques.**
- Recommend quiet activities, such as reading or listening to soothing music in the evening, **to reduce stimulation so client can relax.**
- Instruct in relaxation techniques, music therapy, meditation, and so forth, **to decrease tension, prepare for rest or sleep.**
- Limit evening fluid intake if nocturia is present **to reduce need for nighttime elimination.**
- Discuss and implement effective age-appropriate bedtime rituals (e.g., going to bed at same time each night, drinking warm milk, soothing bath, rocking, story reading, cuddling, favorite blanket or toy) **to enhance client's ability to fall asleep; reinforce that bed is a place to sleep and promote sense of security for child.**
- Provide calm, quiet environment and manage controllable sleep-disrupting factors (e.g., noise, light, room temperature).
- Administer sedatives or other sleep medications, when indicated, noting client's response. Time pain medications for peak effect and duration **to reduce need for redosing during prime sleep hours.**
- Instruct client to get out of bed **if unable to fall asleep**, leave bedroom, engage in relaxing activities and not return to bed until feeling sleepy.
- Review with client the physician's recommendations for medications or surgery (alteration of facial structures, tracheot-

---

Information that appears in brackets has been added by the authors to clarify and enhance the use of nursing diagnoses.

omy) and/or apneic oxygenation therapy—continuous positive airway pressure, such as Respironics—**when sleep apnea is the cause for sleep disturbance, as documented by sleep disorder studies.**

Nursing Priority No. 4.

To promote wellness (Teaching/Discharge Considerations):

- Review possibility of next-day drowsiness or "rebound" insomnia and temporary memory loss **that may be associated with prescription sleep medications.**
- Discuss use and appropriateness of over-the-counter sleep medications or herbal supplements. Note possible side effects and drug interactions.
- Refer to support group or counselor **to help deal with psychological stressors (e.g., grief, sorrow, chronic pain).** (Refer to NDs Grieving; chronic Sorrow; chronic Pain.)
- Encourage family counseling **to help deal with concerns arising from parasomnias.**
- Identify appropriate safety precautions (e.g., securing doors, windows, and stairways; placing client bedroom on first floor), and attach audible alarm to bedroom door **to alert parents when child is sleepwalking.**
- Refer to sleep specialist or sleep laboratory **when problem is unresponsive to customary interventions.**

Documentation Focus

Assessment/Reassessment

- Assessment findings, including specifics of current and past sleep pattern and effects on lifestyle and level of functioning
- Medications, interventions tried, previous therapies
- Family history of similar problem

Planning

- Plan of care and who is involved in planning
- Teaching plan

Implementation/Evaluation

- Client's response to interventions, teaching, and actions performed
- Attainment or progress toward desired outcome(s)
- Modifications to plan of care

Information that appears in brackets has been added by the authors to clarify and enhance the use of nursing diagnoses.

Discharge Planning

- Long-term needs and who is responsible for actions to be taken
- Specific referrals made

Sample Nursing Outcomes & Interventions Classifications (NOC/NIC)

NOC—Sleep
NIC—Sleep Enhancement

disturbed SLEEP PATTERN

[Diagnostic Division: Activity/Rest]

Definition: Time-limited interruptions of sleep amount and quality due to external factors.

Related Factors

Environmental barrier (e.g., ambient temperature/humidity; daylight/darkness exposure, ambient noise, unfamiliar setting); immobilization

Nonrestorative sleep pattern (i.e., due to caregiving responsibilities, parenting practices, sleep partner)

Insufficient privacy; disruption caused by sleep partner

Defining Characteristics

Subjective

Difficulty initiating sleep; unintentional awakening
Feeling unrested; dissatisfaction with sleep

Objective

Alteration in sleep pattern
Difficulty in daily functioning

Desired Outcomes/Evaluation Criteria—Client Will:

- Identify individually appropriate interventions to promote sleep.
- Report improved sleep.
- Report increased sense of well-being and feeling rested.

Information that appears in brackets has been added by the authors to clarify and enhance the use of nursing diagnoses.

Actions/Interventions

Nursing Priority No. 1.

To assess causative/contributing factors:

- Identify presence of factors known to interfere with sleep, including current illness, hospitalization; new baby or sick family member in home. **Sleep problems can arise from internal and external factors and may require assessment over time to differentiate specific cause(s).**
- Ascertain presence of short-term alteration in sleep patterns, such as can occur with travel (jet lag), sharing bed with new sleep partner, fighting with family member, crisis at work, loss of job, death in family. **Helps identify circumstances that are known to interrupt sleep acutely, but not necessarily long term.**
- Note environmental factors, such as unfamiliar or uncomfortable room; excessive noise and light, uncomfortable temperature; frequent medical and monitoring interventions; and roommate actions—snoring, watching television late at night, wanting to talk. **These factors can reduce client's ability to rest and sleep at a time when more rest is needed. *Note:* Clients in critical care units are known to experience lack of sleep or frequent disruptions, often compounding their illness.**

Nursing Priority No. 2.

To evaluate sleep and degree of dysfunction:

- Assess client's usual sleep patterns and compare with current sleep disturbance, relying on client/significant other (SO) report of problem **to ascertain intensity and duration of problems.**
- Listen to reports of sleep quality (e.g., "short," "interrupted") and response from lack of good sleep (feeling foggy, sleepy, and woozy; fighting sleep; fatigue). **Helps clarify client's perception of sleep quantity and quality and response to inadequate sleep.**
- Determine client's sleep expectations. **Individual may have faulty beliefs or attitudes about sleep and/or unrealistic sleep expectations (e.g., "I must get 8 hr of sleep every night or I can't accomplish anything").**
- Observe for physical signs of fatigue (e.g., restlessness, hand tremors, thick speech, drooping eyes, inattention, lack of interest in activities).
- Incorporate screening information into in-depth sleep diary or testing if needed **to evaluate the type and etiology of sleep disturbance and to identify useful treatment options.**

Information that appears in brackets has been added by the authors to clarify and enhance the use of nursing diagnoses.

 Acute Care  Collaborative Community/Home Care Cultural

Nursing Priority No. 3.

To assist client to establish optimal sleep/rest pattern:

- Manage environment for hospitalized client:

  Adjust ambient lighting **to maintain daytime light and nighttime dark.**

  Request visitors to leave, close room door, post "Quiet, patient sleeping" sign, as indicated, **to provide privacy.**

  Encourage usual bedtime routines such as washing face and hands and brushing teeth.

  Provide bedtime care such as straightening bed sheets, changing damp linens or gown, back massage **to promote physical comfort.**

  Turn on soft music, calm TV program, or quiet environment, as client prefers **to enhance relaxation.**

  Minimize sleep-disrupting factors (e.g., shut room door, adjust room temperature as needed, reduce talking and other disturbing noises such as phones, beepers, alarms) **to promote readiness for sleep and improve sleep duration and quality.**

  Perform monitoring and care activities without waking client whenever possible. **Allows for longer periods of uninterrupted sleep, especially during night.**

  Avoid or limit use of physical restraints in accordance with client's needs and facility policy.

- Refer to physician or sleep specialist as indicated **for specific interventions and/or therapies, including medications, biofeedback.**
- Refer to NDs Insomnia and Sleep Deprivation for related interventions and rationale.

Nursing Priority No. 4.

To promote wellness (Teaching/Discharge Considerations):

- Assure client that occasional sleeplessness should not threaten health and that resolving time-limited situation can restore healthful sleep. **Knowledge that occasional insomnia is universal and usually not harmful may promote relaxation and relief from worry, which can perpetuate the problem.**
- Problem-solve immediate needs. **Short-term solutions (e.g., sleeping in different rooms if partner's illness is keeping client awake, acquiring a fan if sleeping quarters too warm or lacks ventilation) may be needed until client adjusts to situation or crisis is resolved, with resulting return to more usual sleep pattern.**
- Encourage appropriate indoor light settings during day and night, especially exposure to bright light or sunlight in the morning, avoidance of daytime napping as appropriate for age and-

---

Information that appears in brackets has been added by the authors to clarify and enhance the use of nursing diagnoses.

situation, being active during day and more passive in evening. **Helps in promotion of normal sleep-wake patterns.**

- Investigate use of aids to block out light and sound, such as sleep mask, room-darkening shades, earplugs, "white noise."
- Discuss use and appropriateness of over-the-counter sleep medications or herbal supplements **to provide assistance in falling and staying asleep.**

Documentation Focus

Assessment/Reassessment

- Assessment findings, including specifics of current and past sleep pattern, and effects on lifestyle and level of functioning
- Specific interventions, medications, or previously tried therapies

Planning

- Plan of care and who is involved in planning
- Teaching plan

Implementation/Evaluation

- Response to interventions, teaching, and actions performed
- Attainment or progress toward desired outcome(s)
- Modifications to plan of care

Discharge Planning

- Long-term needs and who is responsible for actions to be taken
- Available resources, specific referrals made

Sample Nursing Outcomes & Interventions Classifications (NOC/NIC)

NOC—Sleep
NIC—Sleep Enhancement

impaired SOCIAL INTERACTION

[Diagnostic Division: Social Interaction]

Definition: Insufficient or excessive quantity or ineffective quality of social exchange.

Related Factors

Insufficient knowledge about ways to enhance mutuality
Insufficient skills to enhance mutuality
Communication barrier

Information that appears in brackets has been added by the authors to clarify and enhance the use of nursing diagnoses.

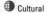

Disturbance of self-concept
Absence of significant other (SO)
Impaired mobility
Therapeutic isolation
Sociocultural dissonance
Environmental barrier
Disturbance in thought processes

Defining Characteristics

Subjective

Discomfort in social situations
Dissatisfaction with social engagement (e.g., belonging, caring, interest, shared history)
Family reports change in interaction (e.g., style, pattern)

Objective

Impaired social functioning
Dysfunctional interaction with others

Desired Outcomes/Evaluation Criteria—Client Will:

- Verbalize awareness of factors causing or promoting impaired social interactions.
- Identify feelings that lead to poor social interactions.
- Express desire for, and be involved in, achieving positive changes in social behaviors and interpersonal relationships.
- Give self positive reinforcement for changes that are achieved.
- Develop effective social support system; use available resources appropriately.

Actions/Interventions

Nursing Priority No. 1.

To assess causative/contributing factors:

- Review social history with client/SO(s) going back far enough in time to note when changes in social behavior or patterns of relating occurred or began: e.g., loss or long-term illness of loved one; failed relationships; loss of occupation, financial, or social or political (power) position; change in status in family hierarchy (job loss, aging, illness); poor coping or adjustment to developmental stage of life, as with marriage, birth or adoption of child, or children leaving home.

Information that appears in brackets has been added by the authors to clarify and enhance the use of nursing diagnoses.

- Ascertain ethnic, cultural, or religious implications for the client **because these impact choice of behaviors and may even script interactions with others.**
- Review medical history, noting stressors of physical or long-term illness (e.g., stroke, cancer, multiple sclerosis, head injury, Alzheimer's disease); mental illness (e.g., schizophrenia); medications or drugs, debilitating accidents, learning disabilities (e.g., sensory integration difficulties, autism spectrum disorder); and emotional disabilities.
- Determine family patterns of relating and social behaviors. Explore possible family scripting of behavioral expectations in the children and how the client was affected. **May result in conforming or rebellious behaviors. Parents are important in teaching their children social skills (e.g., sharing, taking turns, and allowing others to talk without interrupting).**
- Observe client while relating to family/SO(s) **to note prevalent interaction patterns.**
- Encourage client to verbalize feeling of discomfort about social situations. Identify causative factors, if any, recurring precipitating patterns, and barriers to using support systems.

Nursing Priority No. 2.

To assess degree of impairment:

- Encourage client to verbalize perceptions of problem and causes. Active-listen, noting indications of hopelessness, powerlessness, fear, anxiety, grief, anger, feeling unloved or unlovable, problems with sexual identity, hate (directed or not).
- Observe and describe social and interpersonal behaviors in objective terms, noting speech patterns, body language—in the therapeutic setting and in normal areas of daily functioning (if possible)—such as in family, job, social, or entertainment settings. **Helps identify the kinds and extent of problems client is exhibiting.**
- Determine client's use of coping skills and defense mechanisms. **Affects ability to be involved in social situations.**
- Evaluate possibility of client being the victim of or using destructive behaviors against self or others. (Refer to NDs risk for other-/self-directed Violence.) **Problems with communication lead to frustration and anger, leaving the individual with few coping skills, and may result in destructive behaviors.**

Information that appears in brackets has been added by the authors to clarify and enhance the use of nursing diagnoses.

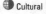

- Interview family, SO(s), friends, spiritual leaders, coworkers, as appropriate, **to obtain observations of client's behavioral changes and effects on others.**
- Note effects of changes on socioeconomic level, ethnic and religious practices.

Nursing Priority No. 3.

To assist client/SO(s) to recognize/make positive changes in impaired social and interpersonal interactions:

- Establish therapeutic relationship using positive regard for the client, Active-listening, and providing safe environment for self-disclosure.
- Have client list behaviors that cause discomfort. **Once recognized, client can choose to change as he or she learns to listen and communicate in socially acceptable ways.**
- Have family/SO(s) list client's behaviors that are causing discomfort for them. **Family needs to understand that the client is unable to use social skills that have not been learned.**
- Review/list negative behaviors observed previously by caregivers, coworkers, and so forth.
- Compare lists and validate reality of perceptions. Help client prioritize those behaviors needing change.
- Explore with client and role-play means of making agreed-on changes in social interactions and behaviors.
- Role-play random social situations in therapeutically controlled environment with "safe" therapy group. Have group note behaviors, both positive and negative, and discuss these and any changes needed.
- Role-play changes and discuss impact. Include family/SO(s), as indicated. **Enhances comfort with new behaviors.**
- Provide positive reinforcement for improvement in social behaviors and interactions. **Encourages continuation of desired behaviors and efforts for change.**
- Participate in multidisciplinary client-centered conferences to evaluate progress. Involve everyone associated with client's care, family members, SO(s), and therapy group.
- Work with client to alleviate underlying negative self-concepts **because they often impede positive social interactions. Attempts at trying to connect with another can become devastating to self-esteem and emotional well-being.**
- Involve neurologically impaired client in individual and/or group interactions or special classes, as situation allows.
- Refer for family therapy, as indicated, **because social behaviors and interpersonal relationships involve more than the affected individual.**

Information that appears in brackets has been added by the authors to clarify and enhance the use of nursing diagnoses.

Nursing Priority No. 4.

To promote wellness (Teaching/Discharge Considerations):

- Encourage client to keep a daily journal in which social interactions of each day can be reviewed and the comfort/discomfort experienced noted with possible causes or precipitating factors. **Helps client identify responsibility for own behavior(s) and learn new skills that can be used to enhance social interactions.**
- Assist the client to develop positive social skills through practice of skills in real social situations accompanied by a support person. Provide positive feedback during interactions with client.
- Seek community programs for client involvement that promote positive behaviors the client is striving to achieve.
- Encourage classes, reading materials, community support groups, and lectures for self-help in alleviating negative self-concepts that lead to impaired social interactions.
- Involve client in a music-based program, if available (e.g., The Listening Program). **There is a direct correlation between the musical portion of the brain and the language area, and the use of these programs may result in better communication skills.**
- Encourage ongoing family or individual therapy as long as it is promoting growth and positive change. (However, be alert to possibility of therapy being used as a crutch.)
- Provide for occasional follow-up, as appropriate, **for reinforcement of positive behaviors after professional relationship has ended.**
- Refer to psychiatric clinical nurse specialist for additional assistance when indicated.

Documentation Focus

Assessment/Reassessment

- Individual findings, including factors affecting interactions, nature of social exchanges, specifics of individual behaviors, type of learning disability present
- Cultural or religious beliefs and expectations
- Perceptions and response of others

Planning

- Plan of care and who is involved in the planning
- Teaching plan

Information that appears in brackets has been added by the authors to clarify and enhance the use of nursing diagnoses.

Implementation/Evaluation
- Responses to interventions, teaching, and actions performed
- Attainment or progress toward desired outcome(s)
- Modifications to plan of care

Discharge Planning
- Long-term needs and who is responsible for actions to be taken
- Community resources, specific referrals made

Sample Nursing Outcomes & Interventions Classifications (NOC/NIC)

NOC—Social Interaction Skills
NIC—Socialization Enhancement

SOCIAL ISOLATION

[Diagnostic Division: Social Interaction]

Definition: Aloneness experienced by the individual and perceived as imposed by others and as a negative or threatening state.

Related Factors

Factors impacting satisfying personal relationships (e.g., developmental delay); developmentally inappropriate interests
Alteration in physical appearance, mental status
Alteration in wellness
Social behavior incongruent with norms; values incongruent with cultural norms
Insufficient personal resources (e.g., poor achievement, poor insight, affect unavailable and poorly controlled)
Inability to engage in satisfying personal relationships

Defining Characteristics

Subjective

Aloneness imposed by others; feeling different from others
Inability to meet expectations of others; purposelessness
Developmentally inappropriate interests; values incongruent with cultural norms
Insecurity in public; desires to be alone

Information that appears in brackets has been added by the authors to clarify and enhance the use of nursing diagnoses.

Objective

Absence of support system; history of rejection
Sad or flat affect; withdrawn; poor eye contact
Developmental delay
Disabling condition; illness
Preoccupation with own thoughts; repetitive or meaningless actions; hostility
Cultural incongruence; member of a subculture

Desired Outcomes/Evaluation Criteria—Client Will:

- Identify causes and actions to correct isolation.
- Verbalize willingness to be involved with others.
- Participate in activities or programs at level of ability and desire.
- Express increased sense of self-worth.

Actions/Interventions

Nursing Priority No. 1.

To assess causative/contributing factors:

- Determine presence of factors as listed in Related Factors and other concerns (e.g., elderly, female, adolescent, ethnic or racial minority, economically/educationally disadvantaged).
- Note onset of physical or mental illness and whether recovery is anticipated or condition is chronic or progressive. **May affect client's desire to isolate self.**
- Do physical exam, paying particular attention to any illnesses that are identified. **Individuals who are isolated appear to be susceptible to health problems, especially coronary heart disease, although little is understood about why this is true.**
- Identify blocks to social contacts (e.g., physical immobility, sensory deficits, housebound, incontinence). **Client may be unable to go out, embarrassed to be with others, and reluctant to solve these problems.**
- Ascertain implications of cultural values or religious beliefs for the client **because these impact choice of behaviors and may even script interactions with others.**
- Assess factors in client's life that may contribute to sense of helplessness (e.g., loss of spouse/parent). **Client may withdraw and fail to seek out friends who may have previously been in his or her life.**

Information that appears in brackets has been added by the authors to clarify and enhance the use of nursing diagnoses.

- Ascertain client's perception regarding sense of isolation. Differentiate isolation from solitude and loneliness, **which may be acceptable or by choice.**
- Assess client's feelings about self, sense of ability to control situation, sense of hope.
- Note use and effectiveness of coping skills.
- Identify support systems available to the client, including presence of and relationship with extended family.
- Determine drug use (legal and illicit). **Possibility of a relationship between unhealthy behaviors and social isolation or the influence others have on the individual.**
- Identify behavior response of isolation (e.g., excessive sleeping or daydreaming, substance use), **which also may potentiate isolation.**
- Review history and elicit information about traumatic events that may have occurred. (Refer to ND Post-Trauma Syndrome.)

Nursing Priority No. 2.

To alleviate conditions contributing to client's sense of isolation:

- Establish therapeutic nurse-client relationship. **Promotes trust, allowing client to feel free to discuss sensitive matters.**
- Spend time visiting with client and identify other resources available (e.g., volunteer, social worker, chaplain).
- Develop plan of action with client: Look at available resources, support risk-taking behaviors to engage in social interactions, management of personal resources, appropriate medical care or self-care, and so forth. **Learning to manage issues of daily living can increase self-confidence and promote comfort in social settings.**
- Introduce client to those with similar or shared interests and other supportive people. **Provides role models, encourages problem-solving, and possibly making friends that will relieve client's sense of isolation.**
- Provide positive reinforcement when client makes move(s) toward others. **Encourages continuation of efforts.**
- Provide for placement in sheltered community when necessary.
- Assist client to problem-solve solutions to short-term or imposed isolation (e.g., communicable disease measures, including compromised host).
- Encourage open visitation when possible and/or telephone contacts/social media **to maintain involvement with others.**

Information that appears in brackets has been added by the authors to clarify and enhance the use of nursing diagnoses.

- Provide environmental stimuli (e.g., open curtains, pictures, TV, and radio).
- Promote participation in recreational or special interest activities in setting that client views as safe.
- Identify foreign language resources, such as interpreter, newspaper, radio programming, as appropriate.

Nursing Priority No. 3.

To promote wellness (Teaching/Discharge Considerations):

- Assist client to learn or enhance skills (e.g., problem-solving, communication, social skills, self-esteem, activities of daily living).
- Encourage or assist client to enroll in classes, as desired (e.g., assertiveness, vocational, sex education).
- Involve children and adolescents in age-appropriate programs and activities **to promote socialization skills and peer contact.**
- Help client differentiate between isolation and loneliness or aloneness and about ways to prevent slipping into an undesired state.
- Involve client in programs directed at correction and prevention of identified causes of problem (e.g., senior citizen services, daily telephone contact, house sharing, pets, day-care centers, religious or spiritual resources). **Social isolation seems to be growing and may be related to time stressors, watching TV, prolonged Internet use, or fatigue, resulting in individuals finding they do not have a close friend they can share intimate thoughts with.**
- Refer to therapists, as appropriate, **to facilitate grief work, relationship building, and so forth.**

Documentation Focus

Assessment/Reassessment

- Individual findings, including precipitating factors, effect on lifestyle and relationships, and functioning
- Client's perception of situation
- Cultural or religious factors
- Availability and use of resources and support systems

Planning

- Plan of care and who is involved in planning
- Teaching plan

Information that appears in brackets has been added by the authors to clarify and enhance the use of nursing diagnoses.

Implementation/Evaluation

- Responses to interventions, teaching, and actions performed
- Attainment or progress toward desired outcome(s)
- Modifications to plan of care

Discharge Planning

- Long-term needs, referrals made, and who is responsible for actions to be taken
- Available resources, specific referrals made

Sample Nursing Outcomes & Interventions Classifications (NOC/NIC)

NOC—Social Involvement
NIC—Social Enhancement

chronic SORROW

[Diagnostic Division: Ego Integrity]

Definition: Cyclical, recurring, and potentially progressive pattern of pervasive sadness experienced (by a parent, caregiver, individual with chronic illness or disability) in response to continual loss, throughout the trajectory of an illness or disability.

Related Factors

Death of significant other (SO)
Chronic illness or disability (e.g., physical, mental); crises in illness or disability management
Crises related to developmental stage; missed opportunities or milestones
Length of time as a caregiver

Defining Characteristics

Subjective

Overwhelming negative feelings
Sadness (e.g., periodic, recurrent)
Feelings that interfere with well-being (e.g., personal, social)

Desired Outcomes/Evaluation Criteria—Client Will:

- Acknowledge presence and impact of sorrow.
- Demonstrate progress in dealing with grief.

Information that appears in brackets has been added by the authors to clarify and enhance the use of nursing diagnoses.

- Participate in work and/or self-care activities of daily living as able.
- Verbalize a sense of progress toward resolution of sorrow and hope for the future.

Actions/Interventions

Nursing Priority No. 1.

To assess causative/contributing factors:

- Determine current and recent events or conditions contributing to client's state of mind, as listed in Related Factors (e.g., death of loved one, chronic physical or mental illness, disability).
- Look for cues of sadness (e.g., sighing, faraway look, unkempt appearance, inattention to conversation, refusing food). **Chronic sorrow has a cyclical effect, ranging from times of deepening sorrow to times of feeling somewhat better.**
- Determine level of functioning, ability to care for self.
- Note avoidance behaviors (e.g., anger, withdrawal, denial).
- Identify cultural factors or religious conflicts. **Family may experience conflict between the feelings of sorrow and anger because of change in expectation that has occurred (e.g., newborn with a disability when the expectation was for a perfect child, while religious belief is that all children are gifts from God and that the individual/parent is never "given" more than he or she can handle).**
- Ascertain response of family/SO(s) to client's situation. Assess needs of family/SO. **Family may have difficulty dealing with child/ill person because of their own feelings of sorrow and loss, and will do better when their needs are met.**
- Refer to complicated Grieving; caregiver Role Strain; ineffective Coping, as appropriate.

Nursing Priority No. 2.

To assist client to move through sorrow:

- Encourage verbalization about situation **(helpful in beginning resolution and acceptance).** Active-listen feelings and be available for support/assistance.
- Encourage expression of anger, fear, and anxiety. (Refer to appropriate NDs.)
- Acknowledge reality of feelings of guilt/blame, including hostility toward spiritual power. (Refer to ND Spiritual Distress.) **When feelings are validated, client is free to take steps toward acceptance.**

Information that appears in brackets has been added by the authors to clarify and enhance the use of nursing diagnoses.

- Provide comfort and availability as well as caring for physical needs.
- Discuss ways individual has dealt with previous losses. Reinforce use of previously effective coping skills.
- Instruct in, and encourage use of, visualization and relaxation skills.
- Discuss use of medication when depression is interfering with ability to manage life. **Client may benefit from the short-term use of an antidepressant medication to help with dealing with situation.**
- Assist SO to cope with client response. **Family/SO may not be dysfunctional but may be intolerant.**
- Include family/SO in setting realistic goals for meeting individual needs.

Nursing Priority No. 3.

To promote wellness (Teaching/Discharge Considerations):

- Discuss healthy ways of dealing with difficult situations.
- Have client identify familial, religious, and cultural factors that have meaning for him or her. **May help bring loss or distressing situation into perspective and facilitate resolution of grief and sorrow.**
- Encourage involvement in usual activities, exercise, and socialization within limits of physical and psychological state. **Maintaining usual activities may keep individuals from deepening sorrow and depression.**
- Introduce concept of mindfulness (living in the moment). **Promotes feelings of capability and belief that this moment can be dealt with.**
- Refer to other resources (e.g., pastoral care, counseling, psychotherapy, respite-care providers, support groups). **Provides additional help when needed to resolve situation, continue grief work.**

Documentation Focus

Assessment/Reassessment

- Physical and emotional response to conflict, expressions of sadness
- Cultural issues or religious conflicts
- Reactions of family/SO

Planning

- Plan of care and who is involved in planning
- Teaching plan

Information that appears in brackets has been added by the authors to clarify and enhance the use of nursing diagnoses.

Implementation/Evaluation

- Response to interventions, teaching, and actions performed
- Attainment or progress toward desired outcome(s)
- Modifications to plan of care

Discharge Planning

- Long-term needs and who is responsible for actions to be taken
- Available resources, specific referrals made

Sample Nursing Outcomes & Interventions Classifications (NOC/NIC)

NOC—Depression Level
NIC—Hope Inspiration

SPIRITUAL DISTRESS and risk for SPIRITUAL DISTRESS

[Diagnostic Division: Ego Integrity]

Definition: Spiritual Distress: A state of suffering related to the impaired ability to experience and integrate meaning in life through connections with self, others, the world, or a superior being.

Definition: risk for Spiritual Distress: Vulnerable to an impaired ability to experience and integrate meaning and purpose in life through connectedness within self, others, literature, nature, and/or a power greater than oneself, which may compromise health.

Related Factors

Aging; birth of a child
Actively dying; imminent death; death of a significant other (SO); exposure to death
Illness; loss of a body part or function
Increasing dependence on another
Perception of having unfinished business; receiving bad news; life transition; unexpected life event
Loneliness; social alienation; self-alienation; sociocultural deprivation
Treatment regimen
[Challenged belief or value system (e.g., moral or ethical implications of therapy)]

Information that appears in brackets has been added by the authors to clarify and enhance the use of nursing diagnoses.

Risk Factors

Physical
Physical or chronic illness; substance abuse

Psychosocial
Anxiety; depression; low self-esteem
Barrier to experiencing love; ineffective relationships
Change in religious ritual or practice; inability to forgive
Cultural or racial conflict
Loss; separation from support system; stressors

Developmental
Life transition

Environmental
Environmental change; natural disaster

NOTE: A risk diagnosis is not evidenced by signs and symptoms, as the problem has not occurred; rather, nursing interventions are directed at prevention.

Defining Characteristics (Spiritual Distress

Subjective
Anxiety, fear
Fatigue; insomnia
Questioning identity; questioning meaning of suffering or life

Connections to Self
Anger; guilt; insufficient courage
Decrease in serenity;
Feeling of being unloved; inadequate acceptance

Connections With Others
Alienation
Refuses to interact with significant others or spiritual leader
Separation from support system

Connections With Art, Music, Literature, Nature
Disinterest in nature or reading spiritual literature

Connections With Power Greater Than Self
Anger toward power greater than self
Feeling abandoned; hopelessness; perceived suffering

Information that appears in brackets has been added by the authors to clarify and enhance the use of nursing diagnoses.

Inability to pray or participate in religious activities, or to experience the transcendent

Objective

Crying

Connections to Self

Ineffective coping strategies; perceived insufficient meaning in life

Connections With Art, Music, Literature, Nature

Decrease in expression of previous pattern of creativity

Connections With Power Greater Than Self

Inability for introspection; sudden changes in spiritual practice; request for a spiritual leader

Desired Outcomes/Evaluation Criteria—Client Will:

- Identify meaning and purpose in own life that reinforces hope, peace, and contentment.
- Verbalize increased sense of connectedness and hope for future.
- Demonstrate ability to help self and participate in care.
- Participate in activities with others, actively seek relationships.
- Discuss beliefs and values about spiritual issues.
- Verbalize acceptance of self as being worthy, not deserving of illness or situation, and so forth.

Actions/Interventions

Nursing Priority No. 1.

To assess causative/contributing **or risk** factors:

- Ascertain current situation (e.g., natural disaster, death of a spouse, personal injustice).
- Determine client's religious or spiritual orientation, current involvement, presence of conflicts. **Individual spiritual practices or restrictions may affect client care or create conflict between spiritual beliefs and treatment.**
- Note client's reason for living and whether it is directly related to situation (e.g., home and business washed away in a flood, parent whose only child is terminally ill). **Questioning meaning or purpose of life may indicate inner conflict about religious beliefs.**

Information that appears in brackets has been added by the authors to clarify and enhance the use of nursing diagnoses.

- Listen to client's/SO's reports or expressions of concern, anger, alienation from God, belief that illness or situation is a punishment for wrongdoing, and so forth. **Suggests need for spiritual advisor to address client's belief system, if desired.**
- Assess sense of self-concept, worth, ability to enter into loving relationships. **Lack of connectedness with self and others impairs client's ability to trust others or feel worthy of trust from others. Feelings of abandonment may accompany sense of "not being good enough" in face of illness, disaster.**
- Determine sense of futility, feelings of hopelessness and helplessness, lack of motivation to help self. **Indicators that client may see no, or only limited, options, alternatives, or personal choices available and lacks energy to deal with situation.**
- Note expressions of inability to find meaning in life, reason for living. Evaluate suicidal ideation. **Crisis of the spirit or loss of will to live places client at increased risk for inattention to personal well-being or harm to self.**
- Note recent changes in behavior (e.g., withdrawal from others and creative or religious activities, dependence on alcohol or medications). **Helpful in determining severity and duration of situation and possible need for additional referrals, such as substance withdrawal.**
- Observe behavior indicative of poor relationships with others (e.g., manipulative, nontrusting, demanding). **Manipulation is used for management of client's sense of powerlessness because of distrust of others.**
- Ascertain substance use or abuse. **Affects ability to deal with problems in a positive manner.**
- Determine support systems available to client/SO(s) and how they are used. **Provides insight to client's willingness to pursue outside resources.**
- Be aware of influence of care provider's belief system. **(It is still possible to be helpful to client while remaining neutral and refraining from promoting own beliefs.)**

Nursing Priority No. 2.

To assist client/SO(s) to deal with feelings/situation:

- Develop therapeutic nurse-client relationship. Ascertain client's views as to how care provider(s) can be most helpful. Convey acceptance of client's spiritual beliefs and concerns. **Promotes trust and comfort, encouraging client to be open about sensitive matters.**

Information that appears in brackets has been added by the authors to clarify and enhance the use of nursing diagnoses.

- Provide calm, peaceful setting when possible. **Promotes relaxation and enhances opportunity for reflection on situation, discussions with others, meditation.**
- Have client identify and prioritize current or immediate needs. **Helps client focus on what needs to be done and identify manageable steps to take.**
- Encourage client/family to ask questions. **Demonstrates support for individual's willingness to learn.**
- Review coping skills used and their effectiveness in current situation. **Identifies strengths to incorporate into plan and techniques needing revision.**
- Ascertain past coping behaviors **to determine approaches used previously that may be more effective in dealing with current situation.**
- Suggest use of journaling. **Can assist in clarifying values and ideas or recognizing and resolving feelings or situation.**
- Make time for nonjudgmental discussion of philosophical issues or questions about spiritual impact of illness or situation and/or treatment regimen. **Open communication can assist client in reality checks of perceptions and identifying personal options.**
- Problem-solve solutions and identify areas for compromise **that may be useful in resolving possible conflicts.**
- Set limits on acting-out behavior that is inappropriate or destructive. **Promotes safety for client/others and helps prevent loss of self-esteem.**

Nursing Priority No. 3.

To facilitate setting goals and moving forward:

- Involve client in refining healthcare goals and therapeutic regimen, as appropriate. **Enhances commitment to plan, optimizing outcomes.**
- Discuss difference between grief and guilt and help client to identify and deal with each. Point out consequences of actions based on guilt. **Aids client in assuming responsibility for own actions and avoiding acting out of false guilt.**
- Use therapeutic communication skills of reflection and Active-listening. **Helps client find own solutions to concerns.**
- Identify role models (e.g., nurse, individual experiencing similar situation). **Provides opportunities for sharing of experiences, finding hope, and identifying options to deal with situation.**

Information that appears in brackets has been added by the authors to clarify and enhance the use of nursing diagnoses.

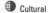

- Assist client to learn use of meditation, prayer, and forgiveness **to heal past hurts.**
- Provide information that anger with God is a normal part of the grieving process. **Realizing these feelings are not unusual can reduce sense of guilt, encourage open expression, and facilitate resolution of conflict.**
- Provide time and privacy to engage in spiritual growth and religious activities (e.g., prayer, meditation, scripture reading, listening to music). **Allows client to focus on self and seek connectedness.**
- Encourage and facilitate outings to neighborhood park, nature walks, or similar outings when able. **Sunshine, fresh air, and activity can stimulate release of endorphins, promoting sense of well-being.**
- ∞ Provide play therapy for child that encompasses spiritual data. **Interactive pleasurable activity promotes open discussion and enhances retention of information. Also provides opportunity for child to practice what has been learned.**
- ∞ Abide by parents' wishes in discussing and implementing child's spiritual support. **Limits confusion for child and prevents conflict of values or beliefs.**
- Refer to appropriate resources (e.g., pastoral or parish nurse, religious counselor, crisis counselor, hospice; psychotherapy; Alcoholics or Narcotics Anonymous). **Useful in dealing with immediate situation and identifying long-term resources for support to help foster sense of connectedness.**
- Refer to NDs ineffective Coping; Powerlessness; Self-Esteem [specify]; Social Isolation; risk for Suicide.

Nursing Priority No. 4.

To promote wellness (Teaching/Discharge Considerations):

- Assist client to develop goals for dealing with life/illness situation. **Enhances commitment to goal, optimizing outcomes.**
- Encourage life-review by client. Help client find a reason for living. **Promotes sense of hope and willingness to continue efforts to improve situation.**
- Role-play new coping techniques **to enhance integration of new skills or necessary changes in lifestyle.**
- Assist client to identify SO(s) and people who could provide support as needed. **Ongoing support is required to enhance sense of connectedness and continue progress toward goals.**
- Encourage family to provide a quiet, calm atmosphere. Be willing to just "be" there and not have a need to "do" some-

---

Information that appears in brackets has been added by the authors to clarify and enhance the use of nursing diagnoses.

thing. **Helps client to think about self in the context of current situation.**

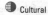

- Encourage individual to become involved in cultural activities of his or her choosing. **Art, music, plays, and other cultural activities provide a means of connecting with self and others.**
- Discuss benefit of family counseling, as appropriate. **Issues of this nature (e.g., situational losses, natural disasters, difficult relationships) affect family dynamics.**
- Assist client to identify spiritual resources that could be helpful (e.g., contact spiritual advisor who has qualifications or experience in dealing with specific problems, such as death and dying, relationship problems, substance abuse, suicide). **Provides answers to spiritual questions, assists in the journey of self-discovery, and can help client learn to accept and forgive self.**

Documentation Focus

Assessment/Reassessment

- Individual findings, including nature of spiritual conflict, effects on SO/family
- Physical and emotional responses to conflict

Planning

- Plan of care and who is involved in planning
- Teaching plan

Implementation/Evaluation

- Responses to interventions, teaching, and actions performed
- Attainment or progress toward desired outcome(s)
- Modifications to plan of care

Discharge Planning

- Long-term needs and who is responsible for actions to be taken
- Available resources, specific referrals made

Sample Nursing Outcomes & Interventions Classifications (NOC/NIC)

NOC—Spiritual Health

NIC—Spiritual Support

Information that appears in brackets has been added by the authors to clarify and enhance the use of nursing diagnoses.

readiness for enhanced SPIRITUAL WELL-BEING

[Diagnostic Division: Ego Integrity]

Definition: A pattern of experiencing and integrating meaning and purpose in life through connectedness with self, others, art, music, literature, nature, and/or a power greater than oneself, which can be strengthened.

Defining Characteristics

Subjective

Connections to Self

Expresses desire for enhanced acceptance, surrender, coping, courage, self-forgiveness, hope, joy, love, serenity (e.g., peace), meaning or purpose in life, satisfaction with philosophy of life

Expresses desire to enhance meditative practice

Connections With Others

Expresses desire to enhance interaction with significant other or spiritual leaders, service to others

Expresses desire to enhance forgiveness from others

Connections With Art, Music, Literature, Nature

Expresses desire to enhance creative energy (e.g., writing poetry, music), spiritual reading, time outdoors

Connections With Powers Greater Than Self

Expresses desire to enhance participation in religious activity, prayerfulness, reverence, mystical experiences

Desired Outcomes/Evaluation Criteria—Client Will:

- Acknowledge the stabilizing and strengthening forces in own life needed for balance and well-being of the whole person.
- Identify meaning and purpose in own life that reinforces hope, peace, and contentment.
- Verbalize a sense of peace or contentment and comfort of spirit.
- Demonstrate behavior congruent with verbalizations that lend support and strength for daily living.

Information that appears in brackets has been added by the authors to clarify and enhance the use of nursing diagnoses.

Actions/Interventions

Nursing Priority No. 1.

To determine spiritual state/motivation for growth:

- Ascertain client's perception of current state and degree of connectedness and expectations. **Provides insight into where client is currently and what his or her hopes for the future may be.**
- Identify motivation and expectations for change.
- Review spiritual and religious history, activities, rituals, and frequency of participation. **Provides basis to build on for growth or change.**
- Determine relational values of support systems to one's spiritual centeredness. **The client's family of origin may have differing beliefs from those espoused by the individual that may be a source of conflict for the client. Comfort can be gained when family and friends share client's beliefs and support search for spiritual knowledge.**
- Explore meaning or interpretation and relationship of spirituality, life, death, and illness to life's journey. **Identifying the meaning of these issues is helpful for the client to use the information in forming a belief system that will enable him or her to move forward and live life to the fullest.**
- Clarify the meaning of one's spiritual beliefs or religious practice and rituals to daily living. **Discussing these issues allows client to explore spiritual needs and decide what fits own view of the world to enhance life.**
- Explore ways that spirituality or religious practices have affected one's life and given meaning and value to daily living. Note consequences as well as benefits. **Understanding that there is a difference between spirituality and religion and how each can be useful will help client begin to view the information in a new way.**
- Discuss life's or God's plan for the individual, if client desires. **Helpful in determining individual goals and choosing specific options.**

Nursing Priority No. 2.

To assist client to integrate values and beliefs to achieve a sense of wholeness and optimum balance in daily living:

- Explore ways beliefs give meaning and value to daily living. **As client develops understanding of these issues, the beliefs will provide support for dealing with current and future concerns.**

Information that appears in brackets has been added by the authors to clarify and enhance the use of nursing diagnoses.

- Clarify reality and appropriateness of client's self-perceptions and expectations. **Necessary to provide firm foundation for growth.**
- Determine influence of cultural beliefs and values. **Most individuals are strongly influenced by the spiritual or religious orientation of their family of origin, which can be a very strong determinant for client's choice of activities and receptiveness to various options.**
- Discuss the importance and value of connections to one's daily life. **The contact that one has with others maintains a feeling of belonging and connection and promotes feelings of wholeness and well-being.**
- Identify ways to achieve connectedness or harmony with self, others, nature, higher power (e.g., meditation, prayer, talking or sharing oneself with others; being out in nature, gardening, walking; attending religious activities). **This is a highly individual and personal decision, and no action is too trivial to be considered.**

Nursing Priority No. 3.

To enhance personal growth and wellness:

- Encourage client to take time to be introspective in the search for peace and harmony. **Finding peace within oneself will carry over to relationships with others and own outlook on life.**
- Discuss use of relaxation or meditative activities (e.g., yoga, tai chi, prayer). **Helpful in promoting general well-being and sense of connectedness with self, nature, or spiritual power.**
- Suggest attendance or involvement in dream-sharing group **to develop and enhance learning of the characteristics of spiritual awareness and facilitate the individual's growth.**
- Identify ways for spiritual or religious expression. **There are multiple options for enhancing spirituality through connectedness with self/others (e.g., volunteering time to community projects, mentoring, singing in the choir, painting, spiritual writings).**
- Encourage participation in desired religious activities, contact with minister or spiritual advisor. **Validating own beliefs in an external way can provide support and strengthen the inner self.**
- Discuss and role-play, as necessary, ways to deal with alternative view or conflict that may occur with family/SO(s), society or cultural group. **Provides opportunity to try out dif-**

Information that appears in brackets has been added by the authors to clarify and enhance the use of nursing diagnoses.

ferent behaviors in a safe environment and be prepared for potential eventualities.

- Provide bibliotherapy, list of relevant resources (e.g., study groups, parish nurse, poetry society), and possible Web sites **for later reference or self-paced learning and ongoing support.**

Documentation Focus

Assessment/Reassessment

- Assessment findings, including client perception of needs and desire for growth or enhancement
- Motivation and expectations for change

Planning

- Plan for growth and who is involved in planning

Implementation/Evaluation

- Response to activities, learning, and actions performed
- Attainment or progress toward desired outcome(s)
- Modifications to plan

Discharge Planning

- Long-term needs, expectations, and plan of action
- Specific referrals made

Sample Nursing Outcomes & Interventions Classifications (NOC/NIC)

NOC—Spiritual Health
NIC—Spiritual Growth Facilitation

impaired STANDING

[Diagnostic Division: Safety]

Definition: Limitation of ability to independently and purposefully attain and/or maintain the body in an upright position from feet to head.

Related Factors

Circulatory perfusion disorder; impaired metabolic functioning; neurological disorder
Emotional disturbance

Information that appears in brackets has been added by the authors to clarify and enhance the use of nursing diagnoses.

Malnutrition; obesity; sarcopenia
Injury to lower extremity
Insufficient endurance or energy
Pain
Prescribed posture; self-imposed relief posture
Surgical procedure

Defining Characteristics

Objective

Impaired ability to adjust position of one or both lower limbs on uneven surface
Impaired ability to attain or maintain a balanced position of the torso; impaired ability to stress torso with body weight
Impaired ability to flex or extend one or both hips
Inability to flex or extend one or both knees
Insufficient muscle strength

Desired Outcomes/Evaluation Criteria—Client Will:

- Verbalize understanding of individual treatment regimen and safety measures.
- Attain and maintain position of standing function that enables activities and prevents complications.
- Participate in activities of daily living (ADLs) and desired activities.

Actions/Interventions

Nursing Priority No. 1.

To identify causative/contributing factors:

- Determine diagnosis that contributes to difficulty with standing balance (e.g., stroke, other neurological disorders [e.g., multiple sclerosis (MS), Parkinson's disease; traumatic brain injury, spinal cord injury with hemi-/paraplegia]; vestibular disorders/vertigo; osteoarthritis, rheumatoid arthritis, degenerative joint disease; back pain conditions; lower-limb amputations; psychiatric conditions including severe depression, dementias). **These conditions can cause postural and balance impairments, muscular weakness, and inadequate range of motion. Impaired standing balance has a detrimental effect on a person's functional ability and increases the risk of falling. For example, sitting and standing balance are major concerns in an amputee's ability to main-**

Information that appears in brackets has been added by the authors to clarify and enhance the use of nursing diagnoses.

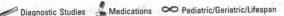

tain the center of gravity over the base of support. Another example: Dizziness and/or unsteadiness and episodes of loss of balance are not infrequent complaints of persons with persistent whiplash-associated disorders.

- Assess client's mental status, noting age, developmental stage, and presence or potential for cognitive dysfunction (e.g., traumatic brain injury, stroke, dementia, extremes of age). **Several studies have suggested that seemingly automatic postural tasks (such as standing balance and walking) require some attention and cognitive processing.**
- Determine fall risk, noting factors that may be present. **Fall risk is high in clients with certain conditions (e.g., advanced age or debilitating disease; vision and hearing loss, diminished depth perception; decreased sensation in feet, artificial joints; trauma to lower extremity; amputation, or other surgery or immobilizer; presence of severe vertigo with postural sway; generalized or specific leg weakness; reaching upward, forward, or laterally outside of standing balance position).**
- Encourage siting before attempting standing, when indicated (e.g., supine client with low blood pressure or dehydration, vertigo, or first attempting to get up after long period on bedrest). **Longer sitting pause times may improve postural stability after rising from a supine position.**

Nursing Priority No. 2.

To assess functional ability:

- Determine functional status in relation to 0 to 4 scale, and note muscle strength and tone, joint mobility, cardiovascular status, balance, and endurance. **Identifies strengths and deficits and may provide information regarding potential for recovery.**
- Determine degree of perceptual or cognitive impairment and ability to follow directions. **Impairments (which may be related to age, chronic or acute disease condition, trauma, surgery, or medications) can necessitate alternative interventions or changes in plan of care.**
- Refer to physician, physical therapy specialists, as indicated **to determine potential for improvement and direction for therapies. May include many different functional and diagnostic studies (e.g., sitting to standing tolerance, muscle strength and movement, American Spinal Injury Association [ASIA] Impairment Scale, Berger Balance Scale, Functional Independence Measure [FIM]).**

Information that appears in brackets has been added by the authors to clarify and enhance the use of nursing diagnoses.

Nursing Priority No. 3.

To promote optimal level of function and prevent complications:

- Assist with/refer for rehabilitation therapies and techniques for implementing standing activities. **Various modalities may be used to gain physiological benefits from standing or modified standing therapy to help preserve joint range of motion, improve muscle flexibility, weight-bearing ability, and bowel and bladder function even when person is not upright.**
- Provide for safety measures as indicated by individual situation, including environmental management and fall prevention. (Refer to ND risk for Falls.)
- Encourage client's participation in self-care activities, and in physical or occupational therapies. **Improves body strength and function, enhances self-concept and sense of independence.**
- Administer pain medications before activity as needed **to permit maximal effort and involvement in activity.**
- Collaborate with nutritionist in providing nutritious foods and needed feeding assistance, maximizing client's abilities in ingesting and swallowing (upright position) **to optimize available energy for activities.**
- Demonstrate and assist with use of assistive devices (e.g., side rails, overhead trapeze, roller pads, safety belt, hydraulic lifts, or chairs) **for position changes and safe transfers.**
- Refer to NDs Activity Intolerance, impaired bed Mobility, impaired wheelchair Mobility, impaired Transfer Ability, impaired Sitting, and impaired Walking for additional interventions.

Nursing Priority No. 4.

To promote wellness (Teaching/Discharge Considerations):

- Encourage client's/significant other's (SO's) involvement in decision making as much as possible. **Enhances commitment to plan, optimizing outcomes.**
- Demonstrate use of mobility devices (e.g., walkers, strollers, scooters, braces, prosthetics) and have client/care provider demonstrate knowledge about and safe use of device. Identify appropriate resources for obtaining and maintaining appliances or equipment. **Safe use of mobility aids promotes client's independence and enhances quality of life and safety for client and caregiver.**
- Refer to support and community services as indicated **to provide care, supervision, companionship, respite services,**

Information that appears in brackets has been added by the authors to clarify and enhance the use of nursing diagnoses.

nutritional and ADL assistance, adaptive devices or changes to living environment, financial assistance, and so forth.

Documentation Focus

Assessment/Reassessment

- Individual findings, including level of function and ability to participate in specific or desired activities

Planning

- Plan of care and who is involved in the planning
- Teaching plan

Implementation/Evaluation

- Responses to interventions, teaching, and actions performed
- Attainment or progress toward desired outcome(s)
- Modifications to plan of care

Discharge Planning

- Discharge and long-term needs, noting who is responsible for each action to be taken
- Specific referrals made
- Sources of and maintenance for assistive devices

Sample Nursing Outcomes & Interventions Classifications (NOC/NIC)

NOC—Knowledge: Body Mechanics
NIC—Exercise Therapy: Muscle Control

STRESS OVERLOAD

[Diagnostic Division: Ego Integrity]

Definition: Excessive amounts and types of demands that require action.

Related Factors

Insufficient resources (e.g., financial, social, knowledge)
Excessive stress; stressors; repeated stressors

Information that appears in brackets has been added by the authors to clarify and enhance the use of nursing diagnoses.

Defining Characteristics

Subjective

Impaired functioning, decision making
Feeling of pressure; increase in impatience, anger
Negative impact from stress (e.g., physical symptoms, psychological distress, feeling sick)
Excessive stress; tension

Objective

Increase in anger behavior

Desired Outcomes/Evaluation Criteria—Client Will:

- Assess current situation accurately.
- Identify ineffective stress-management behaviors and consequences.
- Meet psychological needs as evidenced by appropriate expression of feelings, identification of options, and use of resources.
- Verbalize or demonstrate reduced stress reaction.

Actions/Interventions

Nursing Priority No. 1.

To identify causative/precipitating factors and degree of impairment:

- Ascertain what tragic/difficult events have occurred (e.g., family violence, death of loved one, chronic or terminal illness, workplace stress or loss of job, catastrophic natural or man-made event) over remote and recent past **to assist in determining number, duration, and intensity of events causing perception of overwhelming stress.**
- Ascertain other life events that have recently occurred (e.g., job promotion, moving to different home, getting married/divorced, having a new baby or adding other new family member, traveling, spending holidays with relatives) over recent months. **All such changes, even when desired, can be stressful, and can evoke stress reactions.**
- Evaluate client's report of physical or emotional problems (e.g., fatigue, aches and pains, irritable bowel, skin rashes, frequent colds, sleeplessness, crying spells, anger, feeling

Information that appears in brackets has been added by the authors to clarify and enhance the use of nursing diagnoses.

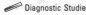

overwhelmed or numb, compulsive behaviors) **that can be representing body's response to stress.**

- Determine client's/significant other's (SO's) understanding of events, noting differences in viewpoints.
- Note client's gender, age, and developmental level of functioning. **Although everyone experiences stress and stressors, women, children, young adults, divorced and separated persons, and persons in roles or occupations requiring constant multitasking tend to have higher stress-related symptoms. Multiple stressors can weaken the immune system and tax physical and emotional coping mechanisms in persons of any age, but particularly the elderly.**
- Note cultural values or religious beliefs that may affect client's expectation for self in dealing with situation and expectations placed on client by SO(s)/family. **It is important to look at how they define family (can be nuclear, extended, or clan), who are the primary caregivers, and what are their social goals.**
- Identify client locus of control: internal (expressions of responsibility for self and ability to control outcomes: "I didn't quit smoking") or external (expressions of lack of control over self and environment: "Nothing ever works out"). **Knowing client's locus of control will help in developing a plan of care reflecting client's ability to realistically make changes that will help to manage stress better.**
- Assess emotional responses and coping mechanisms being used.
- Determine stress feelings and self-talk client is engaging in. **Negative self-talk, all-or-nothing or pessimistic thinking, exaggeration, or unrealistic expectations all contribute to stress overload.**
- Assess degree of mastery client has exhibited in life. **Passive individual may have more difficulty being assertive and standing up for rights.**
- Determine presence or absence and nature of resources (e.g., whether family/SO(s) are supportive, lack of money, problems with relationship or social functioning).
- Note change in relationships with SO(s). **Conflict in the family, loss of a family member, divorce can result in a change in support client is accustomed to and impair ability to manage situation.**
- Evaluate stress level, using appropriate tool (e.g., Stress & Depression, Self-Assessment Tool) to help identify areas of

---

Information that appears in brackets has been added by the authors to clarify and enhance the use of nursing diagnoses.

most distress. **While most stress seems to come from disastrous events in individual's life, positive events can also be stressful.**

Nursing Priority No. 2.

To assist client to deal with current situation:

- Active-listen concerns and provide empathetic presence, using talk and silence as needed.
- Provide for or encourage restful environment where possible.
- Discuss situation or condition in simple, concise manner. Devote time for listening. **May help client express emotions, grasp situation, and feel more in control.**
- Deal with the immediate issues first (e.g., treatment of acute physical or psychological illness, meet safety needs, removal from traumatic or violent environment).
- Assist client in determining whether he or she can change stressor or response. **May help client to sort out things over which he or she has control and/or determine responses that can be modified.**
- Allow client to react in own way without judgment. Provide support and diversion as indicated.
- Help client to focus on strengths, to set limits on acting-out behaviors, and to learn ways to express emotions in an acceptable manner. **Promotes internal locus of control, enabling client to maintain self-concept and feel more positive about self.**
- Discuss benefits of a "Stop Doing" in place of a "To Do" list. **May help client identify and take action regarding energy drainers (e.g., internalizing others' criticism, fragmented boundaries, power struggles, unprotected personal time) in order to make room for what energizes and brings him/her closer to achieving goals.**
- Address use of ineffective or dangerous coping mechanisms (e.g., substance use or abuse, self-/other-directed violence) and refer for counseling as indicated.
- Collaborate in treatment of underlying conditions (e.g., physical injury, depression, anger management).

Nursing Priority No. 3.

To promote wellness (Teaching/Discharge Considerations):

- Use client's locus of control to develop individual plan of care **(e.g., for client with internal control, encourage client to take control of own care; for those with external control, begin with small tasks and add as tolerated).**

Information that appears in brackets has been added by the authors to clarify and enhance the use of nursing diagnoses.

- Incorporate strengths, assets, and past coping strategies that were successful for client. **Reinforces that client is able to deal with difficult situations.**
- Provide information about stress and exhaustion phase, which occurs when person is experiencing chronic or unresolved stress. **Release of cortisol can contribute to reduction in immune function, resulting in physical illness, mental disability, and life dysfunction.**
- Review stress management and coping skills that client can use:

  Practice behaviors that may help reduce negative consequences—change thinking by focusing on positives, reframing thoughts, changing lifestyle.

  Take a step back, simplify life; learn to say "no" **to reduce sense of being overwhelmed.**

  Learn to control and redirect anger.

  Develop and practice positive self-esteem skills.

  Rest, sleep, and exercise **to recuperate and rejuvenate self.**

  Participate in self-help actions (e.g., deep breathing and other relaxation exercises, find time to be alone, get involved in recreation or desired activity, plan something fun, develop humor) **to actively relax.**

  Eat right; avoid junk food, excessive caffeine, alcohol, and nicotine **to support general health.**

  Develop spiritual self (e.g., meditate or pray; block negative thoughts; learn to give and take, speak and listen, forgive and move on).

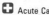

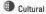

  Interact socially, reach out, nurture self and others **to reduce loneliness or sense of isolation.**
- Review proper medication use to manage exacerbating conditions (e.g., depression, mood disorders).
- Identify community resources (e.g., vocational counseling; educational programs; child/elder care, Women, Infants, or Children [WIC] or food assistance; home or respite care) **that can help client manage lifestyle and environmental stress.**
- Refer for therapy as indicated (e.g., medical treatment, psychological counseling, hypnosis, massage, biofeedback).

Documentation Focus

Assessment/Reassessment

- Individual findings, noting specific stressors, individual's perception of the situation, locus of control

Information that appears in brackets has been added by the authors to clarify and enhance the use of nursing diagnoses.

- Specific cultural or religious factors
- Availability and use of support systems and resources

Planning

- Plan of care and who is involved in planning
- Teaching plan

Implementation/Evaluation

- Responses to interventions, teaching, and actions performed
- Attainment or progress toward desired outcome(s)
- Modifications to plan of care

Discharge Planning

- Long-term needs and who is responsible for actions to be taken
- Specific referrals made

Sample Nursing Outcomes & Interventions Classifications (NOC/NIC)

NOC—Stress Level
NIC—Coping Enhancement

risk for SUDDEN INFANT DEATH SYNDROME

[Diagnostic Division: Safety]

Definition: Vulnerable to unpredicted death of an infant.

[Sudden infant death syndrome (SIDS) is the sudden death of an infant under 1 year of age, which remains unexplained after a thorough case investigation, including performance of a complete autopsy, examination of the death scene, and review of the clinical history. SIDS is a subset of sudden unexpected death in infancy (SUDI), which is the sudden and unexpected death of an infant due to natural or unnatural causes.]

Risk Factors

Modifiable

Delay in or insufficient prenatal care
Infant placed in the prone or side-lying position to sleep

Information that appears in brackets has been added by the authors to clarify and enhance the use of nursing diagnoses.

Soft underlayment (e.g., loose items placed near infant)
Infant overheating or overwrapping
Exposure to smoke

Potentially Modifiable

Young parental age
Low birth weight; prematurity

Nonmodifiable

Male gender
Ethnicity (e.g., African American or Native American)
Season of the year (i.e., winter and fall)
Age 2 to 4 months

> **NOTE:** A risk diagnosis is not evidenced by signs and symptoms as the problem has not occurred; rather, nursing interventions are directed at prevention.

Desired Outcomes/Evaluation Criteria—Parent/Caregiver Will:

- Verbalize understanding of modifiable factors.
- Make changes in environment to reduce risk of death occurring from other factors.
- Follow medically recommended prenatal and postnatal care.

Actions/Interventions

Nursing Priority No. 1.

To assess causative/contributing factors:

- Identify individual risk factors pertaining to situation. **Determines modifiable or potentially modifiable factors that can be addressed.** ***Note:*** **SIDS is the most common cause of sudden unexpected death in infancy (SUDI) between 1 and 6 months, with peak incidence occurring between the second and fourth months. True SIDS has shown a progressive decline since 1992, while SUDI deaths have increased. It is postulated that some deaths previously classified as SIDS are now being more correctly categorized.**
- (Cultural) Determine ethnic/cultural background of family. **Although the overall rate of SIDS in the United States has declined since 1992, disparities in risk factors and SIDS rates remain. African American infants are more than twice as likely to die of SIDS as white infants. American Indian/**

Information that appears in brackets has been added by the authors to clarify and enhance the use of nursing diagnoses.

Alaska Native infants are nearly three times as likely to die of SIDS as white infants. Hispanic and Asian-Pacific Islander infants have the lowest SIDS rates of any racial or ethnic group in the country.

- Note whether mother smoked during pregnancy or is currently smoking. **Smoking is known to negatively affect the fetus prenatally as well as after birth. Some reports indicate an increased risk of SIDS in babies of smoking mothers.**
- Assess extent of prenatal care and extent to which mother followed recommended care measures. **Prenatal care is important for all pregnancies to afford the optimal opportunity for all infants to have a healthy start to life.**
- Note use of alcohol or other drugs/medications during and after pregnancy **that may have a negative impact on the developing fetus or place the infant at risk for death. Enables management to minimize any damaging effects.**

Nursing Priority No. 2.

To promote use of activities to minimize risk of SIDS:

- Recommend that infant be placed on his or her back to sleep, both at nighttime and naptime. **Research confirms that fewer infants die of SIDS when they sleep on their backs, not on tummy or side.**
- Advise all caregivers of the infant regarding the importance of maintaining safe sleeping position in own sleeping place with head and face uncovered. **Anyone who will have responsibility for the care of the child during sleep needs to be reminded of the importance of the back to sleep position.**
- Encourage parents to schedule "tummy time" only while infant is awake. **This activity promotes strengthening of back and neck muscles while parents are close and baby is not sleeping.**
- Encourage early and medically recommended prenatal care and continue with well-baby checkups and immunizations after birth. Include information about signs of premature labor and actions to be taken to avoid problems if possible. **Prematurity presents many problems for the newborn, and keeping babies healthy prevents problems that could put the infant at risk for SIDS. Immunizing infants prevents many illnesses that can also be life threatening.**
- Encourage breastfeeding, if possible. Recommend sitting up in chair when nursing at night. **Breastfeeding has many advantages (e.g., immunological, nutritional, and psychosocial), promoting a healthy infant. Although this does not**

Information that appears in brackets has been added by the authors to clarify and enhance the use of nursing diagnoses.

preclude the occurrence of SIDS, healthy babies are less prone to many illnesses/problems. Note: The risk of the mother falling asleep while feeding infant in bed with resultant accidental suffocation could be of concern.

- Discuss issues of bedsharing and the concerns regarding sudden unexpected infant deaths from accidental entrapment under a sleeping adult or suffocation by becoming wedged in a couch or cushioned chair. **While bedsharing among infants and family members is common in many cultures, there are concerns about accidental death from suffocation, especially when the mother smokes, has recently consumed alcohol, the infant's head is covered by a blanket or quilt, or there are multiple bedsharers.**
- Note cultural beliefs about bedsharing. **Bedsharing is more common among breastfed infants, young unmarried mothers; low-income families where multiple people share a bed; or those from a minority group. (Additional study is needed to better understand bedsharing practices and associated risks and benefits.)**

Nursing Priority No. 3.

To promote wellness (Teaching/Discharge Considerations):

- Discuss known facts about SIDS with parents. **Corrects misconceptions and helps reduce level of anxiety.**
- Avoid overdressing or overheating infants during sleep. **Infants dressed in two or more layers of clothes as they sleep have six times the risk of SIDS as those dressed in fewer layers.**
- Place the baby on a firm mattress in an approved crib. **Avoiding soft mattresses, sofas, cushions, water beds, and other soft surfaces, while not known to prevent SIDS, will minimize chance of suffocation/SUDI.**
- Remove fluffy and loose bedding from sleep area, making sure baby's head and face are not covered during sleep. **Minimizes possibility of suffocation.**
- Discuss the use of apnea monitors. **Apnea monitors have not proved helpful in preventing SIDS but may be used to monitor other medical problems.**
- Recommend public health nurse or similar resource visit new mothers at least once or twice following discharge. **Researchers found that Native American infants whose mothers received such visits were 80% less likely to die from SIDS than those who were never visited.**

Information that appears in brackets has been added by the authors to clarify and enhance the use of nursing diagnoses.

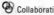

- Ascertain that day-care center/provider(s) are trained in observation and modifying risk factors (e.g., sleeping position) **to reduce risk of death while infant is in their care.**
- Refer parents to local SIDS programs/other resources for learning (e.g., National SIDS/Infant Death Resource Center and similar Web sites) and encourage consultation with healthcare provider if baby shows any signs of illness or behaviors that concern them. **Can provide information and support for risk reduction and correction of treatable problems.**

Documentation Focus

Assessment/Reassessment

- Baseline findings, degree of parental anxiety/concern
- Individual risk factors

Planning

- Plan of care, interventions, and who is involved in planning
- Teaching plan

Implementation/Evaluation

- Parent's responses to interventions, teaching, and actions performed
- Attainment or progress toward desired outcome(s)
- Modifications to plan of care

Discharge Planning

- Long-term needs and actions to be taken
- Support systems available, specific referrals made, and who is responsible for actions to be taken

Sample Nursing Outcomes & Interventions Classifications (NOC/NIC)

NOC—Risk Detection
NIC—Risk Identification

risk for SUFFOCATION

[Diagnostic Division: Safety]

Definition: Vulnerable to inadequate air availability for inhalation.

Information that appears in brackets has been added by the authors to clarify and enhance the use of nursing diagnoses.

Risk Factors

Internal

Alteration in cognitive or motor functioning; emotional disturbance
Alteration in olfactory function
Face/neck disease or injury
Insufficient knowledge of safety precautions

External

Access to empty refrigerator/freezer
Eating large mouthfuls [or pieces] of food; small object in airway
Gas leak; unvented fuel-burning heater; vehicle running in closed garage; smoking in bed
Pacifier around infant's neck; propped bottle in infant's crib
Soft underlayment (e.g., loose items placed near infant); playing with plastic bag
Low-strung clothesline; unattended in water

NOTE: A risk diagnosis is not evidenced by signs and symptoms, as the problem has not occurred; rather, nursing interventions are directed at prevention.

Desired Outcomes/Evaluation Criteria—Client/Caregiver Will:

- Verbalize knowledge of hazards in the environment.
- Identify interventions appropriate to situation.
- Correct hazardous situations to prevent or reduce risk of suffocation.
- Demonstrate cardiopulmonary resuscitation (CPR) skills and how to access emergency assistance.

Actions/Interventions

Nursing Priority No. 1.

To assess causative/contributing factors:

- ∞ Determine age, developmental level, and mentation (e.g., infant/young child, frail elder, person with developmental delay, altered level of consciousness, or cognitive impairments or dementia) **to identify individuals unable to be responsible for or protect self.**

Information that appears in brackets has been added by the authors to clarify and enhance the use of nursing diagnoses.

- Determine client's/significant other's (SO's) knowledge of safety factors or hazards present in the environment **to identify misconceptions and educational needs. Suffocation can be caused by (1) spasm of airway (e.g., food or water going down wrong way, irritant gases, asthma); (2) airway obstruction (e.g., foreign body, tongue falling back in unconscious person, swelling of tissues from burn injury or allergic reaction); (3) airway compression (e.g., tying rope or band tightly around neck, hanging, throttling, smothering); (4) conditions affecting the respiratory mechanism (e.g., epilepsy, tetanus, rabies, nerve diseases causing paralysis of chest wall or diaphragm); (5) conditions affecting respiratory center in brain (e.g., electric shock; stroke or other brain trauma; medications such as morphine, barbiturates); and (6) compression of the chest (e.g., crushing as might occur with cave-in, motor vehicle crash, pressure in a massive crowd).**
- Identify level of concern or awareness and motivation of client/SO(s) to correct safety hazards and improve individual situation. **Lack of commitment, unwillingness to make changes, places dependent individuals at risk.**
- Assess neurological status and note history/presence of conditions (e.g., stroke, cerebral palsy, multiple sclerosis, amyotrophic lateral sclerosis) **that have potential to compromise airway or affect ability to swallow.**
- Determine use of antiepileptics and how well epilepsy is controlled. **Seizure activity (and especially status epilepticus) is a major risk factor for respiratory inhibition or arrest, particularly when consciousness is impaired.**
- Review medication regimen **to note potential for oversedation and respiratory failure (e.g., central nervous system depressants, analgesics, sedatives, antidepressants).**
- Note reports of sleep disturbance and fatigue; **may be indicative of sleep apnea (airway obstruction).**
- Assess for allergies (e.g., medications, foods, environmental) **to which individual could have severe/anaphylactic reaction resulting in respiratory arrest.**
- Be alert to and carefully monitor those individuals who are severely depressed, mentally ill, or aggressive. **These individuals could be at risk for suicide by suffocation (e.g., inhaled carbon monoxide or death by strangling or hanging).** (Refer to ND risk for Suicide.)
- Note signs of respiratory distress (e.g., cough, stridor, wheezing, increased work of breathing) **that could indicate swell-**

Information that appears in brackets has been added by the authors to clarify and enhance the use of nursing diagnoses.

ing or obstruction of airways. Refer to NDs ineffective Airway Clearance; risk for Aspiration; ineffective Breathing Pattern; impaired spontaneous Ventilation, as appropriate, for additional interventions.

Nursing Priority No. 2.

To reverse/correct contributing factors:

- Discuss with client/SO(s) identified environmental or work-related safety hazards and problem-solve methods for resolution (e.g., need for smoke and carbon monoxide alarms, vents for household heater, clean chimney, properly strung clothesline, proper venting of machinery exhaust, monitoring of stored chemicals, bracing trench walls when digging).
- Protect airway at all times, especially if client unable to protect self:

Use proper positioning, suctioning, use of airway adjuncts, as indicated, **for comatose or cognitively impaired individual or client with swallowing impairment or obstructive sleep apnea.**

Provide seizure precautions and antiseizure medication, as indicated.

Administer medications when client is sitting or standing upright and can swallow without difficulty.

Emphasize importance of chewing carefully, taking small amounts of food, and using caution **to prevent aspiration when talking or drinking while eating.**

Provide diet modifications as indicated by specific needs (e.g., developmental level; presence/degree of swallowing disability, impaired cognition) **to reduce risk of aspiration or choking.**

Avoid physical and mechanical restraints, including vest or waist restraint, side rails, choke hold. **Can increase client agitation causing struggle to escape, resulting in entrapment of head and hanging.**

- Emphasize with client/SO the importance of getting help when beginning to choke or feel respiratory distress (e.g., staying with people instead of leaving table, make gestures across throat; making sure someone recognizes the emergency) **in order to provide timely intervention such as abdominal thrusts and calling 911.**
- Refrain from smoking in bed; supervise smoking materials (use, disposal, and storage) for impaired individuals. Keep smoking materials out of reach of children.
- Avoid idling automobile (or using fuel-burning heaters) in closed or unvented spaces.

Information that appears in brackets has been added by the authors to clarify and enhance the use of nursing diagnoses.

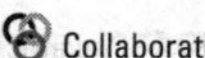 Acute Care 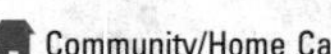 Collaborative Community/Home Care 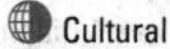 Cultural

- Emphasize importance of periodic evaluation and repair of gas appliances and furnace, automobile exhaust system **to prevent exposure to carbon monoxide.**
- ∞ Review child protective measures:

  Place infant in supine position for sleep. Refer to ND risk for Sudden Infant Death Syndrome.

  Do not prop baby bottles in infant crib.

  Attach pacifier to clothing—not around neck; remove bib before putting baby in bed.

  Store or dispose of plastic bags (e.g., shopping, garbage, dry cleaning, and shipping) out of reach of infants/young children.

  Avoid use of plastic mattress or crib covers.

  Avoid placing infant to sleep on soft surfaces (e.g., beanbag chair, basket with soft sides, soft pillow or comforter, water bed) **that baby can sink into or be unable to free face.**

  Use a crib with slats that are no more than 2 3/8 inches apart **so that baby cannot get head trapped or slip body through slats.**

  Refrain from bedsharing with infant/young child **to prevent accidental smothering.**

  Provide constant supervision of young children in bathtub or swimming pool.

  Make certain that blind and curtain cords, drawstrings on clothing, and so forth, are out of reach of small children **to prevent accidental hanging.**

  Prevent young child/impaired individual from putting objects in mouth (e.g., food such as raw carrots, nuts, seeds, popcorn, hot dogs; toy parts; buttons; balloons; batteries; coins) **that can get lodged in airway and cause choking.**

  Lock or remove lid or door of chests, trunks, old refrigerators or freezers **to prevent child from being trapped in airless environment.**

Nursing Priority No. 3.

To promote wellness (Teaching/Discharge Considerations):

- Review safety factors identified in individual situation and methods for remediation.
- Develop plan with client/caregiver for long-range management of situation to avoid injuries. **Enhances commitment to plan, optimizing outcomes.**
- Review importance of chewing carefully, taking small amounts of food, using caution when talking or drinking while eating. Discuss possibility of choking **because of impaired**

Information that appears in brackets has been added by the authors to clarify and enhance the use of nursing diagnoses.

swallowing or throat muscle relaxation and impaired judgment when drinking alcohol and eating.

- Promote public education in techniques for clearing blocked airways, back blows, Heimlich maneuver, CPR.
- Collaborate in community public health education regarding hazards for children (e.g., appropriate toy size for young child) discussing dangers of "huffing" (inhalants) and playing choking or hanging games with preteens; fire safety drills; bathtub rules; how to spot potential for depression and risk of suicidal gestures in adolescents **to reduce potential for accidental or intentional suffocation.**
- Assist individuals to learn to read package labels and identify safety hazards.
- Promote pool safety, use of approved flotation devices, proper fencing enclosure or alarm system for home pools.
- Discuss safety measures regarding use of heaters, household gas appliances, old or discarded appliances.
- Refer to NDs ineffective Airway Clearance; risk for Aspiration; ineffective Breathing Pattern; impaired Parenting.

Documentation Focus

Assessment/Reassessment

- Individual risk factors, including individual's cognitive status and level of knowledge
- Level of concern and motivation for change
- Equipment or airway adjunct needs

Planning

- Plan of care and who is involved in planning
- Teaching plan

Implementation/Evaluation

- Responses to interventions, teaching, and actions performed
- Attainment or progress toward desired outcome(s)
- Modifications to plan of care

Discharge Planning

- Long-term needs, appropriate preventive measures, and who is responsible for actions to be taken
- Specific referrals made

Information that appears in brackets has been added by the authors to clarify and enhance the use of nursing diagnoses.

Sample Nursing Outcomes & Interventions Classifications (NOC/NIC)

NOC—Risk Control
NIC—Airway Management

risk for SUICIDE

[Diagnostic Division: Safety]

Definition: Vulnerable to self-inflicted, life-threatening injury.

Risk Factors

Behavioral

History of suicide attempt
Purchase of a gun; stockpiling medication
Making or changing a will; giving away possessions
Sudden euphoric recovery from major depression
Impulsiveness; marked change in behavior, attitude, or school performance

Verbal

Threat of killing self; reports desire to die

Situational

Access to weapon
Living alone; retired; economically disadvantaged; relocation; institutionalization
Loss of autonomy or independence
Adolescents living in nontraditional settings (e.g., juvenile detention center, prison, halfway house, group home)

Psychological

Family history of suicide; history of childhood abuse (e.g., physical, psychological, sexual)
Substance abuse
Psychiatric illness or disorder
Guilt
Homosexual youth

Demographic

Age (e.g., elderly people, young adult males, adolescents)
Ethnicity (e.g., Caucasian, Native American)

Information that appears in brackets has been added by the authors to clarify and enhance the use of nursing diagnoses.

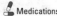

Male gender
Divorced; widowed

Physical
Physical or terminal illness; chronic pain

Social
Loss of important relationship; disruptive family life; insufficient social support; social isolation
Grieving; loneliness
Hopelessness; helplessness
Disciplinary problems; legal difficulty
Cluster suicides

NOTE: A risk diagnosis is not evidenced by signs and symptoms, as the problem has not occurred; rather, nursing interventions are directed at prevention.

Desired Outcomes/Evaluation Criteria—Client Will:

- Acknowledge difficulties perceived in current situation.
- Identify current factors that can be dealt with.
- Be involved in planning course of action to correct existing problems.
- Make decision that suicide is not the answer to the perceived problems.

Actions/Interventions

Nursing Priority No. 1.
To assess causative/contributing factors:

- Identify degree of risk or potential for suicide and seriousness of threat. Use a scale of 1 to 10 and prioritize according to severity of threat, availability of means.
- Note behaviors indicative of intent (e.g., gestures; presence of means, such as guns; threats; giving away possessions; previous attempts; and presence of hallucinations or delusions). **Many people signal their intent, particularly to healthcare providers.**
- Ask directly if person is thinking of acting on thoughts or feelings. **Determines intent. Most people will answer honestly because they actually want help.**

Information that appears in brackets has been added by the authors to clarify and enhance the use of nursing diagnoses.

- Note age and gender. **Risk of suicide is greater in males, teens, and the elderly, but there is a rising awareness of risk in early childhood.**
- Review family history for suicidal behavior. **Individual risk is increased, especially when the person who committed suicide was close to the client.**
- Identify conditions, such as acute or chronic brain syndrome, panic state, hormonal imbalance (e.g., premenstrual syndrome, postpartum psychosis, drug induced) **that may interfere with ability to control own behavior and will require specific interventions to promote safety.**
- Discuss losses client has experienced and meaning of those losses. **Unresolved issues may be contributing to thoughts of hopelessness.**
- Note withdrawal from usual activities, lack of social interactions. **These are classic behaviors of the individual who is feeling depressed and sad and may be having negative thoughts of worthlessness.**
- Assess physical complaints (e.g., sleeping difficulties, lack of appetite). **Sleeping difficulties, lack of appetite can be indicators of depression and suicidal ideation requiring further evaluation.**
- Determine drug use or "self" medication. **The use of drugs and alcohol, especially the combination of alcohol and barbiturates, increases the risk of suicide.**
- Note history of disciplinary problems or involvement with judicial system.
- Assess coping behaviors presently used. **Client's current negative thinking may preclude looking at positive behaviors used in the past that would help in the current situation.**
- Determine presence of significant other (SO)(s)/friends who are available for support.
- Review laboratory findings (e.g., blood alcohol, blood glucose, arterial blood gas, electrolytes, renal function tests), **to identify factors that may affect reasoning ability.**

Nursing Priority No. 2.

To assist clients to accept responsibility for own behavior and prevent suicide:

- Develop therapeutic nurse-client relationship, providing consistent caregiver. **Collaborating with the client to better understand the problem affirms the client's ability to solve the current situation.**

Information that appears in brackets has been added by the authors to clarify and enhance the use of nursing diagnoses.

- Maintain straightforward communication **to avoid reinforcing manipulative behavior.**
- Explain concern for safety and willingness to help client stay safe.
- Encourage expression of feelings and make time to listen to concerns. **Acknowledges reality of feelings and that they are okay. Helps individual sort out thinking and begin to develop understanding of situation and look at other alternatives.**
- Give permission to express angry feelings in acceptable ways and let client know someone will be available to assist in maintaining control. **Promotes acceptance and sense of safety.**
- Acknowledge reality of suicide as an option. Discuss consequences of actions if they follow through on intent. Ask how it will help individual to resolve problems. **Helps to focus on consequences of actions and possibility of other options.**
- Maintain observation of client and check environment for hazards that could be used to commit suicide **to increase client safety or reduce risk of impulsive behavior.**
- Help client identify more appropriate solutions/behaviors (e.g., motor activities/exercise) **to lessen sense of anxiety and associated physical manifestations.**
- Provide directions for actions client can take, avoiding negative statements, such as "Do Nots." **Promotes a positive attitude.**
- Discuss use of psychotropic medication, positive and negative aspects. **While the use of medications is often helpful, there are some drawbacks, including the potential for providing client a means of suicide.**
- Reevaluate potential for suicide periodically at key times (e.g., mood changes, increasing withdrawal), as well as when client is feeling better and discharge planning becomes active. **The highest risk exists when the client has both suicidal ideation and sufficient energy with which to act.**

Nursing Priority No. 3.

To assist client to plan course of action to correct/deal with existing situation:

- Gear interventions to individual involved (e.g., age, relationship, current situation).
- Negotiate contract with client regarding willingness not to do anything lethal for a stated period of time. Specify what caregiver will be responsible for and what client responsibilities are.

Information that appears in brackets has been added by the authors to clarify and enhance the use of nursing diagnoses.

- Specify alternative actions necessary if client is unwilling to negotiate contract. **Client may be willing to agree to other actions (i.e., calling therapist if feelings are overwhelming), even though he or she is not willing to commit to a contract.**

Nursing Priority No. 4.

To promote wellness (Teaching/Discharge Considerations):

- Promote development of internal control by helping client look at new ways to deal with problems.
- Assist with learning problem-solving, assertiveness training, and social skills.
- Engage in physical activity programs. Releases endorphins, **promoting feelings of self-worth and improving sense of well-being.**
- Determine nutritional needs and help client to plan for meeting them.
- Involve family/SO(s) in planning **to improve understanding and support.**
- Refer to formal resources as indicated. **May need referrals to individual, group, or marital psychotherapy, substance abuse treatment program, or social services when situation involves mental illness, family disorganization.**

Documentation Focus

Assessment/Reassessment

- Individual findings, including nature of concern (e.g., suicidal/behavioral risk factors and level of impulse control, plan of action and means to carry out plan)
- Client's perception of situation, motivation for change

Planning

- Plan of care and who is involved in the planning
- Details of contract regarding suicidal ideation or plans
- Teaching plan

Implementation/Evaluation

- Actions taken to promote safety
- Response to interventions, teaching, and actions performed
- Attainment or progress toward desired outcome(s)
- Modifications to plan of care

Information that appears in brackets has been added by the authors to clarify and enhance the use of nursing diagnoses.

Discharge Planning

- Long-term needs and who is responsible for actions to be taken
- Available resources, specific referrals made

Sample Nursing Outcomes & Interventions Classifications (NOC/NIC)

NOC—Suicide Self-Restraint
NIC—Suicide Prevention

delayed SURGICAL RECOVERY and risk for delayed SURGICAL RECOVERY

[Diagnostic Division: Safety]

Definition: delayed Surgical Recovery: Extension of the number of postoperative days required to initiate and perform activities that maintain life, health, and well-being.

Definition: risk for delayed Surgical Recovery: Vulnerable to an extension of the number of postoperative days required to initiate and perform activities that maintain life, health, and well-being, which may compromise health.

Related and Risk Factors

American Society of Anesthesiologists (ASA) Physical Status classification score ≥3
Diabetes mellitus
Edema or trauma at surgical site
Extensive or prolonged surgical procedure
Extremes of age; impaired immobility
History of delayed wound healing; perioperative surgical site infection; surgical site contamination
Persistent nausea or vomiting; malnutrition; obesity
Pain
Pharmaceutical agent

Information that appears in brackets has been added by the authors to clarify and enhance the use of nursing diagnoses.

Postoperative emotional response; psychological disorder in postoperative period

> **NOTE:** A risk diagnosis is not evidenced by signs and symptoms, as the problem has not occurred; rather, nursing interventions are directed at prevention.

Defining Characteristics (delayed Surgical Recovery)

Subjective

Discomfort
Loss of appetite
Postpones resumption of work

Objective

Evidence of interrupted healing of surgical area
Excessive time required for recuperation; inability to resume employment
Impaired mobility; requires assistance for self-care

Desired Outcomes/Evaluation Criteria—Client Will:

- Display complete healing of surgical area.
- Be able to perform desired self-care activities.
- Report increased energy, able to participate in usual (work or employment) activities.

Actions/Interventions

Nursing Priority No. 1.

To assess causative/contributing factors or risk factors:

- Identify vulnerable client (e.g., low socioeconomic status, lack of resources, challenges related to poverty, lack of insurance or transportation, severe trauma or prolonged hospitalization with multiple complicating factors) **who is at higher risk for adverse outcomes.**
- ∞ Determine extent of surgical involvement of organs or tissues, noting age and developmental level, and general state

Information that appears in brackets has been added by the authors to clarify and enhance the use of nursing diagnoses.

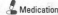

of health **to help determine time that may be required for client to resume activities of daily living (ADLs) and other activities, or expectation of time needed for healing.**

- Note underlying condition or pathology (e.g., cancer, burns, diabetes, hypothyroidism, obesity, steroid therapy, major trauma, infections, radiation therapy, cardiopulmonary disorders, debilitating illness) **that can adversely affect healing and prolong recuperation time. In this population, impaired pulmonary function, hyperglycemia, immobility, and nutritional deficits can compromise wound healing.**
- Determine the length of operative procedure or time under anesthesia (e.g., typical or lengthy); type and severity of perioperative complications (e.g., trauma or other conditions requiring multiple surgeries; heavy bleeding during procedure); type of surgical wound (e.g., clean, clean-contaminated, or grossly contaminated, acutely infected); and development of postoperative complications (e.g., surgical site infection, suture reactions, dehiscence, ventilator-associated pneumonia, deep vein thrombosis [DVT]) **that can affect the pace of healing or prolong recovery.**
- ∞ Determine age, developmental level, and general state of health **to help determine time that may be required for client to resume ADLs and other activities, or expectation of time needed for healing.**
- Evaluate circulation and sensation in surgical area, noting location of incision. **Lack of blood supply at the wound site can slow healing. Note: Areas of the body such as the face and neck receive the most blood supply and heal the fastest, whereas areas such as extremities take longer to heal.**
- Determine nutritional status and current intake **to ascertain if nutrition is adequate to support healing. Client may have preexisting nutritional concerns or may have been fasting perioperatively or experienced nausea, vomiting, and loss of appetite postoperatively..**
- Review client's preoperative medications/other drug regimen **to ascertain that none could impede healing processes (e.g., aspirin and NSAIDs, chemotherapy agents); or increase bleeding time (e.g., alcohol and some herbals such as garlic and ginkgo biloba can also be associated with bleeding complications).**

Information that appears in brackets has been added by the authors to clarify and enhance the use of nursing diagnoses.

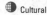

- Perform pain assessment **to ascertain whether pain management is adequate to meet client's needs during recovery.**
- Evaluate client's cognitive and emotional state, noting presence of postoperative changes, including confusion, depression, apathy, expressions of helplessness **to determine need for further assessment of possible physical or psychological interferences.**
- Ascertain attitudes and cultural values of individual about condition. **Family beliefs and cultural values impact rate and expectations for sick role and recovery.**
- Review results of laboratory tests (e.g., complete blood count [CBC], blood/wound cultures, serum glucose; hormones [e.g., cortisol, glucocorticoid, and other hormones associated with inflammation and immune system dysfunction) **to assess for presence and type of infections, immunosuppression, metabolic or endocrine dysfunction, or other conditions affecting body's ability to heal.**
- Note allergies or history of skin reactions. Evaluate use of plastics (e.g., incontinence pads or moisture barriers), tape/adhesives, or latex materials. **Client sensitivity to adhesives and/or latex can cause skin or tissue reactions that delay primary wound healing and cause additional skin/tissue damage.** Refer to NDs impaired Skin Integrity, Latex Allergy Response.
- Note lifestyle factors (e.g., obesity, cigarette smoking, alcohol abuse, lack of exercise/sedentary lifestyle) **that influence circulation and wound healing and can impede recovery.**

Nursing Priority No. 2.

To determine risks or impact of delayed recovery:

- Note length of hospitalization and progress in recovery to date **to compare with expectations for procedure and situation.**
- Determine client's/significant other's (SO's) expectations for recovery and specific stressors related to delay (e.g., return to work or school, home responsibilities, child care, financial difficulties, limited support system).
- Determine energy level and current participation in ADLs. Compare with usual level of function.
- Ascertain whether client usually requires assistance in home setting and who provides it, current availability, and capability.

Information that appears in brackets has been added by the authors to clarify and enhance the use of nursing diagnoses.

- Obtain psychological assessment of client's emotional status, noting potential problems arising from current situation.

Nursing Priority No. 3.

To promote optimal recovery and reduce risk of complications:

- Inspect incisions or wounds routinely, describing changes (e.g., deepening or healing, wound measurements, presence and type of drainage, development of necrosis).
- Practice and instruct client/caregiver(s) in proper hand hygiene and aseptic technique for incisional care **to reduce incidence of contamination and infection.**
- Administer antibiotics as appropriate, and medications to manage postoperative discomforts (e.g., pain, nausea, vomiting) and other concurrent or underlying conditions, such as diabetes, osteoporosis, heart failure, chronic obstructive pulmonary disease (COPD). **Several types of medications may be needed. For example, client may require antibiotics perioperatively, insulin to support tissue repair, or management of chronic pain to improve mobility and tissue recovery.**
- Instruct client/SO in necessary self-care of incisions and specific symptom management. **With short hospital stays, client/SO are usually expected to provide a great deal of postoperative care and monitoring at home.**
- Provide wound care expectations and instructions in verbal and written forms **to facilitate self-care and reduce likelihood of misinterpretation of information when client/SO is providing care at home.**
- Instruct client/SO in routine inspection of incision or wound and to report changes in wound indicative of failure to heal (e.g., deepening wound, local or systemic fever, exudates [noting color, amount, and odor], loss of approximation of wound edges) **to establish comparative baseline and allow for early intervention (e.g., antimicrobial therapy, wound irrigation or packing).**
- Avoid or limit use of plastics or latex materials in wound care, as appropriate. **Can delay healing and cause skin breakdown.**
- Collaborate in treatment and assist with wound care, as indicated. **May require barrier dressings, skin-protective agents, wound vac for open or draining wounds, or surgical débridement.** Refer to/include wound care specialist or stomal therapist, as appropriate, **to address treatment interventions to deal with healing difficulties.**

Information that appears in brackets has been added by the authors to clarify and enhance the use of nursing diagnoses.

- Provide optimal nutrition with adequate protein **to provide a positive nitrogen balance, which aids in healing and contributes to general good health.**
- Encourage adequate fluid and electrolyte intake **to avoid dehydration of tissues and to promote optimal cellular and organ function.**
- Encourage early ambulation and regular exercise **to promote circulation, improve muscle strength and overall endurance, and reduce risks associated with immobility.**
- Recommend pacing (alternating activity with adequate rest periods) **to reduce fatigue and allow weakened muscles and tissues to recuperate.**
- Employ nonpharmacological healing measures, as indicated (e.g., breathing exercises, listening to music, relaxation tapes, biofeedback, hot or cold applications) **to promote relaxation of muscles and tissue healing as well as improve coping and outlook for positive healing experience.**
- Refer for follow-up care, as indicated (e.g., telephone monitoring, home visit, wound care clinic, pain management program).

Nursing Priority No. 4.

To promote wellness (Teaching/Discharge Considerations):

- Demonstrate self-care skills, provide client/SO(s) with health-related information and psychosocial support **to manage symptoms and pain, enhancing well-being.**
- Discuss reality of recovery process in comparison with client's/SO's expectations. **Individuals are often unrealistic regarding energy and time required for healing and own abilities and responsibilities to facilitate process.**
- Involve client/SO(s) in setting incremental goals. **Enhances commitment to plan and reduces likelihood of frustration blocking progress.**
- Refer to physical or occupational therapists, as indicated, **to address exercise program and home-care needs or to identify assistive devices to facilitate independence in ADLs.**
- Identify suppliers for dressings or wound care items and assistive devices as needed.
- Consult dietitian for individual dietary plan **to meet increased nutritional needs that reflect personal situation and resources.**
- Evaluate home situation (e.g., lives alone, bedroom or bathroom on second floor, availability of assistance), where appropriate, **to evaluate for beneficial adjustments, such as**

Information that appears in brackets has been added by the authors to clarify and enhance the use of nursing diagnoses.

moving bedroom to first floor, arranging for commode during recovery, obtaining an in-home emergency call system.

- Discuss alternative placement (e.g., convalescent or rehabilitation center, as appropriate).
- Identify community resources, as indicated (e.g., visiting nurse, home healthcare agency, Meals-on-Wheels, respite care). **Facilitates adjustment to home setting.**
- Recommend support group or self-help program for smoking cessation.
- Refer for counseling or support. **May need additional help to overcome feelings of discouragement, deal with changes in life.**

Documentation Focus

Assessment/Reassessment

- Assessment findings, including wound healing, individual concerns, family involvement, and support factors and availability of resources
- Cultural expectations
- Assistive device use or need

Planning

- Plan of care and who is involved in planning
- Teaching plan

Implementation/Evaluation

- Responses of client/SO(s) to plan, interventions, teaching, and actions performed
- Attainment or progress toward desired outcome(s)
- Modifications to plan of care

Discharge Planning

- Long-range needs and who is responsible for actions to be taken
- Specific referrals made

Sample Nursing Outcomes & Interventions Classifications (NOC/NIC)

NOC—Self-Care: Activities of Daily Living (ADLs)
NIC—Self-Care Assistance

Information that appears in brackets has been added by the authors to clarify and enhance the use of nursing diagnoses.

impaired SWALLOWING

[Diagnostic Division: Food/Fluid]

Definition: Abnormal functioning of the swallowing mechanism associated with deficits in oral, pharyngeal, or esophageal structure or function.

Related Factors

Congenital Deficits

Upper airway anomaly; mechanical obstruction [e.g., edema, tracheostomy tube, tumor]; history of enteral feeding

Neuromuscular impairment [e.g., decreased or absent gag reflex, decreased strength or excursion of muscles involved in mastication, perceptual impairment, facial paralysis]; conditions with significant hypotonia

Respiratory condition; congenital heart disease

Behavioral feeding problem; self-injurious behavior

Failure to thrive; protein-energy malnutrition

Neurological Problems

Nasal or nasopharyngeal cavity defect; oropharynx or upper airway abnormality; laryngeal abnormality/defect; tracheal defect

Esophageal reflux disease; achalasia

Trauma; acquired anatomic defects; cranial nerve involvement

Brain injury (e.g., cerebrovascular impairment, neurological illness, trauma, tumor); neurological problems

Prematurity; developmental delay; cerebral palsy

Defining Characteristics

Subjective

Third Stage: Esophageal

Reports "something stuck"; odynophagia [pain in esophagus on swallowing]

Food refusal; volume limiting

Heartburn; epigastric pain

Nighttime coughing or awakening

Information that appears in brackets has been added by the authors to clarify and enhance the use of nursing diagnoses.

Objective

First Stage: Oral

Inefficient suck or nippling

Prolonged bolus formation; tongue action ineffective in forming bolus; premature entry of bolus

Incomplete lip closure; food pushed out of or falls from mouth

Insufficient chewing

Coughing, choking, or gagging before a swallow

Piecemeal deglutition; abnormal oral phase of swallow study

Inability to clear oral cavity; pooling of bolus in lateral sulci; nasal reflux; drooling

Prolonged meal time with insufficient consumption

Second Stage: Pharyngeal

Food refusal

Alteration in head position; delayed or repetitive swallowing

Inadequate laryngeal elevation; abnormal pharyngeal phase of swallow study

Choking; coughing; gagging sensation; nasal reflux; gurgly voice quality

Fevers of unknown etiology; recurrent pulmonary infection

Third Stage: Esophageal

Difficulty swallowing; abnormal esophageal phase of swallow study

Hyperextension of head [e.g., arching during or after meals]

Repetitive swallowing; bruxism

Unexplained irritability surrounding mealtimes

Acidic-smelling breath; regurgitation; vomitus on pillow; vomiting; hematemesis

Desired Outcomes/Evaluation Criteria—Client Will:

- Pass food and fluid from mouth to stomach safely.
- Maintain adequate hydration as evidenced by good skin turgor, moist mucous membranes, and individually appropriate urine output.
- Achieve and/or maintain desired body weight.

Client/Caregiver Will:

- Verbalize understanding of causative or contributing factors.
- Identify individually appropriate interventions or actions to promote intake and prevent aspiration.

Information that appears in brackets has been added by the authors to clarify and enhance the use of nursing diagnoses.

- Demonstrate feeding methods appropriate to the individual situation.
- Demonstrate emergency measures in the event of choking.

Actions/Interventions

Nursing Priority No. 1.

To assess causative/contributing factors and degree of impairment:

- ∞ Evaluate client's potential for swallowing problems, noting age and medical conditions (e.g., Parkinson's disease, multiple sclerosis, myasthenia gravis, or other neuromuscular conditions). **Swallowing disorders are especially common in the elderly, possibly due to coexistence of variety of neurological, neuromuscular, or other conditions. Infants at risk include those born prematurely or with tracheoesophageal fistula or lip and palate malformation. Persons with traumatic brain injuries often exhibit swallowing impairments, regardless of gender or age.**
- ∞ Determine ability to initiate and sustain effective suck. **Weak suck results in inefficient nippling, suggesting ineffective movement of tongue and mouth muscles, impairing ability to swallow.**
- Assess client's cognitive and sensory-perceptual status. **Sensory awareness, orientation, concentration, motor coordination affect desire and ability to swallow safely and effectively.**
- Note symmetry of facial structures and muscle tone.
- Assess strength and excursion of muscles involved in mastication and swallowing.
- Note voice quality and speech. **Abnormal voice (dysphonia) and abnormal speech patterns (dysarthria) are signs of motor dysfunction of structures involved in oral and pharyngeal swallowing.**
- Inspect oropharyngeal cavity for edema, inflammation, altered integrity of oral mucosa, adequacy of oral hygiene.
- Verify proper fit of dentures, if present.
- Ascertain presence and strength of cough and gag reflex. **Although absence of gag reflex is not necessarily predictive of client's eventual ability to swallow safely, it does increase client's potential for aspiration (overt or silent). Coughing, drooling, double swallowing, decreased ability to move food in mouth, and throat clearing with or after swallowing is indicative of swallowing dysfunction and increases risk for aspiration.**

Information that appears in brackets has been added by the authors to clarify and enhance the use of nursing diagnoses.

- Review medications **that may affect (1) oropharyngeal function (e.g., benzodiazapines, neuroleptics, anticonvulsants, certain sedatives); (2) esophageal function (e.g., nonsteroidal anti-inflammatory agents, iron preparations, tetracycline, calcium channel blockers).**
- Discuss medications that can cause xerostomia (e.g., anticholinergics, opioids, antidepressants, antineoplastics, diuretics), **thus impairing swallowing by means of sedation, pharyngeal weakness, inflammation, dry mouth, and so forth.**
- Note hyperextension of head or arching of neck during or after meals or repetitive swallowing, **suggesting inability to complete swallowing process.**
- Auscultate breath sounds **to evaluate the presence of aspiration.**
- Review laboratory test results for underlying problems (e.g., complete blood count **to screen for infectious or inflammatory conditions** or thyroid or other metabolic and nutritional studies **that can affect swallowing.**
- Prepare for or assist with diagnostic testing of swallowing activity (e.g., reflex cough test, swallowing electromyography, transnasal or esophageal endoscopy, videofluorographic swallow studies; fiber-optic endoscopic examination of swallowing) **to identify the pathophysiology of swallowing disorder.**

Nursing Priority No. 2.

To prevent aspiration and maintain airway patency:

- Identify individual factors that can precipitate aspiration or compromise airway.
- Move client to chair for meals, snacks, and drinks when possible; if client must be in bed, raise head of bed as upright as possible with head in anatomical alignment and slightly flexed forward during feeding. Keep client seated upright or head of bed elevated for 30 to 45 min after feeding, if possible, **to reduce risk of regurgitation or aspiration.**
- Instruct client to cough and expectorate **when secretion management is of concern.**
- Have suction equipment available during initial feeding attempts and as indicated. Suction oral cavity if client cannot clear secretions **to prevent aspiration.**
- Teach client self-suction when appropriate (e.g., drooling, frequent choking, structural changes in mouth or pharynx. **Promotes airway safety and independence and sense of control with managing secretions.**

Information that appears in brackets has been added by the authors to clarify and enhance the use of nursing diagnoses.

Nursing Priority No. 3.

To enhance swallowing ability to meet fluid and caloric body requirements:

- Refer to surgeon, gastroenterologist or neurologist as indicated **for treatment (e.g., reconstructive facial surgery, esophageal dilatation) that may result in improved swallowing.**
- Refer to speech/language pathologist **to identify specific techniques to enhance client efforts and safety measures.**
- Encourage a rest period before meals **to minimize fatigue.**
- Provide analgesics prior to feeding, as indicated, **to enhance comfort, being cautious to avoid decreasing awareness or sensory perception.**
- Focus client's attention on feeding and swallowing activity. Decrease environmental stimuli and talking, **which may be distracting or promote choking during feeding.**
- Determine food preferences of client **to incorporate as possible, enhancing intake.** Present foods in an appealing, attractive manner.
- Ensure temperature (hot or cold versus tepid) of foods and fluid, **which will stimulate sensory receptors.**
- Provide a consistency of food and fluid that is most easily swallowed. **Risk of choking or aspiration is reduced when food can be formed into a bolus before swallowing, such as gelatin desserts prepared with less water than usual; pudding and custard or liquids are thickened (addition of thickening agent, or yogurt, cream soups prepared with less water); thinned purees (hot cereal with added water); thick drinks, such as nectars; fruit juices that have been frozen into "slush" consistency (thin fluids are most difficult to control); medium-soft boiled or scrambled eggs; canned fruit; soft-cooked vegetables.**
- Avoid milk products and chocolate, **which may thicken oral secretions.**
- Feed one consistency and/or texture of food at a time.
- Place food in unaffected side of client's mouth (**when one side of the mouth is affected by condition, e.g., hemiplegia),** and have client use tongue to assist with moving food bolus to swallowing position.
- Manage size of bites (**e.g., small bites of 1/2 tsp or less are usually easier to swallow).** Use a teaspoon or small spoon **to encourage smaller bites.** Cut all solid foods into small pieces.

Information that appears in brackets has been added by the authors to clarify and enhance the use of nursing diagnoses.

- Place food midway in oral cavity **to adequately trigger the swallowing reflex.**
- Provide cognitive cues (e.g., remind client to chew and swallow as indicated) **to enhance concentration and performance of swallowing sequence.** Focus attention on feeding and swallowing activity by decreasing environmental stimuli, **which may be distracting during feeding. Also, if client is talking or laughing while eating, risk of aspiration is increased.**
- Massage the laryngopharyngeal musculature (sides of trachea and neck) gently **to stimulate swallowing.**
- Observe oral cavity after each bite and have client check around cheeks with tongue for remaining food. Remove food if unable to swallow.
- Incorporate client's eating style and pace when feeding **to avoid fatigue and frustration with process.**
- Allow ample time for eating (feeding).
- Remain with client during meal to reduce anxiety and offer assistance.
- Use a glass with a nose cut-out **to avoid posterior head tilting while drinking.** Refrain from pouring liquid into the mouth or "washing food down" with liquid.
- Monitor intake, output, and body weight to evaluate adequacy of fluid and caloric intake.
- Provide positive feedback for client's efforts.
- Provide oral hygiene following each feeding.
- Consider tube feedings or parenteral solutions, as indicated, **for the client unable to achieve adequate nutritional intake.**
- Consult with dysphagia specialist or rehabilitation team, as indicated.
- Refer to lactation counselor or support group (e.g., La Leche League) **for breastfeeding guidance.**
- Refer to NDs ineffective Breastfeeding; ineffective Infant Feeding Pattern, for additional interventions for infants.

Nursing Priority No. 4.

To promote wellness (Teaching/Discharge Considerations):

- Consult with nutritionist **to establish optimum dietary plan.**
- Place medication in gelatin, jelly, or puddings. Consult with pharmacist **to determine if pills may be crushed or if liquids or capsules are available.**
- Assist client and/or SO(s) in learning specific feeding techniques and swallowing exercises.

Information that appears in brackets has been added by the authors to clarify and enhance the use of nursing diagnoses.

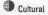

- Encourage continuation of facial exercise program **to maintain or improve muscle strength.**
- Instruct client and/or SO(s) in emergency measures in event of choking **to prevent aspiration or more serious complications.**
- Recommend avoiding food intake within 3 hr of bedtime, eliminating alcohol and caffeine intake, reducing weight if needed, using stress-reduction techniques, and elevating head of bed during sleep **to limit potential for gastric reflux and aspiration.**
- Establish routine schedule for monitoring weight.
- Refer to ND risk for imbalanced Nutrition: less than body requirements.

Documentation Focus

Assessment/Reassessment

- Individual findings, including degree and characteristics of impairment, current weight and recent changes
- Nutritional status
- Effects on lifestyle and socialization

Planning

- Plan of care and who is involved in planning
- Teaching plan

Implementation/Evaluation

- Response to interventions, teaching, and actions performed
- Attainment or progress toward desired outcome(s)
- Modifications to plan of care

Discharge Planning

- Long-term needs and who is responsible for actions to be taken
- Available resources and specific referrals made

Sample Nursing Outcomes & Interventions Classifications (NOC/NIC)

NOC—Swallowing Status
NIC—Swallowing Therapy

Information that appears in brackets has been added by the authors to clarify and enhance the use of nursing diagnoses.

risk for THERMAL INJURY

[Diagnostic Division: Safety]

Definition: Vulnerable to extreme temperature damage to skin and mucous membranes, which may compromise health.

Risk Factors

Alterative in cognitive functioning; neuromuscular impairment, neuropathy
Extremes of age; inadequate supervision
Extremes of environmental temperature; inadequate protective clothing (e.g., flame-retardant sleepwear, glovers, ear coverings)
Fatigue; inattentiveness
Insufficient knowledge of safety precautions (patient, caregiver); unsafe environment
Intoxication (alcohol, drugs); smoking
Treatment regimen

NOTE: A risk diagnosis is not evidenced by signs and symptoms, as the problem has not occurred; rather, nursing interventions are directed at prevention.

Desired Outcomes/Evaluation Criteria—Client/Caregivers Will:

- Be free of damage to skin or mucous membranes associated with extreme temperatures.
- Demonstrate behaviors, lifestyle changes to reduce risk factors and protect from injury.

Actions/Interventions

This ND is a compilation of a number of situations that can result in injury. Refer to specific NDs, such as Hypothermia; risk for Injury; impaired Skin Integrity; impaired Tissue Integrity; risk for Trauma, as appropriate, for more specific interventions.

Nursing Priority No. 1.

To identify causative/precipitating factors related to risk:

- Identify client at risk (e.g., chronic illness conditions with weakness or prolonged immobility; acute or chronic confu-

Information that appears in brackets has been added by the authors to clarify and enhance the use of nursing diagnoses.

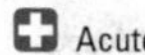

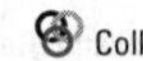

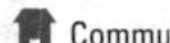

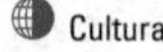

sion, mental illness, dementia, head injury; use of multiple medications; use of alcohol or other drugs; cultural, familial, and socioeconomic factors adversely affecting lifestyle and home; exposure to environmental chemicals).

- Note chronological and developmental age of client. **Infants, young children, disabled, debilitated, aged, or impaired individuals are not able to protect themselves and may not recognize and/or react appropriately in dangerous situations.**
- Evaluate client's/SO's level of cognition, competence, decision-making ability and independence.
- Ascertain if client is using alcohol/other drugs or medications **that could impair ability to act in best interest of self or others.**
- Evaluate client's lifestyle practices, noting reports of risk-prone behavior (e.g., smoking in bed, failure to use safety equipment when working with chemicals, allowing child to play with matches, unprotected exposure to sun or cold environment) **that can place client or others at high risk for injury.**
- Ascertain knowledge of safety needs and injury prevention, as well as motivation to prevent injury. **Information may reveal areas of misinformation, lack of knowledge, need for teaching.**

Nursing Priority No. 2.

To assist client/caregiver to reduce or correct individual risk factors:

- Provide client/significant other (SO) information regarding client's specific situation and consequences of continuing unsafe behaviors **to enhance decision making, clarify expectations and individual needs.**
- Review client's physical and psychological abilities or limitations **to determine adaptations that may be required by current situation.**
- Provide for client's safety while in facility care. **This includes a wide variety of interventions (e.g., apply hot and cold treatments judiciously; prevent/monitor smoking; exercise care in use of all electrical equipment in presence of oxygen; supervise bath temperature in confused individuals, young children, or elderly adults; etc.).**
- Be mindful of skin safety issues during surgical procedures:

  Conduct a fire risk assessment at beginning of each surgical procedure and continuously monitor for changes in risk during procedure. **The highest-risk procedures involve**

Information that appears in brackets has been added by the authors to clarify and enhance the use of nursing diagnoses.

an ignition source (such as electrocautery device), delivery of supplemental oxygen, and the operation of the ignition source near the oxygen (e.g., head, neck, or upper chest surgery).

Provide supplemental oxygen safely, using the lowest concentration possible **to reduce amount of oxygen flowing into surgical field.**

Verify electrical safety of equipment including intact cords, grounds, and medical engineering verification labels.

Place dispersive electrode (electrocautery pad) over largest available muscle mass closest to surgical site, ensuring its contact **to prevent electrical burns.**

Ascertain that alcohol-containing skin prep solutions are not pooled under client or in surgical drapes and had sufficient drying time.

Protect surrounding skin and tissues appropriately when laser equipment is used in surgical procedures. **Prevents inadvertent skin integrity disruption, hair ignition, and adjacent anatomy injury in area of laser beam use.**

Apply eye protection before laser activation. **Eye protection for specific laser wavelength must be used to prevent injury.**

- Implement skin care protocol for client receiving radiation therapy:

Assess skin frequently for side effects of therapy; note breakdown and delayed wound healing. Emphasize importance of reporting open areas to caregiver. **A reddening and/or tanning effect (radiation dermatitis) may develop within the field of radiation.**

Avoid rubbing the skin or use of soap, lotions, creams, ointments, powders, or deodorants on area; avoid applying heat or attempting to wash off marks/tattoos placed on skin to pinpoint location for radiation therapy. May increase dermal reaction.

- Avoid application of lotion or oils to skin of infants receiving phototherapy for hyperbilirubinemia **to prevent dermal injury** and cover male groin with small pad **to protect testes from heat-related injury.**
- Provide or instruct in proper care of skin surfaces during exposure to very cold or hot weather. **Although everyone is at risk for frostbite or sunburn, individuals with impaired sensation or cognition and infants/young children require special attention to deal with extremes in weather.**
- Discuss importance of self-monitoring of factors that can contribute to occurrence of injury (e.g., fatigue, anger). **Client/**

Information that appears in brackets has been added by the authors to clarify and enhance the use of nursing diagnoses.

SO may be able to modify risk through monitoring of actions especially during times when client is likely to be highly stressed.

- Perform home assessment, if indicated, **to address safety issues. Concerns vary widely and may include evaluation of fire alarms or extinguisher function; safe use of oxygen; checking hot water temperature for elderly confused person, or obtaining medical alert device or home health service, etc.**
- Review specific employment concerns or worksite issues and needs (e.g., properly fitting safety equipment, regular use of safety glasses or goggles, safe storage of hazardous substances).
- Discuss need for and sources of supervision (e.g., before- and after-school programs for children, elder day programs, homecare assistance) **when client or care provider is unable or unwilling to attend to safety concerns.**

Nursing Priority No. 3.

To promote wellness (Teaching/Discharge Criteria):

- Identify individual needs and resources for safety education.
- Prevent burn (flame, scalding, chemical, electrical, sunburn) injuries:

Install smoke alarms in kitchen, in every sleeping area, and on every floor of home.

Keep space heaters away from flammable materials and from at-risk persons.

Check all fuel-burning appliances including fireplaces for proper function.

Store combustibles away from all heat-producing appliances.

Prepare and practice an emergency escape plan.

Avoid smoking in bed. Get rid of used cigarettes carefully.

Prevent small children from playing with matches or near open flame or stove.

Turn handles of pots and pans toward side of stove or use back burners.

Set the temperature on water heater to 120°F or use the "low-medium" setting.

Test water temperature before allowing child/impaired person into tub or shower.

Use cool-water humidifiers instead of hot-steam vaporizers.

Store fireworks, cleaning supplies, and other chemicals out of the reach of children.

Wear gloves, safety glasses, and other protective clothing when handling chemicals.

Information that appears in brackets has been added by the authors to clarify and enhance the use of nursing diagnoses.

Avoid storing chemicals in food or drink containers; store in original containers with intact labels.

Check electrical appliances for proper function and follow manufacturer's safety instructions. Discard frayed or damaged electrical cords **to reduce risk of electrical burns.** ***Note:*** **Most electrical injuries that occur in the home are low-voltage burns and almost exclusively involve either the hands or oral cavity.**

Use child safety plugs in all electrical outlets.

Avoid using electrical appliances while showering or wet.

Avoid lengthy or unnecessary sun exposure/ultraviolet tanning, especially with specific disease conditions or treatments (e.g., systemic lupus, tetracycline or psychotropic drug use, radiation therapy) **to reduce risk of sunburn.**

Advise use of high sun protection factor (SPF) sunblock or sunscreen, particularly on young child and/or client with fair skin (prone to burn).

- Provide telephone numbers and other contact numbers as individually indicated (e.g., fire, police, physician).
- Refer to community resources as indicated (e.g., substance recovery, anger management, and parenting classes) **to address conditions that could exacerbate risk of injury to self or others.**
- Refer to or assist with community education programs **to increase awareness of safety measures and available resources.**
- Identify emergency escape plans and routes for home and community to be **prepared in the event of natural or man-made disaster (e.g., fire, toxic chemical release).**

Documentation Focus

Assessment/Reassessment

- Individual risk factors identified
- Client's concerns or difficulty making and following through with plan

Planning

- Plan of care and who is involved in planning
- Teaching plan

Implementation/Evaluation

- Response to interventions, teaching, and actions performed
- Attainment or progress toward outcomes

Information that appears in brackets has been added by the authors to clarify and enhance the use of nursing diagnoses.

Discharge Planning

- Referrals to other resources
- Long-term need and who is responsible for actions

Sample Nursing Outcomes & Interventions Classifications (NOC/NIC)

NOC—Tissue Integrity: Skin & Mucous Membrane
NIC—Skin Surveillance

ineffective THERMOREGULATION

[Diagnostic Division: Safety]

Definition: Temperature fluctuation between hypothermia and hyperthermia.

Related Factors

Trauma; illness
Extremes of age
Fluctuating environmental temperature

Defining Characteristics

Objective

Fluctuations in body temperature above and below the normal range
Tachycardia; hypertension; increase in respiratory rate
Reduction in body temperature below normal range; skin cool to touch; moderate pallor; mild shivering; piloerection; cyanotic nailbeds; slow capillary refill
Increase in body temperature above normal range; skin warm to touch; flushed skin; seizures

Desired Outcomes/Evaluation Criteria—Client/Caregiver Will:

- Verbalize understanding of individual factors and appropriate interventions.
- Demonstrate techniques and behaviors to correct underlying condition or situation.
- Maintain body temperature within normal limits.

Information that appears in brackets has been added by the authors to clarify and enhance the use of nursing diagnoses.

Actions/Interventions

Nursing Priority No. 1.

To identify causative/contributing factors:

- Note extremes of age (e.g., premature neonate, young child, or aging adult) **as this can directly impact ability to maintain or regulate body temperature.**
- Obtain history concerning present symptoms, correlate with previous episodes or family history, and diagnostic studies. **Thermoregulation is a controlled process that maintains the body's core temperature in the range at which most biochemical processes work best (99°F–99.6°F [37.2°C–37.6°C]). Exercise, behavioral impulses, metabolic and hormonal changes influence changes in body temperature, leading to loss or gain of heat.**
- Identify individual factor(s) or underlying condition (e.g., environmental exposure, infectious process, brain injury, effects of drugs or toxins, salt or water depletion, obesity, confined to bed, drug overdose). **Thermoregulation is affected in two ways: (1) endogenous factors (via diseases or conditions of body/organ systems that affect temperature homeostasis) and (2) exogenous factors (via environmental exposures, medications, and nutrition).**
- Monitor laboratory studies (e.g., tests indicative of infection, thyroid or other endocrine tests, organ damage, drug screens) **to identify potential internal causes of temperature imbalances.**

Nursing Priority No. 2.

To assist with measures to correct/treat underlying cause:

- Monitor temperature by appropriate route (e.g., tympanic, rectal, oral), using the same site and device over time and noting variation from client's usual or normal temperature.
- Have cooling and warming equipment and supplies readily available during childbirth and following procedures or surgery.
- Maintain ambient temperature in comfortable range **to prevent or compensate for client's heat production or heat loss (e.g., may need to add or remove clothing or blankets, avoid drafts, reduce or increase room temperature and humidity).**
- Review home management of temperature fluctuations in special population (e.g., newborn infant, person with spinal cord injury, frail elder). **Measures could include use of heating**

Information that appears in brackets has been added by the authors to clarify and enhance the use of nursing diagnoses.

pads, ice bag, radiant heaters or fans; adding or removing clothing or blankets; cool or warm liquids and bath water; occlusive wrap in the delivery room, skin-to-skin contact in newborn; and so forth.

- Initiate emergent and/or immediate interventions such as cooling or warming measures, fluids, electrolytes, nutrients, and medications (e.g., antipyretics, antibiotics, neoplastics), **to restore or maintain body temperature within normal range,** as indicated in NDs Hypothermia; Hyperthermia; risk for imbalanced Body Temperature.
- Administer fluids, electrolytes, and medications, as appropriate, **to restore or maintain body and organ function.**

Nursing Priority No. 3.

To promote wellness (Teaching/Discharge Considerations):

- Review causative or related factors and risk factors, if appropriate, with client/significant other (SO). **Provides information about what, if any, measures can be implemented to protect client from harm or limit potential for problems associated with ineffective thermoregulation.**
- Discuss appropriate dressing with client/caregivers, such as:

  Wearing layers of clothing that can be removed or added as needed

  Donning hat and gloves in cold weather

  Using water-resistant outer gear to protect from wet weather chill

  Dressing in light, loose protective clothing in hot weather
- Review home management of temperature fluctuations in special population (e.g., newborn infant, person with spinal cord injury [SCI], frail elder). **Measures could include use of heating pads, ice bags; radiant heaters or fans; adding or removing clothing or blankets, cool or warm liquids and bath water; occlusive wrap in the delivery room, skin-to-skin contact in newborn, and so forth.**
- Provide oral and written information concerning client's disease processes, current therapies, and postdischarge precautions regarding hypothermia or hyperthermia, as appropriate to situation. **Allows for review of instructions for early intervention and implementation of preventive or corrective measures.**
- Refer to teaching section in NDs risk for imbalanced Body Temperature, Hypothermia, or Hyperthermia, for related interventions as appropriate.

Information that appears in brackets has been added by the authors to clarify and enhance the use of nursing diagnoses.

Documentation Focus

Assessment/Reassessment

- Individual findings, including nature of problem, degree of impairment, or fluctuations in temperature

Planning

- Plan of care and who is involved in planning
- Teaching plan

Implementation/Evaluation

- Responses to interventions, teaching, and actions performed
- Attainment or progress toward desired outcome(s)
- Modifications to plan of care

Discharge Planning

- Long-term needs and who is responsible for actions to be taken
- Specific referrals made

Sample Nursing Outcomes & Interventions Classifications (NOC/NIC)

NOC—Thermoregulation
NIC—Temperature Regulation

impaired TISSUE INTEGRITY and risk for impaired TISSUE INTEGRITY

[Diagnostic Division: Safety]

Definition: impaired Tissue Integrity: Damage to the mucous membrane, cornea, integumentary system, muscular fascia, muscle, tendon, bone cartilage, joint capsule, and/or ligament.

Definition: risk for impaired Tissue Integrity: Vulnerable to damage to the mucous membrane, cornea, integumentary system, muscular fascia, muscle, tendon, bone cartilage, joint capsule, and/or ligament, which may compromise health.

Related and Risk Factors

Alteration in metabolism; imbalanced nutritional state (e.g., obesity, emaciation)

Information that appears in brackets has been added by the authors to clarify and enhance the use of nursing diagnoses.

Alteration in sensation; peripheral neuropathy; impaired mobility
Chemical injury agent (e.g., burn, capsaicin, methylene chloride, mustard agent); high-voltage power supply; mechanical factor
Excessive fluid volume; impaired circulation; insufficient fluid volume
Extremes of age
Extremes of environmental temperature; humidity
Insufficient knowledge about maintaining or protecting tissue integrity
Pharmaceutical agent
Radiation; surgical procedure
[Infection]

> **NOTE:** A risk diagnosis is not evidenced by signs and symptoms, as the problem has not occurred; rather, nursing interventions are directed at prevention.

Defining Characteristics (impaired Tissue Integrity)

Objective

Damaged or destroyed tissue

> **NOTE:** In reviewing this ND, it is apparent there is much overlap with other diagnoses. We have chosen to present generalized interventions. Although there are commonalities to injury situations, we suggest that the reader refer to other primary diagnoses as indicated, such as risk for Bleeding; risk for Contamination; risk for Falls; ineffective Health Maintenance; impaired Home Maintenance; risk for Infection; risk for Injury; impaired physical Mobility; impaired/risk for impaired Parenting; ineffective Protection; risk for Poisoning; impaired/risk for impaired Skin/Tissue Integrity; delayed/risk for delayed Surgical Recovery; risk for Pressure Ulcer; ineffective Tissue Perfusion; risk for Trauma; risk for self and other-directed Violence; for additional interventions.

Desired Outcomes/Evaluation Criteria—Client/Caregiver Will:

- Verbalize understanding of condition and causative **or risk** factors.

Information that appears in brackets has been added by the authors to clarify and enhance the use of nursing diagnoses.

- Identify interventions appropriate for specific condition.
- Demonstrate behaviors and lifestyle changes to promote healing and prevent complications or recurrence.
- Display progressive improvement in wound or lesion healing.

Actions/Interventions

Nursing Priority No. 1.

To identify causative/contributing **or risk** factors:

- Identify underlying conditions or pathology. Assess for individual factors **that can result in tissue damage or can impede healing; for example: (1) trauma that causes internal tissue damage (e.g., burns, high-velocity and penetrating trauma); fractures (especially long-bone fractures) with hemorrhage; (2) external pressures (e.g., from tight dressings, splints or casting, burn eschar); (3) immobility (e.g., long-term bedrest, traction/cast); (4) presence of conditions affecting peripheral circulation and sensation (e.g., atherosclerosis, diabetes, venous insufficiency); (5) lifestyle factors (e.g., smoking, obesity, and sedentary lifestyle); (6) use of medications (e.g., anticoagulants, corticosteroids, immunosuppressives, antineoplastics) that adversely affect healing; (7) malnutrition (deprives the body of protein and calories required for cell growth and repair); and (8) dehydration (impairs transport of oxygen and nutrients).**
- Note age, developmental stage, and gender. **Children, young adults, elderly persons, and men are at greater risk for injury, which may reflect client's ability or desire to protect self, and influences choice of interventions or teaching.**
- Determine mechanism of traumatic injury where indicated (e.g., chemical burn affecting skin, mucous membranes; electrical/high-voltage injury, car crash, gunshot wound; environmental exposure to toxins or extreme temperatures). **Suggests initial treatment options and potential for tissue damage. Note: information should include type of injuring agent (e.g., acid or base with route and length of exposure to offending agent; fire; penetration of contaminated object; possibility of coexisting injuries).**
- Note race or ethnic background, familial history for genetic, sociocultural, and religious factors **that may make individual vulnerable to particular condition or impact treatment.**
- Evaluate skin and mucous membranes for hydration status; note presence and degree of edema (1+ to 4+), urine characteristics and output. **Determines presence of circulatory**

Information that appears in brackets has been added by the authors to clarify and enhance the use of nursing diagnoses.

or metabolic imbalances resulting in fluid deficit or overload that can adversely affect cell or tissue health and organ function. Note: Edematous tissues are prone to breakdown. Refer to NDs risk for imbalanced Fluid Volume, impaired Skin Integrity, risk for Pressure Ulcer.

- Examine eyes for conjunctivitis, hemorrhage, burns, abrasions or lacerations as indicated. Note reports of dry, scratchy eye, vision impairment or pain. **May indicate injury to eye tissues requiring more intensive evaluation and interventions.** (Refer to ND risk for Dry Eye.)
- Determine nutritional status and impact of malnutrition on situation (e.g., pressure points on emaciated and/or elderly client, obesity, lack of activity, slow healing or failure to heal).
- Note evidence of deep organ or tissue involvement in client with wound **(e.g., draining fistula through the integumentary and subcutaneous tissue may signal a bone infection).**
- Note use of prosthetic, diagnostic, or external devices (e.g., artificial limbs, contacts, dentures, endotracheal airways, indwelling catheters, esophageal dilators), **which can cause pressure on/injure delicate tissues or provide entry point for infectious agents.**
- Assess blood supply and sensation (nerve damage) of affected area.
- Note poor hygiene or health practices (e.g., lack of cleanliness, frequent use of enemas, poor dental care) **that may be impacting tissue health.**
- Assess environmental location of home and work or school, as well as recent travel. **Some areas of a country or city may be more susceptible to certain disease conditions or environmental pollutants.**
- Evaluate pulses, calculate ankle-brachial index **to evaluate potential for impairment of circulation to lower extremities. Result less than 0.9 indicates need for close monitoring or more aggressive intervention (e.g., tighter blood glucose and weight control in diabetic client).**
- Refer to NDs (dependent on individual situation) risk for peripheral Neurovascular Dysfunction; risk for Perioperative Positioning Injury; impaired physical/bed Mobility; impaired Skin Integrity; [disturbed visual Sensory Perception]; ineffective peripheral Tissue Perfusion; risk for Trauma; risk for Infection **for related interventions.**

Information that appears in brackets has been added by the authors to clarify and enhance the use of nursing diagnoses.

Nursing Priority No. 2.

To assess degree of impairment: (impaired Tissue Integrity)

- Obtain a history of condition (e.g., pressure, venous, or diabetic wound; eye or oral lesions), including whether condition is acute or recurrent; original site/characteristics of wound; duration of problem and changes that have occurred over time.
- Assess skin and tissues, bony prominences, pressure areas and wounds **for comparative baseline:**

  Note color, texture, and turgor.

  Assess areas of least pigmentation for color changes (e.g., sclera, conjunctiva, nailbeds, buccal mucosa, tongue, palms, and soles of feet).

  Note presence, location, and degree of edema.

  Record size (depth/width), color, location, temperature, texture of wounds or lesions.

  Determine degree and depth of injury or damage to integumentary system (involves epidermis, dermis, and/or underlying tissues), extent of tunneling or undermining, if present.

  Classify burns. Use appropriate measuring tool (e.g., Braden or similar) and staging (I to IV) for ulcers.

  Document with drawings and/or photograph wound, lesion(s), burns, as appropriate.

  Observe for other distinguishing characteristics of surrounding tissue (e.g., exudate; granulation; cyanosis or pallor; tight, shiny skin).

  Describe wound drainage (e.g., amount, color, odor).
- Assist with diagnostic procedures (e.g., x-rays, imaging scans, biopsies, débridement). **May be necessary to determine extent of impairment.**
- Obtain specimens of exudate and lesions for Gram stain, culture and sensitivity, and so forth, when appropriate.
- Determine psychological effects of condition on client/SO(s). **Can be devastating for client's body or self-image and esteem, especially if condition is severe, disfiguring, or chronic, as well as costly and burdensome for SO(s)/caregiver.**

Nursing Priority No. 3.

To correct/minimize impairment and to facilitate healing:

- Inspect lesions or wounds daily, or as appropriate, for changes (e.g., signs of infection, complications, or healing). **Promotes timely intervention and revision of plan of care.**

Information that appears in brackets has been added by the authors to clarify and enhance the use of nursing diagnoses.

- Modify or eliminate factors contributing to condition, if possible. Assist with treatment of underlying condition(s), as appropriate.
- Provide or encourage optimum nutrition (including adequate protein, lipids, calories, trace minerals, and multivitamins) **to promote tissue health/healing** and adequate hydration **to reduce and replenish cellular water loss and enhance circulation.**
- Encourage adequate periods of rest and sleep **to limit metabolic demands, maximize energy available for healing, and meet comfort needs.**
- Provide or assist with oral care (e.g., teaching oral and dental hygiene, avoiding extremes of hot or cold, changing position of endotrachial and nasogastric tubes, lubricating lips) **to prevent damage to mucous membranes.** Refer to ND, impaired oral Mucous Membranes for related interventions.
- Promote early and ongoing mobility. Assist with or encourage position changes, active or passive and assistive exercises in immobile client **to promote circulation and prevent excessive tissue pressure.**
- Collaborate with other healthcare providers (e.g., physician, burn specialist, ophthalmologist, infection or wound specialist, ostomy nurse), as indicated, **to assist with developing plan of care for problematic or potentially serious wounds.**
- Apply appropriate barrier dressings or wound coverings (e.g., semipermeable, occlusive, wet-to-dry, hydrocolloid, hydrogel, polyacrylate moist wound dressing), drainage appliances, and skin-protective agents for open or draining wounds and stomas **to protect the wound and surrounding tissues from excoriating secretions or drainage and to enhance healing.**
- Practice aseptic technique for cleansing, dressing, or medicating lesions. **Reduces risk of infection and/or failure to heal.**
- Use appropriate catheter (e.g., peripheral or central venous) when infusing anticancer or other toxic drugs, and ascertain that IV liquid is patent and infusing well **to prevent infiltration and extravasation with resulting tissue damage.**
- Monitor for correct placement of tubes, catheters, and other devices; assess skin tissues around these devices for effects of tape or fasteners or pressure from the devices **to prevent damage to skin and tissues as a result of pressure, friction, or shear forces.**
- Develop regularly timed repositioning schedule for client with mobility and sensation impairments, using adequate personnel

Information that appears in brackets has been added by the authors to clarify and enhance the use of nursing diagnoses.

and assistive devices as needed; encourage and assist with periodic weight shifts for client in chair **to reduce stress on pressure points and encourage circulation to tissues.**

- Provide appropriate mattress (e.g., foam, flotation, alternating pressure, or air mattress) and appropriate padding devices (e.g., foam boots, heel protectors, ankle rolls), when indicated.
- Limit use of plastic material (e.g., rubber sheet, plastic-backed linen savers) and remove wet or wrinkled linens promptly. **Moisture potentiates skin and underlying tissues, increasing risk of breakdown and infection.**
- Provide or instruct in proper care of extremities during cold or hot weather. **Individuals with impaired sensation or young children/individuals unable to verbalize discomfort require special attention to deal with extremes in weather.**
- Protect client from environmental hazards when vision or hearing or cognitive deficits impact safety.
- Advise smoking cessation and refer for assistance or support, if indicated. **Smoking causes vasoconstriction that interferes with healing.**
- Monitor laboratory studies (e.g., complete blood count, electrolytes, glucose, cultures) **for changes indicative of healing or presence of infection, complications.**

Nursing Priority No. 4.

To promote wellness (Teaching/Discharge Considerations):

- Encourage verbalizations of feelings and expectations regarding condition and potential for recovery of structure and function.
- Help client and family identify effective successful coping mechanisms and implement them **to reduce pain or discomfort and to improve quality of life.**
- Discuss importance of early detection and reporting of changes in condition or any unusual physical discomforts or changes in pain characteristics. **Promotes early intervention and reduces potential for complications.**
- Educate the client/caregivers on proper safety precautions regarding hazardous materials, as indicated:

  Inform client/caregivers of various substances in the home that are potentially dangerous.

  Counsel parents on how to keep chemicals out of the reach of children, cognitively impaired person.

  Consult with local social services agency to evaluate child's home situation.

Information that appears in brackets has been added by the authors to clarify and enhance the use of nursing diagnoses.

Refer client to appropriate agencies for adequate training and protective equipment to protect against hazardous materials/agents in the community or employment setting.

- Emphasize need for adequate nutritional and fluid intake **to optimize healing potential.**
- Instruct in dressing changes (technique and frequency) and proper disposal of soiled dressings **to prevent spread of infectious agent.**
- Review medical regimen (e.g., proper use of topical sprays, creams, ointments, soaks, or irrigations) **to facilitate tissue healing and prevent complications associated with lack of knowledge about maintaining tissue integrity.**
- Emphasize importance of follow-up care, as appropriate (e.g., diabetic foot care clinic, wound care specialist or clinic, enterostomal therapist).
- Identify required changes in lifestyle, occupation, or environment **necessitated by limitations imposed by condition or to avoid causative factors.**
- Refer to community or governmental resources, as indicated (e.g., Public Health Department, Occupational Safety and Health Administration [OSHA], American Burn Association).

Documentation Focus

Assessment/Reassessment

- Individual findings, including history of condition, characteristics of wound or lesion, and evidence of other organ or tissue involvement
- Impact on functioning and lifestyle
- Availability and use of resources

Planning

- Plan of care and who is involved in planning
- Teaching plan

Implementation/Evaluation

- Responses to interventions, teaching, and actions performed
- Attainment or progress toward desired outcome(s)
- Modifications to plan of care

Discharge Planning

- Long-term needs and who is responsible for actions to be taken
- Specific referrals made

Information that appears in brackets has been added by the authors to clarify and enhance the use of nursing diagnoses.

Sample Nursing Outcomes & Interventions Classifications (NOC/NIC)

NOC—Tissue Integrity: Skin & Mucous Membranes
NIC—Wound Care

ineffective peripheral TISSUE PERFUSION and risk for ineffective peripheral TISSUE PERFUSION

[Diagnostic Division: Circulation]

Definition: ineffective Tissue Perfusion: Decrease in blood circulation to the periphery that may compromise health.

Definition: risk for ineffective Tissue Perfusion: Vulnerable to a decrease in blood circulation to the periphery, which may compromise health.

Related Factors (ineffective peripheral Tissue Perfusion):

Diabetes mellitus; hypertension
Insufficient knowledge of disease process or aggravating factors (e.g., smoking, sedentary lifestyle, trauma, obesity, salt intake, immobility)
Sedentary lifestyle; smoking

Risk Factors (in addition to above factors)

Endovascular procedure; trauma
Excessive sodium intake
Insufficient knowledge of risk factors

NOTE: A risk diagnosis is not evidenced by signs and symptoms, as the problem has not occurred; rather, nursing interventions are directed at prevention.

Defining Characteristics (ineffective peripheral Tissue Perfusion)

Subjective

Extremity pain; intermittent claudication
Paresthesia

Information that appears in brackets has been added by the authors to clarify and enhance the use of nursing diagnoses.

Objective

Decrease in or absence of peripheral pulses; ankle-brachial index <0.90; decrease in blood pressure in extremities; femoral bruit

Alteration in skin characteristics (e.g., color, elasticity, hair, moisture, nails, sensation, temperature)

Skin color pales with limb elevation; capillary refill time >3 seconds; color does not return to lowered limb after 1 minute leg elevation

Decrease in pain free distances achieved in the six-minute walk test; distance in the 6-minute walk test below normal range (400 m to 700 m in adults)

Edema

Alteration in motor function

Delay in peripheral wound healing; [ulcerations]

Desired Outcomes/Evaluation Criteria—Client Will:

- Demonstrate increased perfusion as individually appropriate (e.g., skin warm and dry, peripheral pulses present and strong, absence of edema, free of pain or discomfort).
- Verbalize understanding of risk factors or condition, therapy regimen, side effects of medications, and when to contact healthcare provider.
- Demonstrate behaviors and lifestyle changes to improve circulation (e.g., engage in regular exercise, cessation of smoking, weight reduction, disease management).

Actions/Interventions

Nursing Priority No. 1.

To assess causative/contributing factors:

- Note current situation or presence of conditions (e.g., congestive heart failure, lung disorders, major trauma, septic or hypovolemic shock, coagulopathies, sickle cell anemia) **affecting systemic circulation/perfusion.**
- Determine history of conditions associated with thrombus or emboli (e.g., problems with coronary or cerebral circulation, stroke; high-velocity trauma with fractures, abdominal or orthopedic surgery, long periods of immobility; inflammatory diseases; chronic lung disease; diabetes with coexisting peripheral vascular disease; estrogen therapy, cancer and cancer

Information that appears in brackets has been added by the authors to clarify and enhance the use of nursing diagnoses.

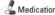

therapies, presence of central venous catheters) **to identify client at higher risk for venous stasis, vessel wall injury, and hypercoagulability.**

- Identify presence of high-risk factors or conditions (e.g., smoking, uncontrolled hypertension, obesity, pregnancy, pelvic tumor, paralysis, hypercholesterolemia, varicose veins, arthritis, sepsis) **that place client at greater risk for developing peripheral vascular disease (including arterial blockage and chronic venous insufficiency) with associated complications.**
- Note location of restrictive clothing, pressure dressings, circular wraps, cast, or traction device **that may restrict circulation to limb.**
- Ascertain impact of condition on functioning and lifestyle. **For example, leg pain may restrict ambulation or person may develop skin ulceration and healing problems that seriously impact quality of life.**

Nursing Priority No. 2.

To evaluate degree of impairment: (ineffective peripheral Tissue Perfusion)

- Assess skin color, temperature, moisture, and whether changes are widespread or localized. **Helps in determining location and type of perfusion problem.**
- Compare skin temperature and color with other limb when assessing extremity circulation. **Helps differentiate type of problem (e.g., deep redness in both hands triggered by vibrating machinery is associated with Raynaud's, while edema, redness, swelling in calf of one leg is associated with localized thrombophlebitis).**
- Assess presence, location, and degree of swelling or edema formation. Measure circumference of extremities, noting differences in size. **Useful in identifying or quantifying edema in involved extremity.**
- Measure capillary refill **to determine adequacy of systemic circulation.**
- Note client's nutritional and fluid status. **Protein-energy malnutrition and weight loss make ischemic tissues more prone to breakdown. Dehydration reduces blood volume and compromises peripheral circulation.**
- Inspect lower extremities for skin texture (e.g., atrophic, shiny appearance, lack of hair; or dry/scaly, reddened skin), and skin breaks or ulcerations **that often accompany diminished peripheral circulation.**

Information that appears in brackets has been added by the authors to clarify and enhance the use of nursing diagnoses.

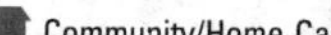

- Palpate arterial pulses (bilateral femoral, popliteal, dorsalis pedis, and posterial tibial) using hand-held Doppler if indicated **to determine level of circulatory blockage.**
- Note whether activity alters pulses **(e.g., client with intermittent claudication may have palpable pulses that disappear after ambulation).**
- Determine pulse equality, as well as intensity (e.g., bounding, normal, diminished, or absent), and compare with unaffected extremity **to evaluate distribution and quality of blood flow and success or failure of therapy.**
- Evaluate extremity pain reports, noting associated symptoms (e.g., cramping or heaviness, discomfort with walking; progressive temperature or color changes; paresthesias).
- Determine time (day or night) that symptoms are worse, precipitating or aggravating events (e.g., walking), and relieving factors (e.g., rest, sitting down with legs in dependent position, oral analgesics) **to help isolate and differentiate problems such as intermittent chronic claudication versus loss of function and pain due to acute sustained ischemia related to loss of arterial blood flow.**
- Assess motor and sensory function. **Problems with ambulation; hypersensitivity; or loss of sensation, numbness, and tingling are changes that can indicate neurovascular dysfunction or limb ischemia.**
- Check for calf tenderness or pain on dorsiflexion of foot (Homans' sign), swelling, and redness. **Indicators of deep vein thrombosis (DVT), although DVT is often present without a positive Homans' sign.**
- Review laboratory studies such as lipid profile, coagulation studies, hemoglobin/hematocrit, renal/cardiac function tests, inflammatory markers (e.g., D dimer, C-reactive protein); and diagnostic studies (e.g., Doppler ultrasound, magnetic resonance angiography, venogram, contrast angiography, resting ankle-brachial index [ABI], leg segmental arterial pressure measurements) **to determine probability, location, and degree of impairment.**

Nursing Priority No. 3.

To maximize tissue perfusion **or reduce risk of perfusion complications:**

- Evaluate reports of extremity pain promptly, noting any associated symptoms (e.g., cramping or heaviness, discomfort with walking, progressive temperature or color changes, paresthesia) **to help isolate and differentiate problems.**

Information that appears in brackets has been added by the authors to clarify and enhance the use of nursing diagnoses.

- Note presence and location of restrictive pressure dressings, circular wraps, cast or traction device **that may impede circulation to limb.**
- Assess skin color and temperature in all extremities **for changes that might indicate circulation problem.**
- Compare skin temperature and color with other limb **if developing problem is suspected.**
- Collaborate in treatment of underlying conditions, such as diabetes, hypertension, cardiopulmonary conditions, blood disorders, traumatic injury, hypovolemia, hypoxemia **to maximize systemic circulation and organ perfusion.**
- Administer medications such as antiplatelet agents, thrombolytics, antibiotics **to improve tissue perfusion or organ function.**
- Administer fluids, electrolytes, nutrients, and oxygen, as indicated, **to promote optimal blood flow, organ perfusion, and function.**
- Assist with or prepare for medical procedures such as endovascular stent placement, surgical revascularization procedures, thrombectomy **to improve peripheral circulation.**
- Assist with application of elasticized tubular support bandages, adhesive elastic or Velcro wraps (e.g., Circ-Aid), medication-impregnated layered bandage (e.g., Unna boot), multilayer bandage regimens, sequential pneumatic compression devices, and custom-fitted compression stockings, as indicated, **to provide graduated compression of lower extremity in presence of venous stasis ulcer.**
- Refer to wound care specialist if arterial or venous ulcerations are present. **In-depth wound care may include débridement and various specialized dressings that provide optimal moisture for healing, prevention of infection, and further injury.**
- Provide interventions **to promote peripheral circulation and limit complications associated with poor perfusion:**

Encourage early ambulation when possible and recommend regular exercise. **Enhances venous return. Studies indicate exercise training may be an effective early treatment for intermittent claudication.**

Recommend or provide foot and ankle exercises when client unable to ambulate freely **to reduce venous pooling and increase venous return.**

Provide pressure-relieving devices for immobilized client (e.g., air mattress, foam or sheepskin padding, bed or foot cradle).

Apply intermittent compression devices or graduated compression stockings (GCSs) to lower extremities **to limit ve-**

Information that appears in brackets has been added by the authors to clarify and enhance the use of nursing diagnoses.

nous stasis, improve venous return, and reduce risk of DVT or tissue ulceration in client who is limited in activity, or otherwise at risk.

Assist or instruct client to change position at timed intervals, rather than using presence of pain as signal to change positions.

Elevate legs when sitting; avoid sharp angulation of the hips or knees.

Avoid massaging the leg in presence of thrombosis.

Avoid, or carefully monitor, use of heat or cold, such as hot water bottle, heating pad, or ice pack.

- Refer to NDs risk for peripheral Neurovascular Dysfunction; risk for impaired Skin Integrity; impaired Tissue Integrity; [disturbed Sensory Perception], for additional interventions as appropriate.

Nursing Priority No. 4.

To promote wellness (Teaching/Discharge Considerations):

- Discuss relevant risk factors (e.g., family history, obesity, age, smoking, hypertension, diabetes, clotting disorders) and potential outcomes of atherosclerosis (e.g., systemic and peripheral vascular disease conditions). **Information necessary for client to make informed choices about remediating risk factors and committing to lifestyle changes.**
- Identify necessary changes in lifestyle and assist client to incorporate disease management into activities of daily living. **Promotes independence, enhances self-concept regarding ability to deal with change and manage own needs.**
- Emphasize need for regular exercise program **to enhance circulation and promote general well-being.**
- Refer to dietitian for well-balanced, low-saturated fat, low-cholesterol diet, or other modifications as indicated.
- Discuss care of dependent limbs/foot care, as appropriate. **When circulation is impaired, changes in sensation place client at risk for development of lesions or ulcerations that are often slow to heal.**
- Discourage sitting or standing for extended periods of time, wearing constrictive clothing, or crossing legs when seated, **which restricts circulation and leads to venous stasis and edema.**
- Provide education about relationship between smoking and peripheral vascular circulation, as indicated. **Smoking contributes to development and progression of peripheral vascular disease and is associated with higher rate of amputation in presence of Buerger's disease.**

Information that appears in brackets has been added by the authors to clarify and enhance the use of nursing diagnoses.

- Educate client/SO in reportable symptoms, including any changes in pain level, difficulty walking, nonhealing wounds **to provide opportunity for timely evaluation and intervention.**
- Emphasize need for regular medical and laboratory follow-up **to evaluate disease progression and response to therapies.**
- Review medication regimen and possible harmful side effects with client/SO. **Client may be on various drugs (e.g., antiplatelet agents, blood viscosity-reducing agents, vasodilators, anticoagulants, or cholesterol-lowering agents) for treatment of the particular vascular disorder. Many of these medications have harmful side effects and require client teaching and ongoing medical monitoring.**
- Emphasize importance of avoiding use of aspirin, some over-the-counter drugs and supplements, or alcohol when taking anticoagulants.
- Refer to community resources such as smoking cessation assistance, weight control program, and exercise group **to provide support for lifestyle changes.**

Documentation Focus

Assessment/Reassessment

- Individual risk factors identified
- Individual findings, noting nature, extent, and duration of problem, effect on independence and lifestyle
- Characteristics of pain, precipitators, and what relieves pain
- Pulse and blood pressure, including above and below suspected lesion as appropriate
- Client concerns or difficulty making and following through with plan

Planning

- Plan of care and who is involved in planning
- Teaching plan

Implementation/Evaluation

- Response to interventions, teaching, and actions performed
- Attainment or progress toward desired outcome(s)
- Modifications to plan of care

Discharge Planning

- Long-term needs and who is responsible for actions to be taken
- Available resources, specific referrals made

Information that appears in brackets has been added by the authors to clarify and enhance the use of nursing diagnoses.

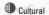

Sample Nursing Outcomes & Interventions Classifications (NOC/NIC)

NOC—Tissue Perfusion: Peripheral
NIC—Circulatory Care: Arterial [or] Venous Insufficiency

risk for decreased cardiac TISSUE PERFUSION

[Diagnostic Division: Activity/Rest—Class 4 Cardiovascular/Pulmonary Responses (00200)]

Definition: Vulnerable to a decrease in cardiac (coronary) perfusion, which may compromise health.

Risk Factors

Coronary artery spasm; cardiovascular surgery; cardiac tamponade
Family history of cardiovascular disease
Hypertension; diabetes mellitus; hypovolemia; hypoxemia; hypoxia
Insufficient knowledge of modifiable risk factors (e.g., smoking, sedentary lifestyle, obesity)
Pharmaceutical agent; substance abuse
Elevated C-reactive protein; hyperlipidemia

NOTE: A risk diagnosis is not evidenced by signs and symptoms, as the problem has not occurred; rather, nursing interventions are directed at prevention.

Desired Outcomes/Evaluation Criteria—Client Will:

- Demonstrate adequate coronary perfusion as individually appropriate (e.g., vital signs within client's normal range, free of chest pain or discomfort).
- Identify individual risk factors.
- Verbalize understanding of treatment regimen.
- Demonstrate behaviors and lifestyle changes to maintain or maximize circulation (e.g., cessation of smoking, relaxation techniques, exercise/dietary program).

Information that appears in brackets has been added by the authors to clarify and enhance the use of nursing diagnoses.

Actions/Interventions

Nursing Priority No. 1.

To identify individual risk factors:

- Note presence of conditions such as congestive heart failure, major trauma with blood loss, recent cardiac surgery or use of ventricular assist device, chronic anemia, sepsis, **which can affect systemic circulation, tissue oxygenation, and organ function.**
- Note client's age and gender when assessing risk for coronary artery spasm or myocardial infarction. **Risk for heart disorders increases with age. Although men are still considered at higher risk for myocardial infarctions and experience them earlier in life, the rate of mortality among women with coronary artery disease is rising.**
- Identify lifestyle issues such as obesity, smoking, high cholesterol, excessive alcohol intake, use of drugs such as cocaine, and physical inactivity, **which can raise client's risk for coronary artery disease and impaired cardiac tissue perfusion.**
- Determine presence of breathing problems, such as obstructive sleep apnea with oxygen desaturation, **which can produce alveolar hypoventilation, respiratory acidosis and hypoxia, resulting in cardiac dysrhythmias and cardiac dysfunction.**
- Determine if client is experiencing usual degree or prolonged stress or may have underlying psychiatric disorder (e.g., anxiety or panic).
- Review client's medications **to note current use of vasoactive drugs such as amiodarone, dopamine, dobutamine, esmolol, lidocaine, nitroglycerin, vasopressin [not a complete listing] that can exert undesirable side effects, increasing myocardial workload and oxygen consumption.**
- Review diagnostic studies (e.g., electrocardiogram, exercise tolerance tests, myocardial perfusion scan; echocardiogram, bubble echocardiogram; angiography, Doppler ultrasound, chest radiography; oxygen saturation, capnometry, or arterial blood gases; electrolytes, lipid profile; blood urea nitrogen/creatinine, cardiac enzymes) **to identify conditions requiring treatment and/or response to therapies.**

Nursing Priority No. 2.

To determine changes in cardiac status:

- Investigate reports of chest pain, noting changes in characteristics of pain **to evaluate for potential myocardial ischemia**

Information that appears in brackets has been added by the authors to clarify and enhance the use of nursing diagnoses.

or inadequate systemic oxygenation or perfusion of organs.

- Monitor vital signs, especially noting blood pressure changes, including hypertension or hypotension, **reflecting systemic vascular resistance problems that alter oxygen consumption and cardiac perfusion.**
- Assess heart sounds and pulses for dysrhythmias. **Can be caused by inadequate myocardial or systemic tissue perfusion, electrolyte or acid-base imbalances.**
- Assess for restlessness, fatigue, changes in level of consciousness, increased capillary refill time, diminished peripheral pulses, and pale, cool skin. **Signs and symptoms of inadequate systemic perfusion, which reflects cardiac function.**
- Inspect for pallor, mottling, cool or clammy skin, and diminished pulses **indicative of systemic vasoconstriction resulting from reduced cardiac output.**
- Investigate reports of difficulty breathing or respiratory rate outside acceptable parameters, **which can be indicative of oxygen exchange problems.**

Nursing Priority No. 3.

To maintain/maximize cardiac perfusion:

- Collaborate in treatment of underlying conditions such as hypovolemia, chronic obstructive pulmonary disease, diabetes, chronic atrial fibrillation **to correct or treat disorders that could influence cardiac perfusion or organ function.**
- Provide supplemental oxygen as indicated **to improve or maintain cardiac and systemic tissue perfusion.**
- Administer fluids and electrolytes as indicated **to maintain systemic circulation and optimal cardiac function.**
- Administer medications (e.g., antihypertensive agents, analgesics, antidysrhythmics, bronchodilators, fibrinolytic agents) **to treat underlying conditions, prevent thromboembolic phenomena, and maintain cardiac tissue perfusion and organ function.**
- Provide periods of undisturbed rest and calming environment **to reduce myocardial workload.**

Nursing Priority No. 4.

To promote wellness (Teaching/Discharge Considerations):

- Discuss cumulative effects of risk factors (e.g., family history, obesity, age, smoking, hypertension, diabetes, clotting disorders) and potential outcomes of atherosclerosis (e.g., systemic and cardiac disease conditions).

Information that appears in brackets has been added by the authors to clarify and enhance the use of nursing diagnoses.

- Review modifiable risk factors **to assist client/significant other (SO) in understanding those areas in which he or she can take action or make healthy-heart choices:**

  Recommend maintenance of normal weight, or weight loss if client is obese. Review specific dietary concerns with client (e.g., reducing animal and dairy fats; increasing plant foods—fruits, vegetables, olive oil, nuts).

  Encourage smoking cessation, when indicated, offering information about smoking-cessation aids and programs.

  Encourage client to engage in regular exercise.

  Discuss cardiac effects of drug use, where indicated (including cocaine, methamphetamines, alcohol).

  Discuss coping and stress tolerance.

  Demonstrate and encourage use of relaxation and stress management techniques.

  Encourage client in high-risk categories (e.g., strong family history, diabetic, prior history of cardiac event) to have regular medical examinations.

- Review medications on regular basis **to manage those that affect cardiac function or those given to prevent blood pressure or thromboembolic problems.**
- Refer to educational/community resources, as indicated. **Client/SO may benefit from support to engage in healthier heart activities (e.g., weight loss, smoking cessation, exercise).**
- Instruct in blood pressure monitoring at home, if indicated; advise purchase of home monitoring equipment. **Facilitates management of hypertension, a major risk factor for damage to blood vessels, which contributes to coronary artery disease.**

Documentation Focus

Assessment/Reassessment

- Individual findings, noting specific risk factors
- Vital signs, cardiac rhythm, presence of dysrhythmias

Planning

- Plan of care and who is involved in planning
- Teaching plan

Implementation/Evaluation

- Response to interventions, teaching, and actions performed
- Attainment or progress toward desired outcome(s)
- Modifications to plan of care

Information that appears in brackets has been added by the authors to clarify and enhance the use of nursing diagnoses.

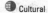

Discharge Planning

- Long-term needs and who is responsible for actions to be taken
- Available resources, specific referrals made

Sample Nursing Outcomes & Interventions Classifications (NOC/NIC)

NOC—Tissue Perfusion: Cardiac
NIC—Cardiac Precautions

risk for ineffective cerebral TISSUE PERFUSION

[Diagnostic Division: Circulation]

Definition: Vulnerable to a decrease in cerebral tissue circulation, which may compromise health.

Risk Factors:

Brain injury (e.g., cerebrrovascular impairment, neurological illness, trauma, tumor); brain neoplasm
Carotid stenosis; aortic atherosclerosis; arterial dissection
Atrial fibrillation; sick sinus syndrome; atrial myxoma
Recent myocardial infarction; akinetic left ventricular segment; dilated cardiomyopathy; mitral stenosis; mechanical prosthetic valve; infective endocarditis; embolism
Coagulopathy (e.g., sickle cell anemia); disseminated intravascular coagulation; abnormal partial thromboplastin time (PTT); abnormal prothrombin time (PT)
Hypertension; hypercholesterolemia
Substance abuse
Pharmaceutical agent; treatment regime

NOTE: A risk diagnosis is not evidenced by signs and symptoms, as the problem has not occurred; rather, nursing interventions are directed at prevention.

Desired Outcomes/Evaluation Criteria—Client Will:

- Display neurological signs within client's normal range.
- Verbalize understanding of condition, therapy regimen, side effects of medications, and when to contact healthcare provider.

Information that appears in brackets has been added by the authors to clarify and enhance the use of nursing diagnoses.

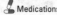

- Demonstrate behaviors and lifestyle changes to improve circulation (e.g., cessation of smoking, relaxation techniques, exercise and dietary program).

Actions/Interventions

Nursing Priority No. 1.

To assess causative/contributing factors:

- Determine history of conditions associated with thrombus or emboli such as stroke, complicated pregnancy, sickle cell disease, fractures (especially long bones and pelvis) **to identify client at higher risk for decreased cerebral perfusion related to bleeding and/or coagulation problems.**
- Note current situation or presence of conditions (e.g., congestive heart failure, major trauma, sepsis, hypertension) **that can affect multiple body systems and systemic circulation/ perfusion.**
- Ascertain potential for presence of acute neurological conditions, such as traumatic brain injuries, tumors, hemorrhage, anoxic brain injury associated with cardiac arrest, and toxic or viral encephalopathies. **These conditions alter the relationship between intracranial volume and pressure, potentially increasing intracranial pressure and decreasing cerebral perfusion.**
- Investigate client reports of headache, particularly when accompanied by a range of progressive neurological deficits. **May accompany cerebral perfusion deficits associated with conditions such as stroke, transient ischemic attack, brain trauma, or cerebral arteriovenous malformations.**
- Ascertain if client has history of cardiac problems (e.g., recent myocardial infarction, heart failure, heart valve dysfunction or replacement, chronic atrial fibrillation).
- Determine presence of cardiac dysrhythmias. **Can be caused by inadequate myocardial perfusion, electrolyte imbalances, or be associated with brain injury (e.g., bradycardia can accompany traumatic injury; stroke can be precipitated by dysrhythmias).**
- Assess level of consciousness, mental status, speech, and behavior. **Clinical symptoms of decreased cerebral perfusion include fluctuations in consciousness and cognitive function.**
- Evaluate blood pressure. **Chronic or severe acute hypertension can precipitate cerebrovascular spasm and stroke. Low blood pressure or severe hypotension causes inadequate perfusion of brain.**

Information that appears in brackets has been added by the authors to clarify and enhance the use of nursing diagnoses.

- Verify proper use of antihypertensive medications. **Individuals may stop medication because of lack of symptoms, presence of undesired side effects, and/or cost of drug, potentiating risk of stroke.**
- Review medication regimen noting use of anticoagulants/antiplatelet agents/other drugs **that could cause intracranial bleeding.**
- Review pulse oximetry or arterial blood gases. **Hypoxia is associated with reduced cerebral perfusion.**
- Review laboratory studies **to identify disorders that increase risk of clotting or bleeding or conditions contributing to decreased cerebral perfusion.**
- Review results of diagnostic studies (e.g., ultrasound or other imaging scans such as echocardiography, computed tomography, or magnetic resonance angiography; diffusion and perfusion magnetic resonance imaging) **to determine location and severity of disorder that can cause or exacerbate cerebral perfusion problem.**

Nursing Priority No. 2.

To maximize tissue perfusion:

- Collaborate in treatment of underlying conditions as indicated.
- Restore or maintain fluid balance **to maximize cardiac output and prevent decreased cerebral perfusion associated with hypovolemia.**
- Manage cardiac dysrhythmias via medication administration, pacemaker insertion.
- Restrict fluids, administer diuretics, as indicated, **to prevent decreased cerebral perfusion associated with fluid imbalance, hypertension, and cerebral edema.**
- Maintain head of bed placement (e.g., 0, 15, 30 degrees) as indicated, **to promote optimal cerebral perfusion.**
- Administer vasoactive medications, as indicated, **to increase cardiac output and/or adequate arterial blood pressure to maintain cerebral perfusion.**
- Administer other medications, as indicated **(e.g., steroids may decrease edema, antihypertensives may manage high blood pressure, anticoagulants may prevent cerebral embolus).**
- Prepare client for surgery, as indicated (e.g., carotid endarterectomy, evacuation of hematoma or space-occupying lesion), **to improve cerebral perfusion.**
- Refer to NDs decreased Cardiac Output; decreased intracranial Adaptive Capacity, for additional interventions.

Information that appears in brackets has been added by the authors to clarify and enhance the use of nursing diagnoses.

Nursing Priority No. 3.

To promote wellness (Teaching/Discharge Considerations):

- Review modifiable risk factors, including hypertension, smoking, diet, physical activity, excessive alcohol intake, illicit drug use, as indicated. **Information can help client make informed choices about remedial risk factors and commit to lifestyle changes, as appropriate.**
- Discuss impact of unmodifiable risk factors such as family history, age, race. **Understanding effects and interrelationship of all risk factors may encourage client to address what can be changed to improve general well-being and reduce individual risk.**
- Assist client to incorporate disease management into activities of daily living. **Promotes independence; enhances self-concept regarding ability to deal with change and manage own needs.**
- Emphasize necessity of routine follow-up and laboratory monitoring, as indicated, **for effective disease management and possible changes in therapeutic regimen.**
- Refer to educational and community resources, as indicated. **Client/significant other (SO) may benefit from instruction and support provided by agencies to engage in healthy activities (e.g., weight loss, smoking cessation, exercise).**

Documentation Focus

Assessment/Reassessment

- Individual findings, noting specific risk factors
- Vital signs, blood pressure, cardiac rhythm
- Medication regimen
- Diagnostic studies, laboratory results

Planning

- Plan of care and who is involved in planning
- Teaching plan

Implementation/Evaluation

- Response to interventions, teaching, and actions performed
- Attainment or progress toward desired outcome(s)
- Modifications to plan of care

Discharge Planning

- Long-term needs and who is responsible for actions to be taken
- Available resources, specific referrals made

Information that appears in brackets has been added by the authors to clarify and enhance the use of nursing diagnoses.

Sample Nursing Outcomes & Interventions Classifications (NOC/NIC)

NOC—Tissue Perfusion: Cerebral
NIC—Cerebral Perfusion Promotion

impaired TRANSFER ABILITY

[Diagnostic Division: Activity/Rest]

Definition: Limitation of independent movement between two nearby surfaces.

Related Factors

Insufficient muscle strength; physical deconditioning; neuromuscular impairment; musculoskeletal impairment
Impaired balance, vision
Pain
Obesity
Insufficient knowledge of transfer techniques; alteration in cognitive functioning
Environmental barrier (e.g., bed height, inadequate space, wheelchair type, treatment equipment, restraints)

Defining Characteristics

Subjective or Objective

Inability to transfer from bed to chair or chair to bed; from chair to car or car to chair; from chair to floor or floor to chair; on or off a toilet or commode; in or out of bathtub or shower; from bed to standing or standing to bed; from chair to standing or standing to chair; from standing to floor or floor to standing; between uneven levels
Note: Specify level of independence using a standardized functional scale. (Refer to ND impaired physical Mobility, for suggested functional level classification.)

Desired Outcomes/Evaluation Criteria—Client/Caregiver Will:

- Verbalize understanding of situation and appropriate safety measures.
- Master techniques of transfer successfully.
- Make desired transfers safely.

Information that appears in brackets has been added by the authors to clarify and enhance the use of nursing diagnoses.

Actions/Interventions

Nursing Priority No. 1.

To assess causative/contributing factors:

- Determine presence of conditions that contribute to transfer problems. **Neuromuscular and musculoskeletal problems (such as multiple sclerosis, fractures with splints or casts, back injuries, knee/hip replacement surgery, amputation, quadriplegia or paraplegia, contractures or spastic muscles); agedness (diminished faculties, multiple medications, painful conditions, decreased balance, muscle mass, tone, or strength), and effects of dementias, brain injury, and so forth, can seriously impact balance and physical and psychological well-being.**
- Evaluate perceptual and cognitive impairments and ability to follow directions. **Plan of care and choice of interventions are dependent on nature of condition—acute, chronic, or progressive.**
- Review medication regimen and schedule **to determine possible side effects or drug interactions impairing balance and/or muscle tone.**

Nursing Priority No. 2.

To assess functional ability:

- Evaluate degree of impairment using functional level classification scale of 0 to 4. **Identifies strengths and deficits (e.g., ability to ambulate with assistive devices or problems with balance, failure to attend to one side, inability to bear weight [client is nonweight-bearing or partial weight-bearing]) and may provide information regarding potential for recovery.**
- Determine presence and degree of perceptual or cognitive impairment and ability to follow directions.
- Note emotional or behavioral responses of client/significant other (SO) to problems of immobility.

Nursing Priority No. 3.

To promote optimal level of movement:

- Assist with treatment of underlying condition causing dysfunction.
- Consult with physical therapist, occupational therapist, or rehabilitation team **to develop general and specific muscle strengthening and range-of-motion exercises, transfer**

Information that appears in brackets has been added by the authors to clarify and enhance the use of nursing diagnoses.

training and techniques, as well as recommendations and provision of balance, gait, and mobility aids or adjunctive devices.

- Use appropriate number of people to assist with transfers and correct equipment (e.g., mechanical lift/sling, gait belt, sitting or standing disk pivot) **to safely transfer the client in a particular situation (e.g., chair to bed, chair to car, in or out of shower or tub).**
- Demonstrate and assist with use of side rails, overhead trapeze, transfer boards, transfer or sit-to-stand hoist, specialty slings, safety grab bars, cane, walker, wheelchair, crutches, as indicated, **to protect client and care providers from injury during transfers and movements.**
- Position devices (e.g., call light, bed-positioning switch) within easy reach on the bed or chair. **Facilitates transfer and allows client to obtain assistance for transfer, as needed.**
- Provide instruction or reinforce information for client and caregivers regarding positioning **to improve or maintain balance when transferring.**
- Monitor body alignment, posture, and balance and encourage wide base of support when standing to transfer.
- Use full-length mirror, as needed, **to facilitate client's view of own postural alignment.**
- Demonstrate and reinforce safety measures, as indicated, such as transfer board, gait belt, supportive footwear, good lighting, clearing floor of clutter **to avoid possibility of fall and subsequent injury.**

Nursing Priority No. 4.

To promote wellness (Teaching/Discharge Considerations):

- Assist client/caregivers to learn safety measures as individually indicated. **Actions (e.g., using correct body mechanics for particular transfer, locking wheelchair before transfer, using properly placed and functioning hoists, ascertaining that floor surface is even and clutter free) are important in facilitating transfers and reducing risk of falls or injury to client and caregiver.**
- Refer to appropriate community resources for evaluation and modification of environment (e.g., shower or tub, uneven floor surfaces, steps, use of ramps, standing tables or lifts).
- Refer also to NDs impaired bed/physical/wheelchair Mobility; Unilateral Neglect; risk for Falls; impaired Walking, for additional interventions.

Information that appears in brackets has been added by the authors to clarify and enhance the use of nursing diagnoses.

Documentation Focus

Assessment/Reassessment
- Individual findings, including level of function and ability to participate in desired transfers
- Mobility aids or transfer devices used

Planning
- Plan of care and who is involved in the planning
- Teaching plan

Implementation/Evaluation
- Responses to interventions, teaching, and actions performed
- Attainment or progress toward desired outcome(s)
- Modifications to plan of care

Discharge Planning
- Discharge and long-term needs, noting who is responsible for each action to be taken
- Specific referrals made
- Sources for and maintenance of assistive devices

Sample Nursing Outcomes & Interventions Classifications (NOC/NIC)

NOC—Transfer Performance
NIC—Self-Care Assistance: Transfer

risk for TRAUMA

[Diagnostic Division: Safety]

Definition: Vulnerable to accidental tissue injury (e.g., wound, burn, fracture), which may compromise health.

Risk Factors

Internal
Alteration in cognitive functioning; emotional disturbance
Alteration in muscle coordination or sensation (resulting form spinal cord injury, diabetes mellitus, etc); weakness; decrease in eye-hand coordination; impaired balance; insufficient vision
Economically disadvantaged

Information that appears in brackets has been added by the authors to clarify and enhance the use of nursing diagnoses.

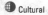

History of trauma (e.g., physical, psychological, sexual)
Insufficient knowledge or safety precautions

External [includes but is not limited to]

Absent or dysfunctional call-for-aid device; bed in high position; struggling with restraints
Absence of stairway gate or window guard; inadequate stair rails; slippery floor; insufficient antislip material in bathroom; use of throw rugs; obstructed passageway; insufficient lighting; unstable chair or ladder
Access to weapon; high crime neighborhood
Children riding in front seat of car; nonuse or misuse of seat restraint; misuse of headgear (e.g., hard hat, motorcycle helmet)
Defective appliance; delay in ignition of gas appliance; grease on stove; electrical hazard (e.g., faulty plug, frayed wire, overloaded outlet/fuse box); unanchored electric wires; gas leak
Exposure to corrosive product or toxic chemical; inadequately stored corrosive (e.g., lye); exposure to radiation
Extremes of environmental temperature; insufficient protection from heat source; bathing in very hot water; pot handle facing front of stove; use of cracked dishware; flammable object (e.g., clothing, toys); wearing loose clothing around open flame; inadequately stored combustible (e.g., matches, oily rags)
Icicles hanging from roof
Playing with dangerous object or explosive
Proximity to vehicle pathway (e.g., driveway, railroad track); unsafe road or walkway; unsafe operation of heavy equipment (e.g., excessive speed, while intoxicated, without required eyewear)
Smoking in bed or near oxygen

NOTE: A risk diagnosis is not evidenced by signs and symptoms, as the problem has not occurred; rather, nursing interventions are directed at prevention.

Desired Outcomes/Evaluation Criteria—Client/Caregiver Will:

- Identify and correct potential risk factors in the environment.
- Demonstrate appropriate lifestyle changes to reduce risk of injury.
- Identify resources to assist in promoting a safe environment.

Information that appears in brackets has been added by the authors to clarify and enhance the use of nursing diagnoses.

- Recognize need for and seek assistance to prevent accidents or injuries.

Actions/Interventions

NOTE: This ND is a compilation of a number of situations that can result in injury. Refer to specific NDs—risk for imbalanced Body Temperature; risk for Contamination; risk for Falls; impaired Home Maintenance; Hyperthermia; Hypothermia; risk for Injury; impaired physical Mobility; risk for impaired Parenting; risk for Poisoning; [disturbed Sensory Perception]; impaired Skin Integrity; risk for Suffocation; risk for Thermal Injury; impaired Tissue Integrity; risk for self-/other-directed Violence; impaired Walking, as appropriate, for more specific interventions.

Nursing Priority No. 1.

To assess causative/contributing factors:

- Determine factors related to individual situation and extent of risk for trauma. **Influences scope and intensity of interventions to manage threat to safety.**
- ∞ Note client's age, gender and developmental stage, decision-making ability, and level of cognition and competence. **Affects client's ability to protect self and/or others, and influences choice of interventions and teaching.**
- Ascertain client's/significant other's (SO's) knowledge of safety needs and injury prevention, and motivation to prevent injury in home, community, and work setting. **Lack of appreciation of significance of individual hazards increases risk of traumatic injury.**
- Note socioeconomic status and availability and use of resources.
- Assess influence of client's lifestyle and stress **that can impair judgment and greatly increase client's potential for injury.**
- Assess mood, coping abilities, personality styles (i.e., temperament, aggression, impulsive behavior, level of self-esteem). **May result in careless actions, or increased risk-taking without consideration of consequences.**
- Evaluate individual's emotional and behavioral response to violence in surroundings (e.g., neighborhood, television, peer group). **May affect client's view of and regard for own/others' safety.**

Information that appears in brackets has been added by the authors to clarify and enhance the use of nursing diagnoses.

- Review potential occupational risk factors (e.g., works with dangerous tools and machinery, electricity, explosives; police, fire, emergency medical service [EMS] officers; working with hazardous chemicals, various inhalants, or radiation).
- Review history of accidents, noting circumstances (e.g., time of day, activities coinciding with accident, who was present, type of injury sustained). **Can provide clues for client's risk for subsequent events and potential for enhanced safety by a change in the people or environment involved (e.g., client may need assistance when getting up at night, or increased playground supervision may be required).**
- Determine potential for abusive behavior by family members/SO(s)/peers.
- Review diagnostic studies and laboratory tests for impairments or imbalances **that may result in or exacerbate conditions, such as confusion, tetany, and pathological fractures.**

Nursing Priority No. 2.

To enhance safety in healthcare environment:

- Screen client for safety concerns (e.g., risk for falls, cognitive, developmental, vision/other sensory impairments upon admission and during stay in healthcare facility. Assess for and report changes in client's functional status. Perform thorough assessments regarding safety issues when planning for client discharge. **Failure to accurately assess and intervene or refer regarding these issues can place the client at needless risk and creates negligence issues for the healthcare practitioner.**
- Review client's therapeutic regimen on a continual basis when under direct care (e.g., vital signs, medications, treatment modalities, infusions, nutrition, physical environment) **to prevent healthcare-related complications.**
- Provide for routine safety needs:

  Provide adequate supervision and frequent observation.

  Place young children, confused client/person with dementia near nurses' station.

  Orient client to environment.

  Make arrangement for call system for bedridden client in home or hospital setting. Demonstrate use and place device within client's reach.

  Provide for appropriate communication tools (e.g., writing implements and paper; alphabet/picture board).

  Encourage client's use of corrective vision and hearing aids.

Information that appears in brackets has been added by the authors to clarify and enhance the use of nursing diagnoses.

Keep bed in low position or place mattress on floor, as appropriate.

Use and pad side rails, as indicated.

Provide seizure precautions.

Lock wheels on bed and movable furniture. Clear travel paths. Provide adequate area lighting.

Assist with activities and transfers, as needed.

Provide well-fitting, nonskid footwear.

Demonstrate and monitor use of assistive devices, such as transfer devices, cane, walker, crutches, wheelchair, safety bars.

Provide supervision while client is smoking.

Provide for appropriate disposal of potentially injurious items (e.g., needles, scalpel blades).

Follow facility protocol and closely monitor use of restraints, when required (e.g., vest, limb, belt, mitten).

- Emphasize with client importance of obtaining assistance when weak or sedated and when problems of balance, coordination, or postural hypotension are present **to reduce risk of syncope and falls.**
- Demonstrate and encourage use of techniques to reduce or manage stress and vent emotions such as anger, hostility **to reduce risk of violence to self/others.**
- Refer to physical or occupational therapist as appropriate **to identify high-risk tasks, conduct site visits, select, create, or modify equipment; and provide education about body mechanics and musculoskeletal injuries, as well as provide needed therapies.**
- Assist with treatments for underlying medical, surgical, or psychiatric conditions **to improve cognition and thinking processes, musculoskeletal function, awareness of own safety needs, and general well-being.**

Nursing Priority No. 3.

To enhance safety for client in community care setting:

- Provide information to caregivers regarding client's specific disease or condition(s) and associated risks.
- Identify interventions and safety devices to promote safe physical environment and individual safety:

Recommend wearing visual or hearing aids **to maximize sensory input.**

Ensure availability of communication devices (e.g., telephone, computer, alarm system or medical emergency alert device).

Information that appears in brackets has been added by the authors to clarify and enhance the use of nursing diagnoses.

Install and maintain electrical and fire safety devices, extinguishers, and alarms.
Review oxygen safety rules.
Identify environmental needs (e.g., decals on glass doors; adequate lighting of stairways, handrails, ramps, bathtub safety tapes) **to reduce risk of falls**, lower temperature on hot water heater **to prevent accidental burns,** etc.
Obtain seat risers for chairs; ergonomic beds or chairs.
Encourage participation in back safety classes, injury-prevention exercises, mobility or transfer device training.
Install childproof cabinets for medications and toxic household substances, use tamper-proof medication containers.
Review proper storage and disposal of volatile liquids; installation of proper ventilation for use when mixing or using toxic substances; use of safety glasses or goggles.
Emphasize importance of appropriate use of car restraints, bicycle, motorcycle, skating, or skiing helmets.
Discuss swimming pool fencing and supervision; attending First Aid and cardiopulmonary resuscitation (CPR) classes.
Obtain trigger locks or gun safes for firearms.

- Initiate appropriate teaching **when reckless behavior is occurring or likely to occur (e.g., smoking in bed, driving without safety belts, working with chemicals without safety goggles).**
- Refer to counseling or psychotherapy, as needed, especially when individual is "accident prone" or self-destructive behavior is noted. (Refer to NDs risk for other-/self-directed Violence.)

Nursing Priority No. 4.

To promote wellness (Teaching/Discharge Considerations):

- Discuss importance of self-monitoring of conditions or emotions that can contribute to occurrence of injury to self/others (e.g., fatigue, anger, irritability). **Client/SO may be able to modify risk through monitoring of actions or postponement of certain actions, especially during times when client is likely to be highly stressed.**
- Encourage use of warm-up and stretching exercises before engaging in athletic activity **to prevent muscle injuries.**
- Recommend use of seat belts; fitted helmets for cyclists, skate-/snowboarders, skiers; approved infant seat in appropriate position in vehicle; avoidance of hitchhiking; substance abuse programs **to promote transportation and recreation safety.**

Information that appears in brackets has been added by the authors to clarify and enhance the use of nursing diagnoses.

- Refer to accident prevention programs (e.g., medication and drug safety, mobility or transfer device training, driving instruction, parenting classes, firearms safety, workplace ergonomics).
- Develop home fire safety program (e.g., family fire drills; use of smoke detectors; yearly chimney cleaning; purchase of fire-retardant clothing, especially children's nightwear; safe use of in-home oxygen; fireworks safety).
- Problem-solve with client/parent to provide adequate child supervision after school, during working hours, on school holidays; or day program for frail or confused elder.
- Explore behaviors related to use of firearms, alcohol, tobacco, and recreational drugs and other substances. **Provides opportunity to review consequences of previously determined risk factors (e.g., potential consequences of illegal activities, effects of smoking on health of family members as well as fire danger; potential for unintentional gunshot injuries, suicide, or homicide; potential for harm related to alcohol and other substances).**
- Identify community resources (e.g., financial, food assistance) **to assist with necessary corrections or improvements and purchases.**
- Recommend involvement in community self-help programs, such as Neighborhood Watch, Helping Hand.
- Promote educational opportunities **geared toward increasing awareness of safety measures (e.g., firearms safety) and resources available to the individual.**
- Seek out and involve businesses in volunteer outreach activities such as building safe playgrounds, community or street cleanup, home repair or improvement for frail elders, and so forth.
- Advocate for and promote solutions for problems of design of buildings, equipment, transportation, and workplace practices **that contribute to accidents.**

Documentation Focus

Assessment/Reassessment

- Individual risk factors, past and recent history of injuries, awareness of safety needs
- Use of safety equipment or procedures
- Environmental concerns, safety issues

Planning

- Plan of care and who is involved in the planning
- Teaching plan

Information that appears in brackets has been added by the authors to clarify and enhance the use of nursing diagnoses.

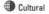

Implementation/Evaluation

- Responses to interventions, teaching, and actions performed
- Attainment or progress toward desired outcome(s)
- Modifications to plan of care

Discharge Planning

- Long-term needs and who is responsible for actions to be taken
- Available resources, specific referrals made

Sample Nursing Outcomes & Interventions Classifications (NOC/NIC)

NOC—Physical Injury Severity
NIC—Environmental Management: Safety

risk for vascular TRAUMA

[Diagnostic Division: Safety]

Definition: Vulnerable to damage to vein and its surrounding tissues related to the presence of a catheter and/or infused solutions, which may compromise health.

Risk Factors

Insertion site; difficulty visualizing artery or vein
Inappropriate catheter type or width; inadequate anchoring of catheter
Irritating solution (e.g., concentration, temperature, pH); rapid infusion rate; length of time catheter is in place

NOTE: A risk diagnosis is not evidenced by signs and symptoms, as the problem has not occurred; rather, nursing interventions are directed at prevention.

Desired Outcomes/Evaluation Criteria—Client Will:

- Identify signs/symptoms to report to healthcare provider.
- Be free of signs/symptoms associated with venipuncture, infusion solution, or local infection.
- Develop plan for home therapy where indicated and demonstrate appropriate procedures.

Information that appears in brackets has been added by the authors to clarify and enhance the use of nursing diagnoses.

Actions/Interventions

Nursing Priority No. 1.

To assess risk factors:

- Determine presence of medical condition(s) requiring IV therapy (e.g., dehydration, trauma, surgery; long-term antibiotic treatment of severe infections; cancer therapies, pain management when oral drugs not effective or practical).
- Note client's age, body size, and weight. **Very young or elderly client is at risk because of lack of subcutaneous tissue surrounding veins, and veins may be fragile or ropy, causing difficulties with insertion. Forearm veins may be difficult to see in obese, edematous, or dark-skinned individual.**
- Identify particular issues such as client's emotional state, including fear of needles, mental or developmental status that might interfere with client's ability to cooperate with procedures, IV site choices that interfere with client's mobility, **to prevent or limit potential for vascular damage.**
- Determine type(s) of solutions being used or planned. **Certain infusates are associated with greater risk of vein irritation and pain (e.g., potassium, contrast media); others are associated with significant risk of tissue injury, especially upon infiltration into surrounding tissues, including certain antibiotics, chemotherapy, or parenteral nutrition.**
- Assess peripheral IV site, when one is already in place, to determine potential for complications. **Reddened, blanched, tight, translucent, or cool skin; swelling; pain; numbness; streak formation; a palpable venous cord or purulent drainage are indicative of problem with IV requiring immediate intervention.**
- Assess central venous access device (CVAD), if present, to determine potential for complications. **Inability to aspirate, slowed or absent solution flow, site pain, engorged veins, or swelling in upper arm, chest wall, neck, or jaw on side of catheter insertion may indicate vein- or catheter-related thrombus, requiring immediate intervention.**

Nursing Priority No. 2.

To reduce potential complications:

- Determine appropriate site choice:

  Inspect and palpate chosen veins to determine size and condition. **Best veins are those that are not scarred, lumpy,**

Information that appears in brackets has been added by the authors to clarify and enhance the use of nursing diagnoses.

or fragile, to improve ease of cannulation and effectiveness of infusion.

Identify extremities or sites that have impaired circulation or injury. **Existing tissue injury, bleeding or edema can inhibit successful IV cannulation and potentiate risk for infiltration of infusates.**

Avoid leg veins in adults **due to potential for thrombophlebitis.**

Avoid anticubital veins when using peripheral catheter **because placement there limits client's movement, and the catheter is easily dislodged.**

Avoid inserting needle in vein valve site. **Damage to this area can cause blood pooling and increase risk of thrombosis.**

- Use best practice approach to IV insertion:

Determine best type of access when IV therapy is initiated. **Peripheral catheter in forearm is recommended for short-duration, nonirritating solutions of less than 7 days. Central line is appropriate for infusing many kinds of solutions over long periods of time or when client has suffered multiple peripheral sticks or one extremity is not available (e.g., amputation, dialysis shunt in one arm).**

Use appropriate needle gauge for chosen vein and solution **to deliver solution at appropriate rate, to promote hemodilution of fluid(s) at the catheter tip, and to reduce mechanical and chemical irritation to vein wall.**

Clean site and inject 1% lidocaine per agency protocol **to reduce risk of infection and pain with needle or cannula insertion.**

Stretch and immobilize skin and tissues **to stabilize vein and prevent rolling, requiring multiple sticks.**

Insert needle bevel up during insertion and hold at 3° to 10° angle **to prevent "blowing" the vein by piercing the back wall.**

Release tourniquet immediately when insertion is complete **to prevent intravascular pressure from causing bleeding into surrounding tissues.**

Observe for hematoma development and/or reports of pain and discomfort during insertion, **indicating vein damage with bleeding into tissues.**

Secure needle or cannula with tape or other securing device **to prevent dislodging and to extend catheter dwell time.**

Information that appears in brackets has been added by the authors to clarify and enhance the use of nursing diagnoses.

Avoid placing tape entirely around arm to anchor catheter; **can impede venous return and cause pooling of fluid, and infiltration or extravasation into surrounding tissues.**

Utilize transparent dressing over insertion site **to protect from external contaminants and to allow easy observation for potential complications.**

- Adhere to recommended infusions, dilutions, and administration rates for medications or irritating substances, such as potassium, **to reduce incidence of tissue irritation and sloughing.**
- Consult with IV/infusion nurse or other medical provider **to problem-solve issues that arise with IVs and/or for interventions for complications.**

Nursing Priority No. 3.

To promote optimum therapeutic effect:

- Observe IV site on a regular basis and instruct client/caregiver to report any discomfort, bruising, redness, swelling, bleeding, or other fluid leaking from site.
- Replace peripheral catheters every 72 to 96 hr (or per agency policy) **to prevent thrombophlebitis and catheter-related infections.**
- Apply pressure to site when IV discontinued for sufficient time **to prevent bleeding, especially in client with coagulopathies or on anticoagulants.**
- Adhere to specific protocols related to infection control. (Refer to ND risk for Infection.)
- Identify community resources and suppliers as indicated **to support home therapy regimen.**

Documentation Focus

Assessment/Reassessment

- Assessment findings pre- and postinsertion, site choice, use of local anesthetic, type and gauge of needle or cannula inserted, number of sticks required, dressing applied
- Type, amount, and rate of solution administered, presence of additives
- Client's response to procedure

Planning

- Plan of care, specific interventions, and who is involved in the planning
- Teaching plan as appropriate

Information that appears in brackets has been added by the authors to clarify and enhance the use of nursing diagnoses.

Implementation/Evaluation

- Attainment or progress toward desired outcome(s)
- Modifications to plan of care

Discharge Planning

- Long-term needs, identifying who is responsible for actions to be taken
- Community resources for equipment and supplies for home therapy
- Specific referrals made

Sample Nursing Outcomes & Interventions classifications (NOC/NIC)

NOC—Risk Control
NIC—Intravenous (IV) Insertion

UNILATERAL NEGLECT

[Diagnostic Division: Neurosensory]

Definition: Impairment in sensory and motor response, mental representation, and spatial attention to the body, and the corresponding environment, characterized by inattention to one side and overattention to the opposite side. Left-side neglect is more severe and persistent than right-side neglect.

Related Factors

Brain injury (e.g., cerebrovascular impairment, neurological illness, trauma, tumor)

Defining Characteristics

Objective

Hemianopsia; marked deviation of the eyes, head, or trunk to stimuli on the non-neglected side
Failure to move eyes, head, limbs, or trunk in the neglected hemisphere; failure to notice people approaching from the neglected side
Disturbance of sound lateralization
Unaware of positioning of neglected limb
Alteration in safety behavior on neglected side
Failure to eat food from portion of plate on neglected side; failure to dress or groom neglected side

---

Information that appears in brackets has been added by the authors to clarify and enhance the use of nursing diagnoses.

Use of vertical half of page only when writing; impaired performance on line cancellation, line bisection, and target cancellation tests; substitution of letters to form alternative words when reading

Omission of drawing on the neglected side; representational neglect (e.g., distortion of drawing on the neglected side)

Perseveration

Transfer of pain sensation to the nonneglected side

Desired Outcomes/Evaluation Criteria—Client/Caregiver Will:

- Acknowledge presence of sensory-perceptual impairment.
- Identify adaptive and protective measures for individual situation.
- Demonstrate behaviors, lifestyle changes necessary to promote physical safety.

Client Will:

- Verbalize positive realistic perception of self incorporating the current dysfunction.
- Perform self-care within level of ability.

Actions/Interventions

Nursing Priority No. 1.

To assess the extent of altered perception and the related degree of disability:

- Identify underlying reason for alterations in sensory, motor, or behavioral perceptions as noted in Related Factors. **The client with injury to either side of the brain may experience spatial neglect, but it more commonly occurs when brain injury affects the right cortical hemisphere, causing left hemiparesis.**
- Ascertain client's/significant other's (SO's) perception of problem/changes, noting differences in perceptions.
- Assess sensory awareness (e.g., response to stimulus of hot and cold, dull and sharp); note problems with awareness of motion and proprioception.
- Observe client's behavior (as noted in Defining Characteristics) **to determine the extent of impairment.**
- Assess ability to distinguish between right and left.
- Note physical signs of neglect (e.g., inability to maintain normal posture; disregard for position of affected limb[s], bumping into objects or walls on the left when ambulating, skin

Information that appears in brackets has been added by the authors to clarify and enhance the use of nursing diagnoses.

irritation/damage on the left side, indicating lack of awareness of injury).

- Explore and encourage verbalization of feelings **to identify meaning of loss and dysfunction to the client and impact it may have on assuming activities of daily living (ADLs).** *Note:* **Expression of loss may be difficult for the client for a variety of reasons. For example, some emotional disturbances and personality changes are caused by the physical effects of brain damage.**
- Assist with/review results of early screening tests. **Tests (often performed at the bedside) may include (and are not limited to) observation to determine if client shows evidence of body neglect such as asymmetric shaving/grooming. Reading test might reveal that client begins reading in the middle of the page, etc.**
- Review results of testing (e.g., computed tomography or magnetic resonance imaging scanning, complete neuropsychological tests) **done to determine cause or type of neglect syndrome (e.g., sensory, motor, representational, personal, spatial, behavioral inattention). Aids in distinguishing neglect from visual field cuts, impaired attention, and planning or visuospatial abilities.**

Nursing Priority No. 2.

To promote optimal comfort and safety for the client in the environment:

- Engage in treatment strategies focused on training of attention to the neglected hemispace:

  Approach client from the unaffected side during acute phase.

  Explain to client that one side is being neglected; repeat as needed.

  Remove excess stimuli from the environment when working with the client **to reduce confusion and reactive stress.**

  Encourage client to turn head and eyes in full rotation and "scan" the environment **to compensate for visual field loss or when neglect therapies include scanning.**

  Position bedside table and objects (e.g., call bell/telephone, tissues) within functional field of vision **to facilitate care.** *Note:* **Therapies may include orienting the client's environment leftward in attempt to help client perceive the neglected space.**

  Position furniture and equipment so travel path is not obstructed. Keep doors wide open or completely closed.

Information that appears in brackets has been added by the authors to clarify and enhance the use of nursing diagnoses.

Remove articles in the environment that may create a safety hazard (e.g., footstool, throw rug).

Orient to environment as often as needed and ensure adequate lighting in the environment **to improve client's interpretation of environmental stimuli.**

Monitor affected body part(s) for positioning and anatomical alignment, pressure points, skin irritation or injury, and dependent edema. **Increased risk of injury and ulcer formation necessitates close observation and timely intervention.**

When moving client, describe location of affected areas of body.

Protect affected body part(s) from pressure, injury, and burns, and help client learn to assume this responsibility.

Assist with ambulation or movement, using appropriate mobility and assistive devices **to promote safety of client and caregiver.**

Provide assistance with ADLs (e.g., feeding, bathing, dressing, grooming, toileting), **which helps client tend to affected side or compensate for client's deficits.**

Refer to ND [disturbed Sensory Perception] for additional interventions, as needed.

- Collaborate with rehabilitation team in strategies (e.g., sensory stimulation techniques such as tapping or stroking, patching one half of each eye, auditory stimulation, wedge prism adaptation techniques, virtual reality technology) **to assist client to overcome or compensate for deficits.**

Nursing Priority No. 3.

To promote wellness (Teaching/Discharge Considerations):

- Encourage client to look at and handle affected side **to stimulate awareness.**
- Bring the affected limb across the midline **for client to visualize during care.**
- Provide tactile stimuli to the affected side by touching/manipulating, stroking, and communicating about the affected side by itself rather than stimulating both sides simultaneously.
- Provide objects of various weight, texture, and size for client to handle **to provide tactile stimulation.**
- Assist client to position the affected extremity carefully and teach to routinely visualize placement of the extremity. Remind with visual cues. If client completely ignores one side

Information that appears in brackets has been added by the authors to clarify and enhance the use of nursing diagnoses.

of the body, use positioning **to improve perception (e.g., position client facing/looking at the affected side).**

- Encourage client to accept affected limb or side as part of self even when it no longer feels like it belongs.
- Use a mirror to help client adjust position **by visualizing both sides of the body.**
- Use descriptive terms to identify body parts rather than "left" and "right"; for example, "Lift this leg" (point to leg) or "Lift your affected leg."
- Encourage client/SO/family members to discuss situation and impact on life/future. **May help verbalize the reality of changes and provides opportunity to explore solutions to problems and special needs.**
- Acknowledge and accept feelings of despondency, grief, and anger. **When feelings are openly expressed, client can deal with them and move forward.** (Refer to ND Grieving, as appropriate.)
- Reinforce to client the reality of the dysfunction and need to compensate.
- Avoid participating in the client's use of denial.
- Encourage family members and SO(s) to treat client normally and not as an invalid, including client in family activities.
- Place nonessential items (e.g., TV, pictures, hairbrush) on affected side during postacute phase once client begins to cross midline **to encourage continuation of behavior.**
- Refer to and encourage client to use rehabilitative services **to enhance independence in functioning.**
- Identify additional community resources to meet individual needs (e.g., Meals-on-Wheels, home-care services) **to maximize independence, allow client to return to community setting.**
- Provide informational material and Web sites **to reinforce teaching and promote self-paced learning.**

Documentation Focus

Assessment/Reassessment

- Individual findings, including extent of altered perception, degree of disability, effect on independence and participation in ADLs
- Results of testing

Planning

- Plan of care and who is involved in the planning
- Teaching plan

Information that appears in brackets has been added by the authors to clarify and enhance the use of nursing diagnoses.

Implementation/Evaluation

- Responses to intervention, teaching, and actions performed
- Attainment or progress toward desired outcome(s)
- Modifications to plan of care

Discharge Planning

- Long-term needs and who is responsible for actions to be taken
- Available resources, specific referrals made

Sample Nursing Outcomes & Interventions Classifications (NOC/NIC)

NOC—Heedfulness of Affected Side
NIC—Unilateral Neglect Management

[acute/chronic] URINARY RETENTION

[Diagnostic Division: Elimination]

Definition: Incomplete emptying of the bladder.

Related Factors

High urethral pressure
Reflex arc inhibition
Strong sphincter; blockage in urinary tract [e.g., benign prostatic hypertrophy (BPH), perineal swelling, trauma]
[Infections; neurological diseases/trauma]
[Pharmaceutical agents (e.g., opiates, atropine, belladonna, psychotropics, antihistamines)]

Defining Characteristics

Subjective

Sensation of bladder fullness
Dribbling of urine
Dysuria

Objective

Bladder distention
Small or frequent voiding; absent urinary output
Residual urine
Overflow incontinence

Information that appears in brackets has been added by the authors to clarify and enhance the use of nursing diagnoses.

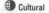

Desired Outcomes/Evaluation Criteria—Client Will:

- Verbalize understanding of causative factors and appropriate interventions for individual situation.
- Demonstrate techniques or behaviors to alleviate or prevent retention.
- Void in sufficient amounts with no palpable bladder distention; experience no postvoid residuals greater than 50 mL; have no dribbling or overflow.

Actions/Interventions

Acute

Nursing Priority No. 1.

To assess causative/contributing factors:

- Note presence of pathological conditions (e.g., urinary tract infection [UTI], neurological disorders or trauma, stone formation, prostate hypertrophy) **that can cause mechanical obstruction, nerve dysfunction, ineffective contraction, or decompensation of detrusor musculature, resulting in ineffective emptying of the bladder and urine retention.**
- Note client's gender and age. **Retention is most common among men, where prostate abnormalities or urethral strictures cause outlet obstruction. In either sex, retention may be due to medications (particularly those with anticholinergic effects, including many over-the-counter drugs); severe fecal impaction (which increases pressure on the bladder); or neurogenic bladder in patients with diabetes, multiple sclerosis, Parkinson's disease, or prior pelvic surgery, resulting in bladder denervation.**
- Investigate reports of sudden loss of ability to pass urine or great difficulty passing urine, pain with urination, blood in urine. **May indicate UTI or bladder outlet obstruction.**
- Obtain urine and review results of urinalysis (e.g., presence of red or white blood cells, nitrates, glucose, bacteria) and culture. Blood may be tested for infection, electrolyte imbalance, and (in men) prostate-specific antigen **to determine presence of treatable conditions.**
- Review medications, noting those that can cause or exacerbate retention (e.g., psychotropics, anesthesia, opiates, sedatives, alpha- and beta-adrenergic blockers, anticholinergics, antihistamines, neuroleptics).
- Examine for fecal impaction, surgical site swelling, postpartal edema, vaginal or rectal packing, enlarged prostate, or other

---

Information that appears in brackets has been added by the authors to clarify and enhance the use of nursing diagnoses.

factors (e.g., recent removal of indwelling catheter with urethral swelling or spasm) **that may produce a blockage of the urethra.**

- Determine anxiety level (e.g., **client may be too embarrassed to void in presence of others).**

Nursing Priority No. 2.

To determine degree of interference/disability:

- Ascertain if client can empty bladder completely, partially, or not at all, in spite of urge to urinate. **Signs of urinary retention caused by (1) blockage of the urethra or (2) disruption of complex system of nerves that connects the urinary tract with the brain.**
- Ascertain whether client has sensation of bladder fullness and determine level of discomfort. **Sensation and discomfort can vary, depending on underlying cause of retention.**
- Determine if there has been any significant urine output in the last 6 to 8 hr; presence of frequent/small voidings; whether dribbling (overflow) is occurring.
- Palpate height of the bladder. Ascertain whether client has sensation of bladder fullness. **Sensation and discomfort can vary, depending on underlying cause of retention. Most people with acute retention also feel pain in lower abdomen (pelvis). Back pain, fever, and painful urination may be present with retention if the cause is UTI.**
- Note recent amount and type of fluid intake. **Adequate fluid intake is necessary for production of healthy output. If client is not voiding despite adequate fluid intake, fluids may be restricted temporarily to prevent bladder overdistention until adequate urine flow is established.**
- Prepare for and assist with urodynamic testing (e.g., cystometrogram **to measure bladder pressure and volume,** bladder scan **to measure retention volume and/or postvoid residual),** or abdominal leak point pressure test.

Nursing Priority No. 3.

To assist in treating/preventing retention:

- Assist in treatments to relieve mechanical obstruction (e.g., bowel impaction; vaginal packing, perineal swelling) **that is restricting urinary flow.**
- Administer medications as indicated (e.g., antibiotics, stool softeners, pain relievers) **to treat underlying cause.**
- Assist client to sit upright on bedpan or commode or stand **to provide functional position of voiding.**

Information that appears in brackets has been added by the authors to clarify and enhance the use of nursing diagnoses.

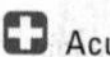
Acute Care

Collaborative
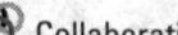
Community/Home Care
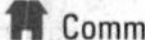
Cultural

- Provide privacy **to reduce retention caused by embarrassment or anxiety.**
- Instruct client with mild or moderate obstructive symptoms to "double void" by urinating, resting on toilet for 3 to 5 min, and then making a second attempt to urinate. **Promotes more efficient bladder evacuation by allowing the detrusor to contract initially, then rest and contract again.**
- Use ice techniques, spirits of wintergreen, stroking inner thigh, running water in sink or warm water over perineum, if indicated, **to stimulate reflex arc.**
- Prepare for more aggressive intervention (e.g., prostatectomy/ other surgeries, as indicated).
- Drain bladder intermittently, using the appropriate catheter (material and size) or catheterize with indwelling catheter **to resolve acute retention.**
- Reduce recurrences by controlling causative or contributing factors when possible (e.g., ice to perineum, use of stool softeners or laxatives, change of medication or dosage).

Nursing Priority No. 4.

To promote wellness (Teaching/Discharge Considerations):

- Emphasize good voiding habits (e.g., four to six times/day). **Repeated holding of urination for prolonged periods can, over time, overstretch and weaken bladder muscles.**
- Encourage client to report problems immediately **so treatment can be instituted promptly.**
- Emphasize need for adequate fluid intake.

Chronic

Nursing Priority No. 1.

To assess causative/contributing factors:

- Review medical history for diagnoses, such as congenital defects, neurological disorders (e.g., multiple sclerosis, polio), prostatic hypertrophy or surgery, birth canal injury or scarring, spinal cord injury with lower motor neuron injury or bladder stones **that may cause detrusor-sphincter dyssynergia (loss of coordination between bladder contraction and external urinary sphincter relaxation), detrusor muscle atrophy, or chronic overdistention because of outlet obstruction.**
- Determine presence of weak or absent sensory and/or motor impulses (as with stroke, spinal injury, or diabetes) **that pre-**

Information that appears in brackets has been added by the authors to clarify and enhance the use of nursing diagnoses.

dispose client to compromised enervation or interpretation of sensory signals resulting in impaired urination.

- Evaluate customary fluid intake.
- Assess client's medication regimen (e.g., psychotropic, antihistamines, atropine, belladonna) **to consult with primary care provider regarding client's continued use of drugs that are known to potentiate urinary retention.**

Nursing Priority No. 2.

To determine degree of interference/disability:

- Ascertain effect of condition on functioning and lifestyle. **Chronic urinary retention can limit client's desired lifestyle (e.g., daily activities, social functioning) and can lead to chronic incontinence and life-threatening complications (e.g., intractable UTIs, kidney failure).**
- Measure amount voided and postvoid residuals.
- Determine frequency and timing of voiding and/or dribbling.
- Note size and force of urinary stream.
- Palpate height of bladder.
- Determine presence of bladder spasms.
- Prepare for and assist with urodynamic testing (e.g., uroflowmetry **to assess voiding speed and urine volume,** cystometrogram **to measure bladder pressure and volume,** bladder scan **to measure retention and/or postvoid residual),** or abdominal leak point pressure test.

Nursing Priority No. 3.

To assist in treating/preventing retention:

- Collaborate in treatment of underlying conditions (e.g., BPH, reducing or eliminating medications responsible for retention, repairing perineal scarring or outlet obstruction) **that may correct or reduce severity of retention and associated overflow or total incontinence.**
- Recommend client void or catheterize on frequent, timed schedule **to maintain low bladder pressures.**
- Maintain consistent fluid intake **to wash out bacteria or avoid infections and limit stone formation.**
- Adjust fluid amount and timing, if indicated, **to prevent bladder distention.**
- Perform and instruct client/SO in Credé's method (client or caregiver applies light pressure or tapping on the bladder) or Valsalva maneuver (client tries to breathe out without letting

Information that appears in brackets has been added by the authors to clarify and enhance the use of nursing diagnoses.

air escape through the nose or mouth), if appropriate, **to stimulate bladder emptying.** ***Note:*** **Client with spinal cord injury and spastic bladder may be able to "trigger" the bladder to contract and avoid having to use a catheter.**

- Establish regular voiding or self-catheterization program **to prevent reflux and increased renal pressures.**
- Consult with urologist and prepare for more aggressive intervention (e.g., reconstructive surgery, lithotripsy, prostatectomy), as indicated, **to remove source of obstruction, reconstruct sphincter, or provide for urinary diversion.**
- Refer for consideration of advanced or research-based therapies (e.g., implanted sacral, tibial, or pelvic electrical stimulating device) **for long-term management of retention.**

Nursing Priority No. 4.

To promote wellness (Teaching/Discharge Considerations):

- Establish regular schedule for bladder emptying whether voiding or using catheter.
- Emphasize need for adequate fluid intake, including use of acidifying fruit juices or ingestion of vitamin C. **Maintains renal function, prevents infection and formation of bladder stones, reduces risk of encrustation around indwelling catheter.**
- Instruct client/SO(s) in clean intermittent self-catheterization techniques **so that more than one individual is able to assist the client in care of elimination needs.**
- Instruct client/SO in care when client has indwelling (urethral or suprapubic catheter) or urinary diversion device (e.g., clean technique, emptying and cleaning of leg bag or drainage bag; irrigation and replacement) **to promote self-care, enhance independence, and prevent complications.**
- Review signs/symptoms of complications requiring medical evaluation/intervention.

Documentation Focus

Assessment/Reassessment

- Individual findings, including nature of problem, degree of impairment, and whether client is incontinent

Planning

- Plan of care and who is involved in planning
- Teaching plan

Information that appears in brackets has been added by the authors to clarify and enhance the use of nursing diagnoses.

Implementation/Evaluation

- Response to interventions, teaching, and actions performed
- Attainment or progress toward desired outcome(s)
- Modifications to plan of care

Discharge Planning

- Long-term needs and who is responsible for actions to be taken
- Specific referrals made

Sample Nursing Outcomes & Interventions Classifications (NOC/NIC)

NOC—Urinary Elimination
NIC—Urinary Retention Care

impaired spontaneous VENTILATION

[Diagnostic Division: Respiration]

Definition: Decreased energy reserves resulting in an inability to maintain independent breathing that is adequate to support life.

Related Factors

Alteration in metabolism; [hypermetabolic state (e.g., infection); nutritional deficits/depletion of energy stores]
Respiratory muscle fatigue

Defining Characteristics

Subjective

Dyspnea
Apprehensiveness

Objective

Increase in metabolism
Increase in heart rate
Restlessness; decrease in cooperation
Increase in accessory muscle use
Decrease in tidal volume
Decrease in partial pressure of oxygen (PO_2), arterial oxygen saturation (SaO_2); increase in partial pressure of carbon dioxide (PCO_2)

Information that appears in brackets has been added by the authors to clarify and enhance the use of nursing diagnoses.

Desired Outcomes/Evaluation Criteria—Client Will:

- Reestablish and maintain effective respiratory pattern via ventilator with absence of retractions or use of accessory muscles, cyanosis, or other signs of hypoxia; and with arterial blood gases (ABGs)/SaO_2 within acceptable range.
- Participate in efforts to wean within individual ability, as appropriate.

Caregiver Will:

- Demonstrate behaviors necessary to maintain respiratory function.

Actions/Interventions

Nursing Priority No. 1.

To determine degree of impairment:

- Identify client with actual or impending respiratory failure (e.g., apnea or slow, shallow breathing; declining mentation or obtunded with need for airway protection).
- Determine presence of conditions that could be associated with hypoventilation. **Causes of (1) central alveolar hypoventilation include congenital defects, drugs, and central nervous system disorders (e.g., stroke, trauma, and neoplasms); (2) obesity hypoventilation syndrome is another well-known cause of hypoventilation; (3) chest wall deformities (e.g., kyphoscoliosis and changes after thoracic surgery) can be associated with alveolar hypoventilation leading to respiratory insufficiency and failure; (4) neuromuscular diseases that can cause alveolar hypoventilation include myasthenia gravis, amyotrophic lateral sclerosis, Guillain-Barré, and muscular dystrophy.**
- Assess spontaneous respiratory pattern, noting rate, depth, rhythm, symmetry of chest movement, use of accessory muscles. **Tachypnea, shallow breathing, demonstrated or reported dyspnea (using a numeric or similar scale); increased heart rate, dysrhythmias; pallor or cyanosis; and intercostal retractions and use of accessory muscles indicate increased work of breathing or impaired gas exchange impairment.**
- Auscultate breath sounds, noting presence or absence and equality of breath sounds, adventitious breath sounds.
- Evaluate ABGs and/or pulse oximetry and capnography **to determine presence and degree of arterial hypoxemia**

Information that appears in brackets has been added by the authors to clarify and enhance the use of nursing diagnoses.

(PaO_2 <55) and hypercapnea (CO_2 >45), resulting in impaired ventilation requiring ventilatory support.

- Obtain or review results of pulmonary function studies (e.g., lung volumes, **inspiratory and expiratory pressures, and forced vital capacity), as appropriate, to assess presence and degree of respiratory insufficiency.**
- Investigate etiology of current respiratory failure **to determine ventilation needs and most appropriate type of ventilatory support.**
- Review serial chest x-rays and imaging magnetic resonance imaging/computed tomography scan results **to diagnose underlying disorder and monitor response to treatment.**
- Note response to current measures and respiratory therapy (e.g., bronchodilators, supplemental oxygen, nebulizer or intermittent positive-pressure breathing treatments).

Nursing Priority No. 2.

To provide/maintain ventilatory support:

- Collaborate with physician, respiratory care practitioners regarding effective mode of ventilation (e.g., noninvasive oxygenation via continuous positive airway pressure (CPAP) and biphasic positive airway pressure [BiPAP]); or intubation and mechanical ventilation (e.g., continuous mandatory, assist control, intermittent mandatory [IMV], pressure support). **Specific mode is determined by client's respiratory requirements, presence of underlying disease process, and the extent to which client can participate in ventilatory efforts.**
- Ensure that ventilator settings and parameters are correct as ordered by client situation, including respiratory rate, fraction of inspired oxygen (FIO_2, expressed as a percentage); tidal volume; peak inspiratory pressure.
- Observe overall breathing pattern, distinguishing between spontaneous respirations and ventilator breaths. **Client may be completely dependent on the ventilator or able to take breaths but have poor oxygen saturation without the ventilator.**
- Verify that client's respirations are in phase with the ventilator. **Decreases work of breathing; maximizes O_2 delivery.**
- Inflate tracheal or endotracheal (ET) tube cuff properly using minimal leak or occlusive technique. Check cuff inflation periodically per facility protocol and whenever cuff is deflated and reinflated **to prevent risk associated with underinflation or overinflation.**

Information that appears in brackets has been added by the authors to clarify and enhance the use of nursing diagnoses.

- Check tubing for obstruction (e.g., kinking or accumulation of water). Drain tubing as indicated; avoid draining toward client or back into the reservoir, **resulting in contamination and providing medium for growth of bacteria.**
- Check ventilator alarms for proper functioning. Do not turn off alarms, even for suctioning. Remove from ventilator and ventilate manually if source of ventilator alarm cannot be quickly identified and rectified. Verify that alarms can be heard in the nurses' station by care providers.
- Verify that oxygen line is in proper outlet/tank; monitor in-line oxygen analyzer or perform periodic oxygen analysis.
- Verify tidal volume set to volume needed for individual situation and proper functioning of spirometer, bellows, or computer readout of delivered volume. Note alterations from desired volume delivery **to determine alteration in lung compliance or leakage through machine/around tube cuff (if used).**
- Monitor airway pressure **for developing complications or equipment problems.**
- Monitor inspiratory and expiratory ratio.
- Promote maximal ventilation of alveoli; check sigh rate intervals (usually $1\frac{1}{2}$ to 2 times tidal volume). **Reduces risk of atelectasis, helps mobilize secretions.**
- Note inspired humidity and temperature; maintain hydration **to liquify secretions, facilitating removal.**
- Auscultate breath sounds periodically. Investigate frequent crackles or rhonchi that do not clear with coughing or suctioning—**suggestive of developing complications (atelectasis, pneumonia, acute bronchospasm, pulmonary edema).**
- Suction only as needed, using lowest pressure possible **to clear secretions and maintain airway.**
- Note changes in chest symmetry. **May indicate improper placement of ET tube, development of barotrauma.**
- Keep resuscitation bag at bedside **to allow for manual ventilation whenever indicated (e.g., if client is removed from ventilator or troubleshooting equipment problems).**
- Administer sedation as required **to synchronize respirations and reduce work of breathing and energy expenditure, as indicated.**
- Administer and monitor response to medications that promote airway patency and gas exchange.
- Refer to NDs ineffective Airway Clearance; ineffective Breathing Pattern; impaired Gas Exchange, for related interventions.

Information that appears in brackets has been added by the authors to clarify and enhance the use of nursing diagnoses.

Nursing Priority No. 3.

To prepare for/assist with weaning process if appropriate:

- Determine physical and psychological readiness to wean, including specific respiratory parameters, absence of infection or cardiac failure, client alert and/or able to sustain spontaneous respiration, nutritional status sufficient to maintain work of breathing.
- Determine mode for weaning. **Pressure support mode or multiple daily T-piece trials may be superior to IMV; low-level pressure support may be beneficial for spontaneous breathing trials; and early extubation and institution of noninvasive positive pressure ventilation may have substantial benefits in alert, cooperative client.**
- Explain weaning activities and techniques, individual plan, and expectations. **Reduces fear of unknown.**
- Elevate head of bed or place in orthopedic chair, if possible, or position **to alleviate dyspnea and to facilitate oxygenation.**
- Coach client in "taking control" of breathing (to take slower, deeper breaths, practice abdominal or pursed-lip breathing, assume position of comfort) **to maximize respiratory function and reduce anxiety.**
- Instruct in or assist client to practice effective coughing techniques. **Necessary for secretion management after extubation.**
- Provide quiet environment, calm approach, undivided attention of nurse. **Promotes relaxation, decreasing energy and oxygen requirements.**
- Involve family/SO(s) as appropriate. Provide diversional activity. **Helps client focus on something other than breathing.**
- Instruct client in use of energy-saving techniques during care activities **to limit oxygen consumption and fatigue.**
- Acknowledge and provide ongoing encouragement for client's efforts. Communicate hope for successful weaning response (even partial). **Enhances commitment to continue activity, maximizing outcomes.**

Nursing Priority No. 4.

To prepare for discharge on ventilator when indicated:

- Ascertain plan for discharge placement (e.g., return home, short-term stay in subacute or rehabilitation center, or permanent placement in long-term care facility).

Information that appears in brackets has been added by the authors to clarify and enhance the use of nursing diagnoses.

- Determine specific equipment needs. Identify resources for equipment needs and maintenance and arrange for delivery prior to client discharge.
- Review layout of home, noting size of rooms, doorways, placement of furniture, number and type of electrical outlets **to identify specific safety needs.**
- Obtain No Smoking signs to be posted in home. Encourage family members to refrain from smoking.
- Have family/SO(s) notify utility companies and fire department about ventilator in home.
- Develop emergency disaster plan to address backup electrical needs and possible evacuation if required.
- Review and provide written or audiovisual materials regarding proper ventilator management, maintenance, and safety **for reference in home setting, enhancing client's/SO's knowledge and level of comfort.**
- Demonstrate airway management techniques and proper equipment cleaning practices.
- Instruct SO(s)/caregivers in other pulmonary physiotherapy measures as indicated (e.g., chest physiotherapy).
- Allow sufficient opportunity for SO(s)/caregivers to practice new skills. Role-play potential crisis situations **to enhance confidence in ability to handle client's needs.**
- Identify signs/symptoms requiring prompt medical evaluation/intervention. **Timely treatment may prevent progression of problem.**
- Provide positive feedback and encouragement for efforts of SO(s)/caregivers. **Promotes continuation of desired behaviors.**
- List names and phone numbers for identified contact persons/resources. **Round-the-clock availability reduces sense of isolation and enhances likelihood of obtaining appropriate information or assistance when needed.**

Nursing Priority No. 5.

To promote wellness (Teaching/Discharge Considerations):

- Discuss impact of specific activities on respiratory status and problem-solve solutions to maximize weaning effort.
- Engage client in specialized exercise program **to enhance respiratory muscle strength and general endurance.**
- Protect client from sources of infection (e.g., monitor health of visitors, roommate, caregivers).
- Recommend involvement in support group; introduce to individuals dealing with similar problems **to provide role models, assistance for problem-solving.**

Information that appears in brackets has been added by the authors to clarify and enhance the use of nursing diagnoses.

- Encourage time out for caregivers **so that they may attend to personal needs, wellness, and growth.**
- Provide opportunities for client/SO(s) to discuss termination of therapy and other end-of-life decisions.
- Refer to individual(s) who are ventilator dependent/have managed home ventilation successfully **to encourage hope for the future.**
- Refer to additional resources (e.g., spiritual advisor, counselor).

Documentation Focus

Assessment/Reassessment

- Baseline findings, subsequent alterations in respiratory function
- Results of diagnostic testing
- Individual risk factors and concerns

Planning

- Plan of care and who is involved in planning
- Teaching plan

Implementation/Evaluation

- Client's/SO's responses to interventions, teaching, and actions performed
- Skill level and assistance needs of SO(s)/family
- Attainment or progress toward desired outcome(s)
- Modifications to plan of care

Discharge Planning

- Discharge plan, including appropriate referrals, action taken, and who is responsible for each action
- Equipment needs and source
- Resources for support persons or home care providers

Sample Nursing Outcomes & Interventions Classifications (NOC/NIC)

NOC—Respiratory Status: Ventilation
NIC—Mechanical Ventilation Management: Invasive

Information that appears in brackets has been added by the authors to clarify and enhance the use of nursing diagnoses.

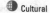

dysfunctional VENTILATORY WEANING RESPONSE

[Diagnostic Division: Respiration]

Definition: Inability to adjust to lowered levels of mechanical ventilator support that interrupts and prolongs the weaning process.

Related Factors

Physiological

Ineffective airway clearance
Alteration in sleep pattern
Inadequate nutrition
Pain
[Muscle weakness or fatigue; inability to control respiratory muscles; immobility]

Psychological

Insufficient knowledge of the weaning process
Uncertainty about ability to wean
Decrease in motivation; low self-esteem
Anxiety; fear; insufficient trust in healthcare professionals
Hopelessness; powerlessness
[Unprepared for weaning attempt]

Situational

Uncontrolled episodic energy demands
Inappropriate pace of weaning process
Insufficient social support
Environmental barrier (e.g., distractions, low nurse-to-patient ratio; unfamiliar healthcare staff)
History of ventilator dependence more than 4 days
History of unsuccessful weaning attempt

Defining Characteristics

Mild

Subjective

Perceived need for increase in oxygen; breathing discomfort; fatigue; warmth
Fear of machine malfunction

Information that appears in brackets has been added by the authors to clarify and enhance the use of nursing diagnoses.

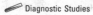

Objective
Restlessness
Mild increase of respiratory rate from baseline
Increase in focus on breathing

Moderate

Subjective
Apprehensiveness

Objective
Increase in blood pressure (<20 mm Hg)/heart rate (<20 beats/min) from baseline
Moderate increase in respiratory rate over baseline; minimal use of respiratory accessory muscles; decrease in air entry on auscultation
Hyperfocused on activities; facial expression of fear
Impaired ability to cooperate or respond to coaching
Diaphoresis
Abnormal skin color (e.g., pale, dusky, cyanosis)

Severe

Objective
Agitation; decrease in level of consciousness
Deterioration in arterial blood gases from baseline
Increase in blood pressure (≥20 mm Hg) or heart rate (≥20 beats/min) from baseline
Significant increase in respiratory rate above baseline; use of significant respiratory accessory muscles; shallow breathing; gasping breaths; paradoxical abdominal breathing
Adventitious breath sounds
Asynchronized breathing with the ventilator
Profuse diaphoresis
Abnormal skin color (e.g., pale, dusky, cyanosis)

Desired Outcomes/Evaluation Criteria—Client Will:

- Actively participate in the weaning process.
- Reestablish independent respiration with arterial blood gases (ABGs) within client's normal range and be free of signs of respiratory failure.
- Demonstrate increased tolerance for activity and participate in self-care within level of ability.

Information that appears in brackets has been added by the authors to clarify and enhance the use of nursing diagnoses.

Actions/Interventions

Nursing Priority No. 1.

To identify contributing factors/degree of dysfunction:

- Determine extent and nature of underlying disorders or factors (e.g., preexisting cardiopulmonary diseases, significant trauma, neuromuscular disorders, multisystem organ failure; ventilator-associated pneumonia; complications from surgical procedures) **that contribute to client's reliance on mechanical support and can affect future weaning efforts.**
- Note length of time client has been receiving ventilator support. Review previous episodes of extubation and reintubation. **Previous unsuccessful weaning attempts (e.g., due to inability to protect airway or clear secretions; oxygen saturation less than 50% on room air) that can influence future weaning interventions.**
- Assess systemic parameters that may affect readiness for weaning using Burns Weaning Assessment Program (BWAP) or similar checklist (e.g., stability of vital signs, factors that increase metabolic rate [e.g., sepsis, fever]; hydration status; need for/recent use of analgesia or sedation; nutritional state; muscle strength; activity level) **to assess systemic parameters that may affect readiness for weaning. *Note:* A recent study of the use of BWAP score in five adult critical care units found that a score of 50 or higher was linked to successful weaning outcomes.**
- Ascertain client's awareness and understanding of weaning process, expectations, and concerns. **Client/significant other (SO) may need specific and repeated instructions during process.**
- Determine psychological readiness, presence and degree of anxiety. **Weaning provokes anxiety regarding ability to breathe on own and likelihood of ventilator dependence. The client must be highly motivated, be able to actively participate in the weaning process, and be physically comfortable enough to work at weaning.**
- Introduce client to individual who has shared similar experiences with successful outcome if desired or indicated **to provide support and encouragement for successful outcome.**
- Review laboratory studies (e.g., complete blood count reflecting number and integrity of red blood cells **[affects oxygen transport]**, serum albumin and electrolyte levels indicating nutritional status **[to confirm sufficient energy to meet demands of spontaneous breathing and weaning]**).

Information that appears in brackets has been added by the authors to clarify and enhance the use of nursing diagnoses.

- Review chest x-ray, pulse oximetry or capnography, and/or ABGs. **Before weaning attempts, chest radiograph should show clear lungs or marked improvement in pulmonary congestion. ABGs should document satisfactory oxygenation on an FIO_2 of 40% or less. Capnometry measures end-tidal carbon dioxide values and can be used to confirm correct placement of endotracheal tube and monitor integrity of ventilation equipment.**

Nursing Priority No. 2.

To support weaning process:

- Discuss with client/SO(s) individual plan and expectations. Assure client of nurse's presence and assistance during weaning attempts. **May reduce client's anxiety about process and ultimate outcome and enhance willingness to work at spontaneous breathing.**
- Consult with dietitian, nutritional support team for adjustments in composition of diet **to support respiratory muscle strength and work of breathing and to prevent excessive production of CO_2, which could alter respiratory drive.**
- Implement weaning protocols and mode (e.g., spontaneous breathing trials, automatic tube compensation [ATC], partial client support [SIMV], or pressure support [PSV] during client's spontaneous breathing) **to optimize the work of breathing and to provide support for spontaneous ventilation.**
- Note response to activity/client care during weaning and limit, as indicated. Provide undisturbed rest or sleep periods. Avoid stressful procedures or situations and nonessential activities. **Prevents excessive oxygen consumption or demand with increased possibility of weaning failure.**
- Time medications during weaning efforts **to minimize sedative effects.**
- Provide quiet room, calm approach, undivided attention of nurse. **Enhances relaxation, conserving energy.**
- Involve SO(s)/family, as appropriate (e.g., sitting at bedside, providing encouragement, and helping monitor client status).
- Provide diversional activity (e.g., watching TV, reading aloud) **to focus attention away from breathing when not actively working at breathing exercises.**
- Auscultate breath sounds periodically; suction airway, as indicated.
- Acknowledge and provide ongoing encouragement for client's efforts.

Information that appears in brackets has been added by the authors to clarify and enhance the use of nursing diagnoses.

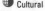

- Minimize setbacks, focus client attention on gains and progress to date **to reduce frustration that may further impair progress.**

Nursing Priority No. 3.

To prepare for discharge on ventilator when indicated:

- Prepare client/SO for alternative actions when client is unable to resume spontaneous ventilation (e.g., tracheostomy with long-term ventilation support in alternate care setting or home, palliative care or end-of-life procedures). **Customized discharge planning for people new to home ventilation is essential. This must include assessment of the environment, assessment of resources, assessment of caregivers, education and training, and a plan of care.**
- Ascertain that all needed equipment is in place, caregivers are trained, and safety concerns have been addressed (e.g., alternative power source, backup equipment, client call or alarm system, established means of client/caregiver communication) **to ease the transfer when client is going home on ventilator.**
- Evaluate caregiver capabilities and burden when client requires long-term ventilator in the home **to determine potential or presence of skill-related problems or emotional issues (e.g., caregiver overload, burnout, or depression).**
- Refer to ND impaired spontaneous Ventilation for additional interventions.

Nursing Priority No. 4.

To promote wellness (Teaching/Discharge Considerations):

- Encourage client/SO(s) to evaluate impact of ventilatory dependence on their lifestyle and what changes they are willing or unwilling to make when client is discharged on ventilator. **Quality-of-life issues must be examined, including issues of privacy and intimacy, and resolved by the ventilator-dependent client and SO(s). All parties need to understand that ventilatory support is a 24-hr job that ultimately affects everyone.**
- Discuss importance of time for self and identify appropriate sources for respite care. (Refer to ND risk for caregiver Role Strain.)
- Emphasize to client/SO(s) importance of monitoring health of visitors and persons involved in care, avoiding crowds during flu season, obtaining immunizations, and so forth, **to protect client from sources of infection.**

Information that appears in brackets has been added by the authors to clarify and enhance the use of nursing diagnoses.

- Encourage client/SO(s) to discuss advance directives and ascertain that all care providers are aware of the plan of care. **Clarifies parameters for emergency situations, termination of therapy, or other end-of-life decisions, as desired.**
- Recommend involvement in support group (may be online); introduce to other ventilator-dependent individuals who are successfully managing home ventilation, if desired, **to answer questions, provide role model, assist with problem-solving, and offer encouragement and hope for the future.**
- Identify conditions requiring immediate medical intervention **to treat developing complications and prevent respiratory failure.**

Documentation Focus

Assessment/Reassessment

- Baseline findings and subsequent alterations
- Results of diagnostic testing or procedures
- Individual risk factors

Planning

- Plan of care, specific interventions, and who is involved in the planning
- Teaching plan

Implementation/Evaluation

- Client response to interventions
- Attainment or progress toward desired outcome(s)
- Modifications to plan of care

Discharge Planning

- Status at discharge, long-term needs and referrals, indicating who is to be responsible for each action
- Equipment needs and supplier

Sample Nursing Outcomes & Interventions Classifications (NOC/NIC)

NOC—Respiratory Status: Ventilation
NIC—Mechanical Ventilatory Weaning

Information that appears in brackets has been added by the authors to clarify and enhance the use of nursing diagnoses.

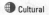

NOTE: NANDA has separated the diagnosis of Violence into its two elements: "other-directed" and "self-directed." However, the interventions in general address both situations and have been left in one block following the definitions and supporting data of those two diagnoses.

risk for other-directed **VIOLENCE**

[Diagnostic Division: Safety]

Definition: Vulnerable to behaviors in which an individual demonstrates that he or she can be physically, emotionally, and/or sexually harmful to others.

Risk Factors

Neurological impairment (e.g., positive electroencephalogram [EEG], head trauma, seizure disorders)
Alteration in cognitive functioning
Cruelty to animals; fire-setting
Prenatal or perinatal complications
Pathological intoxication; [toxic reaction to pharmaceutical agent]
Psychotic disorder; [panic states; rage reactions; manic excitement]
Motor vehicle offense (e.g., traffic violations, use of a motor vehicle to release anger)
Suicidal behavior; impulsiveness; access to weapon
Negative body language (e.g., rigid posture, clenching of fists/jaw, hyperactivity, pacing, threatening stances)
Pattern of other-directed violence (e.g., hitting/kicking/spitting/scratching others, throwing objects/biting someone, attempted rape, rape, sexual molestation; urinating/defecating on a person)
Pattern of threatening violence (e.g., verbal threats against property/people, social threats, cursing, threatening notes/gestures, sexual threats)
Pattern of violent antisocial behavior (e.g., stealing, insistent borrowing, insistent demands for privileges, insistent interrupting, refusal to eat/take medication, ignoring instructions)
Pattern of indirect violence (e.g., tearing objects off walls, urinating/defecating on floor, stamping feet, temper tantrum,

Information that appears in brackets has been added by the authors to clarify and enhance the use of nursing diagnoses.

throwing objects, breaking a window, slamming doors, sexual advances)
History of substance abuse
History of childhood abuse (e.g., physical, psychological, sexual), witnessing family violence

risk for self-directed VIOLENCE

[Diagnostic Division: Safety]

Definition: Vulnerable to behaviors in which an individual demonstrates that he or she can be physically, emotionally, and/or sexually harmful to self.

Risk Factors

Ages 15 to 19, ≥45
Marital status (e.g., single, widowed, divorced)
Employment concern (e.g., unemployed, recent job loss/failure); occupation (e.g., executive, administrator/owner of business, professional, semiskilled worker)
Conflict in interpersonal relationship(s)
Pattern of difficulties in family background (e.g., chaotic or conflictual, history of suicide)
Conflict about sexual orientation; engagement in autoerotic sexual acts
Physical health issue
Mental health issue (e.g., depression, psychosis, severe personality disorder, substance abuse); suicidal ideation, plan; history of multiple suicide attempts; psychological disorder
Insufficient personal resources (e.g., achievement, insight, affect unavailable and poorly controlled); social isolation
Verbal clues (e.g., talking about death, "better off without me," asking about lethal dosages of medication)
Behavioral clues (e.g., writing forlorn love notes, directing angry messages at a significant other (SO) who has rejected the person, giving away personal items, taking out a large life insurance policy)

Desired Outcomes/Evaluation Criteria—[Other-Directed or Self-Directed] Client Will:

- Acknowledge realities of the situation.
- Verbalize understanding of why behavior occurs.

Information that appears in brackets has been added by the authors to clarify and enhance the use of nursing diagnoses.

- Identify precipitating factors.
- Express realistic self-evaluation and increased sense of self-esteem.
- Participate in care and meet own needs in an assertive manner.
- Demonstrate self-control as evidenced by relaxed posture, nonviolent behavior.
- Use resources and support systems in an effective manner.

Actions/Interventions

Addresses both "other-directed" and "self-directed"

Nursing Priority No. 1.

To assess causative/contributing factors:

- Determine underlying dynamics as listed in Risk Factors.
- Ascertain client's perception of self and situation. Note use of defense mechanisms (e.g., denial, projection).
- Observe and listen for early cues of distress or increasing anxiety (e.g., irritability, lack of cooperation, demanding behavior, body posture or expression). **May indicate possibility of loss of control, and intervention at this point can prevent a blowup.**
- Identify conditions such as acute or chronic brain syndrome, panic state, hormonal imbalance (e.g., premenstrual syndrome, postpartal psychosis), drug induced, postanesthesia/postseizure confusion, traumatic brain injury. **These physical conditions may interfere with ability to control own behavior and will need specific interventions to manage.**
- Review laboratory findings (e.g., blood alcohol, blood glucose, arterial blood gases, electrolytes, renal function tests).
- Observe for signs of suicidal/homicidal intent (e.g., perceived morbid or anxious feeling while with the client; warning from the client: "It doesn't matter," "I'd/They'd be better off dead"; mood swings; "accident-prone" or self-destructive behavior; suicidal attempts; possession of alcohol and/or other drug(s) in known substance abuser). (Refer to ND risk for Suicide.)
- Note family history of suicidal or homicidal behavior. **Children who grow up in homes where violence is accepted tend to grow up to use violence as a means of solving problems.**
- Ask directly if the person is thinking of acting on thoughts or feelings **to determine violent intent.**
- Determine availability of homicidal means.
- Assess client coping behaviors already present. **Client may believe there are no alternatives other than violence, es-**

Information that appears in brackets has been added by the authors to clarify and enhance the use of nursing diagnoses.

pecially if individual has come from a family background of violence.

- Identify risk factors and assess for indicators of child abuse or neglect: unexplained or frequent injuries, failure to thrive, and so forth.

Nursing Priority No. 2.

To assist client to accept responsibility for impulsive behavior and potential for violence:

- Develop therapeutic nurse-client relationship. Provide consistent caregiver when possible. **Promotes sense of trust, allowing client to discuss feelings openly.**
- Maintain straightforward communication **to avoid reinforcing manipulative behavior.**
- Discuss motivation for change (e.g., failing relationships, job loss, involvement with judicial system). **Crisis situation can provide impetus for change, but requires timely therapeutic intervention to sustain efforts.**
- Help client recognize that client's actions may be in response to own fear **(may be afraid of own behavior or loss of control),** dependency, and feeling of powerlessness.
- Make time to listen to expressions of feelings. Acknowledge reality of client's feelings and that feelings are okay. (Refer to ND Self-Esteem [specify].)
- Confront client's tendency to minimize situation or behavior. **In domestic violence situations, individual may be remorseful after incident and will apologize and say that it won't happen again.**
- Review factors (feelings and events) involved in precipitating violent behavior.
- Discuss impact of behavior on others and consequences of actions.
- Acknowledge reality of suicide or homicide as an option. Discuss consequences of actions if they were to follow through on intent. Ask how it will help client to resolve problems. **Provides an opportunity for client to look at reality of choices and potential outcomes.**
- Accept client's anger without reacting on emotional basis. Give permission to express angry feelings in acceptable ways and let client know that staff will be available to assist in maintaining control. **Promotes acceptance and sense of safety.**

Information that appears in brackets has been added by the authors to clarify and enhance the use of nursing diagnoses.

- Help client identify more appropriate solutions or behaviors (e.g., motor activities, exercise) **to lessen sense of anxiety and associated physical manifestations.**
- Provide directions for actions client can take, avoiding negatives, such as "Do Nots."

Nursing Priority No. 3.

To assist client in controlling behavior:

- Contract with client regarding safety of self/others.
- Give client as much control as possible within constraints of individual situation. **Enhances self-esteem, promotes confidence in ability to change behavior.**
- Be truthful when giving information and dealing with client. **Builds trust, enhancing therapeutic relationship; prevents manipulative behavior.**
- Identify current and past successes and strengths. Discuss effectiveness of coping techniques used and possible changes. (Refer to ND ineffective Coping.) **Client is often not aware of positive aspects of life, and once recognized, these can be used as a basis for change.**
- Assist client to distinguish between reality and hallucinations or delusions.
- Approach in positive manner, acting as if the client has control and is responsible for own behavior. Be aware, though, that the client may not have control, especially if under the influence of drugs (including alcohol).
- Maintain distance and do not touch client without permission when situation indicates client does not tolerate such closeness (e.g., post-trauma response).
- Remain calm and state limits on inappropriate behavior (including consequences) in a firm manner.
- Direct client to stay in view of staff/caregiver.
- Administer prescribed medications (e.g., anti-anxiety or antipsychotic), taking care not to oversedate client. **The chemistry of the brain is changed by early violence and has been shown to respond to serotonin, as well as related neurotransmitter systems, which play a role in restraining aggressive impulses.**
- Monitor for possible drug interactions, cumulative effects of drug regimen (e.g., anticonvulsants, antidepressants).
- Give positive reinforcement for client's efforts. **Encourages continuation of desired behaviors.**

Information that appears in brackets has been added by the authors to clarify and enhance the use of nursing diagnoses.

- Explore death fantasies when expressed (e.g., "I'll look down and watch them suffer"; "She'll be sorry") or the idea that death is not final (e.g., "I can come back").

Nursing Priority No. 4.

To assist client/SO(s) to correct/deal with existing situation:

- Gear interventions to individual(s) involved, based on age, relationship, and so forth.
- Maintain calm, matter-of-fact, nonjudgmental attitude. **Decreases defensive response.**
- Notify potential victims in the presence of serious homicidal threat in accordance with legal and ethical guidelines. **Various Tarasoff statutes exist in many states requiring mental health professionals to report specific threats to both the individual named and law enforcement.**
- Discuss situation with abused or battered person, providing accurate information about choices and effective actions that can be taken.
- Assist individual to understand that angry, vengeful feelings are appropriate in the situation but need to be expressed and not acted on. (Refer to ND Post-Trauma Syndrome, as psychological responses may be similar.)
- Identify resources available for assistance (e.g., battered women's shelter, social services).

Nursing Priority No. 5.

To promote safety in event of violent behavior:

- Provide a safe, quiet environment and remove items from the client's environment that could be used to inflict harm to self or others.
- Maintain distance from client who is striking out or hitting and take evasive and controlling actions, as indicated.
- Call for additional staff/security personnel.
- Approach aggressive or attacking client from the front, just out of reach, in a commanding posture with palms down.
- Tell client to *STOP*. **This may be sufficient to help client control own actions.**
- Maintain direct, constant eye contact, when appropriate.
- Speak in a low, commanding voice.
- Provide client with a sense that caregiver is in control of the situation **to provide feeling of safety.**
- Maintain clear route for staff and client and be prepared to move quickly.
- Hold client, using restraints or seclusion, when necessary, until client regains self-control.

Information that appears in brackets has been added by the authors to clarify and enhance the use of nursing diagnoses.

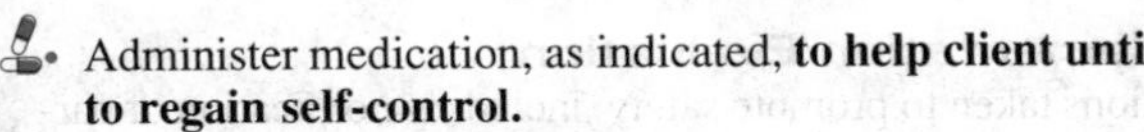

- Administer medication, as indicated, **to help client until able to regain self-control.**

Nursing Priority No. 6.

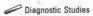

To promote wellness (Teaching/Discharge Considerations):

- Promote client involvement in planning care within limits of situation, allowing for meeting own needs for enjoyment. **Individuals often believe they are not entitled to pleasure and good things in their lives and need to learn how to meet these needs.**
- Assist client to learn assertive rather than manipulative, nonassertive, or aggressive behavior. **Promotes behaviors that help client to engage in positive social activities with others.**
- Discuss reasons for client's behavior with SO(s). Determine desire and commitment of involved parties to sustain current relationships.
- Develop strategies to help parents learn more effective parenting skills (e.g., parenting classes, appropriate ways of dealing with frustrations). **Developing positive relationships has a powerful effect on helping children learn impulse control.**
- Identify support systems (e.g., family/friends, clergy). **In addition to the client, those around him or her need to learn how to be positive role models and display a broader array of skills for resolving problems.**
- Refer to formal resources, as indicated (e.g., individual or group psychotherapy, substance abuse treatment program, social services, safe house facility, parenting classes).
- Refer to NDs impaired Parenting; family Coping [specify]; Post-Trauma Syndrome.

Documentation Focus

Assessment/Reassessment

- Individual findings, including nature of concern (e.g., suicidal or homicidal), behavioral risk factors and level of impulse control, plan of action and means to carry out plan
- Client's perception of situation, motivation for change
- Family history of violence
- Availability and use of resources

Planning

- Plan of care and who is involved in the planning
- Details of contract regarding violence to self/others
- Teaching plan

Information that appears in brackets has been added by the authors to clarify and enhance the use of nursing diagnoses.

Implementation/Evaluation
- Actions taken to promote safety, including notification of parties at risk
- Response to interventions, teaching, and actions performed
- Attainment or progress toward desired outcome(s)
- Modifications to plan of care

Discharge Planning
- Long-term needs and who is responsible for actions to be taken
- Available resources, specific referrals made

Sample Nursing Outcomes & Interventions Classifications (NOC/NIC)

other-directed Violence
NOC—Aggression Self-Control
NIC—Anger Control Assistance

self-directed Violence
NOC—Impulse Self-Control
NIC—Behavior Management: Self-Harm

impaired WALKING

[Diagnostic Division: Activity/Rest]

Definition: Limitation of independent movement within the environment on foot.

Related Factors

Insufficient muscle strength; neuromuscular impairment; musculoskeletal impairment
Decrease in endurance; physical deconditioning
Fear of falling; impaired balance, vision
Pain
Obesity
Alteration in mood; alteration in cognitive functioning
Insufficient knowledge of mobility strategies
Environmental barrier (e.g., stairs, inclines, uneven surfaces, unsafe obstacles, distances, lack of assistive device)

Information that appears in brackets has been added by the authors to clarify and enhance the use of nursing diagnoses.

Defining Characteristics

Subjective or Objective

Impaired ability to walk required distances, walk on an incline/decline, walk on uneven surfaces, to navigate curbs, climb stairs

[Specify level of independence—refer to ND impaired physical Mobility, for suggested functional level classification]

Desired Outcomes/Evaluation Criteria—Client Will:

- Be able to move about within environment as needed or desired within limits of ability or with appropriate adjuncts.
- Verbalize understanding of situation or risk factors and safety measures.

Actions/Interventions

Nursing Priority No. 1.

To assess causative/contributing factors:

- Identify conditions or diagnoses (e.g., advanced age, sensory impairments, pain, obesity, chronic fatigue, cognitive dysfunction, acute illness with weakness; *chronic illness* [e.g., cardiopulmonary disorders, cancer], *musculoskeletal injuries or surgery* [e.g., sprains, fractures, tendon or ligament injury; total joint replacement; surgical repair of fractured bone; amputation], *balance problems* [e.g., inner ear infection, brain injury, stroke], *nerve disorders* [e.g., multiple sclerosis, Parkinson's disease, cerebral palsy], *spinal abnormalities* [disease, trauma, degeneration], *impaired circulation or neuropathies* [e.g., peripheral, diabetic, alcoholic], *degenerative bone or muscle disorders* [e.g., osteoporosis, muscular dystrophy, myositis], *foot conditions* [e.g., plantar warts, bunions, ingrown toenails, pressure ulcers]) **that contribute to walking impairment and identify specific needs and appropriate interventions.**
- Note client's particular symptoms related to walking (e.g., unable to bear weight, cannot walk usual distance, limping, staggering, stiff leg, leg pain, shuffling, asymmetric or unsteady gait, can walk on certain surfaces, but not on others).
- Determine ability to follow directions and note emotional/behavioral responses **that may be affecting client's ability or desire to engage in activity.**

Information that appears in brackets has been added by the authors to clarify and enhance the use of nursing diagnoses.

Nursing Priority No. 2.

To assess functional ability:

- Perform "Timed Up and Go (TUG)" test, as indicated, **to assess client's basic ability to ambulate safely. Factors assessed include sitting balance, ability to transfer from sitting to standing and back to sitting, the pace and stability of ambulation, and the ability to turn without staggering.**
- Determine degree of impairment in relation to suggested functional scale (0 to 4), noting that impairment can be temporary, permanent, or progressive. **Condition may be caused by reversible condition (e.g., weakness associated with acute illness or fractures/surgery with weight-bearing restrictions); or walking impairment can be permanent (e.g., congenital anomalies, amputation, severe rheumatoid arthritis).**
- Assist with or review results of mobility testing (e.g., gait, timing of walking over fixed distance, distance walked over set period of time [endurance], limb movement analysis, leg strength and speed of walking, ambulatory activity monitoring) **for differential diagnosis and to guide treatment interventions.**
- Note emotional and behavioral responses of client/SO(s) to problems of mobility. **Walking impairments can negatively affect self-concept and self-esteem, autonomy, and independence. Social, occupational, and relationship roles can change, leading to isolation, depression, and economic consequences.**

Nursing Priority No. 3.

To promote safe, optimal level of independence in walking:

- Assist with treatment of underlying condition causing dysfunction, as indicated by individual situation.
- Consult with physical therapist, occupational therapist, or rehabilitation team **for individualized mobility program and identify and develop appropriate devices (e.g., shoe insert, leg brace to maintain proper foot alignment for walking, quad cane, hemiwalker).**
- Demonstrate use of and help client become comfortable with adjunctive devices (e.g., individually prescribed and fitted cane, crutches, walking cast or boot, walker, limb prosthesis, mobility scooter) **to maintain joint stability or immobilization or to maintain alignment or balance during movement.**

Information that appears in brackets has been added by the authors to clarify and enhance the use of nursing diagnoses.

- Provide assistance when indicated (e.g., walking on uneven surfaces; client is weak or has to walk a distance; or vision, coordination, or posture are impaired).
- Monitor client's cardiopulmonary tolerance for walking. **Increased pulse rate, chest pain, breathlessness, irregular heartbeat is indicative of need to reduce level of activity.** (Refer to ND Activity Intolerance; decreased Cardiac Output, for related interventions.)
- Encourage adequate rest and gradual increase in walking distance **to reduce fatigue or leg pain associated with walking and improve stamina.** (Refer to NDs Fatigue; risk for peripheral neurovascular Dysfunction.)
- Administer medication, as indicated, **to manage pain and maximize level of functioning.** (Refer to NDs acute/chronic Pain; chronic Pain Syndrome.)
- Implement fall precautions for high-risk clients (e.g., frail or ill elderly, visually or cognitively impaired, person on multiple medications, presence of balance disorders) **to reduce risk of accidental injury.** (Refer to NDs risk for Falls; risk for Disuse Syndrome for related interventions.)
- Provide cueing as indicated. **Client may need reminders (e.g., lift foot higher, look where going, walk tall) to concentrate on/perform tasks of walking, especially when balance or cognition is impaired.**
- Assist client to obtain needed information, such as handicapped sticker for close-in parking, sources for mobility scooter, or special public transportation options, when indicated.

Nursing Priority No. 4.

To promote wellness (Teaching/Discharge Considerations):

- Involve client/SO(s) in care, assisting them to learn ways of managing deficits **to enhance safety for client and SO(s)/caregivers.**
- Identify appropriate resources for obtaining and maintaining appliances, equipment, and environmental modifications **to promote mobility.**
- Evaluate client's home (or work) environment for barriers to walking (e.g., uneven surfaces, many steps, no ramps, long distances between places client needs to walk) **to determine needed changes, make recommendations for client safety.**
- Instruct client/SO in safety measures in home, as individually indicated (e.g., maintaining safe travel pathway, proper lighting, wearing glasses, handrails on stairs, grab bars in bath-

---

Information that appears in brackets has been added by the authors to clarify and enhance the use of nursing diagnoses.

room, using walker instead of cane when tired or when walking on uneven surface) **to reduce risk of falls.**
- Discuss need for emergency call/support system (e.g., Lifeline, HealthWatch) **to provide immediate assistance for falls or other home emergencies when client lives alone.**

Documentation Focus

Assessment/Reassessment
- Individual findings, including level of function and ability to participate in specific or desired activities
- Equipment and assistive device needs

Planning
- Plan of care and who is involved in the planning
- Teaching plan

Implementation/Evaluation
- Responses to interventions, teaching, and actions performed
- Attainment or progress toward desired outcome(s)
- Modifications to plan of care

Discharge Planning
- Discharge and long-term needs, noting who is responsible for each action to be taken
- Specific referrals made
- Sources for and maintenance of assistive devices

Sample Nursing Outcomes & Interventions Classifications (NOC/NIC)

NOC—Ambulation
NIC—Exercise Therapy: Ambulation

WANDERING [specify sporadic or continuous]

[Diagnostic Division: Safety]

Definition: Meandering, aimless, or repetitive locomotion that exposes the individual to harm; frequently incongruent with boundaries, limits, or obstacles.

Information that appears in brackets has been added by the authors to clarify and enhance the use of nursing diagnoses.

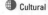

Related Factors

Alteration in cognitive functioning; sedation
Cortical atrophy; psychological disorder
Premorbid behavior (e.g., outgoing, sociable personality)
Separation from familiar environment; overstimulating environment
Physiological state (e.g., hunger, thirst, pain, need to urinate)
Time of day

Defining Characteristics

Objective

Frequent or continuous movement from place to place; pacing
Persistent locomotion in search of something; scanning or searching behavior
Haphazard or fretful locomotion; long periods of locomotion without an apparent destination
Locomotion into unauthorized spaces; trespassing
Locomotion resulting in getting lost; eloping behavior
Impaired ability to locate landmarks in a familiar setting
Locomotion that cannot be easily dissuaded; shadowing a caregiver's locomotion
Hyperactivity
Periods of locomotion interspersed with periods of nonlocomotion (e.g., sitting, standing, sleeping)

Desired Outcomes/Evaluation Criteria—Client Will:

- Be free of injury, or unplanned exits.

Caregiver(s) Will:

- Modify environment, as indicated, to enhance safety.
- Provide for maximal independence of client.

Actions/Interventions

Nursing Priority No. 1.

To assess degree of impairment/stage of disease process:

- Ascertain history of client's memory loss and cognitive changes.
- Assist with or review results of specific testing (e.g., Revised Algase Wandering Scale [RAWS], Need-Driven Dementia-

Information that appears in brackets has been added by the authors to clarify and enhance the use of nursing diagnoses.

Compromised Behavior [NDB], or similar tool), as indicated. **Adjunct tools that quantify wandering in several domains can more easily determine individual risks and safety needs.**

- Evaluate client's mental status during daytime and nighttime, noting when client's confusion is most pronounced and when client sleeps. **Can reveal circumstances under which client is likely to wander.**
- Identify client's reason for wandering, if possible. **Client may demonstrate searching behavior (e.g., looking for lost item) or be experiencing sensations (e.g., hunger, thirst, discomfort) without ability to express the actual need.**
- Note timing and pattern of wandering behavior. **Client attempting to leave at 5 p.m. every day may believe he is going home from work; client may be goal directed (e.g., searching for person or object, escaping from something) or nongoal directed (wandering aimlessly).**
- Monitor client's use or need for assistive devices, such as glasses, hearing aids, cane. **Wandering client is at high risk for falls due to cognitive impairments or forgetting necessary assistive devices or how to properly use them.**
- Determine bowel and bladder elimination pattern, timing of incontinence, presence of constipation **for possible correlation to wandering behavior.**
- Ascertain if client has delusions due to shadows, lights, and noises **to determine necessary changes to environment.**

Nursing Priority No. 2.

To assist client/caregiver to deal with situations:

- Provide a structured daily routine. **Decreases wandering behavior and minimizes caregiver stress.**
- Encourage participation in family activities and familiar routines, such as folding laundry, listening to music, or shared walking time outdoors. **May reduce anxiety, depression, and restlessness.** ***Note:*** **Repetitive activity (e.g., folding laundry, or paperwork) may help client with "lapping," wandering to reduce energy expenditure and fatigue.**
- Offer drink of water or snack, bring client to bathroom on a regular schedule. **Wandering may at times be expressing a need.**
- Provide safe place for client to wander, away from safety hazards (e.g., hot water, kitchen stove, open stairway) and other, noisy clients. Arrange furniture, remove scatter rugs, electrical cords, and other high-risk items **to accommodate safe wandering.**

Information that appears in brackets has been added by the authors to clarify and enhance the use of nursing diagnoses.

- Make sure that doors or gates have alarms or chimes and that alarms are turned on. Provide door and window locks that are not within line of sight or easily opened **to prevent unsafe exits.**
- Provide 24-hr supervision and reality orientation. **Client can be awake at any time and fail to recognize day/night routines.**
- Sit with client and visit or reminisce. Provide TV, radio, music **when client is socially gregarious, enjoys conversation, or reminiscence is calming.**
- Avoid overstimulation from activities or new partner/roommate during rest periods when client is in a facility. **Client who is used to wandering in usual living setting may react with increased agitation and emotional outbreaks when admitted to an unfamiliar setting and restricted from wandering.**
- Use pressure-sensitive bed/chair alarms or door mat **to alert caregivers of movement.**
- Avoid using physical or chemical restraints (sedatives) to control wandering behavior. **May increase agitation, sensory deprivation, and falls; may contribute to wandering behavior.**
- Provide consistent staff as much as possible.
- Provide room near monitoring station; check client location on frequent basis.

Nursing Priority No. 3.

To promote wellness (Teaching/Discharge Considerations):

- Identify problems that are remediable and assist client/significant other (SO) to seek appropriate assistance and access resources. **Encourages problem-solving to improve condition rather than accept the status quo.**
- Provide client ID bracelet or necklace with updated photograph, client name, and emergency contact **to assist with identification efforts, particularly when progressive dementia produces marked changes in client's appearance.**
- Notify neighbors about client's condition and request that they contact client's family or local police if they see client outside alone. **Community awareness can prevent/reduce risk of client being lost or hurt.**
- Register client with community or national resources, such as Alzheimer's Association Safe Return Program, **to assist in identification, location, and safe return of individual with wandering behaviors.**
- Help SO(s) develop plan of care when problem is progressive.

Information that appears in brackets has been added by the authors to clarify and enhance the use of nursing diagnoses.

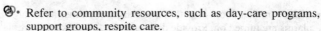

-  Refer to community resources, such as day-care programs, support groups, respite care.
- Refer to NDs acute Confusion; chronic Confusion; [disturbed Sensory Perception (specify)]; risk for Injury; risk for Falls.

Documentation Focus

Assessment/Reassessment

- Assessment findings, including individual concerns, family involvement, and support factors and availability of resources

Planning

- Plan of care and who is involved in planning
- Teaching plan

Implementation/Evaluation

- Responses of client/SO(s) to plan interventions and actions performed
- Attainment or progress toward desired outcome(s)
- Modifications to plan of care

Discharge Planning

- Long-term needs and who is responsible for actions to be taken
- Specific referrals made

Sample Nursing Outcomes & Interventions Classifications (NOC/NIC)

NOC—Safe Wandering
NIC—Elopement Precautions

Information that appears in brackets has been added by the authors to clarify and enhance the use of nursing diagnoses.

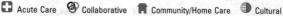

CHAPTER 3

Health Conditions and Client Concerns With Associated Nursing Diagnoses

This chapter presents more than 450 disorders, health conditions, and life situations reflecting all specialty areas, with associated nursing diagnoses written as client problem/need statements that include the "related to" and "evidenced by" components.

This section will facilitate and help validate the assessment and diagnosis steps of the nursing process. Because the nursing process is perpetual and ongoing, other nursing diagnoses may be appropriate based on changing individual situations. Therefore, the nurse must continually assess, identify, and validate new client needs and evaluate subsequent care. Once the appropriate nursing diagnoses have been selected from this chapter, the reader may refer to Chapter 2, which lists the 235 NANDA diagnoses, and review the diagnostic definition, defining characteristics, and related or risk factors for further validation. This step is necessary to determine if the nursing diagnosis is an accurate match, if more data are required, or if another diagnosis needs to be investigated.

To facilitate access to the health conditions or concerns and nursing diagnoses, the client needs have been listed alphabetically and coded to identify nursing specialty areas.

MS: Medical-Surgical
PED: Pediatric
OB: Obstetric
CH: Community/Home
PSY: Psychiatric/Behavioral
GYN: Gynecological

A separate category for geriatrics has not been made because geriatric concerns and conditions are actually subsumed under the other specialty areas, and elderly persons are susceptible to the majority of these problems.

A

Abdominal hysterectomy **MS**

Refer to Hysterectomy

Abdominal perineal resection **MS**

Also refer to Surgery, general

disturbed Body Image may be related to presence of surgical wounds, possibly evidenced by verbalizations of feelings or perceptions, fear of reaction by others, preoccupation with change.

risk for Constipation is possibly evidenced by risk factors of decreased physical activity, slowed gastric motility, abdominal muscle weakness, insufficient fluid intake, change in usual foods and/or eating pattern.*

risk for Sexual dysfunction is possibly evidenced by risk factors of altered body structure or function (radical resection, treatment procedures), vulnerability (psychological concern about response of significant other(s) [SO(s)]), or disruption of sexual response pattern (e.g., erection difficulty).*

Abortion, elective termination **OB**

risk for decisional Conflict is possibly evidenced by risk factors of unclear personal values/beliefs, lack of experience or interference with decision making, information from divergent sources, deficient support system.*

deficient Knowledge [Learning Need] regarding reproduction, contraception, self-care, Rh factor may be related to lack of exposure or recall, misinterpretation of information, possibly evidenced by request for information, statement reflecting misconceptions, inaccurate follow-through of instructions, development of preventable complications.

risk for Moral Distress is possibly evidenced by risk factors of perception of moral or ethical implications of therapeutic procedure, time constraints for decision making.*

Anxiety [specify level] may be related to situational or maturational crises, unmet needs, unconscious conflict about essential values or beliefs, possibly evidenced by increased tension, apprehension, fear of unspecific consequences, sympathetic stimulation, focus on self.

acute Pain/impaired Comfort may be related to aftereffects of procedure, drug effect, possibly evidenced by verbal report, distraction behaviors, changes in muscle tone, changes in vital signs.

risk for [maternal] Injury is possibly evidenced by risk factors of surgical procedure, effects of anesthesia and medications.*

Abortion, spontaneous termination **OB**

risk for Bleeding is possibly evidenced by a risk factor of pregnancy-related complications.*

risk for Spiritual distress is possibly evidenced by risk factors of challenged beliefs/values, blame for loss directed at self or higher power.*

deficient Knowledge [Learning Need] regarding cause of abortion, self-care, contraception, future pregnancy may be related to lack of familiarity with new self or healthcare needs, sources for sup-

*A risk diagnosis is not evidenced by signs and symptoms, as the problem has not occurred; rather, nursing interventions are directed at prevention.

port, possibly evidenced by requests for information and statements of concern or misconceptions, development of preventable complications.

Grieving related to perinatal loss, possibly evidenced by crying, expressions of sorrow, or changes in eating habits or sleep patterns.

risk for Sexual dysfunction is possibly evidenced by risk factors of increasing fear of pregnancy and/or repeat loss, impaired relationship with SO(s), self-doubt regarding own femininity.*

Abruptio placentae **OB**

risk for Shock is possibly evidenced by risk factors of hypotension, hypovolemia.*

Fear related to threat of death (perceived or actual) to fetus and self, possibly evidenced by verbalization of apprehension, increased tension, sympathetic stimulation.

acute Pain may be related to collection of blood between uterine wall and placenta, uterine contractions, possibly evidenced by verbal reports, abdominal guarding, muscle tension, or alterations in vital signs.

risk for disturbed Maternal-Fetal Dyad is possibly evidenced by risk factors of complication of pregnancy, compromised oxygen transport.*

Abscess, brain (acute) **MS**

acute Pain may be related to inflammation, edema of tissues, and is possibly evidenced by reports of headache, restlessness, irritability, and moaning.

risk for Hyperthermia may be related to risk factors of illness [inflammatory process], hypermetabolic state, and dehydration.*

acute Confusion may be related to delirium [cerebral edema, altered perfusion, fever], possibly evidenced by fluctuation in cognition or level of consciousness, increased agitation, restlessness, hallucinations.

risk for Suffocation/Trauma are possibly evidenced by risk factors of disease process [seizure activity], cognitive difficulties.*

Abscess, skin/tissue **CH/MS**

impaired Skin Integrity/impaired Tissue Integrity may be related to immunological deficit, infection, possibly evidenced by disruption of skin, destruction of skin layers or tissues, invasion of body structures.

risk for Infection [spread] possibly evidenced by risk factors of broken skin, traumatized tissues, chronic disease, malnutrition, insufficient knowledge.*

Abuse, physical **CH/PSY**

Also refer to Battered child syndrome

risk for Trauma is possibly evidenced by risk factors of vulnerable client, recipient of verbal threats, history of physical abuse.*

Powerlessness may be related to interpersonal interactions, lifestyle of helplessness as evidenced by verbal expressions of having no control, reluctance to express true feelings, apathy, passivity.

---

*A risk diagnosis is not evidenced by signs and symptoms, as the problem has not occurred; rather, nursing interventions are directed at prevention.

A

chronic low Self-Esteem may be related to situational or maturational crisis, overwhelming threat to self, personal vulnerability, inadequate support systems, possibly evidenced by verbalized concern about ability to deal with current situation, chronic worry, anxiety, depression, poor self-esteem, inability to problem-solve, high illness rate, destructive behavior toward self or others.

Sexual dysfunction may be related to ineffectual or absent role model, vulnerability, physical abuse possibly evidenced by verbalizations, change in sexual behaviors or activities, inability to achieve desired satisfaction.

Abuse, psychological CH/PSY

ineffective Coping may be related to situational or maturational crisis, overwhelming threat to self, personal vulnerability, inadequate support systems, possibly evidenced by verbalized concern about ability to deal with current situation, chronic worry, anxiety, depression, poor self-esteem, inability to problem-solve, high illness rate, destructive behavior toward self or others.

Powerlessness may be related to abusive relationship, lifestyle of helplessness as evidenced by verbal expressions of having no control, reluctance to express true feelings, apathy, passivity.

Sexual dysfunction may be related to ineffectual or absent role model, vulnerability, psychological abuse (harmful relationship), possibly evidenced by reported difficulties, inability to achieve desired satisfaction, conflicts involving values, seeking confirmation of desirability.

Achalasia (cardiospasm) MS

impaired Swallowing may be related to neuromuscular impairment, possibly evidenced by observed difficulty in swallowing or regurgitation.

imbalanced Nutrition: less than body requirements may be related to inability and/or reluctance to ingest adequate nutrients to meet metabolic demands and nutritional needs, possibly evidenced by reported or observed inadequate intake, weight loss, and pale conjunctiva and mucous membranes.

acute Pain may be related to spasm of the lower esophageal sphincter, possibly evidenced by reports of substernal pressure, recurrent heartburn, or gastric fullness (gas pains).

Fear/Anxiety [specify level] may be related to recurrent pain, choking sensation, altered health status, possibly evidenced by verbalizations of distress, apprehension, restlessness, or insomnia.

risk for Aspiration is possibly evidenced by risk factor of regurgitation or spillover of esophageal contents.*

deficient Knowledge [Learning Need] regarding condition, prognosis, self-care, and treatment needs may be related to lack of familiarity with pathology and treatment of condition, possibly evidenced by requests for information, statement of concern, or development of preventable complications.

Acidosis, metabolic MS

Refer to Diabetic ketoacidosis

*A risk diagnosis is not evidenced by signs and symptoms, as the problem has not occurred; rather, nursing interventions are directed at prevention.

Acidosis, respiratory **MS**

Also refer to underlying cause or condition

impaired Gas Exchange may be related to ventilation perfusion imbalance (decreased O_2-carrying capacity of blood, altered O_2 supply, alveolar-capillary membrane changes), possibly evidenced by dyspnea with exertion, tachypnea, changes in mentation, irritability, tachycardia, hypoxia, hypercapnia.

Acne **CH/PED**

impaired Skin Integrity may be related to secretions, infectious process as evidenced by disruptions of skin surface.

disturbed Body Image may be related to change in visual appearance as evidenced by fear of rejection of others, focus on past appearance, negative feelings about body, change in social involvement.

situational low Self-Esteem may be related to adolescence, negative perception of appearance as evidenced by self-negating verbalizations, expressions of helplessness.

Acoustic neuroma **MS**

Also refer to Surgery, general

[disturbed auditory Sensory Perception] may be related to altered sensory reception (compression of eighth cranial nerve), possibly evidenced by unilateral sensorineural hearing loss, tinnitus.

risk for Falls is possibly evidenced by risk factors of hearing difficulties, dizziness, sense of unsteadiness.*

Acquired immune deficiency syndrome **CH**

Refer to AIDS

Acromegaly **CH**

chronic Pain may be related to soft tissue swelling, joint degeneration, peripheral nerve compression possibly evidenced by verbal reports, altered ability to continue previous activities, changes in sleep pattern, fatigue.

disturbed Body Image may be related to biophysical illness or changes, possibly evidenced by verbalization of feelings, concerns, fear of rejection or of reaction of others, negative comments about body, actual change in structure or appearance, change in social involvement.

risk for Sexual dysfunction is possibly evidenced by altered body structure, changes in libido.*

Acute respiratory distress syndrome **MS**

Refer to Respiratory distress syndrome, acute

Adams-Stokes syndrome **CH**

Refer to Dysrhythmia, cardiac

ADD **PED/PSY**

Refer to Attention deficit disorder

Addiction **CH/PSY**

Refer to specific substances; Substance dependence/abuse rehabilitation

---

*A risk diagnosis is not evidenced by signs and symptoms, as the problem has not occurred; rather, nursing interventions are directed at prevention.

A

Addison's disease **MS**

deficient [hypotonic] Fluid Volume may be related to vomiting, diarrhea, increased renal losses, as possibly evidenced by delayed capillary refill, poor skin turgor, dry mucous membranes, report of thirst.

risk for Electrolyte Imbalance is possibly evidenced by risk factors of vomiting, diarrhea, endocrine dysfunction.*

decreased Cardiac Output may be related to hypovolemia and altered electrical conduction (dysrhythmias) and/or diminished cardiac muscle mass, possibly evidenced by alterations in vital signs, changes in mentation, irregular pulse or pulse deficit.

CH

Fatigue may be related to decreased metabolic energy production, altered body chemistry (fluid, electrolyte, and glucose imbalance), as possibly evidenced by unremitting, overwhelming lack of energy, inability to maintain usual routines, decreased performance, impaired ability to concentrate, lethargy, disinterest in surroundings.

disturbed Body Image may be related to changes in skin pigmentation, mucous membranes, loss of axillary or pubic hair, possibly evidenced by verbalization of negative feelings about body and decreased social involvement.

risk for impaired physical Mobility is possibly evidenced by risk factors of neuromuscular impairment (muscle wasting, weakness) and dizziness or syncope.*

imbalanced Nutrition: less than body requirements may be related to glucocorticoid deficiency; abnormal fat, protein, and carbohydrate metabolism; nausea, vomiting, anorexia, possibly evidenced by weight loss, muscle wasting, abdominal cramps, diarrhea, and severe hypoglycemia.

risk for impaired Home Maintenance is possibly evidenced by risk factors of effects of disease process, impaired cognitive functioning, and inadequate support systems.*

Adenoidectomy **PED/MS**

Refer to Tonsillectomy

Adjustment disorder **PED/PSY**

Refer to Anxiety disorders—PED

Adoption/loss of child custody **PSY**

risk for complicated Grieving is possibly evidenced by risk factors of actual loss of child, expectations for future of child and self, thwarted grieving response to loss.*

risk for Powerlessness is possibly evidenced by risk factors of perceived lack of options, no input into decision process, no control over outcome.*

Adrenal crisis, acute **MS**

Also refer to Addison's disease; Shock

deficient [hypotonic] Fluid Volume may be related to failure of regulatory mechanism (damage to or suppression of adrenal gland), in-

---

*A risk diagnosis is not evidenced by signs and symptoms, as the problem has not occurred; rather, nursing interventions are directed at prevention.

ability to concentrate urine, possibly evidenced by decreased venous filling and pulse volume and pressure, hypotension, dry mucous membranes, changes in mentation, decreased serum sodium.

acute Pain may be related to effects of disease process, metabolic imbalances, decreased tissue perfusion, possibly evidenced by reports of severe pain in abdomen, lower back, or legs.

impaired physical Mobility may be related to neuromuscular impairment, decreased muscle strength and control, possibly evidenced by generalized weakness, inability to perform desired activities or movements.

risk for Hyperthermia is possibly evidenced by risk factors of presence of illness, infectious process, dehydration.*

ineffective Protection related to hormone deficiency, drug therapy, nutritional and metabolic deficiencies is possibly evidenced by weakness, anorexia, alteration in perspiration, disorientation.*

Adrenalectomy — MS

ineffective Tissue Perfusion (specify) may be related to hypovolemia and vascular pooling (vasodilation), and is possibly evidenced by diminished pulse, pallor or cyanosis, hypotension, and changes in mentation.

risk for Infection is possibly evidenced by risk factors of inadequate primary defenses (incision, traumatized tissues), suppressed inflammatory response, invasive procedures.*

deficient Knowledge [Learning Need] regarding condition, prognosis, self-care and treatment needs may be related to unfamiliarity with long-term therapy requirements, possibly evidenced by request for information and statement of concern or misconceptions.

Adrenal insufficiency — CH

Refer to Addison's disease

Affective disorder — PSY

Refer to Bipolar disorder; Depressive disorders, major

Affective disorder, seasonal — PSY

Also refer to Depressive disorders, major

[intermittent] ineffective Coping may be related to situational crisis (fall or winter season), disturbance in pattern of tension release, and inadequate resources available, possibly evidenced by verbalizations of inability to cope, changes in sleep pattern (too little or too much), reports of lack of energy, fatigue, lack of resolution of problem, behavioral changes (irritability, discouragement).

imbalanced Nutrition: less than body requirements/risk for Overweight is possibly evidenced by risk factors of eating in response to internal cues other than hunger, alteration in usual coping patterns, change in usual activity level, decreased appetite, lack of energy or interest to prepare food.*

Agoraphobia — PSY

Also refer to Phobia

Anxiety [panic] may be related to contact with feared situation (public place, crowds), possibly evidenced by tachycardia, chest pain, dyspnea, gastrointestinal distress, faintness, sense of impending doom.

---

*A risk diagnosis is not evidenced by signs and symptoms, as the problem has not occurred; rather, nursing interventions are directed at prevention.

Agranulocytosis MS

risk for infection is possibly evidenced by risk factor of suppressed inflammatory response.*

risk for impaired oral Mucous Membrane is possibly evidenced by risk factor of infection.*

risk for imbalanced Nutrition: less than body requirements is possibly evidenced by risk factor of inability to ingest food or fluids.*

AIDS (acquired immunodeficiency syndrome) MS

Also refer to HIV positive

risk for Infection [progression to sepsis/onset of new opportunistic infection] is possibly evidenced by risk factors of depressed immune system, use of antimicrobial agents, inadequate primary defenses, broken skin, traumatized tissue, malnutrition, environmental exposure, invasive techniques, and chronic disease processes.*

risk for deficient Fluid Volume is possibly evidenced by risk factors of excessive losses—copious diarrhea, profuse sweating, vomiting, hypermetabolic state or fever, and restricted intake (nausea, anorexia, lethargy).*

acute Pain/chronic Pain may be related to tissue inflammation or destruction—infections; internal or external cutaneous lesions; rectal excoriation; malignancies; necrosis; peripheral neuropathies, myalgias, and arthralgias, possibly evidenced by verbal reports, self-focusing, or narrowed focus; alteration in muscle tone; paresthesias; paralysis; guarding behaviors; changes in vital signs (acute); restlessness.

ineffective Breathing Pattern/risk for impaired Gas Exchange is possibly evidenced by risk factors of muscular impairment—wasting of respiratory musculature, decreased energy, fatigue, respiratory muscle fatigue; retained secretions—tracheobronchial obstruction; pain.*

CH

imbalanced Nutrition: less than body requirements may be related to altered ability to ingest, digest, and/or absorb nutrients (nausea, vomiting, hyperactive gag reflex, gastrointestinal disturbances, fatigue); increased metabolic rate and nutritional needs (fever, infection); possibly evidenced by weight loss, decreased subcutaneous fat and muscle mass, lack of interest in food, aversion to eating, altered taste sensation, abdominal cramping, hyperactive bowel sounds, diarrhea, sore and inflamed buccal cavity, abnormal laboratory results—vitamin, mineral, and protein deficiencies; electrolyte imbalances.

Fatigue may be related to decreased metabolic energy production, increased energy requirements (hypermetabolic state), overwhelming psychological or emotional demands, altered body chemistry (side effects of medication, chemotherapy), sleep deprivation possibly evidenced by unremitting or overwhelming lack of energy, inability to maintain usual routines, decreased performance, impaired ability to concentrate, lethargy, listlessness, and disinterest in surroundings.

ineffective Protection may be related to chronic disease affecting immune and neurological systems, inadequate nutrition, drug therapies, possibly evidenced by deficient immunity, impaired healing, neuro-

---

*A risk diagnosis is not evidenced by signs and symptoms, as the problem has not occurred; rather, nursing interventions are directed at prevention.

sensory alterations, maladaptive stress response, fatigue, anorexia, disorientation.

A

PSY

Social Isolation may be related to alteration in physical appearance or mental status, altered state of wellness, perceptions of unacceptable social behavior or values, [phobic fear of others (transmission of disease)], possibly evidenced by expressed feelings of aloneness or rejection, absence of supportive SO(s), and withdrawal from usual activities.

chronic Confusion may be related to physiological changes (hypoxemia, central nervous system [CNS] infection by HIV, brain malignancies, and/or disseminated systemic opportunistic infection), altered drug metabolism or excretion, accumulation of toxic elements (renal failure, severe electrolyte imbalance, hepatic insufficiency), possibly evidenced by clinical evidence of organic impairment, altered response to stimuli, memory deficit, and altered personality.

AIDS dementia **CH**

Also refer to Dementia, presenile/senile

chronic Confusion/impaired Memory related to physiological changes (neuronal degeneration), possibly evidenced by inaccurate interpretation of or response to stimuli, progressive or long-standing cognitive impairment, short-term memory deficit, impaired socialization, altered personality, clinical evidence of organic impairment.

ineffective Protection may be related to immune disorder, inadequate nutrition, drug therapies, possibly evidenced by deficient immunity, impaired healing, neurosensory alterations, maladaptive stress response, fatigue, anorexia, disorientation.

Alcohol abuse/withdrawal **CH/MS/PSY**

Refer to Drug overdose, acute [depressants]; Delirium tremens; Substance dependence/abuse rehabilitation

Alcohol intoxication, acute **MS**

Also refer to Delirium tremens

acute Confusion may be related to substance abuse, hypoxemia, and is possibly evidenced by hallucinations, exaggerated emotional response, fluctuation in cognition or level of consciousness, increased agitation.

risk for ineffective Breathing Pattern is possibly evidenced by risk factors of hypoventilation syndrome, neuromuscular dysfunction, fatigue.*

risk for Aspiration is possibly evidenced by risk factors of reduced level of consciousness, depressed cough or gag reflexes, delayed gastric emptying.*

Alcoholism **CH**

Refer to Substance dependence/abuse rehabilitation

Aldosteronism, primary **MS**

deficient Fluid Volume may be related to increased urinary losses, possibly evidenced by dry mucous membranes, poor skin turgor, dilute urine, excessive thirst, weight loss.

---

*A risk diagnosis is not evidenced by signs and symptoms, as the problem has not occurred; rather, nursing interventions are directed at prevention.

impaired physical Mobility may be related to neuromuscular impairment, decreased muscle strength, and pain, possibly evidenced by limited range of motion, slowed movement, limited ability to perform gross/fine motor skills.

risk for decreased Cardiac Output is possibly evidenced by risk factors of altered preload and altered heart rhythm.*

Alkalosis, metabolic **MS**

Refer to underlying cause or condition, e.g., Renal dialysis

Alkalosis, respiratory **MS**

Also refer to underlying cause or condition

impaired Gas Exchange may be related to ventilation-perfusion imbalance (decreased O_2 carrying capacity of blood, altered O_2 supply, alveolar-capillary membrane changes), possibly evidenced by dyspnea, tachypnea, changes in mentation, tachycardia, hypoxia, hypocapnia.

Allergies, seasonal **CH**

Refer to Hay fever

Alopecia **CH**

disturbed Body Image may be related to effects of illness or therapy, aging process, change in appearance, possibly evidenced by verbalization of feelings, concerns, fear of rejection or reaction of others, focus on past appearance, preoccupation with change, feelings of helplessness.

ALS **CH**

Refer to Amyotrophic lateral sclerosis

Alzheimer's disease **CH**

Also refer to Dementia, presenile/senile

risk for Injury/Trauma is possibly evidenced by risk factors of inability to recognize or identify danger in environment, disorientation, confusion, impaired judgment, weakness, muscular incoordination, balancing difficulties, altered perception, seizure activity.*

chronic Confusion related to physiological changes (neuronal degeneration), possibly evidenced by inaccurate interpretation of or response to stimuli, progressive or long-standing cognitive impairment, short-term memory deficit, impaired socialization, altered personality, and clinical evidence of organic impairment.

[disturbed Sensory Perception (specify)] may be related to altered sensory reception, transmission, and/or integration (neurological disease or deficit), socially restricted environment (homebound, institutionalized), sleep deprivation, possibly evidenced by changes in usual response to stimuli, change in problem-solving abilities, exaggerated emotional responses (anxiety, paranoia, hallucinations), inability to tell position of body parts, diminished or altered sense of taste.

Sleep Deprivation may be related to sensory impairment, changes in activity patterns, psychological stress (neurological impairment), possibly evidenced by wakefulness, disorientation (day/night rever-

*A risk diagnosis is not evidenced by signs and symptoms, as the problem has not occurred; rather, nursing interventions are directed at prevention.

sal), increased aimless wandering, inability to identify need or time for sleeping, changes in behavior, lethargy; dark circles under eyes and frequent yawning.

ineffective Health Maintenance may be related to deterioration affecting ability in all areas, including coordination and communication, cognitive impairment, ineffective individual/family coping, possibly evidenced by reported or observed inability to take responsibility for meeting basic health practices, lack of equipment, financial, or other resources, and impairment of personal support system.

PSY

risk for Stress Overload is possibly evidenced by risk factors of inadequate resources, chronic illness, physical demands, threats of violence.*

compromised family Coping/caregiver Role Strain may be related to disruptive behavior of client, family grief about their helplessness watching loved one deteriorate, prolonged disease or disability progression that exhausts the supportive capacity of SO or family, highly ambivalent family relationships.

risk for Relocation Stress Syndrome is possibly evidenced by risk factors of little or no preparation for transfer to a new setting, changes in daily routine, sensory impairment, physical deterioration, separation from support systems.*

Amphetamine abuse **PSY**

Refer to Stimulant abuse

Amputation **MS**

risk for ineffective peripheral Tissue Perfusion is possibly evidenced by risk factors of reduced arterial or venous blood flow, tissue edema, hematoma formation, hypovolemia.*

acute Pain may be related to tissue and nerve trauma, psychological impact of loss of body part, possibly evidenced by reports of incisional or phantom pain, observed guarding or protective behavior, narrowed focus or self-focus, and changes in vital signs.

impaired physical Mobility may be related to loss of limb (primarily lower extremity), altered sense of balance, pain, or discomfort, possibly evidenced by reluctance to attempt movement; impaired coordination; decreased muscle strength, control, and mass.

situational low Self-Esteem may be related to loss of a body part, change in functional abilities, possibly evidenced by verbalization of feelings of powerlessness, grief, preoccupation with loss, negative feelings about body, focus on past strength, function, or appearance; change in usual patterns of responsibility or physical capacity to resume role, fear of rejection or reaction by others, and unwillingness to look at or touch residual limb.

Amyotrophic lateral sclerosis (ALS) **MS**

impaired physical Mobility may be related to muscle wasting, weakness, possibly evidenced by impaired coordination, limited range of motion, and impaired purposeful movement.

---

*A risk diagnosis is not evidenced by signs and symptoms, as the problem has not occurred; rather, nursing interventions are directed at prevention.

A

ineffective Breathing Pattern/impaired spontaneous Ventilation may be related to neuromuscular impairment, decreased energy, fatigue, tracheobronchial obstruction, possibly evidenced by shortness of breath, fremitus, respiratory depth changes, and reduced vital capacity.

impaired Swallowing may be related to muscle wasting and fatigue, possibly evidenced by recurrent coughing or choking, and signs of aspiration.

PSY

Powerlessness [specify level] may be related to chronic and debilitating nature of illness, lack of control over outcome, possibly evidenced by expressions of frustration about inability to care for self and depression over physical deterioration.

Grieving may be related to perceived potential loss of self and physiopsychosocial well-being, possibly evidenced by sorrow, choked feelings, expression of distress, changes in eating habits, sleeping patterns, and altered communication patterns or libido.

CH

impaired verbal Communication may be related to physical barrier (neuromuscular impairment), possibly evidenced by impaired articulation, inability to speak in sentences, and use of nonverbal cues (changes in facial expression).

risk for caregiver Role Strain is possibly evidenced by risk factors of illness severity of care receiver, complexity and amount of homecare needs, duration of caregiving required, caregiver is spouse, family/caregiver isolation, lack of respite or recreation for caregiver.*

Anaphylaxis **CH**

Also refer to Shock

ineffective Airway Clearance may be related to airway spasm (bronchial), laryngeal edema, as possibly evidenced by diminished breath sounds, presence of adventitious sounds, cough ineffective or absent, difficulty vocalizing, wide-eyed.

decreased Cardiac Output may be related to decreased preload, increased capillary permeability (third spacing) and vasodilation, possibly evidenced by tachycardia, palpitations, changes in blood pressure (BP), anxiety, restlessness.

Anemia **CH**

Activity Intolerance may be related to imbalance between O_2 supply (delivery) and demand, possibly evidenced by reports of fatigue and weakness, abnormal heart rate or BP response, decreased exercise or activity level, and exertional discomfort or dyspnea.

imbalanced Nutrition: less than body requirements may be related to failure to ingest or inability to digest food or absorb nutrients necessary for formation of normal red blood cells (RBCs), possibly evidenced by weight loss or weight below normal for age, height, and body build; decreased triceps skinfold measurement; changes in

*A risk diagnosis is not evidenced by signs and symptoms, as the problem has not occurred; rather, nursing interventions are directed at prevention.

gums or oral mucous membranes; decreased tolerance for activity; weakness; and loss of muscle tone.

deficient Knowledge [Learning Need] regarding condition, prognosis, self-care and treatment needs may be related to inadequate understanding or misinterpretation of dietary and physiological needs, possibly evidenced by inadequate dietary intake, request for information, and development of preventable complications.

Anemia, iron-deficiency CH

Also refer to Anemia

Fatigue may be related to anemia, malnutrition, possibly evidenced by feeling tired, inability to maintain usual routines or level of physical activity.

risk for deficient Fluid Volume is possibly evidenced by risk factors of active or chronic blood loss.*

risk for impaired oral Mucous Membrane is possibly evidenced by risk factors of dehydration, malnutrition, vitamin deficiency.*

Anemia, sickle cell MS

impaired Gas Exchange may be related to decreased O_2-carrying capacity of blood, reduced RBC life span or premature destruction, abnormal RBC structure, increased blood viscosity, pulmonary congestion—impairment of surface phagocytosis; predisposition to bacterial pneumonia/pulmonary infarcts, possibly evidenced by dyspnea, use of accessory muscles, cyanosis or signs of hypoxia, tachycardia, changes in mentation, and restlessness.

ineffective Tissue Perfusion: [specify] may be related to stasis, vaso-occlusive nature of sickling, inflammatory response, atrioventricular shunts in pulmonary and peripheral circulation, myocardial damage (small infarcts, iron deposits, fibrosis), possibly evidenced by signs and symptoms dependent on system involved, such as renal (decreased specific gravity and pale urine in face of dehydration), cerebral (paralysis and visual disturbances), peripheral (distal ischemia, tissue infarctions, ulcerations, bone pain), or cardiac (angina, palpitations).

CH

acute Pain/chronic Pain may be related to intravascular sickling with localized vascular stasis, occlusion, infarction or necrosis and deprivation of O_2 and nutrients, accumulation of noxious metabolites, possibly evidenced by reports of localized, generalized, or migratory joint and/or abdominal or back pain, guarding and distraction behaviors (moaning, crying, restlessness), facial grimacing, narrowed focus, and changes in vital signs.

deficient Knowledge [Learning Need] regarding disease process, genetic factors, prognosis, self-care and treatment needs may be related to lack of exposure or recall, misinterpretation of information, unfamiliarity with resources, possibly evidenced by questions, statement of concern or misconceptions, exacerbation of condition, inadequate follow-through of therapy instructions, and development of preventable complications.

---

*A risk diagnosis is not evidenced by signs and symptoms, as the problem has not occurred; rather, nursing interventions are directed at prevention.

A

risk for sedentary Lifestyle is possibly evidenced by risk factors of lack of interest or motivation, lack of resources, lack of training or knowledge of specific exercise needs, safety concerns or fear of injury.*

PED

risk for disproportionate Growth and/or delayed Development are/is possibly evidenced by risk factors of inadequate nutrition, chronic illness.*

compromised family Coping may be related to chronic nature of disease and disability, family disorganization, presence of other crises or situations impacting significant person/parent, lifestyle restrictions, possibly evidenced by SO expressing preoccupation with own reaction and displaying protective behavior disproportionate to client's ability or need for autonomy.

Aneurysm, abdominal aortic (AAA) — MS

Refer to Aortic aneurysm, abdominal (AAA)

Aneurysm, cerebral — MS

Refer to Cerebrovascular accident

Aneurysm, ventricular — MS

decreased Cardiac Output may be related to altered stroke volume, changes in heart rate or rhythm, possibly evidenced by dyspnea, adventitious breath sounds, S_3/S_4 heart sounds, changes in hemodynamic measurements, dysrhythmias.

ineffective Tissue Perfusion [specify] may be related to decreased arterial blood flow, possibly evidenced by BP changes, diminished pulses, edema, dyspnea, dysrhythmias, altered mental status, decreased renal function.

Activity Intolerance may be related to imbalance between oxygen supply and demand, possibly evidenced by weakness, fatigue, abnormal heart rate/BP response to activity, electrocardiogram changes (dysrhythmias, ischemia).

Angina pectoris — MS

acute Pain may be related to decreased myocardial blood flow, increased cardiac workload/O_2 consumption, possibly evidenced by verbal reports, narrowed focus, distraction behaviors (restlessness, moaning), and autonomic responses (diaphoresis, changes in vital signs).

risk for decreased Cardiac Output is possibly evidenced by risk factors of inotropic changes (transient or prolonged myocardial ischemia, effects of medications), alterations in rate, rhythm and electrical conduction.*

Anxiety [specify level] may be related to situational crises, change in health status and/or threat of death, negative self-talk, possibly evidenced by verbalized apprehension, expressed concerns, association of condition with loss of abilities, facial tension, extraneous movements, and focus on self.

CH

Activity Intolerance may be related to imbalance between O_2 supply and demand, possibly evidenced by exertional dyspnea, abnormal

*A risk diagnosis is not evidenced by signs and symptoms, as the problem has not occurred; rather, nursing interventions are directed at prevention.

pulse or BP response to activity, and electrocardiogram (ECG) changes.

deficient Knowledge [Learning Need] regarding condition, prognosis, self-care and treatment needs may be related to lack of exposure, inaccurate or misinterpretation of information, possibly evidenced by questions, request for information, statement of concern, and inaccurate follow-through of instructions.

risk for sedentary Lifestyle is possibly evidenced by risk factors of lack of training or knowledge of specific exercise needs, safety concerns, fear of myocardial injury.*

risk for risk-prone Health Behavior is possibly evidenced by risk factors of condition requiring long-term therapy, changes in lifestyle, multiple stressors, assault to self-concept, altered locus of control.*

Anorexia nervosa **MS**

imbalanced Nutrition: less than body requirements may be related to psychological restrictions of food intake and/or excessive activity laxative abuse, possibly evidenced by weight loss, poor skin turgor, decreased muscle tone, denial of hunger, unusual hoarding or handling of food, amenorrhea, electrolyte imbalance, cardiac irregularities, hypotension.

risk for deficient Fluid Volume is possibly evidenced by risk factors of inadequate intake of food and liquids, chronic or excessive laxative or diuretic use.*

PSY

disturbed Body Image may be related to perceptual developmental changes, possibly evidenced by verbalized perceptions reflecting altered view of body appearance, refusal to verify actual change.

chronic low Self-Esteem may be related to lack of approval, repeated negative reinforcement, perceived lack of respect from others possibly evidenced by reports feelings of shame or guilt, overly conforming, dependent on others' opinions.

impaired Parenting may be related to issues of control in family, situational or maturational crises, history of inadequate coping methods, possibly evidenced by enmeshed family, dissonance among family members, focus on "identified patient," family developmental tasks not being met, family members acting as enablers, ill-defined family rules, functions, or roles.

Antisocial personality disorder **PSY**

risk for other-directed Violence is possibly evidenced by risk factors of contempt for authority or rights of others, inability to tolerate frustration, need for immediate gratification, easy agitation, vulnerable self-concept, inability to verbalize feelings, use of maladjusted coping mechanisms, history of substance abuse.*

ineffective Coping may be related to very low tolerance for external stress, lack of experience of internal anxiety (e.g., guilt, shame), personal vulnerability, unmet expectations, multiple life changes, possibly evidenced by choice of aggression and manipulation to handle problems or conflicts, inappropriate use of defense mechanisms (e.g.,

*A risk diagnosis is not evidenced by signs and symptoms, as the problem has not occurred; rather, nursing interventions are directed at prevention.

A

denial, projection), chronic worry, anxiety, destructive behaviors, high rate of accidents.

chronic low Self-Esteem may be related to lack of positive and/or repeated negative feedback, unmet dependency needs, retarded ego development, dysfunctional family system, possibly evidenced by acting-out behaviors (e.g., substance abuse, sexual promiscuity, feelings of inadequacy, nonparticipation in therapy).

compromised family Coping/disabled family Coping may be related to family disorganization or role changes, highly ambivalent family relationships, client providing little support in turn for the primary person(s), history of abuse or neglect in the home, possibly evidenced by expressions of concern or complaints, preoccupation of primary person with own reactions to situation, display of protective behaviors disproportionate to client's abilities, or need for autonomy.

impaired Social Interaction may be related to inadequate personal resources (shallow feelings), immature interests, underdeveloped conscience, unaccepted social values, possibly evidenced by difficulty meeting expectations of others; lack of belief that rules pertain to self; sense of emptiness or inadequacy covered by expressions of self-conceit, arrogance, or contempt; behavior unaccepted by dominant cultural group.

Anxiety disorder, generalized PSY

Anxiety [specify level]/Powerlessness may be related to real or perceived threat to physical integrity or self-concept (may or may not be able to identify the threat), unconscious conflict about essential values or beliefs and goals of life, unmet needs, negative self-talk, possibly evidenced by sympathetic stimulation, extraneous movements (foot shuffling, hand or arm fidgeting, rocking movements, restlessness), persistent feelings of apprehension and uneasiness, a general anxious feeling that client has difficulty alleviating, poor eye contact, focus on self, impaired functioning, free-floating anxiety, and nonparticipation in decision making.

ineffective Coping may be related to level of anxiety being experienced by the client, personal vulnerability, unmet expectations or unrealistic perceptions, inadequate coping methods and/or support systems, possibly evidenced by verbalization of inability to cope or problem-solve, excessive compulsive behaviors (e.g., smoking, drinking), and emotional or muscle tension, alteration in societal participation, high rate of accidents.

Insomnia may be related to stress, repetitive thoughts, possibly evidenced by reports of difficulty in falling/staying asleep, dissatisfaction with sleep, nonrestorative sleep, lack of energy.

compromised family Coping possibly evidenced by risk factors of inadequate or incorrect information or understanding by a primary person, temporary family disorganization and role changes, prolonged disability that exhausts the supportive capacity of SO(s).*

impaired Social Interaction/Social Isolation may be related to low self-concept, inadequate personal resources, misinterpretation of internal or external stimuli, hypervigilance, possibly evidenced by discomfort in social situations, withdrawal from or reported change in pattern

*A risk diagnosis is not evidenced by signs and symptoms, as the problem has not occurred; rather, nursing interventions are directed at prevention.

of interactions, dysfunctional interactions, expressed feelings of difference from others, sad, dull affect.

Anxiety disorders **PED/PSY**

[severe/panic] Anxiety may be related to situational or maturational crisis, internal transmission and contagion, threat to physical integrity or self-concept, unmet needs, dysfunctional family system, independence conflicts possibly evidenced by somatic complaints, nightmares, excessive psychomotor activity, refusal to attend school, persistent worry or fear of catastrophic doom to family or self.

ineffective Coping may be related to situational or maturational crisis, multiple life changes or losses, personal vulnerability, lack of self-confidence possibly evidenced by inability to problem-solve, persistent or overwhelming fears, inability to meet role expectations, social inhibition, panic attacks.

impaired Social Interaction may be related to excessive self-consciousness, inability to interact with unfamiliar people, altered thought processes possibly evidenced by verbalized or observed discomfort in social situations, inability to receive or communicate a satisfying sense of belonging, caring, or interest; use of unsuccessful social interaction behaviors.

risk for self-directed Violence/risk for Self-Mutilation are possibly evidenced by risk factors of panic states, dysfunctional family, history of self-destructive behaviors, emotional disturbance, increasing motor activity.*

compromised family Coping/disabled family Coping may be related to situational or developmental crisis (e.g., divorce, addition to the family), unrealistic parental expectations, frequent disruptions in living arrangements, high-risk family situations (neglect or abuse, substance abuse), possibly evidenced by SO reports of frustration with clinging behaviors, emotional lability, harsh or punitive response to tyrannical behaviors, disproportionate protective behaviors.

Anxiolytic abuse **PSY**

Refer to Depressant abuse

Aortic aneurysm, abdominal (AAA) **MS**

risk for ineffective Renal Perfusion is possibly evidenced by risk factors of hypertension, hypovolemia, hypoxia.*

acute Pain may be related to physical agent [vascular enlargement—dissection or rupture], possibly evidenced by verbal/coded reports, guarding behavior, facial mask, change in vital signs.

Aortic aneurysm repair, abdominal **MS**

Also refer to Surgery, general

Anxiety related to change in health status, threat of death, surgical intervention, possibly evidenced by expressed concerns, apprehension, increased tension, changes in vital signs.

risk for Bleeding is possibly evidenced by risk factors of aneurysm, treatment-related side effects—surgery, failure of vascular repair.*

*A risk diagnosis is not evidenced by signs and symptoms, as the problem has not occurred; rather, nursing interventions are directed at prevention.

A

risk for ineffective Renal Perfusion/peripheral Tissue Perfusion are possibly evidenced by risk factors of hypertension, treatment-related side effects—surgery, hypovolemia, hypoxia.*

Aortic stenosis **MS**

decreased Cardiac Output may be related to altered contractility, altered preload or afterload possibly evidenced by fatigue, dyspnea, changes in vital signs, jugular vein distension, increased central venous pressure (CVP)/PAWP, and syncope.

risk for impaired Gas Exchange is possibly evidenced by risk factors of alveolar-capillary membrane changes.*

CH

risk for acute Pain is possibly evidenced by risk factors of physical agent [episodic ischemia of myocardial tissues and stretching of left atrium].*

Activity Intolerance may be related to imbalance between O_2 supply and demand [decreased or fixed cardiac output], possibly evidenced by exertional dyspnea, reported fatigue or weakness, and abnormal BP or ECG changes or dysrhythmias in response to activity.

Aplastic anemia **CH**

Also refer to Anemia

ineffective Protection may be related to abnormal blood profile (leukopenia, thrombocytopenia), drug therapies (antineoplastics, antibiotics, nonsteroidal anti-inflammatory drugs, anticonvulsants) as possibly evidenced by fatigue, dyspnea, alteration in clotting.*

Fatigue may be related to anemia, disease states, malnutrition, possibly evidenced by verbalization of overwhelming lack of energy, inability to maintain usual routines or level of physical activity, tired, compromised libido, lethargy, increase in physical complaints.

Appendicitis **MS**

acute Pain may be related to physical agent [distention of intestinal tissues/inflammation], possibly evidenced by verbal reports, guarding behavior, narrowed focus, diaphoresis, changes in vital signs.

risk for deficient Fluid Volume is possibly evidenced by risk factors of excessive losses through normal routes (vomiting), deviations affecting intake of fluids (nausea, anorexia), and factors influencing fluid needs (hypermetabolic state).*

risk for Infection is possibly evidenced by risk factors of tissue destruction [release of pathogenic organisms into peritoneal cavity].*

ARDS **MS**

Refer to Respiratory distress syndrome, acute

Arrhythmia, cardiac **MS/CH**

Refer to Dysrhythmia, cardiac

Arterial occlusive disease, peripheral **CH**

ineffective peripheral Tissue Perfusion may be related to deficient knowledge of disease process, hypertension, smoking, sedentary life-

*A risk diagnosis is not evidenced by signs and symptoms, as the problem has not occurred; rather, nursing interventions are directed at prevention.

style, possibly evidenced by altered skin characteristics, diminished pulses, claudication, delayed peripheral wound healing.

risk for impaired Walking is possibly evidenced by risk factors of limited endurance, pain.*

risk for impaired Skin/Tissue Integrity are possibly evidenced by risk factors of altered circulation or sensation.*

Arthritis, juvenile rheumatoid **PED/CH**

Also refer to Arthritis, rheumatoid

risk for delayed Development is possibly evidenced by risk factors of chronic illness, effects of required therapy.*

Social Isolation risk factors may include delay in accomplishing developmental task, altered state of wellness, and alterations in physical appearance.*

Arthritis, rheumatoid **CH**

acute Pain/chronic Pain may be related to accumulation of fluid, inflammatory process, degeneration of joint, and deformity, possibly evidenced by verbal reports, narrowed focus, guarding or protective behaviors, and physical and social withdrawal.

impaired physical Mobility/impaired Walking may be related to musculoskeletal deformity, pain or discomfort, decreased muscle strength, possibly evidenced by limited range of motion, impaired coordination, reluctance to attempt movement, and decreased muscle strength, control, and mass.

Self-Care Deficit [specify] may be related to musculoskeletal impairment, decreased strength and endurance, limited range of motion, pain on movement, possibly evidenced by inability to manage activities of daily living (ADLs).

disturbed Body Image/ineffective Role Performance may be related to change in body structure or function, impaired mobility or ability to perform usual tasks, focus on past strength, function, or appearance, possibly evidenced by negative self-talk, feelings of helplessness, change in lifestyle or physical abilities, dependence on others for assistance, decreased social involvement.

Arthritis, septic **CH**

acute Pain may be related to joint inflammation, possibly evidenced by verbal or coded reports, guarding behaviors, restlessness, narrowed focus.

impaired physical Mobility may be related to joint stiffness, pain or discomfort, reluctance to initiate movement, possibly evidenced by limited range of motion, slowed movement.

Self-Care deficit [specify] may be related to musculoskeletal impairment, pain or discomfort, decreased strength, impaired coordination, possibly evidenced by inability to perform desired ADLs.

risk for Infection [spread] is possibly evidenced by risk factors of the presence of infectious process, chronic disease states, invasive procedures.*

---

*A risk diagnosis is not evidenced by signs and symptoms, as the problem has not occurred; rather, nursing interventions are directed at prevention.

A

Arthroplasty **MS**

risk for Infection is possibly evidenced by risk factors of breach of primary defenses (surgical incision), stasis of body fluids at operative site, and altered inflammatory response.*

risk for Bleeding is possibly evidenced by risk factors of surgical procedure, trauma to vascular area.*

impaired physical Mobility may be related to decreased strength, pain, musculoskeletal changes, possibly evidenced by impaired coordination and reluctance to attempt movement.

acute Pain may be related to tissue trauma, local edema, possibly evidenced by verbal reports, narrowed focus, guarded movement, diaphoresis, changes in vital signs.

Arthroscopy, knee **MS**

deficient Knowledge [Learning Need] regarding procedure, outcomes, and self-care needs may be related to unfamiliarity with information or resources, misinterpretations, possibly evidenced by questions and requests for information, misconceptions.

risk for impaired Walking is possibly evidenced by risk factors of joint stiffness, discomfort, prescribed movement restrictions, use of assistive devices (crutches) for ambulation.*

Asperger's disorder (now Autism spectrum disorder) **PED/PSY**

impaired Social Interaction may be related to skill deficit about ways to enhance mutuality, communication barriers (poor pragmatic language skills), compulsions, repetitive motor mannerisms, possibly evidenced by observed discomfort in social situations, dysfunctional interactions with others, inability to receive or communicate satisfying sense of belonging.

risk for delayed Development is possibly evidenced by the risk factor of behavior disorder.*

impaired Parenting may be related to developmental delay of child, deficient knowledge of child development, lack of social supports.

risk for Injury is possibly evidenced by risk factors of rituals, repetitive motor mannerisms, poor coordination, vulnerability to manipulation of peers.*

Asthma **MS**

Also refer to Emphysema

ineffective Airway Clearance may be related to increased production and retained pulmonary secretions, bronchospasm, decreased energy, fatigue, possibly evidenced by wheezing, difficulty breathing, changes in depth and rate of respirations, use of accessory muscles, and persistent ineffective cough with or without sputum production.

impaired Gas Exchange may be related to altered delivery of inspired O_2 and air trapping, possibly evidenced by dyspnea, restlessness, reduced tolerance for activity, cyanosis, and changes in arterial blood gases (ABGs) and vital signs.

---

*A risk diagnosis is not evidenced by signs and symptoms, as the problem has not occurred; rather, nursing interventions are directed at prevention.

Anxiety [specify level] may be related to perceived threat of death, possibly evidenced by apprehension, fearful expression, and extraneous movements.

CH

Activity Intolerance may be related to imbalance between O_2 supply and demand, possibly evidenced by fatigue and exertional dyspnea.

risk for Contamination is possibly evidenced by risk factors of presence of atmospheric pollutants, environmental contaminants in the home (e.g., smoking or secondhand tobacco smoke).

Athlete's foot — CH

impaired Skin Integrity may be related to fungal invasion, humidity, secretions, possibly evidenced by disruption of skin surface, reports of painful itching.

risk for Infection [spread] is possibly evidenced by risk factors of multiple breaks in skin, exposure to moist and warm environment.*

Atrial fibrillation — CH

Also refer to Dysrhythmia, cardiac

Activity Intolerance may be related to imbalance between oxygen supply and demand, possibly evidenced by dyspnea, dizziness, presyncope, or syncopal episodes.

risk for ineffective cerebral Tissue Perfusion is possibly evidenced by risk factors of arterial fibrillation, embolism, thrombolytic therapy (microemboli).*

Atrial flutter — CH

Refer to Dysrhythmia, cardiac

Atrial tachycardia — CH

Refer to Dysrhythmia, cardiac

Attention deficit disorder (ADD) — PED/PSY

ineffective Coping may be related to situational or maturational crisis, retarded ego development, low self-concept, possibly evidenced by easy distraction by extraneous stimuli, shifting between uncompleted activities.

chronic low Self-Esteem may be related to retarded ego development, lack of positive or repeated negative feedback, negative role models, possibly evidenced by lack of eye contact, derogatory self-comments, hesitance to try new tasks, inadequate level of confidence.

deficient Knowledge [Learning Need] regarding condition, prognosis, therapy may be related to misinformation or misinterpretations, unfamiliarity with resources, possibly evidenced by verbalization of problems or misconceptions, poor school performance, unrealistic expectations of medication regimen.

Autism spectrum disorder — PED/PSY

impaired Social Interaction may be related to abnormal response to sensory input or inadequate sensory stimulation, organic brain dysfunction, delayed development of secure attachment or trust, lack of intuitive skills to comprehend and accurately respond to social cues,

---

*A risk diagnosis is not evidenced by signs and symptoms, as the problem has not occurred; rather, nursing interventions are directed at prevention.

B

disturbance in self-concept, possibly evidenced by lack of responsiveness to others, lack of eye contact or facial responsiveness, treating persons as objects, lack of awareness of feelings in others, indifference or aversion to comfort, affection, or physical contact, failure to develop cooperative social play and peer friendships in childhood.

impaired verbal Communication may be related to inability to trust others, withdrawal into self, organic brain dysfunction, abnormal interpretation or response to and/or inadequate sensory stimulation, possibly evidenced by lack of interactive communication mode, no use of gestures or spoken language, absent or abnormal nonverbal communication, lack of eye contact or facial expression, peculiar patterns of speech (form, content, or speech production), and impaired ability to initiate or sustain conversation despite adequate speech.

risk for Self-Mutilation is possibly evidenced by risk factors of organic brain dysfunction; inability to trust others; disturbance in self-concept; inadequate sensory stimulation or abnormal response to sensory input (sensory overload); history of physical, emotional, or sexual abuse and response to demands of therapy; realization of severity of condition.*

disturbed Personal Identity may be related to organic brain dysfunction, lack of development of trust, maternal deprivation, fixation at presymbiotic phase of development, possibly evidenced by lack of awareness of the feelings or existence of others, increased anxiety resulting from physical contact with others, absent or impaired imitation of others, repeating what others say, persistent preoccupation with parts of objects, obsessive attachment to objects, marked distress over changes in environment, autoerotic or ritualistic behaviors, self-touching, rocking, swaying.

compromised /disabled family Coping may be related to family members unable to express feelings; excessive guilt, anger, or blaming among family members regarding child's condition; ambivalent or dissonant family relationships; prolonged coping with problem exhausting supportive ability of family members, possibly evidenced by denial of existence or severity of disturbed behaviors, preoccupation with personal emotional reaction to situation, rationalization that problem will be outgrown, attempts to intervene with child are achieving increasingly ineffective results, family withdraws from or becomes overly protective of child.

Barbiturate abuse **CH/PSY**

Refer to Depressant abuse

Battered child syndrome **PED/CH**

Also refer to Abuse

risk for Trauma is possibly evidenced by risk factors of dependent position in relationship(s), vulnerability (e.g., congenital problems, chronic illness), history of previous abuse or neglect, lack of or non-use of support systems by caregiver(s).*

interrupted Family Processes/impaired Parenting may be related to poor role model, unrealistic expectations, presence of stressors, and lack

*A risk diagnosis is not evidenced by signs and symptoms, as the problem has not occurred; rather, nursing interventions are directed at prevention.

of support, possibly evidenced by verbalization of negative feelings, inappropriate caretaking behaviors, and evidence of physical or psychological trauma to child.

PSY

chronic low Self-Esteem may be related to deprivation and negative feedback of family members, personal vulnerability, feelings of abandonment, possibly evidenced by lack of eye contact, withdrawal from social contacts, discounting own needs, nonassertive or passive, indecisive or overly conforming behaviors.

Post-Trauma Syndrome may be related to sustained or recurrent physical or emotional abuse, possibly evidenced by acting-out behavior, development of phobias, poor impulse control, and emotional numbness.

ineffective Coping may be related to situational or maturational crisis, overwhelming threat to self, personal vulnerability, inadequate support systems, possibly evidenced by verbalized concern about ability to deal with current situation, chronic worry, anxiety, depression, poor self-esteem, inability to problem-solve, high illness rate, destructive behavior toward self or others.

Benign prostatic hyperplasia **CH/MS**

[acute/chronic] Urinary Retention/overflow urinary Incontinence may be related to mechanical obstruction (enlarged prostate), decompensation of detrusor musculature, inability of bladder to contract adequately, possibly evidenced by frequency, hesitancy, inability to empty bladder completely, incontinence or dribbling, nocturia, bladder distention, residual urine.

acute Pain may be related to mucosal irritation, bladder distention, colic, urinary infection, and radiation therapy, possibly evidenced by verbal reports (bladder or rectal spasm), narrowed focus, altered muscle tone, grimacing, distraction behaviors, restlessness, and changes in vital signs.

risk for deficient Fluid Volume/Electrolyte Imbalance are possibly evidenced by risk factors of postobstructive diuresis, renal or endocrine dysfunction.*

Fear/Anxiety [specify level] may be related to change in health status (possibility of surgical procedure, malignancy); embarrassment or loss of dignity associated with genital exposure before, during, and after treatment; and concern about sexual ability, possibly evidenced by increased tension, apprehension, worry, expressed concerns regarding perceived changes, and fear of unspecific consequences.

Bipolar disorder **PSY**

risk for other-directed Violence is possibly evidenced by risk factors of irritability, impulsive behavior, delusional thinking, angry response when ideas are refuted or wishes denied, manic excitement, with possible indicators of threatening body language or verbalizations, increased motor activity, overt and aggressive acts, hostility.*

imbalanced Nutrition: less than body requirements may be related to inadequate intake in relation to metabolic expenditures, possibly evidenced by body weight 20% or more below ideal weight, observed

*A risk diagnosis is not evidenced by signs and symptoms, as the problem has not occurred; rather, nursing interventions are directed at prevention.

inadequate intake, inattention to mealtimes, and distraction from task of eating, laboratory evidence of nutritional deficits or imbalances.

B

risk for Poisoning [lithium toxicity] is possibly evidenced by risk factors of narrow therapeutic range of drug, client's ability (or lack of) to follow through with medication regimen and monitoring, and denial of need for information or therapy.*

Insomnia may be related to psychological stress, lack of recognition of fatigue or need to sleep, hyperactivity, possibly evidenced by denial of need to sleep, interrupted nighttime sleep, one or more nights without sleep, changes in behavior and performance, increasing irritability, restlessness, and dark circles under eyes.

[disturbed Sensory Perception (specify)]/Stress Overload may be related to decrease in sensory threshold, endogenous chemical alteration, psychological stress, sleep deprivation, possibly evidenced by increased distractibility and agitation, anxiety, disorientation, poor concentration, auditory or visual hallucination, bizarre thinking, and motor incoordination.

interrupted Family Processes may be related to situational crises (illness, economics, change in roles), euphoric mood and grandiose ideas or actions of client, manipulative behavior and limit testing, client's refusal to accept responsibility for own actions, possibly evidenced by statements of difficulty coping with situation, lack of adaptation to change, or not dealing constructively with illness, ineffective family decision-making process, failure to send and receive clear messages, and inappropriate boundary maintenance.

Bone cancer **MS/CH**

Also refer to Myeloma, multiple; Amputation

acute Pain may be related to bone destruction, pressure on nerves, possibly evidenced by verbal or coded report, protective behavior, changes in vital signs.

risk for Trauma is possibly evidenced by risk factors of increased bone fragility, general weakness, balancing difficulties.*

Bone marrow transplantation **MS/CH**

Also refer to Transplantation, recipient

risk for Injury is possibly evidenced by risk factors of immune dysfunction or suppression, abnormal blood profile, action of donor T cells.*

deficient Diversional Activity may be related to hospitalization or length of treatment, restriction of visitors, limitation of activities, possibly evidenced by expressions of boredom, restlessness, withdrawal, and requests for something to do.

risk for imbalanced Nutrition: less that body requirements is possibly evidenced by risk factors of increased metabolic needs for healing, altered ability to ingest nutrients—nausea, vomiting, anorexia, taste changes, oral lesions.*

Borderline personality disorder **PSY**

risk for self-directed/other-directed Violence/Self-Mutilation are possibly evidenced by risk factors of use of projection as a major defense mechanism, pervasive problems with negative transference, feelings

*A risk diagnosis is not evidenced by signs and symptoms, as the problem has not occurred; rather, nursing interventions are directed at prevention.

of guilt or need to "punish" self, distorted sense of self, inability to cope with increased psychological or physiological tension in a healthy manner.*

Anxiety [severe to panic] may be related to unconscious conflicts (experience of extreme stress), perceived threat to self-concept, unmet needs, possibly evidenced by easy frustration and feelings of hurt, abuse of alcohol or other drugs, transient psychotic symptoms, and performance of self-mutilating acts.

chronic low Self-Esteem/disturbed Personal Identity may be related to lack of positive feedback, unmet dependency needs, retarded ego development or fixation at an earlier level of development, possibly evidenced by difficulty identifying self or defining self-boundaries, feelings of depersonalization, extreme mood changes, lack of tolerance of rejection or of being alone, unhappiness with self, striking out at others, performance of ritualistic self-damaging acts, and belief that punishing self is necessary.

Social Isolation may be related to immature interests, unaccepted social behavior, inadequate personal resources, and inability to engage in satisfying personal relationships, possibly evidenced by alternating clinging and distancing behaviors, difficulty meeting expectations of others, experiencing feelings of difference from others, expressing interests inappropriate to developmental age, and exhibiting behavior unaccepted by dominant cultural group.

Botulism (food-borne) **MS**

deficient Fluid Volume may be related to active losses—vomiting, diarrhea, decreased intake—nausea, dysphagia, possibly evidenced by reports of thirst, dry skin and mucous membranes, decreased BP and urine output, change in mental state, increased hematocrit (Hct).

impaired physical Mobility may be related to neuromuscular impairment, possibly evidenced by limited ability to perform gross or fine motor skills.

Anxiety [specify level]/Fear may be related to threat of death, interpersonal transmission, possibly evidenced by expressed concerns, apprehension, awareness of physiological symptoms, focus on self.

risk for impaired spontaneous Ventilation is possibly evidenced by risk factors of neuromuscular impairment, presence of infectious process.*

CH

Contamination may be related to lack of proper precautions in food storage or preparation as evidenced by gastrointestinal and neurological effects of exposure to biological agent.

Bowel obstruction **MS**

Refer to Ileus

Brain tumor **MS**

acute Pain may be related to pressure on brain tissues, possibly evidenced by reports of headache, facial mask of pain, narrowed focus, and changes in vital signs.

---

*A risk diagnosis is not evidenced by signs and symptoms, as the problem has not occurred; rather, nursing interventions are directed at prevention.

impaired Memory may be related to altered circulation to and/or destruction of brain tissue, possibly evidenced by memory loss, personality changes, impaired ability to make decisions or conceptualize, and inaccurate interpretation of environment.

[disturbed Sensory Perception (specify)] may be related to altered sensory reception/integration, possibly evidenced by changes in sensory acuity, change in behavior pattern, poor concentration/problem-solving abilities, disorientation.

risk for deficient Fluid Volume is possibly evidenced by risk factors of recurrent vomiting from irritation of vagal center in medulla and decreased intake.*

Self-Care Deficit [specify] may be related to sensory or neuromuscular impairment interfering with ability to perform tasks, possibly evidenced by unkempt and disheveled appearance, body odor, and verbalization or observation of inability to perform ADLs.

Breast cancer — MS/CH

Also refer to Cancer

Anxiety [specify level] may be related to change in health status, threat of death, stress, interpersonal transmission, possibly evidenced by expressed concerns, apprehension, uncertainty, focus on self, diminished productivity.

deficient Knowledge [Learning Need] regarding diagnosis, prognosis, and treatment options may be related to lack of exposure or unfamiliarity with information resources, information misinterpretation, cognitive limitation, anxiety, possibly evidenced by verbalizations, statements of misconceptions, inappropriate behaviors.

disturbed Body Image may be related to surgical procedure, alteration in self-perception and is possibly evidenced by absence of body part, focus on past appearance, fear of rejection by others.*

risk for Sexual Dysfunction is possibly evidenced by risk factors of health-related changes, medical treatments, concern about relationship with SO.*

Bronchitis — CH

ineffective Airway Clearance may be related to excessive, thickened mucus secretions, possibly evidenced by presence of rhonchi, tachypnea, and ineffective cough.

Activity Intolerance [specify level] may be related to imbalance between O_2 supply and demand, general weakness, exhaustion—interruption in usual sleep pattern due to cough, discomfort, dyspnea, possibly evidenced by reports of fatigue, dyspnea, and abnormal vital sign response to activity.

acute Pain may be related to inflammation of lung parenchyma, persistent cough, cellular reactions to circulating toxins, aching associated with fever, possibly evidenced by reports of pleuritic chest pain, guarding affected area, distraction behaviors, and restlessness.

Bronchopneumonia — MS/CH

Also refer to Bronchitis

ineffective Airway Clearance may be related to tracheal bronchial inflammation, edema formation, increased sputum production, pleuritic

---

*A risk diagnosis is not evidenced by signs and symptoms, as the problem has not occurred; rather, nursing interventions are directed at prevention.

pain, decreased energy, fatigue, possibly evidenced by changes in rate and depth of respirations, abnormal breath sounds, use of accessory muscles, dyspnea, cyanosis, effective or ineffective cough—with or without sputum production.

impaired Gas Exchange may be related to alveolar-capillary membrane changes—inflammatory effects, ventilation-perfusion mismatch—collection of secretions affecting O_2 exchange across alveolar membrane, and hypoventilation, altered release of oxygen at cellular level—fever, shifting oxyhemoglobin curve, possibly evidenced by restlessness, changes in mentation, dyspnea, tachycardia, pallor, cyanosis, and ABGs or oximetry evidence of hypoxia.

risk for Infection [spread] is possibly evidenced by risk factors of decreased ciliary action, stasis of secretions, presence of existing infection, immunosuppression, chronic disease, malnutrition.*

Bulimia nervosa **PSY/MS**

Also refer to Anorexia nervosa

impaired Dentition may be related to dietary habits, poor oral hygiene, chronic vomiting, possibly evidenced by erosion of tooth enamel, multiple caries, abraded teeth.

impaired oral Mucous Membrane may be related to malnutrition or vitamin deficiency, poor oral hygiene, chronic vomiting, possibly evidenced by sore, inflamed buccal mucosa, swollen salivary glands, ulcerations of mucosa, reports of constant sore mouth or throat.

risk for deficient Fluid Volume/risk for Bleeding are possibly evidenced by risk factors of consistent self-induced vomiting, chronic or excessive laxative or diuretic use, esophageal erosion or tear (Mallory-Weiss syndrome).*

deficient Knowledge [Learning Need] regarding condition, prognosis, complication, treatment may be related to lack of exposure or recall, unfamiliarity with information about condition, learned maladaptive coping skills, possibly evidenced by verbalization of misconception of relationship of current situation and binging and purging behaviors, distortion of body image, verbalized need for information, desire to change behaviors.

Burns (dependent on type, degree, and severity of the injury) **MS/CH**

risk for deficient Fluid Volume/risk for Bleeding are possibly evidenced by risk factors of loss of fluids through wounds, capillary damage and evaporation, hypermetabolic state, insufficient intake, hemorrhagic losses.*

risk for ineffective Airway Clearance is possibly evidenced by risk factors of tracheobronchial obstruction—mucosal edema and loss of ciliary action with smoke inhalation; circumferential full-thickness burns of the neck, thorax, and chest, with compression of the airway or limited chest excursion, trauma—direct upper airway injury by flame, steam, chemicals, or gases; fluid shifts, pulmonary edema, decreased lung compliance.*

risk for Infection is possibly evidenced by risk factors of loss of protective dermal barrier, traumatized tissue, necrosis, decreased he-

*A risk diagnosis is not evidenced by signs and symptoms, as the problem has not occurred; rather, nursing interventions are directed at prevention.

moglobin (Hb), suppressed inflammatory response, environmental exposure, invasive procedures.*

acute Pain/chronic Pain may be related to destruction of skin, tissues, and nerves; edema formation, and manipulation of injured tissues, possibly evidenced by verbal reports, narrowed focus, distraction and guarding behaviors, facial mask of pain, and changes in vital signs.

C

risk for imbalanced Nutrition: less than body requirements is possibly evidenced by risk factors of hypermetabolic state as much as 50% to 60% higher than normal proportional to the severity of injury, protein catabolism, anorexia, restricted oral intake.*

Post-Trauma Syndrome may be related to life-threatening event, possibly evidenced by reexperiencing the event, repetitive dreams or nightmares, psychic or emotional numbness, and sleep disturbance.

ineffective Protection may be related to extremes of age, inadequate nutrition, anemia, impaired immune system, possibly evidenced by impaired healing, deficient immunity, fatigue, anorexia.

PED

deficient Diversional Activity may be related to long-term hospitalization, frequent lengthy treatments, and physical limitations, possibly evidenced by expressions of boredom, restlessness, withdrawal, and requests for something to do.

risk for delayed Development is possibly evidenced by risk factors of effects of physical disability, separation from SO(s), and environmental deficiencies.*

Bursitis — CH

acute Pain/chronic Pain may be related to inflammation of affected joint, possibly evidenced by verbal reports, guarding behavior, and narrowed focus.

impaired physical Mobility may be related to inflammation and swelling of joint and pain, possibly evidenced by diminished range of motion, reluctance to attempt movement, and imposed restriction of movement by medical treatment.

Calculi, urinary — CH/MS

acute Pain may be related to increased frequency or force of ureteral contractions, tissue trauma, edema formation, cellular ischemia, possibly evidenced by reports of sudden, severe, colicky pain, guarding and distraction behaviors, self-focus, and changes in vital signs.

impaired urinary Elimination may be related to stimulation of the bladder by calculi, renal or ureteral irritation, mechanical obstruction of urinary flow, inflammation, possibly evidenced by urgency and frequency, oliguria, hematuria.

risk for deficient Fluid Volume is possibly evidenced by risk factors of stimulation of renal-intestinal reflexes—nausea, vomiting, and diarrhea, changes in urinary output, postobstructive diuresis.*

risk for Infection is possibly evidenced by risk factors of stasis of urine, insufficient fluid intake.*

deficient Knowledge [Learning Need] regarding condition, prognosis, self-care, and treatment needs may be related to lack of exposure or recall and information misinterpretation, possibly evidenced by re-

*A risk diagnosis is not evidenced by signs and symptoms, as the problem has not occurred; rather, nursing interventions are directed at prevention.

quests for information, statements of concern, and recurrence or development of preventable complications.

Cancer MS

Also refer to Chemotherapy

Fear/Death Anxiety may be related to situational crises, threat to or change in health or socioeconomic status, role functioning, interaction patterns, threat of death, separation from family, interpersonal transmission of feelings, possibly evidenced by expressed concerns, feelings of inadequacy or helplessness, insomnia, increased tension, restlessness, focus on self, sympathetic stimulation.

Grieving may be related to potential loss of physiological well-being (body part or function), change in lifestyle, perceived potential death, possibly evidenced by anger, sadness, withdrawal, choked feelings, changes in eating or sleep patterns, activity level, libido, and communication patterns.

acute Pain/chronic Pain may be related to the disease process (compression of nerve tissue, infiltration of nerves or their vascular supply, obstruction of a nerve pathway, inflammation), or side effects of therapeutic agents, possibly evidenced by verbal reports, self-focusing or narrowed focus, alteration in muscle tone, facial mask of pain, distraction or guarding behaviors, autonomic responses, and restlessness.

Fatigue may be related to decreased metabolic energy production, increased energy requirements (hypermetabolic state), overwhelming psychological or emotional demands, and altered body chemistry—side effects of medications, chemotherapy, radiation therapy, biotherapy—possibly evidenced by unremitting or overwhelming lack of energy, inability to maintain usual routines, decreased performance, impaired ability to concentrate, lethargy, listlessness, and disinterest in surroundings.

impaired Home Maintenance may be related to debilitation, lack of resources, and/or inadequate support systems, possibly evidenced by verbalization of problem, request for assistance, and lack of necessary equipment or aids.

PSY/PED

risk for interrupted Family Processes possibly evidenced by risk factors of situational or transitional crises—long-term illness, change in roles or economic status; developmental—anticipated loss of a family member.*

readiness for enhanced family Coping possibly evidenced by verbalizations of impact of crisis on own values, priorities, goals, or relationships.

Candidiasis CH

Also refer to Thrush

impaired Skin/Tissue Integrity may be related to infectious lesions, possibly evidenced by disruption of skin surfaces and mucous membranes.

acute Pain/impaired Comfort may be related to exposure of irritated skin and mucous membranes to excretions (urine, feces), possibly

*A risk diagnosis is not evidenced by signs and symptoms, as the problem has not occurred; rather, nursing interventions are directed at prevention.

evidenced by verbal or coded reports, restlessness, or guarding behaviors.

risk for Sexual Dysfunction is possibly evidenced by risk factors of the presence of infectious process and vaginal discomfort.*

C

Cannabis abuse **CH**

Refer to Stimulant abuse

Cardiac catheterization **MS**

Anxiety [specify level] may be related to threat to or change in health status, stress, family heredity possibly evidenced by expressed concerns, apprehension, uncertainty, focus on self.

risk for decreased Cardiac Output is possibly evidenced by risk factors of altered heart rate and rhythm (vasovagal response, ventricular dysrhythmias), decreased myocardial contractility (ischemia).*

risk for decreased cardiac Tissue Perfusion is possibly evidenced by risk factors of coronary artery spasm, hypovolemia, hypoxia, [thrombosis, emboli].*

risk for adverse Reaction to Iodinated Contrast Media is possibly evidenced by risk factors of underlying disease—heart disease, concurrent use of medications (e.g., beta blockers, metformin), history of allergies.*

Cardiac surgery **MS/PED**

risk for decreased Cardiac Output is possibly evidenced by risk factors of altered myocardial contractility secondary to temporary factors (ventricular wall surgery, recent myocardial infarction, response to certain medications or drug interactions), altered preload (hypovolemia), and afterload (systemic vascular resistance), altered heart rate or rhythm (dysrhythmias).*

risk for deficient Fluid Volume/risk for Bleeding are possibly evidenced by risk factors of intraoperative bleeding with inadequate blood replacement; bleeding related to insufficient heparin reversal, fibrinolysis, or platelet destruction; or volume depletion effects of intraoperative or postoperative diuretic therapy.*

risk for impaired Gas Exchange is possibly evidenced by risk factors of alveolar-capillary membrane changes (atelectasis), intestinal edema, inadequate function or premature discontinuation of chest tubes, and diminished O_2-carrying capacity of the blood.*

acute Pain/impaired Comfort may be related to tissue inflammation or trauma, edema formation, intraoperative nerve trauma, and myocardial ischemia, possibly evidenced by reports of incisional discomfort, pain in chest and donor site; paresthesia or pain in hand, arm, shoulder; anxiety, restlessness, irritability; distraction behaviors; and changes in heart rate and BP.

impaired Skin/Tissue Integrity related to mechanical trauma (surgical incisions, puncture wounds) and edema evidenced by disruption of skin surface and tissues.

Cardiogenic shock **MS**

Refer to Shock, cardiogenic

*A risk diagnosis is not evidenced by signs and symptoms, as the problem has not occurred; rather, nursing interventions are directed at prevention.

Cardiomyopathy **CH/MS**

decreased Cardiac Output may be related to altered contractility, possibly evidenced by dyspnea, fatigue, chest pain, dizziness, syncope.

Activity Intolerance may be related to imbalance between O_2 supply and demand, possibly evidenced by weakness, fatigue, dyspnea, abnormal heart rate and BP response to activity, ECG changes.

ineffective Role Performance may be related to changes in physical health, stress, demands of job/life, possibly evidenced by change in usual patterns of responsibility, role strain, change in capacity to resume role.

Carotid endarterectomy **MS**

Also refer to Surgery, general

risk for ineffective cerebral Tissue Perfusion is possibly evidenced by risk factors of carotid stenosis, embolism, thrombolytic therapy.*

Carpal tunnel syndrome **CH/MS**

acute Pain/chronic Pain may be related to pressure on median nerve, possibly evidenced by verbal reports, reluctance to use affected extremity, guarding behaviors, expressed fear of re-injury, altered ability to continue previous activities.

impaired physical Mobility may be related to neuromuscular impairment and pain, possibly evidenced by decreased hand strength, weakness, limited range of motion, and reluctance to attempt movement.

risk for peripheral neurovascular Dysfunction is possibly evidenced by risk factors of mechanical compression (e.g., brace, repetitive tasks or motions), immobilization.*

deficient Knowledge [Learning Need] regarding condition, prognosis, treatment, and safety needs may be related to lack of exposure or recall, information misinterpretation, possibly evidenced by questions, statements of concern, request for information, inaccurate follow-through of instructions, development of preventable complications.

Casts **CH/MS**

Also refer to Fractures

risk for peripheral neurovascular Dysfunction is possibly evidenced by risk factors of presence of fracture(s), mechanical compression (cast), tissue trauma, immobilization, vascular obstruction.*

risk for impaired Skin Integrity is possibly evidenced by risk factors of pressure of cast, moisture or debris under cast, objects inserted under cast to relieve itching, and altered sensation or circulation.*

Self-Care Deficit [specify] may be related to impaired ability to perform self-care tasks, possibly evidenced by statements of need for assistance and observed difficulty in performing ADLs.

Cataract **CH**

[disturbed visual Sensory Perception] may be related to altered sensory reception or status of sense organs, and therapeutically restricted environment (surgical procedure, patching), possibly evidenced by diminished acuity, visual distortions, and change in usual response to stimuli.

*A risk diagnosis is not evidenced by signs and symptoms, as the problem has not occurred; rather, nursing interventions are directed at prevention.

risk for Trauma is possibly evidenced by risk factors of poor vision, reduced hand-eye coordination.*

Anxiety [specify level]/Fear may be related to alteration in visual acuity, threat of permanent loss of vision/independence, possibly evidenced by expressed concerns, apprehension, and feelings of uncertainty.

deficient Knowledge [Learning Need] regarding ways of coping with altered abilities, therapy choices, lifestyle changes may be related to lack of exposure or recall, misinterpretation, or cognitive limitations, possibly evidenced by requests for information, statement of concern, inaccurate follow-through of instructions, development of preventable complications.

Cat scratch disease — CH

acute Pain may be related to effects of circulating toxins (fever, headache, and lymphadenitis), possibly evidenced by verbal reports, guarding behavior, and changes in vital signs.

Hyperthermia may be related to inflammatory process, possibly evidenced by increased body temperature, flushed warm skin, tachypnea, tachycardia.

Celiac disease — CH

imbalanced Nutrition: less than body requirements may be related to inability to absorb nutrients (mucosal damage, loss of villi, proliferation of crypt cells, shortened transit time through gastrointestinal tract), possibly evidenced by weight loss, abdominal distention, steatorrhea, evidence of anemia, vitamin deficiencies.

Diarrhea may be related to irritation, malabsorption, possibly evidenced by abdominal pain, hyperactive bowel sounds, at least three loose stools per day.

risk for deficient Fluid Volume is possibly evidenced by risk factors of mild to massive steatorrhea, diarrhea.*

Cellulitis — CH/MS

risk for Infection [abscess, bacteremia] is possibly evidenced by risk factors of broken skin, chronic disease, presence of pathogens, insufficient knowledge to avoid exposure to pathogens.*

acute Pain/impaired Comfort may be related to inflammatory process, circulating toxins possibly evidenced by reports of localized pain or headache, guarding behaviors, restlessness, changes in vital signs.

impaired Tissue Integrity may be related to trauma, inflammation and/or invasion of tissues by infectious bacterial agent, or altered circulation, possibly evidenced by redness, warmth, edema, tenderness or pain under the surface of skin, or deep in tissues.

Cerebrovascular accident (CVA) — MS

ineffective cerebral Tissue Perfusion may be related to interruption of blood flow (occlusive disorder, hemorrhage, cerebral vasospasm, or edema), possibly evidenced by altered level of consciousness, changes in vital signs, changes in motor or sensory responses, restlessness, memory loss, as well as sensory, language, intellectual, and emotional deficits.

---

*A risk diagnosis is not evidenced by signs and symptoms, as the problem has not occurred; rather, nursing interventions are directed at prevention.

impaired physical Mobility may be related to neuromuscular involvement (weakness, paresthesia, flaccid or hypotonic paralysis, spastic paralysis), perceptual or cognitive impairment, possibly evidenced by inability to purposefully move involved body parts, limited range of motion, impaired coordination, and/or decreased muscle strength or control.

impaired verbal [and/or written] Communication may be related to impaired cerebral circulation, neuromuscular impairment, loss of facial/oral muscle tone and control, generalized weakness, fatigue, possibly evidenced by impaired articulation; inability to speak (dysarthria); inability to modulate speech, find and/or name words, identify objects; and/or inability to comprehend written or spoken language, inability to produce written communication.

Self-Care Deficit [specify] may be related to neuromuscular impairment, decreased strength or endurance, loss of muscle control or coordination, perceptual or cognitive impairment, pain, discomfort, and depression, possibly evidenced by stated or observed inability to perform ADLs, requests for assistance, disheveled appearance, and incontinence.

risk for impaired Swallowing is possibly evidenced by risk factors of muscle paralysis or perceptual impairment.*

risk for Unilateral Neglect is possibly evidenced by risk factors of sensory loss of part of visual field with perceptual loss of corresponding body segment.*

CH

impaired Home Maintenance may be related to condition of individual family member, insufficient finances, family organization or planning, unfamiliarity with resources, and inadequate support systems, possibly evidenced by members expressing difficulty in managing home in a comfortable manner, requesting assistance with home maintenance, disorderly surroundings, and overtaxed family members.

situational low Self-Esteem/disturbed Body Image/ineffective Role Performance may be related to functional impairment, loss, focus on past function/strength, and cognitive or perceptual changes, possibly evidenced by actual change in function, self-negating verbalizations, reports perceptions reflecting altered view of body function.

Grieving may be related to loss of processes of body [neuromuscular impairments], loss of job/role function, status/independence, possibly evidenced by psychological distress, despair, anger, disorganization.

Cervix, dysfunctional **OB**

Refer to Dilation of cervix, premature

Cesarean birth **OB**

Also refer to Cesarean birth, unplanned; Cesarean birth, postpartal

deficient Knowledge [Learning Need] regarding surgical procedure and expectation, postoperative routines and therapy, and self-care needs may be related to lack of information/misinterpretation, possibly evidenced by statements of concern, questions, and misconceptions.

*A risk diagnosis is not evidenced by signs and symptoms, as the problem has not occurred; rather, nursing interventions are directed at prevention.

risk for deficient Fluid Volume/risk for Bleeding are possibly evidenced by risk factors of restrictions of oral intake, blood loss; pregnancy-related complications.*

risk for impaired Attachment is possibly evidenced by risk factors of separation, existing health conditions of mother or infant, lack of privacy.*

C

Cesarean birth, postpartal **OB**

Also refer to Postpartal period

risk for impaired Attachment is possibly evidenced by risk factors of developmental transition or gain of a family member, situational crisis (e.g., surgical intervention, physical complications interfering with initial acquaintance and interaction, negative self-appraisal).*

acute Pain/impaired Comfort may be related to surgical trauma, effects of anesthesia, hormonal effects, bladder or abdominal distention, possibly evidenced by verbal reports (e.g., incisional pain, cramping, afterpains, spinal headache), guarding or distraction behaviors, irritability, facial mask of pain.

risk for situational low Self-Esteem is possibly evidenced by risk factors of perceived "failure" at life event, maturational transition, perceived loss of control in unplanned delivery.*

risk for Injury is possibly evidenced by risk factors of biochemical or regulatory functions (e.g., orthostatic hypotension, development of pregnancy-induced hypertension or eclampsia), effects of anesthesia, thromboembolism, abnormal blood profile (anemia or excessive blood loss, rubella sensitivity, Rh incompatibility), tissue trauma.*

risk for Infection is possibly evidenced by risk factors of tissue trauma, broken skin, decreased Hb, invasive procedures and/or increased environmental exposure, prolonged rupture of amniotic membranes, malnutrition.*

Self-Care Deficit [specify] may be related to effects of anesthesia, decreased strength and endurance, physical discomfort, possibly evidenced by verbalization of inability to perform desired ADL(s).

Cesarean birth, unplanned **OB**

Also refer to Cesarean birth, postpartal

deficient Knowledge [Learning Need] regarding underlying procedure, pathophysiology, and self-care needs may be related to incomplete or inadequate information, possibly evidenced by request for information, verbalization of concerns or misconceptions, and inappropriate or exaggerated behavior.

Anxiety [specify level] may be related to actual or perceived threat to mother/fetus, emotional threat to self-esteem, unmet needs or expectations, interpersonal transmission, possibly evidenced by increased tension, apprehension, feelings of inadequacy, sympathetic stimulation, narrowed focus, restlessness.

Powerlessness may be related to interpersonal interaction, perception of illness-related regimen, lifestyle of helplessness, possibly evidenced by verbalization of lack of control, lack of participation in care or decision making, passivity.

*A risk diagnosis is not evidenced by signs and symptoms, as the problem has not occurred; rather, nursing interventions are directed at prevention.

risk for disturbed Maternal-Fetal Dyad is possibly evidenced by risk factors of compromised oxygen transport, complication of pregnancy.*

risk for labor Pain is possibly evidenced by risk factors of increased or prolonged contractions, psychological reaction.*

risk for Infection is possibly evidenced by risk factors of invasive procedures, rupture of amniotic membranes, break in skin, decreased Hb, exposure to pathogens.*

Chemotherapy MS/CH

Also refer to Cancer

risk for deficient Fluid Volume is possibly evidenced by risk factors of gastrointestinal losses (vomiting, diarrhea), interference with adequate intake (stomatitis, anorexia), losses through abnormal routes (indwelling tubes, wounds, fistulas), hypermetabolic state.*

imbalanced Nutrition: less than body requirements may be related to inability to ingest adequate nutrients—nausea, stomatitis, gastric irritation, taste distortions, and fatigue; hypermetabolic state, poorly controlled pain, possibly evidenced by weight loss (wasting), aversion to eating, reported altered taste sensation, sore and inflamed buccal cavity, diarrhea and/or constipation.

impaired oral Mucous Membrane may be related to side effects of therapeutic agents or radiation, dehydration, and malnutrition, possibly evidenced by ulcerations, leukoplakia, decreased salivation, and reports of pain.

disturbed Body Image may be related to anatomical or structural changes, loss of hair and weight, possibly evidenced by negative feelings about body, preoccupation with change, feelings of helplessness or hopelessness, and change in social environment.

ineffective Protection may be related to inadequate nutrition, drug or radiation therapy, abnormal blood profile, disease state (cancer), possibly evidenced by impaired healing, deficient immunity, anorexia, fatigue.

readiness for enhanced Hope is possibly evidenced by expressed desire to enhance belief in possibilities and sense of meaning to life.

Cholecystectomy MS

acute Pain may be related to interruption in skin and tissue layers with mechanical closure (sutures or staples) and invasive procedures (including T-tube, nasogastric [NG] tube), possibly evidenced by verbal reports, guarding or distraction behaviors, and changes in vital signs.

ineffective Breathing Pattern may be related to pain, muscular impairment, decreased energy, fatigue, possibly evidenced by fremitus, tachypnea, and decreased respiratory depth and vital capacity, holding breath, reluctance to cough.

risk for deficient Fluid Volume/risk for Bleeding is possibly evidenced by risk factors of losses from vomiting or NG aspiration, medically restricted intake, altered coagulation.*

Cholelithiasis CH

acute Pain may be related to obstruction or ductal spasm, inflammatory process, tissue ischemia, necrosis, possibly evidenced by verbal re-

*A risk diagnosis is not evidenced by signs and symptoms, as the problem has not occurred; rather, nursing interventions are directed at prevention.

ports, guarding or distraction behaviors, self- or narrowed focus, and changes in vital signs.

risk for imbalanced Nutrition: less than body requirements is possibly evidenced by risk factors of self-imposed or prescribed dietary restrictions, nausea and vomiting, dyspepsia, pain; loss of nutrients; impaired fat digestion—obstruction of bile flow.*

deficient Knowledge [Learning Need] regarding pathophysiology, therapy choices, and self-care needs may be related to lack of information or recall, misinterpretation, possibly evidenced by verbalization of concerns, questions, and recurrence of condition.

C

Chronic obstructive lung disease CH/MS

ineffective Airway Clearance may be related to bronchospasm, increased production of tenacious secretions, retained secretions, and decreased energy, fatigue, possibly evidenced by presence of wheezes, crackles, tachypnea, dyspnea, changes in depth of respirations, use of accessory muscles, persistent cough, and chest x-ray findings.

impaired Gas Exchange may be related to altered O_2 delivery (obstruction of airways by secretions or bronchospasm, air trapping) and alveoli destruction, possibly evidenced by dyspnea, restlessness, confusion, abnormal ABG values—hypoxia, hypercapnia, changes in vital signs, and reduced tolerance for activity.

Activity Intolerance may be related to imbalance between O_2 supply and demand and generalized weakness, possibly evidenced by verbal reports of fatigue, exertional dyspnea, and abnormal vital sign response.

imbalanced Nutrition: less than body requirements may be related to inability to ingest adequate nutrients (dyspnea, fatigue, medication side effects, sputum production, anorexia), possibly evidenced by weight loss, reported altered taste sensation, decreased muscle mass or subcutaneous fat, poor muscle tone, and aversion to eating/lack of interest in food.

risk for Infection is possibly evidenced by risk factors of decreased ciliary action, stasis of secretions, and debilitated state or malnutrition.*

Circumcision PED

deficient Knowledge [Learning Need] regarding surgical procedure, prognosis, and treatment may be related to lack of exposure, misinterpretation, unfamiliarity with information resources, possibly evidenced by request for information, verbalization of concern/misconceptions, inaccurate follow-through of instructions.

acute Pain may be related to trauma to/edema of tender tissues, possibly evidenced by crying, changes in sleep pattern, refusal to eat.

impaired urinary Elimination may be related to tissue injury or inflammation or development of urethral fistula, possibly evidenced by edema, difficulty voiding.

risk for Bleeding is possibly evidenced by risk factors of decreased clotting factors immediately after birth, previously undiagnosed problems with bleeding or clotting.*

*A risk diagnosis is not evidenced by signs and symptoms, as the problem has not occurred; rather, nursing interventions are directed at prevention.

risk for Infection is possibly evidenced by risk factors of immature immune system, invasive procedure, tissue trauma, environmental exposure.*

Cirrhosis MS/CH

C

Also refer to Substance dependence/abuse rehabilitation; Hepatitis, acute viral

risk for impaired Liver Function are possibly evidenced by risk factors of viral infection, alcohol abuse.*

imbalanced Nutrition: less than body requirements may be related to inability to ingest or absorb nutrients (anorexia, nausea, indigestion, early satiety), abnormal bowel function, impaired storage of vitamins, possibly evidenced by aversion to eating, observed lack of intake, poor muscle tone, muscle wasting, weight loss, and imbalances in nutritional studies.

excess Fluid Volume may be related to compromised regulatory mechanism (e.g., syndrome of inappropriate antidiuretic hormone, decreased plasma proteins, malnutrition) and excess sodium and/or fluid intake, possibly evidenced by generalized or abdominal edema, weight gain, dyspnea, BP changes, positive hepatojugular reflex, change in mentation, altered electrolytes, changes in urine specific gravity, and pleural effusion.

risk for impaired Skin Integrity is possibly evidenced by risk factors of altered circulation and metabolic state, poor skin turgor, skeletal prominence, presence of edema or ascites, and accumulation of bile salts in skin.*

risk for Bleeding is possibly evidenced by risk factors of abnormal blood profile, altered clotting factors—decreased production of prothrombin, fibrinogen, and factors VIII, IX, and X; impaired vitamin K absorption; release of thromboplastin, portal hypertension, development of esophageal varices.*

risk for acute Confusion is possibly evidenced by risk factors of alcohol abuse, increased serum ammonia level, and inability of liver to detoxify certain enzymes or drugs.*

Self-Esteem [specify]/disturbed Body Image may be related to biophysical changes, altered physical appearance, uncertainty of prognosis, changes in role function, personal vulnerability, self-destructive behavior (alcohol-induced disease), possibly evidenced by verbalization of changes in lifestyle, fear of rejection/reaction of others, negative feelings about body or abilities, and feelings of helplessness, hopelessness, powerlessness.

ineffective Protection may be related to abnormal blood profile (altered clotting factors), portal hypertension, development of esophageal varices as evidenced by fatigue, anorexia, itching, disorientation.*

Cocaine hydrochloride poisoning, acute MS

Also refer to Stimulant abuse; Substance dependence/abuse rehabilitation

ineffective Breathing Pattern may be related to pharmacological effects on respiratory center of the brain, possibly evidenced by tachypnea, altered depth of respiration, shortness of breath, and abnormal ABGs.

*A risk diagnosis is not evidenced by signs and symptoms, as the problem has not occurred; rather, nursing interventions are directed at prevention.

risk for decreased Cardiac Output is possibly evidenced by risk factors of drug effect on myocardium (degree dependent on drug purity and quality used), alterations in electrical rate, rhythm, or conduction, preexisting myocardiopathy.*

C

CH

risk for impaired Liver Function is possibly evidenced by risk factors of cocaine abuse and direct effects of cocaine on the myocardium.*

imbalanced Nutrition: less than body requirements may be related to anorexia, insufficient or inappropriate use of financial resources, and is possibly evidenced by reported inadequate intake, weight loss or less than normal weight gain, lack of interest in food, poor muscle tone, signs or laboratory evidence of vitamin deficiencies.

risk for Infection is possibly evidenced by risk factors of injection techniques, impurities of drugs, localized trauma/nasal septum damage, malnutrition, altered immune state.*

PSY

ineffective Coping may be related to personal vulnerability, negative role modeling, inadequate support systems, ineffective or inadequate coping skills with substitution of drug, possibly evidenced by use of harmful substance despite evidence of undesirable consequences.

[disturbed Sensory Perception (specify)] may be related to exogenous chemical, altered sensory reception, transmission, or integration (hallucination), altered status of sense organs, possibly evidenced by responding to internal stimuli from hallucinatory experiences, bizarre thinking, anxiety, panic, changes in sensory acuity (sense of smell or taste).

Coccidioidomycosis (San Joaquin/Valley Fever) — CH

acute Pain may be related to inflammation, possibly evidenced by verbal reports, distraction behaviors, narrowed focus.

Fatigue may be related to decreased energy production, states of discomfort, possibly evidenced by reports of overwhelming lack of energy, inability to maintain usual routine, emotional lability or irritability, impaired ability to concentrate, decreased endurance or libido.

deficient Knowledge [Learning Need] regarding nature and course of disease, therapy and self-care needs may be related to lack of information, possibly evidenced by statements of concern and questions.

Colitis, ulcerative — MS

Diarrhea may be related to inflammation or malabsorption of the bowel, presence of toxins, segmental narrowing of the lumen, possibly evidenced by increased bowel sounds and peristalsis, frequent watery stools (acute phase), changes in stool color, abdominal pain, urgency, cramping.

acute Pain/chronic Pain may be related to inflammation of the intestines, hyperperistalsis, prolonged diarrhea, and anal/rectal irritation, fissures, fistulas, possibly evidenced by verbal reports, guarding or distraction behaviors—restlessness, or self-focusing.

*A risk diagnosis is not evidenced by signs and symptoms, as the problem has not occurred; rather, nursing interventions are directed at prevention.

risk for deficient Fluid Volume is possibly evidenced by risk factors of excessive losses through normal routes—severe frequent diarrhea, vomiting; capillary plasma loss; hypermetabolic state—inflammation, fever; restricted intake—nausea, anorexia.*

CH

imbalanced Nutrition: less than body requirements may be related to altered intake or absorption of nutrients—medically restricted intake, fear that eating may cause diarrhea; and hypermetabolic state, possibly evidenced by weight loss, decreased subcutaneous fat and muscle mass, poor muscle tone, hyperactive bowel sounds, steatorrhea, pale conjunctiva and mucous membranes, aversion to eating.

ineffective Coping may be related to chronic nature and indefinite outcome of disease, multiple stressors repeated over time, situational crisis, personal vulnerability, severe pain, inadequate sleep, lack of or ineffective support systems, possibly evidenced by verbalization of inability to cope, discouragement, anxiety, preoccupation with physical self, chronic worry, emotional tension, depression, recurrent exacerbation of symptoms.

risk for Powerlessness is possibly evidenced by risk factors of unresolved dependency conflicts, feelings of insecurity or resentment, repression of anger and aggressive feelings, lacking a sense of control in stressful situations, sacrificing own wishes for others, retreat from aggression or frustration.*

Colostomy **MS**

risk for impaired Skin Integrity is possibly evidenced by risk factors of absence of sphincter at stoma, character and flow of effluent and flatus from stoma, reaction to product or removal of adhesive, improperly fitting or care of appliance.*

risk for Diarrhea/Constipation are possibly evidenced by risk factors of interruption or alteration of normal bowel function/placement of ostomy, changes in dietary or fluid intake, and effects of medication.*

CH

deficient Knowledge [Learning Need] regarding changes in physiological function, and self-care and treatment needs may be related to lack of exposure or recall, information misinterpretation, possibly evidenced by questions, statement of concern, and inaccurate follow-through of instruction or performance of ostomy care, development of preventable complications.

disturbed Body Image may be related to biophysical changes (presence of stoma, loss of control of bowel elimination) and psychosocial factors (altered body structure, disease process—cancer, colitis, and associated treatment regimen, possibly evidenced by verbalization of change in perception of self, negative feelings about body, fear of rejection/reaction of others, not touching or looking at stoma, and refusal to participate in care.

impaired Social Interaction may be related to fear of embarrassing situation secondary to altered bowel control with loss of contents, odor,

*A risk diagnosis is not evidenced by signs and symptoms, as the problem has not occurred; rather, nursing interventions are directed at prevention.

possibly evidenced by reduced participation and verbalized or observed discomfort in social situations.

risk for Sexual Dysfunction is possibly evidenced by risk factors of altered body structure and function, radical resection and treatment procedures, vulnerability, psychological concern about response of SO(s), and disruption of sexual response pattern—erection difficulty.*

C

Coma **MS**

risk for Suffocation is possibly evidenced by risk factors of cognitive impairment/loss of protective reflexes and purposeful movement.*

risk for deficient Fluid Volume/imbalanced Nutrition: less than body requirements are possibly evidenced by risk factors of inability to ingest food or fluids, increased needs—hypermetabolic state.*

[total] Self-Care Deficit may be related to cognitive impairment and absence of purposeful activity, evidenced by inability to perform ADLs.

risk for ineffective cerebral Tissue Perfusion is possibly evidenced by risk factors of head trauma, substance abuse, embolism, cerebral aneurysm, brain tumor/neoplasm.*

risk for Infection is possibly evidenced by risk factors of stasis of body fluids (oral, pulmonary, urinary), invasive procedures, and nutritional deficits.*

Coma, diabetic **MS**

Refer to Diabetic ketoacidosis; Coma

Complex regional pain syndrome **MS**

acute Pain/chronic Pain may be related to continued nerve stimulation, possibly evidenced by verbal reports, distraction or guarding behaviors, narrowed focus, changes in sleep patterns, and altered ability to continue previous activities.

ineffective peripheral Tissue Perfusion may be related to reduction of arterial blood flow (arteriole vasoconstriction), possibly evidenced by extremity pain, altered skin characteristics, diminished pulses, and edema.

[disturbed tactile Sensory Perception] may be related to altered sensory reception (neurological deficit, pain), possibly evidenced by change in usual response to stimuli, abnormal sensitivity of touch, physiological anxiety, and irritability.

risk for ineffective Role Performance is possibly evidenced by risk factors of situational crisis, chronic disability, debilitating pain.*

risk for compromised family Coping is possibly evidenced by risk factors of temporary family disorganization and role changes and prolonged disability that exhausts the supportive capacity of SO(s).*

Concussion, brain **CH**

acute Pain may be related to trauma to or edema of cerebral tissue, possibly evidenced by reports of headache, guarding or distraction behaviors, and narrowed focus.

---

*A risk diagnosis is not evidenced by signs and symptoms, as the problem has not occurred; rather, nursing interventions are directed at prevention.

risk for deficient Fluid Volume is possibly evidenced by risk factors of vomiting, decreased intake, and hypermetabolic state (fever).*

risk for impaired Memory is possibly evidenced by risk factor of neurological disturbances.*

deficient Knowledge [Learning Need] regarding condition, treatment safety needs, and potential complications may be related to lack of recall, misinterpretation, cognitive limitation, possibly evidenced by questions or statement of concerns, development of preventable complications.

C

Conduct disorder (childhood, adolescence) **PSY/PED**

risk for self-directed Violence/risk for other-directed Violence are possibly evidenced by risk factors of retarded ego development, antisocial character, poor impulse control, dysfunctional family system, loss of significant relationships, history of suicidal or acting-out behaviors.*

defensive Coping may be related to inadequate coping strategies, maturational crisis, multiple life changes or losses, lack of control of impulsive actions, and personal vulnerability, possibly evidenced by inappropriate use of defense mechanisms, inability to meet role expectations, poor self-esteem, failure to assume responsibility for own actions, hypersensitivity to slight or criticism, and excessive smoking, drinking, or drug use.

ineffective Impulse Control may be related to chronic low self-esteem, anger, disorder of development, mood, personality possibly evidenced by acting without thinking, irritability, temper outbursts.

chronic low Self-Esteem may be related to life choices perpetuating failure, personal vulnerability, possibly evidenced by self-negating verbalizations, anger, rejection of positive feedback, frequent lack of success in life events.

CH

compromised family Coping/disabled family Coping may be related to excessive guilt, anger, or blaming among family members regarding child's behavior; parental inconsistencies; disagreements regarding discipline, limit setting, and approaches; and exhaustion of parental resources (prolonged coping with disruptive child), possibly evidenced by unrealistic parental expectations, rejection or overprotection of child; and exaggerated expressions of anger, disappointment, or despair regarding child's behavior or ability to improve or change.

impaired Social Interaction may be related to retarded ego development, developmental state (adolescence), lack of social skills, low self-concept, dysfunctional family system, and neurological impairment, possibly evidenced by dysfunctional interaction with others (difficulty waiting turn in games or group situations, not seeming to listen to what is being said), difficulty playing quietly and maintaining attention to task or play activity, often shifting from one activity to another and interrupting or intruding on others.

Congestive heart failure **MS**

Refer to Heart failure, chronic

*A risk diagnosis is not evidenced by signs and symptoms, as the problem has not occurred; rather, nursing interventions are directed at prevention.

C

Conn's syndrome MS/CH

Refer to Aldosteronism, primary

Constipation CH

Constipation may be related to weak abdominal musculature, gastrointestinal obstructive lesions, pain on defecation, diagnostic procedures, pregnancy, possibly evidenced by change in character and frequency of stools, feeling of abdominal or rectal fullness or pressure, changes in bowel sounds, abdominal distention.

impaired Comfort may be related to abdominal fullness or pressure, straining to defecate, and trauma to delicate tissues, possibly evidenced by verbal reports, reluctance to defecate, and distraction behaviors.

deficient Knowledge [Learning Need] regarding dietary needs, bowel function, and medication effect may be related to lack of information, misconceptions, possibly evidenced by development of problem and verbalization of concerns or questions.

Coronary artery bypass surgery MS

risk for decreased Cardiac Output is possibly evidenced by risk factors of decreased myocardial contractility, diminished circulating volume (preload), alterations in electrical conduction, and increased systemic vascular resistance (SVR) (afterload).*

acute Pain may be related to direct chest tissue and bone trauma, invasive tubes and lines, donor site incision, tissue inflammation and edema formation, intraoperative nerve trauma, possibly evidenced by verbal reports, changes in vital signs, and distraction behaviors (restlessness), irritability.

[disturbed Sensory Perception (specify)] may be related to restricted environment (postoperative or acute), sleep deprivation, effects of medications, continuous environmental sounds and activities, and psychological stress of procedure, possibly evidenced by disorientation, alterations in behavior, exaggerated emotional responses, and visual or auditory distortions.

CH

ineffective Role Performance may be related to situational crises (dependent role), recuperative process, uncertainty about the future, possibly evidenced by delay or alteration in physical capacity to resume role, change in usual role or responsibility, change in self or others' perception of role.

Crohn's disease MS/CH

Also refer to Colitis, ulcerative

imbalanced Nutrition: less than body requirements may be related to intestinal pain after eating, decreased transit time through bowel, fear that eating may cause diarrhea, possibly evidenced by weight loss, decreased subcutaneous fat and muscle mass, poor muscle tone, aversion to eating, and observed lack of intake.

Diarrhea may be related to inflammation, irritation—particular dietary intake, malabsorption of the bowel, presence of toxins, segmental narrowing of the lumen, possibly evidenced by hyperactive bowel

*A risk diagnosis is not evidenced by signs and symptoms, as the problem has not occurred; rather, nursing interventions are directed at prevention.

sounds, increased peristalsis, cramping, and frequent loose liquid stools.

deficient Knowledge [Learning Need] regarding condition, nutritional needs, and prevention of recurrence may be related to misinterpretation of information, lack of recall, unfamiliarity with resources, possibly evidenced by statements of concern, questions, inaccurate follow-through of instructions, and development of preventable complications or exacerbation of condition.

C

Croup — PED/CH

ineffective Airway Clearance may be related to presence of thick, tenacious mucus and swelling or spasms of the epiglottis, possibly evidenced by harsh, brassy cough; tachypnea, use of accessory breathing muscles, and presence of wheezes.

deficient Fluid Volume may be related to decreased ability or aversion to swallowing, presence of fever, and increased respiratory losses, possibly evidenced by dry mucous membranes, poor skin turgor, and scanty, concentrated urine.

Croup, membranous — PED/CH

Also refer to Croup

risk for Suffocation is possibly evidenced by risk factors of inflammation of larynx with formation of false membrane.*

Anxiety [specify level]/Fear may be related to change in environment, perceived threat to self (difficulty breathing), and transmission of anxiety of adults, possibly evidenced by restlessness, facial tension, glancing about, and sympathetic stimulation.

C-Section — OB

Refer to Cesarean birth; Cesarean birth, unplanned

Cushing's syndrome — CH/MS

risk for excess Fluid Volume is possibly evidenced by risk factor of compromised regulatory mechanism (fluid and sodium retention).*

risk for Infection is possibly evidenced by risk factors of immunosuppressed inflammatory response, skin and capillary fragility, and negative nitrogen balance.*

imbalanced Nutrition: less than body requirements may be related to inability to utilize nutrients (disturbance of carbohydrate metabolism), possibly evidenced by decreased muscle mass and increased resistance to insulin.

Self-Care Deficit [specify] may be related to muscle wasting, generalized weakness, fatigue, and demineralization of bones, possibly evidenced by statements of or observed inability to complete or perform ADLs.

disturbed Body Image may be related to change in structure or appearance (effects of disease process, drug therapy), possibly evidenced by negative feelings about body, feelings of helplessness, and changes in social involvement.

Sexual Dysfunction may be related to loss of libido, impotence, and cessation of menses, possibly evidenced by verbalization of concerns and/or dissatisfaction with and alteration in relationship with SO.

---

*A risk diagnosis is not evidenced by signs and symptoms, as the problem has not occurred; rather, nursing interventions are directed at prevention.

risk for Trauma [fractures] is possibly evidenced by risk factors of increased protein breakdown, negative protein balance, demineralization of bones.*

CVA **MS/CH**

Refer to Cerebrovascular accident

D

Cystic fibrosis **CH/PED**

ineffective Airway Clearance may be related to excessive production of thick mucus and decreased ciliary action, possibly evidenced by abnormal breath sounds, ineffective cough, cyanosis, and altered respiratory rate and depth.

risk for Infection is possibly evidenced by risk factors of stasis of respiratory secretions and development of atelectasis.*

imbalanced Nutrition: less than body requirements may be related to impaired digestive process and absorption of nutrients, possibly evidenced by failure to gain weight, muscle wasting, and retarded physical growth.

deficient Knowledge [Learning Need] regarding pathophysiology of condition, medical management, and available community resources may be related to insufficient information, misconceptions, possibly evidenced by statements of concern and questions, inaccurate follow-through of instructions, development of preventable complications.

compromised family Coping may be related to chronic nature of disease and disability, inadequate or incorrect information or understanding by a primary person, possibly evidenced by significant person attempting assistive or supportive behaviors with less than satisfactory results, protective behavior disproportionate to client's abilities, or need for autonomy.

Cystitis **CH**

acute Pain may be related to inflammation and bladder spasms, possibly evidenced by verbal reports, distraction behaviors, and narrowed focus.

impaired urinary Elimination may be related to inflammation or irritation of bladder, possibly evidenced by frequency, nocturia, and dysuria.

deficient Knowledge [Learning Need] regarding condition, treatment, and prevention of recurrence may be related to inadequate information, misconceptions, possibly evidenced by statements of concern and questions, recurrent infections.

Cytomegalic inclusion disease **CH**

Refer to Cytomegalovirus infection

Cytomegalovirus (CMV) infection **CH**

[risk for disturbed visual Sensory Perception] is possibly evidenced by risk factor of inflammation of the retina.*

risk for fetal Infection is possibly evidenced by risk factors of transplacental exposure, contact with blood or body fluids.*

Deep Vein Thrombosis (DVT) **CH/MS**

Refer to Thrombophlebitis

*A risk diagnosis is not evidenced by signs and symptoms, as the problem has not occurred; rather, nursing interventions are directed at prevention.

Degenerative joint disease CH

Refer to Arthritis, rheumatoid

Dehiscence (abdominal) MS

impaired Skin Integrity may be related to altered circulation, altered nutritional state (obesity, malnutrition), and physical stress on incision, possibly evidenced by poor or delayed wound healing and disruption of skin surface or wound closure.

risk for Infection is possibly evidenced by risk factors of inadequate primary defenses (separation of incision, traumatized intestines, environmental exposure).*

risk for impaired Tissue Integrity is possibly evidenced by risk factor of exposure of abdominal contents to external environment.*

Fear/[severe] Anxiety may be related to crises, perceived threat of death, possibly evidenced by fearfulness, restless behaviors, and sympathetic stimulation.

deficient Knowledge [Learning Need] regarding condition, prognosis, and treatment needs may be related to lack of information or recall, misinterpretation of information, possibly evidenced by development of preventable complication, requests for information, and statement of concern.

Dehydration PED/CH

deficient Fluid Volume [specify] may be related to etiology as defined by the specific situation, possibly evidenced by dry mucous membranes, poor skin turgor, decreased pulse volume and pressure, and thirst.

risk for impaired oral Mucous Membrane is possibly evidenced by risk factors of dehydration and decreased salivation.*

deficient Knowledge [Learning Need] regarding fluid needs may be related to lack of information, misinterpretation, possibly evidenced by questions, statement of concern, and inadequate follow-through of instructions, development of preventable complications.

Delirium tremens (acute alcohol withdrawal) MS/PSY

[severe] Anxiety/[panic] Fear may be related to cessation of alcohol intake, physiological withdrawal, threat to self-concept, perceived threat of death, possibly evidenced by increased tension, apprehension, feelings of inadequacy, shame, self-disgust, or remorse; fear of unspecified consequences, identifies object of fear.

[disturbed Sensory Perception (specify)] may be related to exogenous factors—alcohol consumption and sudden cessation; endogenous—electrolyte imbalance, elevated ammonia and blood urea nitrogen (BUN); sleep deprivation, and psychological stress, possibly evidenced by disorientation, restlessness, irritability, exaggerated emotional responses, bizarre thinking, and visual or auditory distortions or hallucinations.

risk for decreased Cardiac Output is possibly evidenced by risk factors of direct effect of alcohol on heart muscle, altered SVR, presence of dysrhythmias.*

---

*A risk diagnosis is not evidenced by signs and symptoms, as the problem has not occurred; rather, nursing interventions are directed at prevention.

risk for Trauma is possibly evidenced by risk factors of alterations in balance, reduced muscle coordination, cognitive impairment, and involuntary clonic/tonic muscle activity.*

imbalanced Nutrition: less than body requirements may be related to poor dietary intake, effects of alcohol on organs involved in digestion, interference with absorption or metabolism of nutrients and amino acids, possibly evidenced by reports of inadequate food intake, altered taste sensation, lack of interest in food, debilitated state, decreased subcutaneous fat and muscle mass, signs or laboratory findings of mineral and electrolyte deficiency.

D

Delivery, precipitous/out of hospital OB

Also refer to Labor, precipitous; Labor, stage I (active phase); Labor stage II (expulsion)

risk for deficient Fluid Volume is possibly evidenced by risk factors of presence of nausea, vomiting, lack of intake, excessive vascular loss.*

risk for Infection is possibly evidenced by risk factors of broken or traumatized tissue, increased environmental exposure, rupture of amniotic membranes.*

risk for fetal Injury is possibly evidenced by risk factors of rapid descent and pressure changes, compromised circulation, environmental exposure.*

Delusional disorder PSY

risk for self-directed Violence/risk for other-directed Violence are possibly evidenced by risk factors of perceived threats of danger, increased feelings of anxiety, acting out in an irrational manner.*

[severe] Anxiety may be related to inability to trust, possibly evidenced by rigid delusional system, frightened of other people and own hostility.

Powerlessness may be related to lifestyle of helplessness, feelings of inadequacy, interpersonal interaction, possibly evidenced by verbal expressions of no control or influence over situation(s), use of paranoid delusions, aggressive behavior to compensate for lack of control.

impaired Social Interaction may be related to mistrust of others, delusional thinking, lack of knowledge or skills to enhance mutuality, possibly evidenced by discomfort in social situations, difficulty in establishing relationships with others, expression of feelings of rejection, no sense of belonging.

Dementia, presenile/senile CH/PSY

Also refer to Alzheimer's disease

impaired Memory may be related to neurological disturbances, possibly evidenced by observed experiences of forgetting, inability to determine if a behavior was performed, inability to perform previously learned skills, inability to recall factual information or recent or past events.

Fear may be related to decreases in functional abilities, public disclosure of disabilities, further mental or physical deterioration, possibly evidenced by social isolation, apprehension, irritability, defensiveness, suspiciousness, aggressive behavior.

---

*A risk diagnosis is not evidenced by signs and symptoms, as the problem has not occurred; rather, nursing interventions are directed at prevention.

Self-Care Deficit [specify] may be related to cognitive decline, physical limitations, frustration over loss of independence, depression, possibly evidenced by impaired ability to perform ADLs.

risk for Trauma is possibly evidenced by risk factors of changes in muscle coordination or balance, impaired judgment, seizure activity.*

risk for sedentary Lifestyle is possibly evidenced by risk factors of lack of interest or motivation, lack of resources, lack of training or knowledge of specific exercise needs, safety concerns or fear of injury.*

risk for caregiver Role Strain is possibly evidenced by risk factors of illness severity of care receiver, duration of caregiving required, complexity or amount of caregiving tasks, care receiver exhibiting deviant or bizarre behavior; family/caregiver isolation, lack of respite or recreation, spouse is caregiver.*

Grieving may be related to awareness of something "being wrong," predisposition for anxiety and feelings of inadequacy, family perception of potential loss of loved one, possibly evidenced by expressions of distress, anger at potential loss, choked feelings, crying, alteration in activity level, communication patterns, eating habits, and sleep patterns.

Depressant abuse **CH/PSY**

Also refer to Drug overdose, acute (depressants)

ineffective Denial may be related to weak, underdeveloped ego, unmet self-needs, possibly evidenced by inability to admit impact of condition on life, minimizes symptoms or problem, refuses healthcare attention.

ineffective Coping may be related to weak ego, possibly evidenced by abuse of chemical agents, lack of goal-directed behavior, inadequate problem-solving, destructive behavior toward self.

imbalanced Nutrition: less than body requirements may be related to use of substance in place of nutritional food, possibly evidenced by loss of weight, pale conjunctiva and mucous membranes, electrolyte imbalances, anemias.

risk for Injury is possibly evidenced by risk factors of changes in sleep, decreased concentration, loss of inhibitions.*

Depression, postpartum **OB/PSY**

Also refer to Depressive disorders

risk for impaired Attachment is possibly evidenced by risk factors of anxiety associated with the parent role, inability to meet personal needs, perceived guilt regarding relationship with infant.*

Fatigue may be related to stress, sleep deprivation, depression as evidenced by reports overwhelming lack of energy, inability to maintain usual routines, increase in physical complaints.

situational low Self-Esteem may be related to developmental changes, disturbed body image, possibly evidenced by evaluation of self as unable to deal with situation, self-negating verbalizations, reports helplessness.

---

*A risk diagnosis is not evidenced by signs and symptoms, as the problem has not occurred; rather, nursing interventions are directed at prevention.

Depressive disorders, major depression, dysthymia **PSY**

risk for self-directed Violence is possibly evidenced by risk factors of depressed mood and feeling of worthlessness and hopelessness.*

[moderate to severe] Anxiety may be related to stress, unconscious conflict about essential values or goals of life, unmet needs, threat to self-concept, interpersonal transmission or contagion, possibly evidenced by feelings of inadequacy, sleep disturbances, fatigue, difficulty concentrating, diminished productivity/ability to problem-solve, rumination.

Insomnia may be related to biochemical alterations (decreased serotonin), unresolved fears and anxieties, and inactivity, possibly evidenced by difficulty in falling or remaining asleep, early morning awakening or awakening later than desired, reports of not feeling rested, physical signs (e.g., dark circles under eyes, excessive yawning).

Social Isolation/impaired Social Interaction may be related to alterations in mental status or thought processes (depressed mood), inadequate personal resources, decreased energy, inertia, difficulty engaging in satisfying personal relationships, feelings of worthlessness, low self-concept, inadequacy or absence of significant purpose in life, and knowledge or skill deficit about social interactions, possibly evidenced by decreased involvement with others, expressed feelings of difference from others, remaining in home/room/bed, refusing invitations or suggestions for social involvement, and dysfunctional interaction with peers, family, and/or others.

interrupted Family Processes may be related to situational crises of illness of family member with change in roles or responsibilities, developmental crises (e.g., loss of family member or relationship), possibly evidenced by statements of difficulty coping with situation, family system not meeting needs of its members, difficulty accepting or receiving help appropriately, ineffective family decision-making process, and failure to send and to receive clear messages.

risk for impaired Religiosity is possibly evidenced by risk factors of ineffective support or coping, lack of social interaction, depression.*

Dermatitis, seborrheic **CH**

impaired Skin Integrity may be related to chronic inflammatory condition of the skin, possibly evidenced by disruption of skin surface with dry or moist scales, yellowish crusts, erythema, and fissures.

Diabetes, gestational **OB**

Also refer to Diabetes mellitus

risk for unstable Blood Glucose Level is possibly evidenced by risk factors of pregnancy, dietary intake, lack of diabetes management, inadequate blood glucose monitoring.*

risk for disturbed Maternal-Fetal Dyad is possibly evidenced by risk factors of impaired glucose metabolism, compromised oxygen transport—changes in circulation; treatment-related side effects.*

deficient Knowledge [Learning Need] regarding diabetic condition, prognosis, and treatment needs may be related to lack of resources or exposure to information, misinformation, possibly evidenced by

---

*A risk diagnosis is not evidenced by signs and symptoms, as the problem has not occurred; rather, nursing interventions are directed at prevention.

questions, statements of misconceptions, inaccurate follow-through of instructions, development of preventable complications.

Diabetes mellitus **CH/PED**

deficient Knowledge [Learning Need] regarding disease process, treatment, and individual care needs may be related to unfamiliarity with information, lack of recall, misinterpretation, possibly evidenced by requests for information, statements of concern, misconceptions, inadequate follow-through of instructions, or development of preventable complications.

risk for unstable Blood Glucose Level is possibly evidenced by risk factors of lack of adherence to diabetes management, medication management, inadequate blood glucose monitoring, physical activity level, health status, stress, rapid growth periods.*

risk-prone Health Behavior may be related to inadequate comprehension, multiple stressors, as evidenced by minimization of health status change, failure to achieve optimal sense of control.

risk for Infection is possibly evidenced by risk factors of decreased leukocyte function, circulatory changes, and delayed healing.*

[risk for disturbed Sensory Perception (specify)] is possibly evidenced by risk factors of endogenous chemical alteration (glucose, insulin, and/or electrolyte imbalance).*

compromised family Coping may be related to inadequate or incorrect information or understanding by primary person(s), other situational or developmental crises or situations the significant person(s) may be facing, lifelong condition requiring behavioral changes impacting family, possibly evidenced by family expressions of confusion about what to do, verbalizations that they are having difficulty coping with situation, family does not meet physical or emotional needs of its members; SO(s) preoccupied with personal reaction (e.g., guilt, fear), display protective behavior disproportionate (too little or too much) to client's abilities or need for autonomy.

Diabetic ketoacidosis **CH/MS**

deficient Fluid Volume [specify] may be related to hyperosmolar urinary losses, gastric losses and inadequate intake, possibly evidenced by increased urinary output, dilute urine; reports of weakness, thirst, sudden weight loss, hypotension, tachycardia, delayed capillary refill, dry mucous membranes, poor skin turgor.

unstable Blood Glucose Level may be related to medication management, lack of diabetes management, inadequate blood glucose monitoring, presence of infection, possibly evidenced by elevated serum glucose level, presence of ketones in urine, nausea, weight loss, blurred vision, irritability.

Fatigue may be related to decreased metabolic energy production, altered body chemistry (insufficient insulin), increased energy demands (hypermetabolic state—infection), possibly evidenced by overwhelming lack of energy, inability to maintain usual routines, decreased performance, impaired ability to concentrate, listlessness.

risk for Infection possibly evidenced by risk factors of high glucose levels, decreased leukocyte function, stasis of body fluids, invasive procedures, alterations in circulation.*

---

*A risk diagnosis is not evidenced by signs and symptoms, as the problem has not occurred; rather, nursing interventions are directed at prevention.

Dialysis, general **CH**

Also refer to Dialysis, peritoneal; Hemodialysis

imbalanced Nutrition: less than body requirements may be related to inadequate ingestion of nutrients—dietary restrictions, anorexia, nausea, vomiting, stomatitis, sensation of feeling full with continuous ambulatory peritoneal dialysis; loss of peptides and amino acids (building blocks for proteins) during dialysis, possibly evidenced by reported inadequate intake, aversion to eating, altered taste sensation, poor muscle tone, weakness, sore and inflamed buccal cavity, pale conjunctiva and mucous membranes.

Grieving may be related to actual or perceived loss, chronic and/or fatal illness, and thwarted grieving response to a loss, possibly evidenced by verbal expression of distress or unresolved issues, denial of loss, altered eating habits, sleep and dream patterns, activity levels, libido, crying, labile affect; feelings of sorrow, guilt, and anger.

disturbed Body Image/situational low Self-Esteem may be related to situational crisis and chronic illness with changes in usual roles and body image, possibly evidenced by verbalization of changes in lifestyle, focus on past function, negative feelings about body, feelings of helplessness and powerlessness, extension of body boundary to incorporate environmental objects (e.g., dialysis setup), change in social involvement, overdependence on others for care, not taking responsibility for self-care, lack of follow-through, and self-destructive behavior.

Self-Care Deficit [specify] may be related to perceptual or cognitive impairment (accumulated toxins), intolerance to activity, decreased strength and endurance, pain, discomfort, possibly evidenced by reported inability to perform ADLs, disheveled or unkempt appearance, strong body odor.

Powerlessness may be related to illness-related regimen and healthcare environment, possibly evidenced by verbal expression of having no control, depression over physical deterioration, nonparticipation in care, anger, and passivity.

compromised family Coping/disabled family Coping may be related to inadequate or incorrect information or understanding by a primary person, temporary family disorganization and role changes, client providing little support in turn for the primary person, and prolonged disease and disability progression that exhausts the supportive capacity of significant persons, possibly evidenced by expressions of concern or reports about response of SO(s)/family to client's health problem, preoccupation of SO(s) with own personal reactions, display of intolerance or rejection, and protective behavior disproportionate (too little or too much) to client's abilities or need for autonomy.

Dialysis, peritoneal **MS/CH**

Also refer to Dialysis, general

risk for excess Fluid Volume is possibly evidenced by risk factors of inadequate osmotic gradient of dialysate, fluid retention—malpositioned, kinked, or clotted catheter; bowel distention, peritonitis, scarring of peritoneum; excessive oral or IV intake.*

*A risk diagnosis is not evidenced by signs and symptoms, as the problem has not occurred; rather, nursing interventions are directed at prevention.

risk for Trauma is possibly evidenced by risk factors of improper placement during insertion or manipulation of catheter.*

acute Pain/impaired Comfort may be related to catheter irritation, improper catheter placement, presence of edema, abdominal distention, inflammation or infection, rapid infusion or infusion of cold or acidic dialysate, possibly evidenced by verbal reports, guarding or distraction behaviors, and self-focus.

risk for Infection [peritoneal] is possibly evidenced by risk factors of contamination of catheter or infusion system, skin contaminants, sterile peritonitis (response to composition of dialysate).*

risk for ineffective Breathing Pattern is possibly evidenced by risk factors of increased abdominal pressure restricting diaphragmatic excursion, rapid infusion of dialysate, pain or discomfort, inflammatory process—atelectasis/pneumonia.*

D

Diaper rash **PED**

Refer to Candidiasis

Diarrhea **PED/CH**

deficient Knowledge [Learning Need] regarding causative and contributing factors, and therapeutic needs may be related to lack of information, misconceptions, possibly evidenced by statements of concern, questions, and development of preventable complications.

risk for deficient Fluid Volume is possibly evidenced by risk factors of excessive losses through gastrointestinal tract, altered intake.*

acute Pain may be related to abdominal cramping and irritation or excoriation of skin, possibly evidenced by verbal reports, facial grimacing, and changes in vital signs.

impaired Skin Integrity may be related to effects of excretions on delicate tissues, possibly evidenced by reports of discomfort and disruption of skin surface or destruction of skin layers.

Digitalis toxicity **MS/CH**

decreased Cardiac Output may be related to altered myocardial contractility or electrical conduction, properties of digitalis (long half-life and narrow therapeutic range), concurrent medications, age and general health status, and electrolyte and acid-base balance, possibly evidenced by changes in rate, rhythm, or conduction (development or worsening of dysrhythmias); changes in mentation, worsening of heart failure, elevated serum drug levels.

risk for imbalanced Fluid Volume is possibly evidenced by risk factors of excessive losses from vomiting or diarrhea, decreased intake, nausea, decreased plasma proteins, malnutrition, continued use of diuretics; excess sodium and fluid retention.*

deficient Knowledge [Learning Need] regarding condition therapy and self-care needs may be related to information misinterpretation and lack of recall, possibly evidenced by inaccurate follow-through of instructions and development of preventable complications.

Dilation and curettage (D and C) **OB/GYN**

Also refer to Abortion, elective termination; Abortion, spontaneous termination

---

*A risk diagnosis is not evidenced by signs and symptoms, as the problem has not occurred; rather, nursing interventions are directed at prevention.

deficient Knowledge [Learning Need] regarding surgical procedure, possible postprocedural complications, and therapeutic needs may be related to lack of exposure or unfamiliarity with information, possibly evidenced by requests for information and statements of concern, misconceptions.

D

Dilation of cervix, premature — OB

Also refer to Labor, preterm

Anxiety [specify level] may be related to situational crisis, threat of death or fetal loss, possibly evidenced by increased tension, apprehension, feelings of inadequacy, sympathetic stimulation, and repetitive questioning.

risk for disturbed Maternal-Fetal Dyad is possibly evidenced by risk factors of surgical intervention, use of tocolytic drugs.*

risk for fetal Injury is possibly evidenced by risk factors of premature delivery, surgical procedure.*

Grieving may be related to perceived potential fetal loss, possibly evidenced by expression of distress, guilt, anger, choked feelings.

Dislocation/subluxation of joint — CH

acute Pain may be related to lack of continuity of bone/joint, muscle spasms, edema, possibly evidenced by verbal or coded reports, guarded or protective behaviors, narrowed focus, changes in vital signs.

risk for Injury is possibly evidenced by risk factors of nerve impingement, improper fitting of splint device.*

impaired physical Mobility may be related to immobilization device, activity restrictions, pain, edema, decreased muscle strength, possibly evidenced by limited range of motion, limited ability to perform motor skills, gait changes.

Disseminated intravascular coagulation (DIC) — MS

risk for deficient Fluid Volume is possibly evidenced by risk factors of failure of regulatory mechanism (coagulation process) and active loss—hemorrhage.*

ineffective Tissue Perfusion [specify] may be related to alteration of arterial or venous flow (microemboli throughout circulatory system, and hypovolemia), possibly evidenced by changes in respiratory rate and depth, changes in mentation, decreased urinary output, and development of acral cyanosis or focal gangrene.

Anxiety [specify level]/Fear may be related to sudden change in health status/threat of death, interpersonal transmission or contagion, possibly evidenced by sympathetic stimulation, restlessness, focus on self, and apprehension.

risk for impaired Gas Exchange is possibly evidenced by risk factors of reduced O_2-carrying capacity, development of acidosis, fibrin deposition in microcirculation, and ischemic damage of lung parenchyma.*

acute Pain may be related to bleeding into joints/muscles, with hematoma formation, and ischemic tissues with areas of acral cyanosis or focal gangrene, possibly evidenced by verbal reports, narrowed fo-

*A risk diagnosis is not evidenced by signs and symptoms, as the problem has not occurred; rather, nursing interventions are directed at prevention.

cus, alteration in muscle tone, guarding or distraction behaviors, restlessness, changes in vital signs.

Dissociative disorders **PSY**

[severe] Anxiety/[panic] Fear may be related to a maladaptation or ineffective coping continuing from early life, unconscious conflict(s), threat to self-concept, unmet needs, or phobic stimulus, possibly evidenced by maladaptive response to stress (e.g., dissociating self or fragmentation of the personality), increased tension, feelings of inadequacy, and focus on self, projection of personal perceptions onto the environment.

risk for self-directed Violence/risk for other-directed Violence is possibly evidenced by risk factors of dissociative state/conflicting personalities, depressed mood, panic states, and suicidal or homicidal behaviors.*

disturbed Personal Identity may be related to psychological conflicts (dissociative state), childhood trauma or abuse, threat to physical integrity or self-concept, and underdeveloped ego, possibly evidenced by alteration in perception or experience of the self, loss of one's own sense of reality or the external world, poorly differentiated ego boundaries, confusion about sense of self, confusion regarding purpose or direction in life, memory loss, presence of more than one personality within the individual.

compromised family Coping may be related to multiple stressors repeated over time, prolonged progression of disorder that exhausts the supportive capacity of significant person(s), family disorganization and role changes, high-risk family situation, possibly evidenced by family/SO(s) describing inadequate understanding or knowledge that interferes with assistive or supportive behaviors, relationship and marital conflict.

Diverticulitis **CH**

acute Pain may be related to inflammation of intestinal mucosa, abdominal cramping, and presence of fever or chills, possibly evidenced by verbal reports, guarding or distraction behaviors, changes in vital signs, and narrowed focus.

Diarrhea/Constipation may be related to altered structure or function and presence of inflammation, possibly evidenced by signs and symptoms dependent on specific problem (e.g., increase or decrease in frequency of stools and change in consistency).

deficient Knowledge [Learning Need] regarding disease process, potential complications, therapeutic and self-care needs may be related to lack of information/misconceptions, possibly evidenced by statements of concern, request for information, and development of preventable complications.

risk for Powerlessness is possibly evidenced by risk factors of chronic nature of disease process and recurrent episodes despite cooperation with medical regimen.*

Down syndrome **PED/CH**

Also refer to Mental retardation

risk for disproportionate Growth and/or delayed Development possibly evidenced by risk factor of genetic disorder.

---

*A risk diagnosis is not evidenced by signs and symptoms, as the problem has not occurred; rather, nursing interventions are directed at prevention.

risk for Trauma is possibly evidenced by risk factors of cognitive difficulties and poor muscle tone or coordination, weakness.*

imbalanced Nutrition: less than body requirements may be related to poor muscle tone and protruding tongue, possibly evidenced by weak and ineffective sucking or swallowing and observed lack of adequate intake with weight loss or failure to gain.

interrupted Family Processes may be related to situational or maturational crises requiring incorporation of new skills into family dynamics, possibly evidenced by confusion about what to do, verbalized difficulty coping with situation, unexamined family myths.

risk for complicated Grieving is possibly evidenced by risk factors of loss of "the perfect child," chronic condition requiring long-term care, and unresolved feelings.*

risk for impaired Attachment is possibly evidenced by risk factors of ill infant/child who is unable to effectively initiate parental contact due to altered behavioral organization, inability of parents to meet personal needs.*

Social Isolation is possibly evidenced by risk factors of withdrawal from usual social interactions and activities, assumption of total child care, and becoming overindulgent or overprotective.*

Drug overdose, acute (depressants) **MS/PSY**

Also refer to Substance dependence/abuse rehabilitation

ineffective Breathing Pattern/impaired Gas Exchange may be related to neuromuscular impairment or CNS depression, decreased lung expansion, possibly evidenced by changes in respirations, cyanosis, and abnormal ABGs.

risk for Trauma/risk for Suffocation/risk for Poisoning are possibly evidenced by risk factors of CNS depression or agitation, hypersensitivity to the drug(s), psychological stress.*

risk for self-directed Violence/risk for other-directed Violence are possibly evidenced by risk factors of suicidal behaviors, toxic reactions to drug(s).*

risk for Infection is possibly evidenced by risk factors of drug injection techniques, impurities in injected drugs, localized trauma; malnutrition, altered immune state.*

Drug withdrawal **CH/MS**

[disturbed Sensory Perception (specify)] may be related to biochemical imbalance, altered sensory integration possibly evidenced by sensory distortions, poor concentration, irritability, hallucinations.

risk for Injury is possibly evidenced by risk factors of CNS agitation (depressants).*

risk for Suicide is possibly evidenced by risk factors of alcohol or other substance abuse, legal or disciplinary problems, depressed mood (stimulants).*

acute Pain/impaired Comfort may be related to biochemical changes associated with cessation of drug use, possibly evidenced by reports of muscle aches, fever, diaphoresis, rhinorrhea, lacrimation, malaise.

Self-Care Deficit (specify) may be related to perceptual or cognitive impairment, therapeutic management (restraints), possibly evidenced by inability to meet own physical needs.

---

*A risk diagnosis is not evidenced by signs and symptoms, as the problem has not occurred; rather, nursing interventions are directed at prevention.

Insomnia may be related to cessation of substance use, fatigue possibly evidenced by reports of insomnia/hypersomnia, decreased ability to function, increased irritability.

Fatigue may be related to altered body chemistry (drug withdrawal), sleep deprivation, malnutrition, poor physical condition possibly evidenced by verbal reports of overwhelming lack of energy, inability to maintain usual level of physical activity, inability to restore energy after sleep, compromised concentration.

Duchenne's muscular dystrophy — PED/CH

Refer to Muscular dystrophy [Duchenne's]

DVT — CH/MS

Refer to Thrombophlebitis

Dysmenorrhea — GYN

acute Pain may be related to exaggerated uterine contractibility, possibly evidenced by verbal reports, guarding or distraction behaviors, narrowed focus, and changes in vital signs.

ineffective Coping may be related to chronic, recurrent nature of problem, anticipatory anxiety, and inadequate coping methods, possibly evidenced by muscular tension, headaches, general irritability, chronic depression, and verbalization of inability to cope, report of poor self-concept.

Dysrhythmia, cardiac — MS

risk for decreased Cardiac Output is possibly evidenced by risk factors of altered electrical conduction and reduced myocardial contractility.*

deficient Knowledge [Learning Need] regarding medical condition and therapy needs may be related to lack of information or recall, misinterpretation, and unfamiliarity with information resources, possibly evidenced by questions, statement of misconception, failure to improve on previous regimen, and development of preventable complications.

risk for Poisoning, [digitalis toxicity] is possibly evidenced by risk factors of limited range of therapeutic effectiveness, lack of education or proper precautions, reduced vision, cognitive limitations.*

Eating disorders — CH/PSY

Refer to Anorexia nervosa; Bulimia nervosa; Obesity

Eclampsia — OB

Also refer to Pregnancy-induced hypertension

Anxiety [specify level]/Fear may be related to situational crisis, threat of change in health status or death (self/fetus), separation from support system, interpersonal contagion possibly evidenced by expressed concerns, apprehension, increased tension, decreased self-assurance, difficulty concentrating.

risk for maternal Injury is possibly evidenced by risk factors of tissue edema, hypoxia, tonic/clonic convulsions, abnormal blood profile and/or clotting factors.*

---

*A risk diagnosis is not evidenced by signs and symptoms, as the problem has not occurred; rather, nursing interventions are directed at prevention.

impaired physical Mobility may be related to prescribed bedrest, discomfort, anxiety possibly evidenced by difficulty turning, postural instability.

risk for Self-Care Deficit [specify] is possibly evidenced by risk factors of weakness, discomfort, physical restrictions.*

Ectopic pregnancy (tubal) **OB**

Also refer to Abortion, spontaneous termination

acute Pain may be related to distention or rupture of fallopian tube, possibly evidenced by verbal reports, guarding or distraction behaviors, facial mask of pain, diaphoresis, changes in vital signs.

risk for deficient Fluid Volume/risk for Bleeding are possibly evidenced by risk factors of pregnancy-related complications, hemorrhagic losses and decreased or restricted intake.*

Anxiety [specify level]/Fear may be related to threat of death and possible loss of ability to conceive, possibly evidenced by increased tension, apprehension, sympathetic stimulation, restlessness, and focus on self.

Eczema (dermatitis) **CH**

acute Pain/impaired Comfort may be related to cutaneous inflammation and irritation, possibly evidenced by verbal reports, irritability, and scratching.

risk for Infection is possibly evidenced by risk factors of broken skin and tissue trauma.*

Social Isolation may be related to alterations in physical appearance, possibly evidenced by expressed feelings of rejection and decreased interaction with peers.

Edema, pulmonary **MS**

excess Fluid Volume may be related to decreased cardiac functioning, excessive fluid/sodium intake, possibly evidenced by dyspnea, presence of crackles (rales), pulmonary congestion on x-ray, restlessness, anxiety, and increased CVP and pulmonary pressures.

impaired Gas Exchange may be related to altered blood flow and decreased alveolar/capillary exchange (fluid collection or shifts into interstitial space or alveoli), possibly evidenced by hypoxia, restlessness, and confusion.

Anxiety [specify level]/Fear may be related to perceived threat of death (inability to breathe), possibly evidenced by responses ranging from apprehension to panic state, restlessness, and focus on self.

Electroconvulsive therapy **PSY**

Decisional Conflict may be related to lack of relevant or multiple and divergent sources of information, mistrust of regimen or healthcare personnel, sense of powerlessness, support system deficit.

acute Confusion may be related to CNS effects of electric shock, medications, and anesthesia, possibly evidenced by fluctuation in cognition, agitation.

impaired Memory may be related to neurological disturbance, possibly evidenced by reported or observed experiences of forgetting, difficulty recalling recent events or factual information.

---

*A risk diagnosis is not evidenced by signs and symptoms, as the problem has not occurred; rather, nursing interventions are directed at prevention.

Emphysema **CH/MS**

impaired Gas Exchange may be related to alveolar-capillary membrane changes and destruction, possibly evidenced by dyspnea, restlessness, changes in mentation, abnormal ABG values.

ineffective Airway Clearance may be related to increased production or retained tenacious secretions, decreased energy level, and muscle wasting, possibly evidenced by abnormal breath sounds (rhonchi), ineffective cough, changes in rate and depth of respirations, and dyspnea.

Activity Intolerance may be related to imbalance between O_2 supply and demand, possibly evidenced by reports of fatigue, weakness, exertional dyspnea, and abnormal vital sign response to activity.

imbalanced Nutrition: less than body requirements may be related to inability to ingest food (shortness of breath, anorexia, generalized weakness, medication side effects), possibly evidenced by lack of interest in food, reported altered taste, loss of muscle mass and tone, fatigue, and weight loss.

risk for Infection is possibly evidenced by risk factors of inadequate primary defenses (stasis of body fluids, decreased ciliary action), chronic disease process, and malnutrition.*

Powerlessness may be related to illness-related regimen and healthcare environment, possibly evidenced by verbal expression of having no control, depression over physical deterioration, nonparticipation in therapeutic regimen, anger, and passivity.

Encephalitis **MS**

risk for ineffective cerebral Tissue Perfusion is possibly evidenced by risk factors of cerebral edema altering or interrupting cerebral arterial or venous blood flow, hypovolemia, exchange problems at cellular level (acidosis).*

Hyperthermia may be related to increased metabolic rate, illness, and dehydration, possibly evidenced by increased body temperature, flushed, warm skin; and increased pulse and respiratory rates.

acute Pain may be related to inflammation or irritation of the brain and cerebral edema, possibly evidenced by verbal reports of headache, photophobia, distraction behaviors, restlessness, and changes in vital signs.

risk for Trauma/risk for Suffocation risk factors may include clonic/tonic activity, altered sensorium, cognitive impairment, generalized weakness.*

Endocarditis **MS**

risk for decreased Cardiac Output is possibly evidenced by risk factors of inflammation of lining of heart and structural change in valve leaflets.*

Anxiety [specify level] may be related to change in health status and threat of death, possibly evidenced by apprehension, expressed concerns, and focus on self.

acute Pain may be related to generalized inflammatory process and effects of embolic phenomena, possibly evidenced by verbal reports, narrowed focus, distraction behaviors, and changes in vital signs.

*A risk diagnosis is not evidenced by signs and symptoms, as the problem has not occurred; rather, nursing interventions are directed at prevention.

risk for Activity Intolerance may be related to imbalance between O_2 supply and demand, debilitating condition.*

risk for ineffective Tissue Perfusion [specify] is possibly evidenced by risk factors of embolic interruption of arterial flow (embolization of thrombi or valvular vegetations).*

Endometriosis GYN

acute Pain/chronic Pain may be related to pressure of concealed bleeding, formation of adhesions, possibly evidenced by verbal reports (pain between or with menstruation), guarding or distraction behaviors, and narrowed focus.

Sexual Dysfunction may be related to pain secondary to presence of adhesions, possibly evidenced by verbalization of problem, and altered relationship with partner.

deficient Knowledge [Learning Need] regarding pathophysiology of condition and therapy needs may be related to lack of information/misinterpretations, possibly evidenced by statements of concern and misconceptions.

Enteral feeding MS/CH

imbalanced Nutrition: less than body requirements may be related to conditions that interfere with nutrient intake or increase nutrient need or metabolic demand—cancer and associated treatments, anorexia, surgical procedures, dysphagia, or decreased level of consciousness, possibly evidenced by body weight 10% or more under ideal, decreased subcutaneous fat or muscle mass, poor muscle tone, changes in gastric motility and stool characteristics.

risk for Infection is possibly evidenced by risk factors of invasive procedure with surgical placement of feeding tube, malnutrition, chronic disease, improper preparation, handling, or contamination of the feeding solution.*

risk for Aspiration is possibly evidenced by risk factors of presence of feeding tube, bolus tube feedings, increased intragastric pressure, delayed gastric emptying, medication administration.*

risk for imbalanced Fluid Volume is possibly evidenced by risk factors of active loss or failure of regulatory mechanisms specific to underlying disease process or trauma, inability to obtain or ingest fluids.*

Fatigue may be related to decreased metabolic energy production; increased energy requirements—hypermetabolic state, healing process; altered body chemistry—medications, chemotherapy; and is possibly evidenced by overwhelming lack of energy, inability to maintain usual routines/accomplish routine tasks, lethargy, impaired ability to concentrate.

Enteritis MS/CH

Refer to Colitis, ulcerative; Crohn's disease

Epididymitis MS

acute Pain may be related to inflammation, edema formation, and tension on the spermatic cord, possibly evidenced by verbal reports, guarding or distraction behaviors (restlessness), and changes in vital signs.

*A risk diagnosis is not evidenced by signs and symptoms, as the problem has not occurred; rather, nursing interventions are directed at prevention.

risk for Infection, [spread] is possibly evidenced by risk factors of presence of inflammation, infectious process, insufficient knowledge to avoid spread of infection.*

deficient Knowledge [Learning Need] regarding pathophysiology, outcome, and self-care needs may be related to lack of information, misinterpretations, possibly evidenced by statements of concern, misconceptions, and questions.

Epilepsy CH

Refer to Seizure disorder

Erectile dysfunction CH

Sexual Dysfunction may be related to altered body function possibly evidenced by reports of disruption of sexual response pattern, inability to achieve desired satisfaction.

situational low Self-Esteem may be related to functional impairment; rejection of other(s) possibly evidenced by self-negating verbalizations.

Failure to thrive, infant/child PED

imbalanced Nutrition: less than body requirements may be related to inability to ingest, digest, or absorb nutrients (defects in organ function or metabolism, genetic factors), physical deprivation, psychosocial factors, possibly evidenced by lack of appropriate weight gain or weight loss, poor muscle tone, pale conjunctiva, and laboratory tests reflecting nutritional deficiency.

risk for disproportionate Growth and/or delayed Development is possibly evidenced by risk factors of maladaptive feeding behavior, economically disadvantaged, caregiver mental health issue, or presence of abuse (physical, psychological, sexual).

risk for impaired Parenting is possibly evidenced by risk factors of lack of knowledge, inadequate bonding, unrealistic expectations for self or infant, and lack of appropriate response of child to relationship.*

deficient Knowledge [Learning Need] regarding pathophysiology of condition, nutritional needs, growth and development expectations, and parenting skills may be related to lack of information, misinformation or misinterpretation, possibly evidenced by verbalization of concerns, questions, and misconceptions, or development of preventable complications.

Fatigue syndrome, chronic CH

Fatigue may be related to disease state, inadequate sleep, possibly evidenced by verbalization of unremitting and overwhelming lack of energy, inability to maintain usual routines, listlessness, compromised concentration.

chronic Pain may be related to chronic physical disability, possibly evidenced by verbal reports of headache, sore throat, arthralgias, abdominal pain, muscle aches, altered ability to continue previous activities, changes in sleep pattern.

Self-Care Deficit [specify] may be related to tiredness, pain/discomfort, possibly evidenced by reports of inability to perform desired ADLs.

---

*A risk diagnosis is not evidenced by signs and symptoms, as the problem has not occurred; rather, nursing interventions are directed at prevention.

F

risk for ineffective Role Performance is possibly evidenced by risk factors of health alterations, stress.*

Femoral popliteal bypass **MS**

Also refer to Surgery, general

risk for ineffective peripheral Tissue Perfusion is possibly evidenced by risk factors of interruption of arterial blood flow, hypovolemia.*

risk for peripheral neurovascular Dysfunction is possibly evidenced by risk factors of vascular obstruction, immobilization, mechanical compression, dressings.*

impaired Walking may be related to surgical incisions, dressings, possibly evidenced by inability to walk desired distance, climb stairs, negotiate inclines.

F

Fetal alcohol syndrome **PED**

risk for Injury [CNS damage] is possibly evidenced by risk factors of external chemical factors (alcohol intake by mother), placental insufficiency, fetal drug withdrawal in utero or postpartum, and prematurity.*

disorganized infant Behavior may be related to prematurity, environmental overstimulation, lack of containment or boundaries, possibly evidenced by change from baseline physiological measures, tremors, startles, twitches, hyperextension of arms and legs, deficient self-regulatory behaviors, deficient response to visual or auditory stimuli.

risk for impaired Parenting is possibly evidenced by risk factors of mental and/or physical illness, inability of mother to assume the overwhelming task of unselfish giving and nurturing, presence of stressors (financial or legal problems), lack of available or ineffective role model, interruption of bonding process, lack of appropriate response of child to relationship.*

PSY

ineffective [maternal] Coping may be related to personal vulnerability, low self-esteem, inadequate coping skills, and multiple stressors (repeated over period of time), possibly evidenced by inability to meet basic needs, fulfill role expectations, or problem-solve, and excessive use of drug(s).

dysfunctional Family Processes may be related to lack of or insufficient support from others, mother's drug problem and treatment status, together with poor coping skills, lack of family stability, overinvolvement of parents with children and multigenerational addictive behaviors, possibly evidenced by abandonment, rejection, neglectful relationships with family members, and decisions and actions by family that are detrimental.

Fetal demise **OB**

Grieving may be related to death of fetus/infant (wanted or unwanted), possibly evidenced by verbal expressions of distress, anger, loss, crying, alteration in eating habits or sleep pattern.

situational low Self-Esteem may be related to perceived "failure" at a life event, possibly evidenced by negative self-appraisal in response to life event in a person with a previous positive self-evaluation,

*A risk diagnosis is not evidenced by signs and symptoms, as the problem has not occurred; rather, nursing interventions are directed at prevention.

verbalization of negative feelings about the self (helplessness, uselessness), difficulty making decisions.

risk for Spiritual Distress is possibly evidenced by risk factors of loss of loved one, low self-esteem, poor relationships, challenged belief and value system (birth is supposed to be the beginning of life, not of death), and intense suffering.*

Fibromyalgia syndrome, primary **CH**

acute Pain/chronic Pain may be related to idiopathic diffuse condition possibly evidenced by reports of achy pain in fibrous tissues (muscles, tendons, ligaments), muscle stiffness or spasm, disturbed sleep, guarding behaviors, fear of re-injury or exacerbation, restlessness, irritability, self-focusing, reduced interaction with others.

Fatigue may be related to disease state, stress, anxiety, depression, sleep deprivation, possibly evidenced by verbalization of overwhelming lack of energy, inability to maintain usual routines or desired level of physical activity, feeling tired, having feelings of guilt for not keeping up with responsibilities, having an increase in physical complaints, being listless.

risk for Hopelessness is possibly evidenced by risk factors of chronic debilitating physical condition, prolonged activity restriction (possibly self-induced) creating isolation, lack of specific therapeutic cure, prolonged stress.*

Fractures **MS/CH**

Also refer to Casts; Traction

risk for Trauma [additional injury] is possibly evidenced by risk factors of loss of skeletal integrity, movement of skeletal fragments, use of traction apparatus, etc.*

acute Pain may be related to muscle spasms, movement of bone fragments, soft tissue trauma, edema, traction or immobility device, stress, and anxiety, possibly evidenced by verbal reports, distraction behaviors, self-focusing or narrowed focus, facial mask of pain, guarding or protective behavior, alteration in muscle tone, and changes in vital signs.

risk for peripheral neurovascular Dysfunction is possibly evidenced by risk factors of reduction or interruption of blood flow (direct vascular injury, tissue trauma, excessive edema, thrombus formation, hypovolemia).*

impaired physical Mobility may be related to musculoskeletal impairment, pain, discomfort, restrictive therapies (extremity immobilization, bedrest), and psychological immobility, possibly evidenced by inability to purposefully move within the physical environment, imposed restrictions, reluctance to attempt movement, limited range of motion, and decreased muscle strength or control.

risk for impaired Gas Exchange is possibly evidenced by risk factors of altered blood flow, blood or fat emboli, alveolar-capillary membrane changes (interstitial pulmonary edema, congestion).*

deficient Knowledge [Learning Need] regarding healing process, therapy requirements, potential complications, and self-care needs may be related to lack of exposure or recall, misinterpretation of infor-

*A risk diagnosis is not evidenced by signs and symptoms, as the problem has not occurred; rather, nursing interventions are directed at prevention.

mation, possibly evidenced by statements of concern, questions, and misconceptions.

Frostbite **MS/CH**

impaired Tissue Integrity may be related to altered circulation and thermal injury, possibly evidenced by damaged or destroyed tissue.

acute Pain may be related to diminished circulation with tissue ischemia or necrosis, and edema formation, possibly evidenced by verbal reports, guarding or distraction behaviors, narrowed focus, and changes in vital signs.

risk for Infection is possibly evidenced by risk factors of traumatized tissue or tissue destruction, altered circulation, and compromised immune response in affected area.*

G

Gallstones **CH**

Refer to Cholelithiasis

Gangrene, dry **MS**

ineffective peripheral Tissue Perfusion may be related to interruption in arterial flow, possibly evidenced by cool skin temperature, change in color (black), atrophy of affected part, and presence of pain.

acute Pain may be related to tissue hypoxia and necrotic process, possibly evidenced by verbal reports, guarding or distraction behaviors, narrowed focus, and changes in vital signs.

Gas, lung irritant **MS/CH**

ineffective Airway Clearance may be related to irritation and inflammation of airway, possibly evidenced by marked cough, abnormal breath sounds (wheezes), dyspnea, and tachypnea.

risk for impaired Gas Exchange is possibly evidenced by risk factors of irritation and inflammation of alveolar membrane (dependent on type of agent and length of exposure).*

Anxiety [specify level] may be related to change in health status and threat of death, possibly evidenced by verbalizations, increased tension, apprehension, and sympathetic stimulation.

Gastritis, acute **MS**

acute Pain may be related to irritation or inflammation of gastric mucosa, possibly evidenced by verbal reports, guarding or distraction behaviors, and changes in vital signs.

risk for deficient Fluid Volume/risk for Bleeding are possibly evidenced by risk factors of excessive losses through vomiting and diarrhea, reluctance to ingest or restrictions of oral intake, gastrointestinal disorder, continued bleeding.*

Gastritis, chronic **CH**

risk for imbalanced Nutrition: less than body requirements is possibly evidenced by risk factors of inability to ingest adequate nutrients (prolonged nausea, vomiting, anorexia, epigastric pain).*

deficient Knowledge [Learning Need] regarding pathophysiology, psychological factors, therapy needs, and potential complications may be related to lack of information or recall, unfamiliarity with infor-

*A risk diagnosis is not evidenced by signs and symptoms, as the problem has not occurred; rather, nursing interventions are directed at prevention.

mation resources, information misinterpretation, possibly evidenced by verbalization of concerns, questions, and continuation of problem or development of preventable complications.

Gastroenteritis **MS**

Diarrhea may be related to toxins, contaminants, travel, infectious process, parasites possibly evidenced by at least three loose, liquid stools/day, hyperactive bowel sounds, abdominal pain.

risk for deficient Fluid Volume is possibly evidenced by risk factors of excessive losses (diarrhea, vomiting), hypermetabolic state (infection), decreased intake (nausea, anorexia), extremes of age or weight.*

risk for Infection [transmission] is possibly evidenced by risk factors of insufficient knowledge to prevent contamination (inappropriate hand hygiene and food handling).*

Gastroesophageal reflux disease (GERD) **CH**

acute Pain/chronic Pain may be related to acidic irritation of mucosa, muscle spasm, recurrent vomiting, possibly evidenced by reports of heartburn, distraction behaviors.

impaired Swallowing may be related to GERD, esophageal defects, achalasia possibly evidenced by reports of heartburn or epigastric pain, "something stuck" when swallowing, food refusal or volume limiting, nighttime coughing or awakening.

risk for imbalanced Nutrition: less than body requirements is possibly evidenced by risk factors of limiting intake, recurrent vomiting.*

risk for Insomnia is possibly evidenced by risk factors of nighttime heartburn, regurgitation of stomach contents.*

risk for Aspiration is possibly evidenced by risk factors of incompetent lower esophageal sphincter, regurgitation of gastric acid.*

Gender identity disorder **PSY**

(For individuals experiencing persistent and marked distress regarding uncertainty about issues relating to personal identity, e.g., sexual orientation and behavior.)

Anxiety [specify level] may be related to unconscious or conscious conflicts about essential values and beliefs (ego-dystonic gender identification), threat to self-concept, unmet needs, possibly evidenced by increased tension, helplessness, hopelessness, feelings of inadequacy, uncertainty, insomnia and focus on self, and impaired daily functioning.

ineffective Role Performance/disturbed Personal Identity may be related to crisis in development in which person has difficulty knowing or accepting to which sex he or she belongs or is attracted, or has a sense of discomfort and inappropriateness about anatomical sex characteristics, possibly evidenced by confusion about sense of self, purpose or direction in life, sexual identification or preference, verbalization of desire to be or insistence that person is the opposite sex, change in self-perception of role, and conflict in roles.

ineffective Sexuality Pattern may be related to ineffective or absent role models and conflict with sexual orientation and/or preferences, lack of or impaired relationship with an SO, possibly evidenced by ver-

*A risk diagnosis is not evidenced by signs and symptoms, as the problem has not occurred; rather, nursing interventions are directed at prevention.

balizations of discomfort with sexual orientation or role, and lack of information about human sexuality.

compromised family Coping/disabled family Coping may be related to inadequate or incorrect information or understanding, SO unable to perceive or to act effectively in regard to client's needs, temporary family disorganization and role changes, and client providing little support in turn for primary person.*

readiness for enhanced family Coping is possibly evidenced by expression of the desire to acknowledge growth impact of crisis/situation, to enhance connection with others who have experienced a similar situation.

Genetic disorder **CH/OB**

Anxiety may be related to presence of specific risk factors (e.g., exposure to teratogens), situational crisis, threat to self-concept, conscious or unconscious conflict about essential values and life goals, possibly evidenced by increased tension, apprehension, uncertainty, feelings of inadequacy, expressed concerns.

deficient Knowledge [Learning Need] regarding purpose and process of genetic counseling may be related to lack of awareness of ramifications of diagnosis, process necessary for analyzing available options, and information misinterpretation, possibly evidenced by verbalization of concerns, statement of misconceptions, request for information.

risk for interrupted Family Processes is possibly evidenced by risk factors of situational crisis, individual/family vulnerability, difficulty reaching agreement regarding options.*

Spiritual Distress may be related to intense inner conflict about the outcome, normal grieving for the loss of the "perfect" child, anger that is often directed at God or greater power, religious beliefs and moral convictions, possibly evidenced by verbalization of inner conflict about beliefs, questioning of the moral and ethical implications of therapeutic choices, viewing situation as punishment, anger, hostility, and crying.

risk for complicated Grieving is possibly evidenced by risk factors of preloss psychological symptoms, predisposition for anxiety and feelings of inadequacy, frequency of major life events.*

Gigantism **CH**

Refer to Acromegaly

Glaucoma **CH**

[disturbed visual Sensory Perception] may be related to altered sensory reception—increased intraocular pressure, atrophy of optic nerve head, possibly evidenced by progressive loss of visual field.

Anxiety [specify level] may be related to change in health status, presence of pain, possibility or reality of loss of vision, unmet needs, and negative self-talk, possibly evidenced by apprehension, uncertainty, and expressed concern regarding changes in life event.

Glomerulonephritis **PED**

excess Fluid Volume may be related to failure of regulatory mechanism (inflammation of glomerular membrane inhibiting filtration), possi-

---

*A risk diagnosis is not evidenced by signs and symptoms, as the problem has not occurred; rather, nursing interventions are directed at prevention.

bly evidenced by weight gain, edema or anasarca, intake greater than output, and BP changes.

acute Pain may be related to effects of circulating toxins and edema or distention of renal capsule, possibly evidenced by verbal reports, guarding or distraction behaviors, and changes in vital signs.

imbalanced Nutrition: less than body requirements may be related to anorexia and dietary restrictions, possibly evidenced by aversion to eating, reported altered taste, weight loss, and decreased intake.

deficient Diversional Activity may be related to treatment modality or restrictions, fatigue, and malaise, possibly evidenced by statements of boredom, restlessness, and irritability.

risk for disproportionate Growth is possibly evidenced by risk factors of infection, malnutrition, chronic illness.*

G

Goiter CH

disturbed Body Image may be related to visible swelling in neck, possibly evidenced by verbalization of feelings, fear of reaction of others, actual change in structure, change in social involvement.

Anxiety may be related to change in health status and progressive growth of mass perceived threat of death.

risk for imbalanced Nutrition: less than body requirements is possibly evidenced by risk factors of decreased ability to ingest or difficulty swallowing.*

risk for ineffective Airway Clearance is possibly evidenced by risk factors of tracheal compression or obstruction.*

Gonorrhea CH

Also refer to Sexually transmitted infection (STI)

risk for Infection [dissemination, bacteremia] is possibly evidenced by risk factors of presence of infectious process in highly vascular area and lack of recognition of disease process.*

acute Pain may be related to irritation or inflammation of mucosa and effects of circulating toxins, possibly evidenced by verbal reports of genital or pharyngeal irritation, perineal or pelvic pain, guarding or distraction behaviors.

deficient Knowledge [Learning Need] regarding disease cause, transmission, therapy, and self-care needs may be related to lack of information, misinterpretation, denial of exposure, possibly evidenced by statements of concern, questions, misconceptions, and inaccurate follow-through of instructions, development of preventable complications.

Gout CH

acute Pain may be related to inflammation of joint(s), possibly evidenced by verbal reports, guarding or distraction behaviors, and changes in vital signs.

impaired physical Mobility may be related to joint pain and inflammation, possibly evidenced by reluctance to attempt movement, limited range of motion, and therapeutic restriction of movement.

deficient Knowledge [Learning Need] regarding cause, treatment, and prevention of condition may be related to lack of information or misinterpretation, possibly evidenced by statements of con-

*A risk diagnosis is not evidenced by signs and symptoms, as the problem has not occurred; rather, nursing interventions are directed at prevention.

cern, questions, misconceptions, and inaccurate follow-through of instructions.

Guillain-Barré syndrome (acute polyneuritis) **MS**

risk for ineffective Breathing Pattern/Airway Clearance are possibly evidenced by risk factors of weakness or paralysis of respiratory muscles, impaired gag or swallow reflexes, decreased energy, fatigue.*

[disturbed Sensory Perceptual (specify)] may be related to altered sensory reception, transmission, or integration (altered status of sense organs, sleep deprivation), therapeutically restricted environment, endogenous chemical alterations (electrolyte imbalance, hypoxia), and psychological stress, possibly evidenced by reported or observed change in usual response to stimuli, altered communication patterns, and measured change in sensory acuity and motor coordination.

impaired physical Mobility may be related to neuromuscular impairment, pain or discomfort, possibly evidenced by impaired coordination, partial or complete paralysis, decreased muscle strength and control.

Anxiety [specify level]/Fear may be related to situational crisis, change in health status, or threat of death, possibly evidenced by increased tension, restlessness, helplessness, apprehension, uncertainty, fearfulness, focus on self, and sympathetic stimulation.

risk for Disuse Syndrome is possibly evidenced by risk factors of paralysis and pain.*

Hallucinogen abuse **CH/PSY**

Also refer to Substance dependence/abuse rehabilitation

Anxiety [specify level]/Fear may be related to situational crisis, threat to or change in health status, perceived threat of death, inexperience or unfamiliarity with effects of drug, possibly evidenced by assumptions of "losing my mind or control," apprehension, preoccupation with feelings of impending doom, sympathetic stimulation.

Self-Neglect may be related to substance use, executive processing ability, possibly evidenced by inadequate personal/environmental hygiene, nonadherence to health activities.

Self-Care Deficit (specify) may be related to perceptual or cognitive impairment, therapeutic management (restraints), possibly evidenced by inability to meet own physical needs.

Hay fever **CH**

impaired Comfort may be related to irritation or inflammation of upper airway mucous membranes and conjunctiva, possibly evidenced by verbal reports, irritability, and restlessness.

deficient Knowledge [Learning Need] regarding underlying cause, appropriate therapy, and required lifestyle changes may be related to lack of information, possibly evidenced by statements of concern, questions, and misconceptions.

Heart failure, chronic **MS**

decreased Cardiac Output may be related to altered myocardial contractility, inotropic changes; alterations in rate, rhythm, and electrical

*A risk diagnosis is not evidenced by signs and symptoms, as the problem has not occurred; rather, nursing interventions are directed at prevention.

conduction; and structural changes (valvular defects, ventricular aneurysm), possibly evidenced by tachycardia, dysrhythmias, changes in BP, extra heart sounds, decreased urine output, diminished peripheral pulses, cool, ashen skin; orthopnea, crackles; dependent or generalized edema and chest pain.

excess Fluid Volume may be related to reduced glomerular filtration rate (GFR), increased antidiuretic hormone production, and sodium and water retention, possibly evidenced by orthopnea and abnormal breath sounds, S_3 heart sound, jugular vein distention, positive hepatojugular reflex, weight gain, hypertension, oliguria, generalized edema.

risk for impaired Gas Exchange is possibly evidenced by risk factors of alveolar-capillary membrane changes (fluid collection or shifts into interstitial space or alveoli).*

H

CH

Activity Intolerance may be related to imbalance between O_2 supply and demand, generalized weakness, and prolonged bedrest, sedentary lifestyle, possibly evidenced by reported or observed weakness, fatigue, changes in vital signs, presence of dysrhythmias, dyspnea, pallor, and diaphoresis.

risk for impaired Skin Integrity is possibly evidenced by risk factors of prolonged chair or bedrest, edema, vascular pooling, decreased tissue perfusion.*

deficient Knowledge [Learning Need] regarding cardiac function/disease process, therapy and self-care needs may be related to lack of information or misinterpretation, possibly evidenced by questions, statements of concern, misconceptions, development of preventable complications or exacerbations of condition.

Heatstroke **MS**

Hyperthermia may be related to prolonged exposure to hot environment, vigorous activity with failure of regulating mechanism of the body, possibly evidenced by high body temperature, flushed, hot skin, tachycardia, and seizure activity.

decreased Cardiac Output may be related to functional stress of hypermetabolic state, altered circulating volume and venous return, and direct myocardial damage secondary to hyperthermia, possibly evidenced by decreased peripheral pulses, dysrhythmias, tachycardia, and changes in mentation.

Hemodialysis **MS/CH**

Also refer to Dialysis, general

risk for Injury [loss of vascular access] is possibly evidenced by risk factors of clotting or thrombosis, infection, disconnection, and hemorrhage.*

risk for deficient Fluid Volume/risk for Bleeding are possibly evidenced by risk factors of excessive fluid losses or shifts via ultrafiltration, fluid restrictions, altered coagulation, disconnection of shunt.*

*A risk diagnosis is not evidenced by signs and symptoms, as the problem has not occurred; rather, nursing interventions are directed at prevention.

risk for excess Fluid Volume is possibly evidenced by risk factors of rapid or excessive fluid intake—IV, blood, plasma expanders, saline given to support BP during procedure.*
ineffective Protection may be related to chronic disease state, drug therapy, abnormal blood profile, inadequate nutrition, possibly evidenced by altered clotting, impaired healing, deficient immunity, fatigue, anorexia.

Hemophilia PED

risk for Bleeding/deficient [isotonic] Fluid Volume are possibly evidenced by risk factors of impaired coagulation/hemorrhagic losses.*
acute Pain/chronic Pain risk factors may include nerve compression from hematomas, nerve damage, or hemorrhage into joint space.*
risk for impaired physical Mobility is possibly evidenced by risk factors of joint hemorrhage, swelling, degenerative changes, and muscle atrophy.*
ineffective Protection may be related to abnormal blood profile, possibly evidenced by altered clotting.
compromised family Coping may be related to prolonged nature of condition that exhausts the supportive capacity of significant person(s), possibly evidenced by protective behaviors disproportionate to client's abilities or need for autonomy.

H

Hemorrhoidectomy MS/CH

acute Pain may be related to edema or swelling, and tissue trauma, possibly evidenced by verbal reports, guarding or distraction behaviors, focus on self, and changes in vital signs.
risk for Urinary Retention is possibly evidenced by risk factors of perineal trauma, edema or swelling, and pain.*
deficient Knowledge [Learning Need] regarding therapeutic treatment and potential complications may be related to lack of information or misconceptions, possibly evidenced by statements of concern and questions.

Hemorrhoids CH/OB

acute Pain may be related to inflammation and edema of prolapsed varices, possibly evidenced by verbal reports, and guarding or distraction behaviors.
Constipation may be related to pain on defecation and reluctance to defecate, possibly evidenced by frequency less than usual pattern, and hard, formed stools.

Hemothorax MS

Also refer to Pneumothorax
risk for Trauma/risk for Suffocation are possibly evidenced by risk factors of concurrent disease or injury process, dependence on external device (chest drainage system), and lack of safety education or precautions.*
Anxiety [specify level] may be related to change in health status and threat of death, possibly evidenced by increased tension, restlessness, expressed concern, sympathetic stimulation, and focus on self.

*A risk diagnosis is not evidenced by signs and symptoms, as the problem has not occurred; rather, nursing interventions are directed at prevention.

Hepatitis, acute viral MS/CH

impaired Liver Function related to viral infection as evidenced by jaundice, hepatic enlargement, abdominal pain, marked elevations in serum liver function tests.

Fatigue may be related to decreased metabolic energy production, discomfort, altered body chemistry—changes in liver function, effect on target organs, possibly evidenced by reports of lack of energy, inability to maintain usual routines, decreased performance, and increased physical complaints.

imbalanced Nutrition: less than body requirements may be related to inability to ingest adequate nutrients—nausea, vomiting, anorexia, hypermetabolic state, altered absorption and metabolism, possibly evidenced by aversion to eating or lack of interest in food, altered taste sensation, observed lack of intake, and weight loss.

acute Pain/impaired Comfort may be related to inflammation and swelling of the liver, arthralgias, urticarial eruptions, and pruritus, possibly evidenced by verbal reports, guarding or distraction behaviors, focus on self, and changes in vital signs.

risk for Infection is possibly evidenced by risk factors of inadequate secondary defenses and immunosuppression, malnutrition, insufficient knowledge to avoid exposure to pathogens.*

risk for impaired Tissue Integrity is possibly evidenced by risk factors of bile salt accumulation in the tissues.*

risk for impaired Home Management is possibly evidenced by risk factors of debilitating effects of disease process and inadequate support systems (family, financial, role model).*

deficient Knowledge [Learning Need] regarding disease process and transmission, treatment needs, and future expectations may be related to lack of information or recall, misinterpretation, unfamiliarity with resources, possibly evidenced by questions, statement of concerns, misconceptions, inaccurate follow-through of instructions, or development of preventable complications.

Hernia, hiatal CH

chronic Pain may be related to regurgitation of acidic gastric contents, possibly evidenced by verbal reports, facial grimacing, and focus on self.

deficient Knowledge [Learning Need] regarding pathophysiology, prevention of complications and self-care needs may be related to lack of information, misconceptions, possibly evidenced by statements of concern, questions, and recurrence of condition.

Herniated nucleus pulposus (ruptured intervertebral disk) CH/MS

acute Pain/chronic Pain may be related to nerve compression or irritation and muscle spasms, possibly evidenced by verbal reports, guarding or distraction behaviors, preoccupation with pain, self-focus or narrowed focus, changes in vital signs when pain is acute, altered muscle tone or function, changes in eating or sleeping patterns and libido, physical or social withdrawal.

impaired physical Mobility may be related to pain (muscle spasms), discomfort, therapeutic restrictions—bedrest, traction, or braces;

*A risk diagnosis is not evidenced by signs and symptoms, as the problem has not occurred; rather, nursing interventions are directed at prevention.

H

muscular impairment, and depressive mood state, possibly evidenced by reports of pain on movement, reluctance to attempt or difficulty with purposeful movement, decreased muscle strength, impaired coordination, and limited range of motion.

deficient Diversional Activity may be related to length of recuperation period and therapy restrictions, physical limitations, pain, and depression, possibly evidenced by statements of boredom, disinterest, "nothing to do," restlessness, irritability, withdrawal.

Heroin withdrawal **CH/MS**

acute Pain/impaired Comfort may be related to cessation of drug, muscle tremors/twitching, possibly evidenced by reports of muscle aches, hot or cold flashes, diaphoresis, lacrimation, rhinorrhea, drug cravings.

[severe] Anxiety may be related to CNS hyperactivity possibly evidenced by apprehension, pervasive anxious feelings, jittery, restlessness, weakness, insomnia, anorexia.

risk for ineffective Health Management possibly evidenced by risk factors of protracted withdrawal, economic difficulties, family or social support deficits, perceived barriers or benefits.*

Herpes, herpes simplex **CH**

acute Pain may be related to presence of localized inflammation and open lesions, possibly evidenced by verbal reports, distraction behaviors, and restlessness.

risk for [secondary] Infection is possibly evidenced by risk factors of broken or traumatized tissue, altered immune response, and untreated infection or treatment failure.*

risk for Sexual Dysfunction is possibly evidenced by risk factors of lack of knowledge, values conflict, and/or fear of transmitting the disease.*

Herpes zoster (shingles) **CH**

acute Pain may be related to inflammation and local lesions along sensory nerve(s), possibly evidenced by verbal reports, guarding or distraction behaviors, narrowed focus, restlessness, and changes in vital signs.

deficient Knowledge [Learning Need] regarding pathophysiology, therapeutic needs, and potential complications may be related to lack of information, misinterpretation, possibly evidenced by statements of concern, questions, and misconceptions.

High-altitude pulmonary edema (HAPE) **MS**

Also refer to Mountain sickness, acute

impaired Gas Exchange may be related to ventilation perfusion imbalance, alveolar-capillary membrane changes, altered O_2 supply, possibly evidenced by dyspnea, confusion, cyanosis, tachycardia, abnormal ABGs.

excess Fluid Volume may be related to compromised regulatory mechanism, possibly evidenced by shortness of breath, anxiety, edema, abnormal breath sounds, pulmonary congestion.

---

*A risk diagnosis is not evidenced by signs and symptoms, as the problem has not occurred; rather, nursing interventions are directed at prevention.

High-altitude sickness **MS**

Refer to Mountain sickness, acute; High-altitude pulmonary edema

HIV infection **CH**

Also refer to AIDS

risk-prone Health Behavior may be related to life-threatening, stigmatizing condition or disease, assault to self-esteem, altered locus of control, inadequate support systems, possibly evidenced by verbalization of nonacceptance or denial of diagnosis, failure to take action that prevents health problems.

deficient Knowledge [Learning Need] regarding disease, prognosis, and treatment needs may be related to lack of exposure or recall, information misinterpretation, unfamiliarity with information resources, or cognitive limitation, possibly evidenced by statement of misconception, request for information, inappropriate or exaggerated behaviors (hostile, agitated, hysterical, apathetic), inaccurate follow-through of instructions, or development of preventable complications.

risk for ineffective Health Management is possibly evidenced by risk factors of complexity of healthcare system and access to care, economic difficulties; complexity of therapeutic regimen—confusing or difficult dosing schedule, duration of regimen; mistrust of regimen and/or healthcare personnel, client and provider interactions; health beliefs or cultural influences, perceived seriousness, susceptibility, or benefits of therapy; decisional conflicts, powerlessness.*

risk for complicated Grieving is possibly evidenced by risk factors of preloss psychological symptoms, predisposition for anxiety and feelings of inadequacy, frequency of major life events.*

Hodgkin's disease **CH/MS**

Also refer to Cancer; Chemotherapy

Anxiety [specify level]/Fear may be related to threat of self-concept and threat of death, possibly evidenced by apprehension, insomnia, focus on self, and increased tension.

deficient Knowledge [Learning Need] regarding diagnosis, pathophysiology, treatment, and prognosis may be related to lack of information/misinterpretation, possibly evidenced by statements of concern, questions, and misconceptions.

acute Pain/impaired Comfort may be related to manifestations of inflammatory response (fever, chills, night sweats) and pruritus, possibly evidenced by verbal reports, distraction behaviors, and focus on self.

risk for ineffective Breathing Pattern/Airway Clearance are possibly evidenced by risk factors of tracheobronchial obstruction (enlarged mediastinal nodes and/or airway edema).*

Hospice/End-of-life care **CH**

acute Pain/chronic Pain may be related to biological, physical, psychological agent, chronic physical disability, possibly evidenced by verbal or coded report, preoccupation with pain, changes in appetite/

*A risk diagnosis is not evidenced by signs and symptoms, as the problem has not occurred; rather, nursing interventions are directed at prevention.

eating, sleep pattern, altered ability to continue desired activities, guarded or protective behaviors, restlessness, irritability, narrowed focus—altered time perception, impaired thought processes.

Activity Intolerance/Fatigue may be related to generalized weakness, bedrest or immobility, pain, progressive disease state or debilitating condition, depressive state, imbalance between O_2 supply and demand, possibly evidenced by inability to maintain usual routine, verbalized lack of desire or interest in activity, decreased performance, lethargy.

Grieving/Death Anxiety may be related to anticipated loss of physiological well-being, change in body function, perceived threat of death or dying process, possibly evidenced by changes in communication pattern, denial of potential loss; choked feelings, anger, fear of loss of physical or mental abilities; negative death images or unpleasant thoughts about any event related to death or dying; anticipated pain related to dying; powerlessness over issues related to dying, worrying about impact of one's own death on SO(s), being the cause of other's grief and suffering, concerns of overworking the caregiver as terminal illness incapacitates.

H

compromised family Coping/disabled family Coping/caregiver Role Strain may be related to prolonged disease/disability progression, temporary family disorganization and role changes, unrealistic expectations, inadequate or incorrect information or understanding by primary person, possibly evidenced by client expressing despair about family reactions or lack of involvement, history of poor relationship between caregiver and care receiver; altered caregiver health status; SO attempting assistive or supportive behaviors with less than satisfactory results, apprehension about future regarding caregiver's ability to provide care; SO describing preoccupation about personal reactions; displaying intolerance, abandonment, rejection; family behaviors that are detrimental to well-being.

risk for Spiritual Distress is possibly evidenced by risk factors of physical or psychological stress, energy-consuming anxiety; situational losses; blocks to self-love, low self-esteem, inability to forgive.*

risk for Moral Distress is possibly evidenced by risk factors of conflict among decision makers, cultural conflicts, end-of-life decisions, loss of autonomy, physical distance of decision makers.*

Hydrocephalus PED/MS

ineffective cerebral Tissue Perfusion may be related to decreased arterial or venous blood flow (compression of brain tissue), possibly evidenced by changes in mentation, restlessness, irritability, reports of headache, pupillary changes, and changes in vital signs.

[disturbed visual Sensory Perception] may be related to pressure on sensory or motor nerves, possibly evidenced by reports of double vision, development of strabismus, nystagmus, pupillary changes, and optic atrophy.

risk for impaired physical Mobility is possibly evidenced by risk factors of neuromuscular impairment, decreased muscle strength, and impaired coordination.*

---

*A risk diagnosis is not evidenced by signs and symptoms, as the problem has not occurred; rather, nursing interventions are directed at prevention.

risk for decreased intracranial Adaptive Capacity is possibly evidenced by risk factors of brain injury, changes in perfusion pressure or intracranial pressure.*

CH

risk for Infection is possibly evidenced by risk factors of invasive procedure, presence of shunt.*

deficient Knowledge [Learning Need] regarding condition, prognosis, and long-term therapy needs and medical follow-up may be related to lack of information, misperceptions, possibly evidenced by questions, statement of concern, request for information, and inaccurate follow-through of instruction, or development of preventable complications.

Hyperactivity disorder — PED/PSY

ineffective Impulse Control may be related to compunction, possibly evidenced by acting without thinking, temper outbursts.

defensive Coping may be related to mild neurological deficits, dysfunctional family system, abuse or neglect, possibly evidenced by denial of obvious problems, projection of blame or responsibility, grandiosity, difficulty in reality testing perceptions.

impaired Social Interaction may be related to retarded ego development, negative role models, neurological impairment, possibly evidenced by having discomfort in social situations, interrupting or intruding on others, having difficulty waiting turn in games or group activities, having difficulty maintaining attention to task.

disabled family Coping may be related to excessive guilt, anger, or blaming among family members, parental inconsistencies, disagreements regarding discipline, limit-setting approaches, exhaustion of parental expectations, possibly evidenced by unrealistic parental expectations, rejection or overprotection of child, exaggerated expression of feelings, despair regarding child's behavior.

Hyperbilirubinemia — PED

neonatal Jaundice may be related to difficulty transitioning to extrauterine life, feeding pattern not well established, abnormal weight loss, possibly evidenced by abnormal blood profile—elevated BUN, yellow-orange skin/sclera.

risk for Injury [effects of treatment] is possibly evidenced by risk factors of physical properties of phototherapy and effects on body regulatory mechanisms, invasive procedure (exchange transfusion), abnormal blood profile, chemical imbalances.*

deficient Knowledge [Learning Need] regarding condition prognosis, treatment and safety needs may be related to lack of exposure or recall and information misinterpretation, possibly evidenced by questions, statement of concern, and inaccurate follow-through of instructions, or development of preventable complications.

Hyperemesis gravidarum — OB

deficient Fluid Volume may be related to excessive gastric losses and reduced intake, possibly evidenced by dry mucous membranes, decreased, concentrated urine, decreased pulse volume and pressure, thirst, and hemoconcentration.

---

*A risk diagnosis is not evidenced by signs and symptoms, as the problem has not occurred; rather, nursing interventions are directed at prevention.

risk for Electrolyte Imbalance is possibly evidenced by risk factors of vomiting, dehydration.*

imbalanced Nutrition: less than body requirements may be related to inability to ingest, digest, or absorb nutrients (prolonged vomiting), possibly evidenced by reported inadequate food intake, lack of interest in food or aversion to eating, and weight loss.

risk for ineffective Coping is possibly evidenced by risk factors of situational or maturational crisis (pregnancy, change in health status, projected role changes, concern about outcome).*

Hypertension **CH**

deficient Knowledge [Learning Need] regarding condition, therapeutic regimen, and potential complications may be related to lack of information or recall, misinterpretation, cognitive limitations, and/or denial of diagnosis, possibly evidenced by statements of concern, questions, and misconceptions, inaccurate follow-through of instructions, and lack of BP control.

risk-prone Health Behavior may be related to condition requiring change in lifestyle, altered locus of control, and absence of feelings, denial of illness, possibly evidenced by verbalization of nonacceptance of health status change and lack of movement toward independence.

risk for Activity Intolerance is possibly evidenced by risk factors of generalized weakness, imbalance between oxygen supply and demand.*

risk for Sexual Dysfunction is possibly evidenced by risk factors of side effects of medication.*

MS

risk for decreased Cardiac Output is possibly evidenced by risk factors of increased afterload (vasoconstriction), fluid shifts, hypovolemia, myocardial ischemia, ventricular hypertrophy or rigidity.*

acute Pain may be related to increased cerebrovascular pressure, possibly evidenced by verbal reports (throbbing pain located in suboccipital region, present on awakening and disappearing spontaneously after being up and about), reluctance to move head, avoidance of bright lights and noise, increased muscle tension.

Hypertension, pulmonary **CH/MS**

Refer to Pulmonary hypertension

Hyperthyroidism **CH**

Also refer to Thyrotoxicosis

Fatigue may be related to hypermetabolic imbalance with increased energy requirements, irritability of CNS, and altered body chemistry, possibly evidenced by verbalization of overwhelming lack of energy to maintain usual routine, decreased performance, emotional lability or irritability, and impaired ability to concentrate.

Anxiety [specify level] may be related to increased stimulation of the CNS (hypermetabolic state, pseudocatecholamine effect of thyroid hormones), possibly evidenced by increased feelings of apprehen-

*A risk diagnosis is not evidenced by signs and symptoms, as the problem has not occurred; rather, nursing interventions are directed at prevention.

sion, overexcitement or distress, irritability or emotional lability, shakiness, restless movements, tremors.

risk for imbalanced Nutrition: less than body requirements is possibly evidenced by risk factors of inability to ingest adequate nutrients for hypermetabolic rate and constant activity level, impaired absorption of nutrients—vomiting, diarrhea, hyperglycemia, relative insulin insufficiency.*

risk for Dry Eye is possibly evidenced by risk factors of periorbital edema, altered protective mechanisms of eye—reduced ability to blink, eye dryness.*

Hypoglycemia **CH**

acute Confusion may be related to inadequate glucose for cellular brain function and effects of endogenous hormone activity, possibly evidenced by increased restlessness, misperceptions, or fluctuation in cognition/level of consciousness.

risk for unstable Blood Glucose Level is possibly evidenced by risk factors of dietary intake, lack of adherence to diabetes management, inadequate blood glucose monitoring, medication management.*

deficient Knowledge [Learning Need] regarding pathophysiology of condition, therapy, and self-care needs may be related to lack of information or recall, misinterpretations, possibly evidenced by development of hypoglycemia and statements of questions, misconceptions.

Hypoparathyroidism (acute) **MS**

risk for Injury is possibly evidenced by risk factors of neuromuscular excitability or tetany and formation of renal stones.*

acute Pain may be related to recurrent muscle spasms and alteration in reflexes, possibly evidenced by verbal reports, distraction behaviors, and narrowed focus.

risk for ineffective Airway Clearance is possibly evidenced by risk factor of spasm of the laryngeal muscles.*

Anxiety [specify level] may be related to threat to, or change in, health status, physiological responses.

Hypothermia (systemic) **CH**

Also refer to Frostbite

Hypothermia may be related to exposure to cold environment, inadequate clothing, age extremes (very young or elderly), damage to hypothalamus, consumption of alcohol or medications causing vasodilation, possibly evidenced by reduction in body temperature below normal range, shivering, cool skin, pallor.

deficient Knowledge [Learning Need] regarding risk factors, treatment needs, and prognosis may be related to lack of information or recall, misinterpretation, possibly evidenced by statement of concerns, misconceptions, occurrence of problem, and development of complications.

Hypothyroidism **CH**

Also refer to Myxedema

impaired physical Mobility may be related to weakness, fatigue, muscle aches, altered reflexes, and mucin deposits in joints and interstitial

---

*A risk diagnosis is not evidenced by signs and symptoms, as the problem has not occurred; rather, nursing interventions are directed at prevention.

H

spaces, possibly evidenced by decreased muscle strength or control, and impaired coordination.

Fatigue may be related to decreased metabolic energy production, possibly evidenced by verbalization of unremitting or overwhelming lack of energy, inability to maintain usual routines, impaired ability to concentrate, decreased libido, irritability, listlessness, decreased performance, increase in physical complaints.

[disturbed Sensory Perception (specify)] may be related to mucin deposits and nerve compression, possibly evidenced by paresthesias of hands and feet or decreased hearing.

Constipation may be related to decreased physical activity, slowed peristalsis, possibly evidenced by frequency less than usual pattern, decreased bowel sounds, hard dry stools, and development of fecal impaction.

Hysterectomy GYN/MS

Also refer to Surgery, general

acute Pain may be related to tissue trauma and abdominal incision, edema or hematoma formation, possibly evidenced by verbal reports, guarding or distraction behaviors, and changes in vital signs.

risk for impaired urinary Elimination/[acute] Urinary Retention are possibly evidenced by risk factors of mechanical trauma, surgical manipulation, presence of localized edema or hematoma, or nerve trauma with temporary bladder atony.*

ineffective Sexuality Pattern/risk for Sexual Dysfunction are possibly evidenced by risk factors of concerns regarding altered body function or structure, perceived changes in femininity, changes in hormone levels, loss of libido, and changes in sexual response pattern.*

risk for complicated Grieving is possibly evidenced by risk factors of preloss psychological symptoms, predisposition for anxiety and feelings of inadequacy, frequency of major life events. *

Ileocolitis MS/CH

Refer to Crohn's disease

Ileostomy MS/CH

Refer to Colostomy

Ileus MS

acute Pain may be related to distention or edema, and ischemia of intestinal tissue, possibly evidenced by verbal reports, guarding or distraction behaviors, narrowed focus, and changes in vital signs.

Diarrhea/Constipation may be related to presence of obstruction or changes in peristalsis, possibly evidenced by changes in frequency and consistency or absence of stool, alterations in bowel sounds, presence of pain, and cramping.

risk for deficient Fluid Volume is possibly evidenced by risk factors of increased intestinal losses (vomiting and diarrhea) and decreased intake.*

Impetigo PED/CH

impaired Skin Integrity may be related to presence of infectious process and pruritus, possibly evidenced by open or crusted lesions.

*A risk diagnosis is not evidenced by signs and symptoms, as the problem has not occurred; rather, nursing interventions are directed at prevention.

acute Pain may be related to inflammation and pruritus, possibly evidenced by verbal reports, distraction behaviors, and self-focusing.
risk for [secondary] Infection is possibly evidenced by risk factors of broken skin, traumatized tissue, altered immune response, and virulence and contagious nature of causative organism.*
risk for Infection [transmission] is possibly evidenced by risk factors of virulent nature of causative organism, insufficient knowledge to prevent infection of others.*

Infection, prenatal **OB**

Also refer to AIDS
risk for maternal/fetal Infection is possibly evidenced by risk factors of inadequate primary defenses (e.g., broken skin, stasis of body fluids), inadequate secondary defenses (e.g., decreased Hb, immunosuppression), inadequate acquired immunity, environmental exposure, malnutrition, rupture of amniotic membranes.*
deficient Knowledge regarding treatment/prevention, prognosis of condition may be related to lack of exposure to information and/or unfamiliarity with resources, misinterpretation possibly evidenced by verbalization of problem, inaccurate follow-through of instructions, development of preventable complications or continuation of infectious process.
impaired Comfort may be related to body response to infective agent, properties of infection (e.g., skin or tissue irritation, development of lesions), possibly evidenced by verbal reports, restlessness, withdrawal from social contacts.

Infection, wound **MS/CH**

risk for Infection [sepsis] is possibly evidenced by risk factors of presence of infection, broken skin, traumatized tissues, chronic disease (e.g., diabetes, anemia), stasis of body fluids, invasive procedures, altered immune response.*
impaired Skin Integrity/impaired Tissue Integrity may be related to altered circulation, presence of infection, wound drainage, nutritional deficit, possibly evidenced by delayed healing, damaged tissues, invasion of body structures.
risk for delayed Surgical Recovery is possibly evidenced by risk factors of presence of infection, activity restrictions or limitations, nutritional deficiencies.*

Inflammatory bowel disease **CH**

Refer to Colitis, ulcerative; Crohn's disease

Infertility **CH**

situational low Self-Esteem may be related to functional impairment (inability to conceive), unrealistic self-expectations, sense of failure possibly evidenced by self-negating verbalizations, expressions of helplessness, perceived inability to deal with situation.
chronic Sorrow may be related to perceived physical disability (inability to conceive) possibly evidenced by expressions of anger, disappointment, emptiness, self-blame, helplessness, sadness, feelings interfering with client's ability to achieve maximum well-being.

*A risk diagnosis is not evidenced by signs and symptoms, as the problem has not occurred; rather, nursing interventions are directed at prevention.

risk for Spiritual Distress is possibly evidenced by risk factors of energy-consuming anxiety, low self-esteem, deteriorating relationship with SO, viewing situation as deserved or punishment for past behaviors.*

Influenza CH

acute Pain/impaired Comfort may be related to inflammation and effects of circulating toxins, possibly evidenced by verbal reports, distraction behaviors, and narrowed focus.

risk for deficient Fluid Volume is possibly evidenced by risk factors of excessive gastric losses, hypermetabolic state, and altered intake.*

Hyperthermia may be related to effects of circulating toxins and dehydration, possibly evidenced by increased body temperature, warm, flushed skin, and tachycardia.

risk for ineffective Breathing Pattern is possibly evidenced by risk factors of response to infectious process, decreased energy, fatigue.*

Insulin shock MS/CH

Refer to Hypoglycemia

Intestinal obstruction MS

Refer to Ileus

K

Irritable bowel syndrome CH

acute Pain may be related to abnormally strong intestinal contractions, increased sensitivity of intestine to distention, hypersensitivity to hormones gastrin and cholecystokinin, skin or tissue irritation, perirectal excoriation, possibly evidenced by verbal reports, guarding behavior, expressive behavior (restlessness, moaning, irritability).

Constipation may be related to motor abnormalities of longitudinal muscles and changes in frequency and amplitude of contractions, dietary restrictions, stress, possibly evidenced by change in bowel pattern, decreased frequency, sensation of incomplete evacuation, abdominal pain, distention.

Diarrhea may be related to motor abnormalities of longitudinal muscles and changes in frequency and amplitude of contractions, possibly evidenced by precipitous passing of liquid stool on rising or immediately after eating, rectal urgency, incontinence, bloating.

Kawasaki disease PED

Hyperthermia may be related to increased metabolic rate and dehydration, possibly evidenced by increased body temperature greater than normal range, flushed skin, increased respiratory rate, and tachycardia.

acute Pain may be related to inflammation and edema or swelling of tissues, possibly evidenced by verbal reports, restlessness, guarding behaviors, and narrowed focus.

impaired Skin Integrity may be related to inflammatory process, altered circulation, and edema formation, possibly evidenced by disruption of skin surface, including macular rash and desquamation.

impaired oral Mucous Membrane may be related to inflammatory process, dehydration, and mouth breathing, possibly evidenced by pain, hyperemia, and fissures of lips.

---

*A risk diagnosis is not evidenced by signs and symptoms, as the problem has not occurred; rather, nursing interventions are directed at prevention.

risk for decreased Cardiac Output is possibly evidenced by risk factors of structural changes, inflammation of coronary arteries and alterations in rate, rhythm, or conduction.*

Kidney stone(s) **CH**

Refer to Calculi, urinary

Labor, induced/augmented **OB**

deficient Knowledge [Learning Need] regarding procedure, treatment needs, and possible outcomes may be related to lack of exposure/recall, information misinterpretation, and unfamiliarity with information resources, possibly evidenced by questions, statements of concern/misconception, and exaggerated behaviors.

risk for maternal Injury is possibly evidenced by risk factors of adverse effects or response to therapeutic interventions.*

risk for impaired fetal Gas Exchange is possibly evidenced by risk factors of altered placental perfusion or cord prolapse.*

labor Pain may be related to altered characteristics of chemically stimulated contractions, cervical dilation, psychological concerns, possibly evidenced by verbal reports, increased muscle tone, distraction or guarding behaviors, and narrowed focus.

Labor, precipitous **OB**

Anxiety [specify level] may be related to situational crisis, threat to self or fetus, interpersonal transmission, possibly evidenced by increased tension; being scared, fearful, restless, jittery; sympathetic stimulation.

risk for impaired Skin Integrity/impaired Tissue Integrity is possibly evidenced by risk factors of mechanical factors (e.g., pressure, shearing forces). *

labor Pain may be related to occurrence of rapid, strong uterine contractions; psychological issues, possibly evidenced by verbalizations of inability to use learned pain-management techniques, sympathetic stimulation, distraction behaviors (e.g., moaning, restlessness).

Labor, preterm **OB/CH**

Activity Intolerance may be related to muscle or cellular hypersensitivity, possibly evidenced by continued uterine contractions or irritability.

risk for Poisoning is possibly evidenced by risk factors of dose-related toxic or side effects of tocolytics.*

risk for fetal Injury is possibly evidenced by risk factors of delivery of premature or immature infant.*

Anxiety [specify level] may be related to situational crisis, perceived or actual threats to self or fetus, and inadequate time to prepare for labor, possibly evidenced by increased tension, restlessness, expressions of concern, and changes in vital signs.

deficient Knowledge [Learning Need] regarding preterm labor treatment needs and prognosis may be related to lack of information and misinterpretation, possibly evidenced by questions, statements of concern, misconceptions, inaccurate follow-through of instruction, and development of preventable complications.

---

*A risk diagnosis is not evidenced by signs and symptoms, as the problem has not occurred; rather, nursing interventions are directed at prevention.

L

Labor, stage I (active phase) **OB**

labor Pain/impaired Comfort may be related to contraction-related hypoxia, dilation of tissues, and pressure on adjacent structures combined with stimulation of both parasympathetic and sympathetic nerve endings, possibly evidenced by verbal reports, guarding or distraction behaviors (restlessness), muscle tension, and narrowed focus.

impaired urinary Elimination may be related to altered intake, dehydration, fluid shifts, hormonal changes, hemorrhage, severe intrapartal hypertension, mechanical compression of bladder, and effects of regional anesthesia, possibly evidenced by changes in amount or frequency of voiding, urinary retention, slowed progression of labor, and reduced sensation.

risk for ineffective [individual/couple] Coping is possibly evidenced by risk factors of situational crises, personal vulnerability, use of ineffective coping mechanisms, inadequate support systems, and pain.*

Labor, stage II (expulsion) **OB**

labor Pain may be related to strong uterine contractions, tissue stretching/dilation and compression of nerves by presenting part of the fetus, and bladder distention, possibly evidenced by verbalizations, facial grimacing, guarding or distraction behaviors (restlessness), narrowed focus, and diaphoresis.

Cardiac Output [fluctuation] may be related to changes in SVR, fluctuations in venous return (repeated or prolonged Valsalva's maneuvers, effects of anesthesia or medications, dorsal recumbent position occluding the inferior vena cava and partially obstructing the aorta), possibly evidenced by decreased venous return, changes in vital signs (BP, pulse), urinary output, fetal bradycardia.

risk for impaired fetal Gas Exchange is possibly evidenced by risk factors of mechanical compression of head or cord, maternal position or prolonged labor affecting placental perfusion, and effects of maternal anesthesia, hyperventilation.*

impaired Skin Integrity/impaired Tissue Integrity may be related to untoward stretching or lacerations of delicate tissues (precipitous labor, hypertonic contractile pattern, adolescence, large fetus), and application of forceps.*

risk for Fatigue is possibly evidenced by risk factors of pregnancy, stress, anxiety, sleep deprivation, increased physical exertion, anemia, environmental humidity or temperature, lights.*

Laminectomy, cervical **MS**

Also refer to Laminectomy, lumbar

risk for perioperative Positioning Injury is possibly evidenced by risk factors of immobilization, muscle weakness, obesity, advanced age.*

risk for ineffective Airway Clearance is possibly evidenced by risk factors of retained secretions, pain, muscle weakness.*

risk for impaired Swallowing is possibly evidenced by risk factors of operative edema, pain, neuromuscular impairment.*

---

*A risk diagnosis is not evidenced by signs and symptoms, as the problem has not occurred; rather, nursing interventions are directed at prevention.

Laminectomy, lumbar

MS

Also refer to Surgery, general

ineffective Tissue Perfusion [specify] may be related to diminished or interrupted blood flow—edema of operative site, hematoma formation, hypovolemia, possibly evidenced by paresthesia, numbness, decreased range of motion or muscle strength.

risk for [spinal] Trauma is possibly evidenced by risk factors of temporary weakness of spinal column, balancing difficulties, changes in muscle tone or coordination.*

acute Pain may be related to traumatized tissues—surgical manipulation, harvesting bone graft, localized inflammation, and edema, possibly evidenced by altered muscle tone, verbal reports, and distraction or guarding behaviors, changes in vital signs, diaphoresis, pallor.

impaired physical Mobility may be related to imposed therapeutic restrictions, neuromuscular impairment, and pain, possibly evidenced by limited range of motion, decreased muscle strength or control, impaired coordination, and reluctance to attempt movement.

risk for [acute] Urinary Retention is possibly evidenced by risk factors of pain and swelling in operative area and reduced mobility/restrictions of position.*

Laryngectomy

MS

Also refer to Cancer; Chemotherapy

ineffective Airway Clearance may be related to partial or total removal of the glottis, temporary or permanent change to neck breathing, edema formation, and copious and thick secretions, possibly evidenced by dyspnea or difficulty breathing, changes in rate and depth of respiration, use of accessory respiratory muscles, weak or ineffective cough, abnormal breath sounds, and cyanosis.

impaired Skin Integrity/impaired Tissue Integrity may be related to surgical removal of tissues and grafting, effects of radiation or chemotherapeutic agents, altered circulation or reduced blood supply, compromised nutritional status, edema formation, and pooling or continuous drainage of secretions, possibly evidenced by disruption of skin and tissue surface and destruction of skin and tissue layers.

impaired oral Mucous Membrane may be related to dehydration or absence of oral intake, decreased saliva production, poor or inadequate oral hygiene, pathological condition (oral cancer), mechanical trauma (oral surgery), difficulty swallowing and pooling or drooling of secretions, and nutritional deficits, possibly evidenced by xerostomia (dry mouth), oral discomfort, thick, mucoid saliva, decreased saliva production, dry and crusted or coated tongue, inflamed lips, absent teeth and gums, poor dental health and halitosis.

CH

impaired verbal Communication may be related to anatomical deficit (removal of vocal cords), physical barrier (tracheostomy tube), and required voice rest, possibly evidenced by inability to speak, change in vocal characteristics, and impaired articulation.

*A risk diagnosis is not evidenced by signs and symptoms, as the problem has not occurred; rather, nursing interventions are directed at prevention.

risk for Aspiration is possibly evidenced by risk factors of impaired swallowing, facial and neck surgery, presence of tracheostomy, tube feedings.*

Laryngitis **CH/PED**

Refer to Croup

Latex allergy **CH**

Latex Allergy Response may be related to hypersensitivity to natural latex rubber protein, possibly evidenced by contact dermatitis—erythema, blisters; delayed hypersensitivity—eczema, irritation; or hypersensitivity—generalized edema, wheezing, bronchospasm, hypotension, cardiac arrest.

Anxiety [specify level]/Fear may be related to threat of death, possibly evidenced by expressed concerns, hypervigilance, restlessness, focus on self.

risk for risk-prone Health Behavior is possibly evidenced by risk factor of health status requiring change in occupation.*

Lead poisoning, acute **PED/CH**

Also refer to Lead poisoning, chronic

Contamination may be related to flaking or peeling paint (young children), improperly lead-glazed ceramic pottery, unprotected contact with lead (e.g., battery manufacture or recycling, bronzing, soldering or welding), imported herbal products or medicinals, possibly evidenced by abdominal cramping, headache, irritability, decreased attentiveness, constipation, tremors.

risk for Trauma is possibly evidenced by risk factors of loss of coordination, altered level of consciousness, clonic or tonic muscle activity, neurological damage.*

risk for deficient Fluid Volume is possibly evidenced by risk factors of excessive vomiting, diarrhea, or decreased intake.*

deficient Knowledge [Learning Need] regarding sources of lead and prevention of poisoning may be related to lack of information/misinterpretation, possibly evidenced by statements of concern, questions, and misconceptions.

Lead poisoning, chronic **CH**

Also refer to Lead poisoning, acute

Contamination may be related to flaking or peeling paint (young children), improperly lead-glazed ceramic pottery, unprotected contact with lead (e.g., battery manufacture or recycling, bronzing, soldering or welding), imported herbal products or medicinals, possibly evidenced by chronic abdominal pain, headache, personality changes, cognitive deficits, seizures, neuropathy.

imbalanced Nutrition: less than body requirements may be related to decreased intake (chemically induced changes in the gastrointestinal tract), possibly evidenced by anorexia, abdominal discomfort, reported metallic taste, and weight loss.

chronic Pain may be related to deposition of lead in soft tissues and bone, possibly evidenced by verbal reports, distraction behaviors, and focus on self.

*A risk diagnosis is not evidenced by signs and symptoms, as the problem has not occurred; rather, nursing interventions are directed at prevention.

risk for delayed Development/disproportionate Growth are possibly evidenced by risk factors of lead poisoning, chronic illness.*

Leukemia, acute **MS**

Also refer to Chemotherapy

risk for Infection is possibly evidenced by risk factors of inadequate secondary defenses (alterations in mature white blood cells [WBCs], increased number of immature lymphocytes, immunosuppression, and bone marrow suppression), invasive procedures, and malnutrition.*

Anxiety [specify level]/Fear may be related to change in health status, threat of death, and situational crisis, possibly evidenced by sympathetic stimulation, apprehension, feelings of helplessness, focus on self, and insomnia.

Activity Intolerance [specify level] may be related to reduced energy stores, increased metabolic rate, imbalance between O_2 supply and demand—anemia, hypoxia; therapeutic restrictions—isolation, bedrest; effect of drug therapy, possibly evidenced by generalized weakness, reports of fatigue and exertional dyspnea, abnormal heart rate or BP response.

acute Pain may be related to physical agents (infiltration of tissues/organs/CNS, expanding bone marrow) and chemical agents (antileukemic treatments), psychological manifestations—anxiety, fear possibly evidenced by verbal reports (abdominal discomfort, arthralgia, bone pain, headache), distraction behaviors, narrowed focus, and changes in vital signs.

risk for deficient Fluid Volume/risk for Bleeding is possibly evidenced by risk factors of excessive losses (vomiting, diarrhea, coagulopathy), decreased intake (nausea, anorexia), increased fluid need (hypermetabolic state/fever), predisposition for kidney stone formation, tumor lysis syndrome.*

Leukemia, chronic **MS**

risk for Infection is possibly evidenced by risk factors of inadequate secondary defenses (alterations in mature WBCs, increased number of immature lymphocytes, immunosuppression, and bone marrow suppression), invasive procedures, and malnutrition.*

ineffective Protection may be related to abnormal blood profiles, drug therapy—cytotoxic agents, steroids, or radiation treatments possibly evidenced by deficient immunity, impaired healing, altered clotting, weakness.

Fatigue may be related to disease state, anemia possibly evidenced by verbalizations, inability to maintain usual routines, listlessness.

imbalanced Nutrition: less than body requirements may be related to inability to ingest nutrients, possibly evidenced by lack of interest in food, anorexia, weight loss, abdominal fullness, pain.

Long-term care **CH**

Also refer to condition(s) requiring or contributing to need for facility placement

Anxiety [specify level]/Fear may be related to change in health status, role functioning, interaction patterns, socioeconomic status, environment; unmet needs, recent life changes, and loss of friends/SO(s),

*A risk diagnosis is not evidenced by signs and symptoms, as the problem has not occurred; rather, nursing interventions are directed at prevention.

possibly evidenced by apprehension, restlessness, insomnia, repetitive questioning, pacing, purposeless activity, expressed concern regarding changes in life events, and focus on self.

Grieving may be related to perceived, actual, or potential loss of physiopsychosocial well-being, personal possessions, and SO(s), as well as cultural beliefs about aging and debilitation, possibly evidenced by denial of feelings, depression, sorrow, guilt, alterations in activity level, sleep patterns, eating habits, and libido.

risk for Poisoning [drug toxicity] is possibly evidenced by risk factors of effects of aging (reduced metabolism, impaired circulation, precarious physiological balance, presence of multiple diseases and organ involvement), and use of multiple prescribed and over-the-counter drugs.*

impaired Memory may be related to neurological disturbances, hypoxia, fluid imbalance, possibly evidenced by inability to recall events/factual information, reports experience of forgetting.

Insomnia may be related to internal factors (illness, psychological stress, inactivity) and external factors (environmental changes, facility routines), possibly evidenced by reports of difficulty in falling asleep/not feeling rested, interrupted sleep, awakening earlier than desired, change in behavior or performance, increasing irritability, and listlessness.

L

risk for Sexual Dysfunction is possibly evidenced by risk factors of biopsychosocial alteration of sexuality, interference in psychological/physical well-being, self-image, and lack of privacy/SO(s).*

risk for Relocation Stress Syndrome is possibly evidenced by risk factors of temporary or permanent move that may be voluntary or involuntary, lack of predeparture counseling, multiple losses, feeling of powerlessness, lack of or inappropriate use of support system, changes in psychosocial or physical health status.*

risk for impaired Religiosity is possibly evidenced by risk factors of life transition, ineffective support or coping, lack of social interaction, depression.*

Lupus erythematosus, systemic (SLE) CH

Fatigue may be related to inadequate energy production or increased energy requirements (chronic inflammation), overwhelming psychological or emotional demands, states of discomfort, and altered body chemistry (including effects of drug therapy), possibly evidenced by reports of unremitting and overwhelming lack of energy, inability to maintain usual routines, decreased performance, lethargy, and decreased libido.

acute Pain may be related to widespread inflammatory process affecting connective tissues, blood vessels, serosal surfaces and mucous membranes, possibly evidenced by verbal reports, guarding or distraction behaviors, self-focusing, and changes in vital signs.

impaired Skin /Tissue Integrity may be related to chronic inflammation, edema formation, and altered circulation, possibly evidenced by presence of skin rash or lesions, ulcerations of mucous membranes, and photosensitivity.

*A risk diagnosis is not evidenced by signs and symptoms, as the problem has not occurred; rather, nursing interventions are directed at prevention.

disturbed Body Image may be related to presence of chronic condition with rash, lesions, ulcers, purpura, mottled erythema of hands, alopecia, loss of strength, and altered body function, possibly evidenced by hiding body parts, negative feelings about body, feelings of helplessness, and change in social involvement.

Lyme disease **CH/MS**

acute Pain/chronic Pain may be related to systemic effects of toxins, presence of rash, urticaria, and joint swelling or inflammation, possibly evidenced by verbal reports, guarding behaviors, autonomic responses, and narrowed focus.

Fatigue may be related to increased energy requirements, altered body chemistry, and states of discomfort evidenced by reports of overwhelming lack of energy, inability to maintain usual routines, decreased performance, lethargy, and malaise.

risk for decreased Cardiac Output is possibly evidenced by risk factors of alteration in cardiac rate, rhythm, or conduction.*

Macular degeneration **CH**

[disturbed visual Sensory Perception] may be related to altered sensory reception, possibly evidenced by reported or measured change in sensory acuity, change in usual response to stimuli.

Anxiety [specify level]/Fear may be related to situational crisis, threat to or change in health status and role function, possibly evidenced by expressed concerns, apprehension, feelings of inadequacy, diminished productivity, impaired attention.

risk for impaired Social Interaction possibly evidenced by risk factors of limited physical mobility, environmental barriers.*

Mallory-Weiss syndrome **MS**

Also refer to Achalasia

risk for deficient Fluid Volume is possibly evidenced by risk factors of excessive vascular losses, presence of vomiting, and reduced intake.*

deficient Knowledge [Learning Need] regarding causes, treatment, and prevention of condition may be related to lack of information or misinterpretation, possibly evidenced by statements of concern, questions, and recurrence of problem.

Mastectomy **MS**

impaired Skin Integrity/impaired Tissue Integrity may be related to surgical removal of skin and tissue, altered circulation, presence of edema, drainage, changes in skin elasticity and sensation, and tissue destruction (radiation), possibly evidenced by disruption of skin surface and destruction of skin layers and subcutaneous tissues.

impaired physical Mobility may be related to neuromuscular impairment, pain, and edema formation, possibly evidenced by reluctance to attempt movement, limited range of motion, and decreased muscle mass and strength.

dressing Self-Care Deficit may be related to temporary decreased range of motion of one or both arms, possibly evidenced by statements of inability to perform or complete self-care tasks.

---

*A risk diagnosis is not evidenced by signs and symptoms, as the problem has not occurred; rather, nursing interventions are directed at prevention.

disturbed Body Image/situational low Self-Esteem may be related to loss of body part denoting femininity, fear of rejection or reaction of others, behaviors inconsistent with self-value system, possibly evidenced by not looking at or touching area, having self-negating verbalizations, being preoccupied with loss, and having a change in social involvement or relationship.

risk for complicated Grieving is possibly evidenced by risk factors of preloss psychological symptoms, predisposition for anxiety and feelings of inadequacy, frequency of major life events.*

Mastitis — OB/GYN

acute Pain may be related to erythema and edema of breast tissues, possibly evidenced by verbal reports, guarding or distraction behaviors, self-focusing, changes in vital signs.

risk for Infection [spread/abscess formation] is possibly evidenced by risk factors of traumatized tissues, stasis of fluids, and insufficient knowledge to prevent complications.*

deficient Knowledge [Learning Need] regarding pathophysiology, treatment, and prevention may be related to lack of information or misinterpretation, possibly evidenced by statements of concern, questions, and misconceptions.

risk for ineffective Breastfeeding is possibly evidenced by risk factors of inability to feed on affected side or interruption in breastfeeding.*

M

Mastoidectomy — PED/MS

risk for Infection [spread] is possibly evidenced by risk factors of preexisting infection, surgical trauma, and stasis of body fluids in close proximity to brain.*

acute Pain may be related to inflammation, tissue trauma, and edema formation, possibly evidenced by verbal reports, distraction behaviors, restlessness, self-focusing, and changes in vital signs.

[disturbed auditory Sensory Perception] may be related to presence of surgical packing, edema, and surgical disturbance of middle ear structures, possibly evidenced by reported/tested hearing loss in affected ear.

Measles — CH/PED

acute Pain may be related to inflammation of mucous membranes, conjunctiva, and presence of extensive skin rash with pruritus, possibly evidenced by verbal reports, distraction behaviors, self-focusing, and changes in vital signs.

Hyperthermia may be related to presence of viral toxins and inflammatory response, possibly evidenced by increased body temperature, flushed, warm skin, and tachycardia.

risk for [secondary] Infection is possibly evidenced by risk factors of altered immune response and traumatized dermal tissues.*

deficient Knowledge [Learning Need] regarding condition, transmission, and possible complications may be related to lack of information, misinterpretation, possibly evidenced by statements of concern, questions, misconceptions, and development of preventable complications.

---

*A risk diagnosis is not evidenced by signs and symptoms, as the problem has not occurred; rather, nursing interventions are directed at prevention.

Melanoma, malignant MS/CH

Also refer to Cancer; Chemotherapy

Meningitis, acute meningococcal MS

risk for Infection [spread] is possibly evidenced by risk factors of hematogenous dissemination of pathogen, stasis of body fluids, suppressed inflammatory response (medication-induced), and exposure of others to pathogens.*

risk for ineffective cerebral Tissue Perfusion is possibly evidenced by risk factors of cerebral edema altering or interrupting cerebral arterial or venous blood flow, hypovolemia, exchange problems at cellular level (acidosis).*

Hyperthermia may be related to infectious process (increased metabolic rate) and dehydration, possibly evidenced by increased body temperature, warm, flushed skin; and tachycardia.

acute Pain may be related to inflammation or irritation of the meninges with spasm of extensor muscles (neck, shoulders, and back), possibly evidenced by verbal reports, guarding or distraction behaviors, narrowed focus, photophobia, and changes in vital signs.

risk for Trauma/Suffocation is possibly evidenced by risk factors of alterations in level of consciousness, possible development of clonic/tonic muscle activity (seizures), and generalized weakness, prostration, ataxia, vertigo.*

Meniscectomy MS/CH

impaired Walking may be related to pain, joint instability, and imposed medical restrictions of movement, possibly evidenced by impaired ability to move about environment as needed or desired.

deficient Knowledge [Learning Need] regarding postoperative expectations, prevention of complications, and self-care needs may be related to lack of information, possibly evidenced by statements of concern, questions, and misconceptions.

Menopause GYN

ineffective Thermoregulation may be related to fluctuation of hormonal levels, possibly evidenced by skin flushed/warm to touch, diaphoresis, night sweats, cold hands or feet.

Fatigue may be related to change in body chemistry, lack of sleep, depression, possibly evidenced by reports of lack of energy, being tired, having an inability to maintain usual routines, decreased performance.

risk for Sexual Dysfunction is possibly evidenced by risk factors of perceived altered body function, changes in physical response, myths or inaccurate information, impaired relationship with SO.*

risk for stress urinary Incontinence is possibly evidenced by risk factors of degenerative changes in pelvic muscles and structural support.*

readiness for enhanced Health Management possibly evidenced by expressed desire for management of life cycle changes, increased control of health practice.

---

*A risk diagnosis is not evidenced by signs and symptoms, as the problem has not occurred; rather, nursing interventions are directed at prevention.

Mental delay (formerly mental retardation) **CH**

Also refer to Down syndrome

impaired verbal Communication may be related to developmental delay, impairment of cognitive and motor abilities, possibly evidenced by impaired articulation, difficulty with phonation, and inability to modulate speech or find appropriate words (dependent on degree of retardation).

risk for Self-Care Deficit [specify] is possibly evidenced by risk factors of impaired cognitive ability and motor skills.*

risk for Overweight or Obesity is possibly evidenced by risk factors of decreased metabolic rate coupled with impaired cognitive development, dysfunctional eating patterns, and sedentary activity level.*

risk for sedentary Lifestyle is possibly evidenced by risk factors of lack of interest or motivation, lack of resources, lack of training or knowledge of specific exercise needs, safety concerns, fear of injury.*

impaired Social Interaction may be related to impaired thought processes, communication barriers, and knowledge or skill deficit about ways to enhance mutuality, possibly evidenced by dysfunctional interactions with peers, family, and/or SO(s), and verbalized or observed discomfort in social situation.

compromised family Coping may be related to chronic nature of condition and degree of disability that exhausts supportive capacity of SO(s), other situational or developmental crises or situations SO(s) may be facing, unrealistic expectations of SO(s), possibly evidenced by preoccupation of SO with personal reaction, SO(s) withdraw(s) or enter(s) into limited interaction with individual, protective behavior disproportionate (too much or too little) to client's abilities or need for autonomy.

impaired Home Maintenance may be related to impaired cognitive functioning, insufficient finances/family organization or planning, lack of knowledge, and inadequate support systems, possibly evidenced by requests for assistance, expression of difficulty in maintaining home, disorderly surroundings, and overtaxed family members.

risk for Sexual Dysfunction is possibly evidenced by risk factors of biopsychosocial alteration of sexuality, ineffectual or absent role models, misinformation or lack of knowledge, lack of SO(s), and lack of appropriate behavior control.*

Metabolic syndrome **CH/MS**

risk for unstable Blood Glucose Level is possibly evidenced by risk factors of dietary intake, weight gain, physical activity level.*

sedentary Lifestyle may be related to deficient knowledge of health benefits of physical exercise, lack of interest/motivation or resources, possibly evidenced by verbalized preference for activities low in physical activity, choice of a daily routine lacking physical exercise.

compromised family Coping may be related to chronic nature of condition and degree of disability that exhausts supportive capacity of SO(s), other situational or developmental crises or situations SO(s) may be facing, unrealistic expectations of SO(s), possibly evidenced by preoccupation of SO with personal reaction, SO(s) withdraw(s) or enter(s) into limited interaction with individual, protective behav-

*A risk diagnosis is not evidenced by signs and symptoms, as the problem has not occurred; rather, nursing interventions are directed at prevention.

ior disproportionate (too much or too little) to client's abilities or need for autonomy.

impaired Home Maintenance may be related to impaired cognitive functioning, insufficient finances and family organization or planning, lack of knowledge, and inadequate support systems, possibly evidenced by requests for assistance, expression of difficulty in maintaining home, disorderly surroundings, and overtaxed family members.

risk for ineffective Tissue Perfusion [specify] is possibly evidenced by risk factors of arterial plaque formation (elevated triglycerides, low levels of HDL), prothrombotic state, proinflammatory state.*

Miscarriage — OB

Refer to Abortion, spontaneous termination

Mitral stenosis — MS/CH

Activity Intolerance may be related to imbalance between O_2 supply and demand, possibly evidenced by reports of fatigue, weakness, exertional dyspnea, and tachycardia.

impaired Gas Exchange may be related to altered blood flow, possibly evidenced by restlessness, hypoxia, and cyanosis (orthopnea/paroxysmal nocturnal dyspnea).

decreased Cardiac Output may be related to impeded blood flow as evidenced by jugular vein distention, peripheral or dependent edema, orthopnea, paroxysmal nocturnal dyspnea.

deficient Knowledge [Learning Need] regarding pathophysiology, therapeutic needs, and potential complications may be related to lack of information or recall, misinterpretation, possibly evidenced by statements of concern, questions, inaccurate follow-through of instructions, and development of preventable complications.

Mononucleosis, infectious — CH

Fatigue may be related to decreased energy production, states of discomfort, and increased energy requirements (inflammatory process), possibly evidenced by reports of overwhelming lack of energy, inability to maintain usual routines, lethargy, and malaise.

acute Pain/impaired Comfort may be related to inflammation of lymphoid and organ tissues, irritation of oropharyngeal mucous membranes, and effects of circulating toxins, possibly evidenced by verbal reports, distraction behaviors, and self-focusing.

Hyperthermia may be related to inflammatory process, possibly evidenced by increased body temperature, warm, flushed skin, and tachycardia.

deficient Knowledge [Learning Need] regarding disease transmission, self-care needs, medical therapy, and potential complications may be related to lack of information, misinterpretation, possibly evidenced by statements of concern, misconceptions, and inaccurate follow-through of instructions.

Mood disorders — PSY

Refer to Depressive disorders

*A risk diagnosis is not evidenced by signs and symptoms, as the problem has not occurred; rather, nursing interventions are directed at prevention.

Mountain sickness, acute (AMS) **CH/MS**

acute Pain may be related to reduced O_2 tension, possibly evidenced by reports of headache.

Fatigue may be related to stress, increased physical exertion, sleep deprivation, possibly evidenced by overwhelming lack of energy, inability to restore energy even after sleep, compromised concentration, decreased performance.

risk for deficient Fluid Volume is possibly evidenced by risk factors of increased water loss (e.g., overbreathing dry air), exertion, or altered fluid intake (nausea).*

Multiple personality **PSY**

Refer to Dissociative disorders

Multiple sclerosis **CH**

Fatigue may be related to decreased energy production or increased energy requirements to perform activities, psychological or emotional demands, pain or discomfort, medication side effects, possibly evidenced by verbalization of overwhelming lack of energy, inability to maintain usual routine, decreased performance, impaired ability to concentrate, increase in physical complaints.

[disturbed visual, kinesthetic, tactile Sensory Perception] may be related to delayed or interrupted neuronal transmission, possibly evidenced by impaired vision, diplopia, disturbance of vibratory or position sense, paresthesias, numbness, and blunting of sensation.

impaired physical Mobility may be related to neuromuscular impairment; discomfort or pain; sensoriperceptual impairments; decreased muscle strength, control and/or mass; deconditioning, as evidenced by limited ability to perform motor skills; limited range of motion; gait changes, postural instability.

Powerlessness/Hopelessness may be related to illness-related regimen, unpredictability of disease, and lifestyle of helplessness, possibly evidenced by verbal expressions of having no control or influence over the situation, depression over physical deterioration that occurs despite client compliance with regimen, nonparticipation in care or decision making when opportunities are provided, passivity, decreased verbalization and affect, isolating behaviors.

impaired Home Maintenance may be related to effects of debilitating disease, impaired cognitive and/or emotional functioning, insufficient finances, and inadequate support systems, possibly evidenced by reported difficulty, observed disorderly surroundings, and poor hygienic conditions.

compromised family Coping/disabled family Coping may be related to situational crises/temporary family disorganization and role changes, client providing little support in turn for SO(s), prolonged disease or disability progression that exhausts the supportive capacity of SO(s), feelings of guilt, anxiety, hostility, despair, and highly ambivalent family relationships, possibly evidenced by client expressing or confirming concern or report about SO's response to client's illness, SO(s) preoccupied with own personal reactions, intolerance, abandonment, neglectful care of the client, and distortion of reality regarding client's illness.

*A risk diagnosis is not evidenced by signs and symptoms, as the problem has not occurred; rather, nursing interventions are directed at prevention.

Mumps **PED/CH**

acute Pain may be related to presence of inflammation, circulating toxins, and enlargement of salivary glands, possibly evidenced by verbal reports, guarding or distraction behaviors, self-focusing, and changes in vital signs.

Hyperthermia may be related to inflammatory process (increased metabolic rate) and dehydration, possibly evidenced by increased body temperature, warm, flushed skin, and tachycardia.

risk for deficient Fluid Volume is possibly evidenced by risk factors of hypermetabolic state and painful swallowing, with decreased intake.*

Muscular dystrophy (Duchenne's) **PED/CH**

impaired physical Mobility may be related to musculoskeletal impairment or weakness, possibly evidenced by decreased muscle strength, control, and mass, limited range of motion, and impaired coordination.

risk for delayed Development is possibly evidenced by risk factors of genetic disorder/chronic illness, learning disability.*

risk for Overweight/Obesity is possibly evidenced by risk factors of sedentary lifestyle and dysfunctional eating patterns.*

compromised family Coping may be related to situational crisis, emotional conflicts around issues about hereditary nature of condition and prolonged disease or disability that exhausts supportive capacity of family members, possibly evidenced by preoccupation with personal reactions regarding disability and displaying protective behavior disproportionate (too little or too much) to client's abilities or need for autonomy.

Myasthenia gravis **MS**

ineffective Breathing Pattern/ineffective Airway Clearance may be related to neuromuscular weakness and decreased energy, fatigue, possibly evidenced by dyspnea, changes in rate and depth of respiration, ineffective cough, and adventitious breath sounds.

impaired verbal Communication may be related to neuromuscular weakness, fatigue, and physical barrier (intubation), possibly evidenced by facial weakness, impaired articulation, hoarseness, and inability to speak.

impaired Swallowing may be related to neuromuscular impairment of laryngeal or pharyngeal muscles, and muscular fatigue, possibly evidenced by reported or observed difficulty swallowing, coughing, choking, and evidence of aspiration.

Anxiety [specify level]/Fear may be related to situational crisis, threat to self-concept, change in health or socioeconomic status or role function; separation from support systems, lack of knowledge, and inability to communicate, possibly evidenced by expressed concerns, increased tension, restlessness, apprehension, sympathetic stimulation, crying, focus on self, uncooperative behavior, withdrawal, anger, and noncommunication.

CH

deficient Knowledge [Learning Need] regarding drug therapy, potential for crisis (myasthenic or cholinergic), and self-care management may

*A risk diagnosis is not evidenced by signs and symptoms, as the problem has not occurred; rather, nursing interventions are directed at prevention.

be related to inadequate information, misinterpretation, possibly evidenced by statements of concern, questions, and misconceptions; development of preventable complications.

impaired physical Mobility may be related to neuromuscular impairment, possibly evidenced by reports of progressive fatigability with repetitive or prolonged muscle use, impaired coordination, and decreased muscle strength/control.

[disturbed visual Sensory Perception] may be related to neuromuscular impairment, possibly evidenced by visual distortions (diplopia) and motor incoordination.

Myeloma, multiple **MS/CH**

Also refer to Cancer

acute Pain/chronic Pain may be related to destruction of tissues or bone, side effects of therapy, possibly evidenced by verbal or coded reports, guarding or protective behaviors, changes in appetite or weight, sleep; reduced interaction with others.

impaired physical Mobility may be related to loss of integrity of bone structure, pain, deconditioning, depressed mood, possibly evidenced by verbalizations, limited range of motion, slowed movement, gait changes.

ineffective Protection may be related to cancer, drug therapies, radiation treatments, inadequate nutrition, possibly evidenced by weakness, alteration in clotting, neurosensory impairment.*

M

Myocardial infarction **MS**

Also refer to Myocarditis

acute Pain may be related to ischemia of myocardial tissue, possibly evidenced by verbal reports, guarding or distraction behaviors (restlessness), facial mask of pain, self-focusing, and diaphoresis, changes in vital signs.

Anxiety [specify level]/Fear may be related to threat of death, threat of change of health status, role functioning and lifestyle; interpersonal transmission or contagion, possibly evidenced by increased tension, fearful attitude, apprehension, expressed concerns or uncertainty, restlessness, sympathetic stimulation, and somatic complaints.

risk for decreased Cardiac Output is possibly evidenced by risk factors of changes in rate and electrical conduction, reduced preload/increased SVR and altered muscle contractility/depressant effects of some medications, infarcted or dyskinetic muscle, structural defects.*

CH

risk for sedentary Lifestyle is possibly evidenced by risk factors of lack of resources, lack of training or knowledge of specific exercise needs, safety concerns, fear of injury.*

Myocarditis **MS**

Also refer to Myocardial infarction

Activity Intolerance may be related to imbalance in O_2 supply and demand (myocardial inflammation or damage), cardiac depressant effects of certain drugs, and enforced bedrest, possibly evidenced by

*A risk diagnosis is not evidenced by signs and symptoms, as the problem has not occurred; rather, nursing interventions are directed at prevention.

reports of fatigue, exertional dyspnea, tachycardia and palpitations in response to activity, ECG changes—dysrhythmias, and generalized weakness.

risk for decreased Cardiac Output is possibly evidenced by risk factors of altered contractility, altered stroke volume.*

deficient Knowledge [Learning Need] regarding pathophysiology of condition, outcomes, treatment, and self-care needs and lifestyle changes may be related to lack of information, misinterpretation, possibly evidenced by statements of concern, misconceptions, inaccurate follow-through of instructions, and development of preventable complications.

Myringotomy PED/MS

Refer to Mastoidectomy

Myxedema CH

Also refer to Hypothyroidism

disturbed Body Image may be related to change in structure or function (loss of hair, thickening of skin, masklike facial expression, enlarged tongue, menstrual and reproductive disturbances), possibly evidenced by negative feelings about body, feelings of helplessness, and change in social involvement.

Overweight may be related to decreased metabolic rate and activity level, possibly evidenced by weight gain greater than ideal for height and frame.

risk for decreased Cardiac Output is possibly evidenced by risk factors of alteration in heart rhythm, altered contractility.*

Narcolepsy CH

Insomnia may be related to medical condition, possibly evidenced by hypersomnia, reports of unsatisfying nighttime sleep, vivid visual or auditory illusions or hallucinations at onset of sleep, sleep interrupted by vivid or frightening dreams.

risk for Trauma is possibly evidenced by risk factors of sudden loss of muscle tone, momentary paralysis (cataplexy), sudden inappropriate sleep episodes.*

risk for chronic low Self-Esteem is possibly evidenced by risk factors of negative evaluation of self, personal vulnerability, chronic physical condition, impaired work or social performance, problems with social relationships, reduced quality of life.*

Necrotizing cellulitis, fasciitis MS

Also refer to Cellulitis, Sepsis

Hyperthermia may be related to inflammatory process, response to circulatory toxins, possibly evidenced by body temperature above normal range; flushed, warm skin: tachycardia, altered mental status.

impaired Tissue Integrity ischemia, possibly evidenced by damaged or destroyed tissue, dermal gangrene.

Neglect/Abuse CH/PSY

Refer to Abuse; Battered child syndrome

*A risk diagnosis is not evidenced by signs and symptoms, as the problem has not occurred; rather, nursing interventions are directed at prevention.

Neonatal, normal newborn PED

risk for impaired Gas Exchange is possibly evidenced by risk factors of prenatal or intrapartal stressors, excess production of mucus, or cold stress.*

risk for Hypothermia is possibly evidenced by risk factors of large body surface in relation to mass, limited amounts of insulating subcutaneous fat, nonrenewable sources of brown fat and few white fat stores, thin epidermis with close proximity of blood vessels to the skin, inability to shiver, and movement from a warm uterine environment to a much cooler environment.*

risk for impaired Attachment is possibly evidenced by risk factors of developmental transition (gain of a family member), anxiety associated with the parent role, lack of privacy (healthcare interventions, intrusive family/visitors).*

risk for imbalanced Nutrition: less than body requirements is possibly evidenced by risk factors of rapid metabolic rate, high caloric requirement, increased insensible water losses through pulmonary and cutaneous routes, fatigue, and a potential for inadequate or depleted glucose stores.*

risk for Infection is possibly evidenced by risk factors of inadequate secondary defenses (inadequate acquired immunity, e.g., deficiency of neutrophils and specific immunoglobulins), and inadequate primary defenses (e.g., environmental exposure, broken skin, traumatized tissues, decreased ciliary action).*

Neonatal, premature newborn PED

N

impaired Gas Exchange may be related to alveolar-capillary membrane changes (inadequate surfactant levels), altered blood flow (immaturity of pulmonary arteriole musculature), altered O_2 supply (immaturity of CNS and neuromuscular system, tracheobronchial obstruction), altered O_2-carrying capacity of blood (anemia), and cold stress, possibly evidenced by respiratory difficulties, inadequate oxygenation of tissues, and acidemia.

ineffective Breathing Pattern/ineffective infant Feeding Pattern may be related to immaturity of the respiratory center, poor positioning, drug-related depression and metabolic imbalances, decreased energy, fatigue, possibly evidenced by dyspnea, tachypnea, periods of apnea, nasal flaring and use of accessory muscles, cyanosis, abnormal ABGs, and tachycardia.

risk for ineffective Thermoregulation is possibly evidenced by risk factors of immature CNS development (temperature regulation center), decreased ratio of body mass to surface area, decreased subcutaneous fat, limited brown fat stores, inability to shiver or sweat, poor metabolic reserves, muted response to hypothermia, and frequent medical or nursing manipulations and interventions.*

risk for deficit Fluid Volume is possibly evidenced by risk factors of extremes of age and weight, excessive fluid losses (thin skin, lack of insulating fat, increased environmental temperature, immature kidney, and failure to concentrate urine).*

risk for disorganized infant Behavior is possibly evidenced by risk factors of prematurity (immaturity of CNS system, hypoxia), lack of

*A risk diagnosis is not evidenced by signs and symptoms, as the problem has not occurred; rather, nursing interventions are directed at prevention.

containment or boundaries, pain, overstimulation, separation from parents.*

Nephrectomy MS

acute Pain may be related to surgical tissue trauma with mechanical closure (suture), possibly evidenced by verbal reports, guarding or distraction behaviors, self-focusing, and changes in vital signs.

risk for deficient Fluid Volume is possibly evidenced by risk factors of excessive vascular losses and restricted intake.*

ineffective Breathing Pattern may be related to incisional pain with decreased lung expansion, possibly evidenced by tachypnea, fremitus, changes in respiratory depth and chest expansion, and changes in ABGs.

Constipation may be related to reduced dietary intake, decreased mobility, gastrointestinal obstruction (paralytic ileus), and incisional pain with defecation, possibly evidenced by decreased bowel sounds, reduced frequency/amount of stool, and hard, formed stool.

Nephrolithiasis MS/CH

Refer to Calculi, urinary

Nephrotic syndrome MS/CH

excess Fluid Volume may be related to compromised regulatory mechanism with changes in hydrostatic or oncotic vascular pressure and increased activation of the renin-angiotensin-aldosterone system, possibly evidenced by edema, anasarca, effusions, ascites, weight gain, intake greater than output, and BP changes.

imbalanced Nutrition: less than body requirements may be related to excessive protein losses and inability to ingest adequate nutrients (anorexia), possibly evidenced by weight loss and muscle wasting (may be difficult to assess due to edema), lack of interest in food, and observed inadequate intake.

risk for Infection is possibly evidenced by risk factors of chronic disease and steroidal suppression of inflammatory responses.*

risk for impaired Skin Integrity is possibly evidenced by risk factors of presence of edema and activity restrictions.*

Neuralgia, trigeminal CH

acute Pain may be related to neuromuscular impairment with sudden violent muscle spasm, possibly evidenced by verbal reports, guarding or distraction behaviors, self-focusing, and changes in vital signs.

deficient Knowledge [Learning Need] regarding control of recurrent episodes, medical therapies, and self-care needs may be related to lack of information or recall and misinterpretation, possibly evidenced by statements of concern, questions, and exacerbation of condition.

Neuritis CH

acute Pain/chronic Pain may be related to nerve damage usually associated with a degenerative process, possibly evidenced by verbal reports, guarding or distraction behaviors, self-focusing, and changes in vital signs.

*A risk diagnosis is not evidenced by signs and symptoms, as the problem has not occurred; rather, nursing interventions are directed at prevention.

deficient Knowledge [Learning Need] regarding underlying causative factors, treatment, and prevention may be related to lack of information, misinterpretation, possibly evidenced by statements of concern, questions, and misconceptions.

Nicotine withdrawal **CH**

readiness for enhanced Health Management possibly evidenced by expressed desire to seek higher level of wellness.

risk for Overweight is possibly evidenced by risk factor of eating in response to internal cues.*

risk for ineffective Health Management is possibly evidenced by risk factors of economic difficulties, lack of support systems, continued environmental exposure.*

Nonketotic hyperglycemic-hyperosmolar coma **MS**

deficient Fluid Volume may be related to excessive renal losses, inadequate oral intake, extremes of age, presence of infection, possibly evidenced by sudden weight loss, dry skin and mucous membranes, poor skin turgor, hypotension, increased pulse, fever, change in mental status (confusion to coma).

imbalanced Nutrition: less than body requirements may be related to decreased preload (hypovolemia), altered heart rhythm (hyper- or hypokalemia), possibly evidenced by decreased hemodynamic pressures (e.g., CVP), ECG changes, dysrhythmias.

decreased Cardiac Output may be related to inadequate utilization of nutrients (insulin deficiency), decreased oral intake, hypermetabolic state, possibly evidenced by recent weight loss, imbalance between glucose and insulin levels.

risk for Trauma is possibly evidenced by risk factors of weakness, cognitive limitations or altered consciousness, loss of large- or small-muscle coordination (risk for seizure activity).*

Obesity **CH**

Overweight may be related to food intake that exceeds body needs, psychosocial factors, socioeconomic status, possibly evidenced by weight of 20% or more over optimum body weight, excess body fat by skinfold or other measurements, reported or observed dysfunctional eating patterns, intake more than body requirements.

sedentary Lifestyle may be related to lack of interest or motivation, lack of resources, lack of training or knowledge of specific exercise needs, safety concerns, fear of injury, possibly evidenced by demonstration of physical deconditioning, choice of a daily routine lacking physical exercise.

Activity Intolerance may be related to imbalance between O_2 supply and demand, and sedentary lifestyle, possibly evidenced by fatigue or weakness, exertional discomfort, and abnormal heart rate or BP response.

risk for Sleep Deprivation is possibly evidenced by risk factors of inadequate daytime activity, discomfort, sleep apnea.*

PSY

disturbed Body Image/chronic low Self-Esteem may be related to view of self in contrast to societal values; family or subcultural encour-

*A risk diagnosis is not evidenced by signs and symptoms, as the problem has not occurred; rather, nursing interventions are directed at prevention.

agement of overeating; control, sex, and love issues; perceived failure at ability to control weight, possibly evidenced by negative feelings about body; fear of rejection or reaction of others; feeling of hopelessness, powerlessness; and lack of follow-through with treatment plan.

impaired Social Interaction may be related to self-concept disturbance, absence of or ineffective supportive SO(s), limited mobility, possibly evidenced by reluctance to participate in social gatherings, verbalized or observed discomfort in social situations, dysfunctional interactions with others, feelings of rejection.

Obsessive-compulsive disorder — PSY

[severe] Anxiety may be related to earlier life conflicts possibly evidenced by repetitive actions, recurring thoughts, decreased social and role functioning.

impaired Skin Integrity/impaired Tissue Integrity is possibly evidenced by risk factor of repetitive behaviors related to cleansing (e.g., hand washing, brushing teeth, showering).*

risk for ineffective Role Performance is possibly evidenced by risk factors of psychological stress, health-illness problems.*

Opioid abuse — CH/PSY

Refer to Depressant abuse

Organic brain syndrome — CH

Refer to Alzheimer's disease

Osteoarthritis (degenerative joint disease) — CH

Refer to Arthritis, rheumatoid

(Although this is a degenerative process versus the inflammatory process of rheumatoid arthritis, nursing concerns are the same.)

Osteomyelitis — MS/CH

acute Pain may be related to inflammation and tissue necrosis, possibly evidenced by verbal reports, guarding or distraction behaviors, self-focus, and changes in vital signs.

Hyperthermia may be related to increased metabolic rate and infectious process, possibly evidenced by increased body temperature and warm, flushed skin.

ineffective [bone] Tissue Perfusion may be related to inflammatory reaction with thrombosis of vessels, destruction of tissue, edema, and abscess formation, possibly evidenced by bone necrosis, continuation of infectious process, and delayed healing.

risk for impaired Walking is possibly evidenced by risk factors of inflammation and tissue necrosis, pain, joint instability.*

deficient Knowledge [Learning Need] regarding pathophysiology of condition, long-term therapy needs, activity restriction, and prevention of complications may be related to lack of information, misinterpretation, possibly evidenced by statements of concern, questions, and misconceptions, and inaccurate follow-through of instructions.

---

*A risk diagnosis is not evidenced by signs and symptoms, as the problem has not occurred; rather, nursing interventions are directed at prevention.

O

Osteoporosis **CH**

risk for Trauma is possibly evidenced by risk factors of loss of bone density and integrity increasing risk of fracture with minimal or no stress.*

acute Pain/chronic Pain may be related to vertebral compression on spinal nerve, muscles, and ligaments; spontaneous fractures, possibly evidenced by verbal reports, guarding or distraction behaviors, self-focus, and changes in sleep pattern.

impaired physical Mobility may be related to pain and musculoskeletal impairment, possibly evidenced by limited range of motion, reluctance to attempt movement, expressed fear of re-injury, and imposed restrictions or limitations.

Palsy, cerebral (spastic hemiplegia) **PED/CH**

impaired physical Mobility may be related to muscular weakness or hypertonicity, increased deep tendon reflexes, tendency to contractures, and underdevelopment of affected limbs, possibly evidenced by decreased muscle strength, control, mass; limited range of motion; and impaired coordination.

compromised family Coping may be related to permanent nature of condition, situational crisis, emotional conflicts, temporary family disorganization, and incomplete information or understanding of client's needs, possibly evidenced by verbalized anxiety or guilt regarding client's disability, inadequate understanding and knowledge base, and displaying protective behaviors disproportionate (too little or too much) to client's abilities or need for autonomy.

risk for disproportionate Growth and/or delayed Development are possibly evidenced by risk factors of congenital disorder/brain injury, seizure disorder, or visual/hearing impairment.*

P

Pancreatitis **MS**

acute Pain may be related to obstruction of pancreatic or biliary ducts, chemical contamination of peritoneal surfaces by pancreatic exudate, autodigestion of pancreas, extension of inflammation to the retroperitoneal nerve plexus, possibly evidenced by verbal reports, guarding or distraction behaviors, self-focusing, grimacing, changes in vital signs, and alteration in muscle tone.

risk for deficient Fluid Volume/risk for Bleeding are possibly evidenced by risk factors of excessive gastric losses (vomiting, nasogastric [NG] suctioning), increase in size of vascular bed (vasodilation, effects of kinins), third-space fluid transudation, ascites formation, alteration of clotting process.*

risk for unstable Blood Glucose Level is possibly evidenced by risk factors of compromised physical health status, excessive stress, ineffective medication management.*

imbalanced Nutrition: less than body requirements may be related to vomiting, decreased oral intake, prescribed dietary restrictions, altered ability to digest nutrients (loss of digestive enzymes), possibly evidenced by reported inadequate food intake, aversion to eating, reported altered taste sensation, weight loss, and reduced muscle mass.

---

*A risk diagnosis is not evidenced by signs and symptoms, as the problem has not occurred; rather, nursing interventions are directed at prevention.

risk for Infection is possibly evidenced by risk factors of inadequate primary defenses (stasis of body fluids, altered peristalsis, change in pH secretions), immunosuppression, nutritional deficiencies, tissue destruction, and chronic disease.*

Panic disorder PSY

Fear may be related to unfounded morbid dread of a seemingly harmless object/situation, possibly evidenced by physiological symptoms, mental/cognitive behaviors indicative of panic, withdrawal from/total avoidance of situations placing client in contact with feared object.

[severe to panic] Anxiety may be related to unidentified stressors, limitations placed on ritualistic behavior, possibly evidenced by episodes of immobilizing apprehension, behaviors indicative of panic, expressed feelings of terror or inability to cope.

Paranoid personality disorder PSY

risk for self-directed Violence/risk for other-directed Violence are possibly evidenced by risk factors of perceived threats of danger, paranoid delusions, and increased feelings of anxiety.*

[severe] Anxiety may be related to inability to trust (has not mastered task of trust versus mistrust), possibly evidenced by rigid delusional system (serves to provide relief from stress that justifies the delusion), frightened of other people and own hostility.

Powerlessness may be related to feelings of inadequacy, lifestyle of helplessness, maladaptive interpersonal interactions (e.g., misuse of power, force, abusive relationships), sense of severely impaired self-concept, and belief that individual has no control over situation(s), possibly evidenced by paranoid delusions, use of aggressive behavior to compensate, and expressions of recognition of damage paranoia has caused self and others.

[disturbed Sensory Perception (specify)] may be related to psychological stress, possibly evidenced by change in behavior pattern/usual response to stimuli.

compromised family Coping may be related to temporary or sustained family disorganization or role changes, prolonged progression of condition that exhausts the supportive capacity of SO(s), possibly evidenced by family system not meeting physical, emotional, or spiritual needs of its members; inability to express or to accept wide range of feelings, inappropriate boundary maintenance, SO(s) describe(s) preoccupation with personal reactions.

Paraplegia MS/CH

Also refer to Quadriplegia

impaired Transfer Ability may be related to loss of muscle function and control, injury to upper extremity joints (overuse).

[disturbed kinesthetic/tactile Sensory Perception] may be related to neurological deficit with loss of sensory reception and transmission, psychological stress, possibly evidenced by reported or measured change in sensory acuity, change in usual response to stimuli, anxiety, disorientation, bizarre thinking; exaggerated emotional responses.

*A risk diagnosis is not evidenced by signs and symptoms, as the problem has not occurred; rather, nursing interventions are directed at prevention.

reflex urinary Incontinence/impaired urinary Elimination may be related to disruption of bladder innervation bladder atony, fecal impaction possibly evidenced by bladder distention, retention, incontinence or overflow, urinary tract infections, kidney stone formation, renal dysfunction.

situational low Self-Esteem may be related to situational crisis, loss of body functions, change in physical abilities, perceived loss of self/identity, possibly evidenced by negative feelings about body or self, feelings of helplessness, powerlessness, delay in taking responsibility for self-care or participation in therapy, and change in social involvement.

Sexual Dysfunction may be related to loss of sensation, altered function, and vulnerability, possibly evidenced by seeking of confirmation of desirability, verbalization of concern, alteration in relationship with SO, and change in interest in self or others.

Parathyroidectomy — MS

acute Pain may be related to presence of surgical incision and effects of calcium imbalance (bone pain, tetany), possibly evidenced by verbal reports, guarding or distraction behaviors, self-focus, and changes in vital signs.

risk for excess Fluid Volume is possibly evidenced by risk factors of preoperative renal involvement, stress-induced release of antidiuretic hormone, and changing calcium and electrolyte levels.*

risk for ineffective Airway Clearance is possibly evidenced by risk factors of edema formation and laryngeal nerve damage.*

deficient Knowledge [Learning Need] regarding postoperative care, complications, and long-term needs may be related to lack of information or recall, misinterpretation, possibly evidenced by statements of concern, questions, and misconceptions.

P

Parenteral feeding — MS/CH

imbalanced Nutrition: less than body requirements may be related to conditions that interfere with nutrient intake or increase nutrient need or metabolic demand—cancer and associated treatments, anorexia, surgical procedures, dysphagia, or decreased level of consciousness, possibly evidenced by body weight 10% or more under ideal, decreased subcutaneous fat or muscle mass, for poor muscle tone.

risk for Infection is possibly evidenced by risk factors of insertion of venous catheter, malnutrition, chronic disease, or improper preparation or handling of feeding solution.*

risk for Injury [multifactor] is possibly evidenced by risk factors of catheter-related complications (air emboli or septic thrombophlebitis).*

risk for imbalanced Fluid Volume is possibly evidenced by risk factors of active loss or failure of regulatory mechanisms specific to underlying disease process or trauma, complications of therapy—high glucose solutions/hyperglycemia—hyperosmolar nonketotic coma and severe dehydration; inability to obtain or ingest fluids.*

Fatigue may be related to decreased metabolic energy production, increased energy requirements—hypermetabolic state, healing process; altered body chemistry—medications, chemotherapy; possibly

*A risk diagnosis is not evidenced by signs and symptoms, as the problem has not occurred; rather, nursing interventions are directed at prevention.

evidenced by overwhelming lack of energy, inability to maintain usual routines/accomplish routine tasks, lethargy, impaired ability to concentrate.

Parkinson's disease **CH**

impaired Walking may be related to neuromuscular impairment (muscle weakness, tremors, bradykinesia) and musculoskeletal impairment (joint rigidity), possibly evidenced by inability to move about the environment as desired, increased occurrence of falls.

impaired Swallowing may be related to neuromuscular impairment, muscle weakness, possibly evidenced by reported or observed difficulty in swallowing, drooling, evidence of aspiration (choking, coughing).

impaired verbal Communication may be related to muscle weakness and incoordination, possibly evidenced by impaired articulation, difficulty with phonation, and changes in rhythm and intonation.

risk for Stress Overload is possibly evidenced by risk factors of inadequate resources, chronic illness, physical demands.*

caregiver Role Strain may be related to illness, severity of care receiver, psychological or cognitive problems in care receiver, caregiver is spouse, duration of caregiving required, lack of respite or recreation for caregiver, possibly evidenced by feeling stressed, depressed, worried; lack of resources or support; family conflict.

Pelvic inflammatory disease **OB/GYN/CH**

risk for Infection [spread] is possibly evidenced by risk factors of presence of infectious process in highly vascular pelvic structures, delay in seeking treatment.*

acute Pain may be related to inflammation, edema, and congestion of reproductive and pelvic tissues, possibly evidenced by verbal reports, guarding or distraction behaviors, self-focus, and changes in vital signs.

Hyperthermia may be related to inflammatory process and hypermetabolic state, possibly evidenced by increased body temperature; warm, flushed skin; and tachycardia.

risk for situational low Self-Esteem is possibly evidenced by risk factors of perceived stigma of physical condition (infection of reproductive system).*

deficient Knowledge [Learning Need] regarding cause, complications of condition, therapy needs, and transmission of disease to others may be related to lack of information, misinterpretation, possibly evidenced by statements of concern, questions, misconceptions, and development of preventable complications.

Periarteritis nodosa **MS/CH**

Refer to Polyarteritis [nodosa]

Pericarditis **MS**

acute Pain may be related to tissue inflammation and presence of effusion, possibly evidenced by verbal reports of pain affected by movement or position, guarding or distraction behaviors, self-focus, and changes in vital signs.

*A risk diagnosis is not evidenced by signs and symptoms, as the problem has not occurred; rather, nursing interventions are directed at prevention.

Activity Intolerance may be related to imbalance between O_2 supply and demand (restriction of cardiac filling and ventricular contraction, reduced cardiac output), possibly evidenced by reports of weakness, fatigue, exertional dyspnea, abnormal heart rate or BP response, and signs of heart failure.

risk for decreased Cardiac Output is possibly evidenced by risk factors of accumulation of fluid (effusion), restricted cardiac filling and contractility.*

Anxiety [specify level] may be related to change in health status and perceived threat of death, possibly evidenced by increased tension, apprehension, restlessness, and expressed concerns.

Perinatal loss/death of child OB/CH

Grieving may be related to death of fetus or infant, possibly evidenced by verbal expressions of distress, anger, loss, guilt; crying; change in eating habits or sleep.

situational low Self-Esteem may be related to perceived failure at a life event, inability to meet personal expectations, possibly evidenced by negative self-appraisal in response to situation or personal actions, expressions of helplessness, hopelessness, evaluation of self as unable to deal with situation.

risk for ineffective Role Performance is possibly evidenced by risk factors of stress, family conflict, inadequate support system.*

risk for interrupted Family Processes is possibly evidenced by risk factors of situational crisis, developmental transition [loss of child], family roles shift.*

risk for Spiritual Distress is possibly evidenced by risk factors of blame for loss directed at self or higher power, intense suffering, alienation from SO or support systems. *

Peripheral arterial occlusive disease CH

Refer to Arterial occlusive disease, peripheral

Peripheral vascular disease (atherosclerosis) CH

ineffective peripheral Tissue Perfusion may be related to reduction or interruption of arterial or venous blood flow, possibly evidenced by changes in skin temperature and color, lack of hair growth, BP and pulse changes in extremity, presence of bruits, and reports of claudication.

Activity Intolerance may be related to imbalance between O_2 supply and demand, possibly evidenced by reports of muscle fatigue, weakness, and exertional discomfort (claudication).

risk for impaired Skin/Tissue Integrity are possibly evidenced by risk factors of impaired circulation, alteration in sensation.*

Peritonitis MS

risk for Infection [spread/septicemia] is possibly evidenced by risk factors of inadequate primary defenses (broken skin, traumatized tissue, altered peristalsis), inadequate secondary defenses (immunosuppression), and invasive procedures.*

deficient Fluid Volume [mixed] may be related to fluid shifts from extracellular, intravascular, and interstitial compartments into intestines

*A risk diagnosis is not evidenced by signs and symptoms, as the problem has not occurred; rather, nursing interventions are directed at prevention.

and/or peritoneal space, excessive gastric losses (vomiting, diarrhea, NG suction), fever, hypermetabolic state, and restricted intake, possibly evidenced by dry mucous membranes; poor skin turgor; delayed capillary refill; weak peripheral pulses; diminished urinary output; dark, concentrated urine; hypotension; and tachycardia.

acute Pain may be related to chemical irritation of parietal peritoneum, trauma to tissues, abdominal distention—accumulation of fluid in abdominal or peritoneal cavity, possibly evidenced by verbal reports, muscle guarding, rebound tenderness, distraction behaviors, facial mask of pain, self-focus, changes in vital signs.

risk for imbalanced Nutrition: less than body requirements is possibly evidenced by risk factors of nausea, vomiting, intestinal dysfunction, metabolic abnormalities, increased metabolic needs.*

Pheochromocytoma — MS

Anxiety [specify level] may be related to excessive physiological (hormonal) stimulation of the sympathetic nervous system, situational crises, threat to or change in health status, possibly evidenced by apprehension, shakiness, restlessness, focus on self, fearfulness, diaphoresis, and sense of impending doom.

deficient Fluid Volume [mixed] may be related to excessive gastric losses (vomiting, diarrhea), hypermetabolic state, diaphoresis, and hyperosmolar diuresis, possibly evidenced by hemoconcentration, dry mucous membranes, poor skin turgor, thirst, and weight loss.

decreased Cardiac Output/ineffective Tissue Perfusion [specify] may be related to altered preload—decreased blood volume, altered SVR, and increased sympathetic activity (excessive secretion of catecholamines), possibly evidenced by cool, clammy skin; change in BP (hypertension, postural hypotension), visual disturbances, severe headache, and angina.

deficient Knowledge [Learning Need] regarding pathophysiology of condition, outcome, preoperative and postoperative care needs may be related to lack of information or recall, possibly evidenced by statements of concern, questions, and misconceptions.

Phlebitis — CH

Refer to Thrombophlebitis

Phobia — PSY

Also refer to Anxiety disorder, generalized

Fear may be related to learned irrational response to natural or innate origins (phobic stimulus), unfounded morbid dread of a seemingly harmless object or situation, possibly evidenced by sympathetic stimulation and reactions ranging from apprehension to panic, withdrawal from or total avoidance of situations that place individual in contact with feared object.

impaired Social Interaction may be related to intense fear of encountering feared object, activity or situation; and anticipated loss of control, possibly evidenced by reported change of style or pattern of interaction, discomfort in social situations, and avoidance of phobic stimulus.

*A risk diagnosis is not evidenced by signs and symptoms, as the problem has not occurred; rather, nursing interventions are directed at prevention.

Placenta previa **OB**

risk for deficient Fluid Volume is possibly evidenced by risk factors of excessive vascular losses (vessel damage and inadequate vasoconstriction).*

impaired fetal Gas Exchange may be related to altered blood flow, altered O_2-carrying capacity of blood (maternal anemia), and decreased surface area of gas exchange at site of placental attachment, possibly evidenced by changes in fetal heart rate or activity and release of meconium.

Fear may be related to threat of death (perceived or actual) to self or fetus, possibly evidenced by verbalization of specific concerns, increased tension, sympathetic stimulation.

risk for deficient Diversional Activity is possibly evidenced by risk factors of imposed activity restrictions, bedrest.*

Pleurisy **CH**

acute Pain may be related to inflammation or irritation of the parietal pleura, possibly evidenced by verbal reports, guarding or distraction behaviors, self-focus, and changes in vital signs.

ineffective Breathing Pattern may be related to pain on inspiration, possibly evidenced by decreased respiratory depth, tachypnea, and dyspnea.

risk for Infection [pneumonia] is possibly evidenced by risk factors of stasis of pulmonary secretions, decreased lung expansion, and ineffective cough.*

Pneumonia **CH/MS**

Refer to Bronchitis; Bronchopneumonia

Pneumothorax **MS**

Also refer to Hemothorax

ineffective Breathing Pattern may be related to decreased lung expansion (fluid and air accumulation), musculoskeletal impairment, pain, inflammatory process, possibly evidenced by dyspnea, tachypnea, altered chest excursion, respiratory depth changes, use of accessory muscles and nasal flaring, cough, cyanosis, and abnormal ABGs.

risk for decreased Cardiac Output is possibly evidenced by risk factors of compression or displacement of cardiac structures.*

acute Pain may be related to irritation of nerve endings within pleural space by foreign object (chest tube), possibly evidenced by verbal reports, guarding or distraction behaviors, self-focus, and changes in vital signs.

Polyarteritis (nodosa) **MS/CH**

ineffective Tissue Perfusion [specify] may be related to reduction or interruption of blood flow, possibly evidenced by organ tissue infarctions, changes in organ function, and development of organic psychosis.

Hyperthermia may be related to widespread inflammatory process, possibly evidenced by increased body temperature and warm, flushed skin.

acute Pain may be related to inflammation, tissue ischemia, and necrosis of affected area, possibly evidenced by verbal reports, guarding or distraction behaviors, self-focus, and changes in vital signs.

---

*A risk diagnosis is not evidenced by signs and symptoms, as the problem has not occurred; rather, nursing interventions are directed at prevention.

P

Grieving may be related to perceived loss of self, possibly evidenced by expressions of sorrow and anger, altered sleep and/or eating patterns, changes in activity level, and libido.

Polycythemia vera **CH**

Activity Intolerance may be related to imbalance between O_2 supply and demand, possibly evidenced by reports of fatigue, weakness.

ineffective Tissue Perfusion [specify] may be related to reduction or interruption of arterial or venous blood flow (insufficiency, thrombosis, or hemorrhage), possibly evidenced by pain in affected area, impaired mental ability, visual disturbances, and color changes of skin or mucous membranes.

Polyradiculitis **MS**

Refer to Guillain-Barré syndrome

Postoperative recovery period **MS**

ineffective Breathing Pattern may be related to neuromuscular and perceptual or cognitive impairment, decreased lung expansion and energy, and tracheobronchial obstruction, possibly evidenced by changes in respiratory rate and depth, reduced vital capacity, apnea, cyanosis, and noisy respirations.

risk for imbalanced Body Temperature is possibly evidenced by risk factors of exposure to cool environment, effect of medications/anesthetic agents, extremes of age or weight, and dehydration.*

risk for acute Confusion is possibly evidenced by risk factors of pharmaceutical agents—anesthesia, pain.

risk for deficient Fluid Volume is possibly evidenced by risk factors of restriction of oral intake, loss of fluid through abnormal routes (indwelling tubes, drains) and normal routes (vomiting, loss of vascular integrity, changes in clotting ability), extremes of age and weight.*

acute Pain may be related to disruption of skin, tissue, and muscle integrity; musculoskeletal/bone trauma; and presence of tubes and drains, possibly evidenced by verbal reports, alteration in muscle tone, facial mask of pain, distraction or guarding behaviors, narrowed focus, and changes in vital signs.

impaired Skin/Tissue Integrity may be related to mechanical interruption of skin and tissues, altered circulation, effects of medication, accumulation of drainage, and altered metabolic state, possibly evidenced by disruption of skin surface, skin layers, and tissues.

risk for Infection possibly evidenced by risk factors of broken skin, traumatized tissues, stasis of body fluids, presence of pathogens or contaminants, environmental exposure, and invasive procedures.*

Postpartal period **OB/CH**

readiness for enhanced Family Processes possibly evidenced by expressing willingness to enhance family dynamics.

risk for deficient Fluid Volume/risk for Bleeding are possibly evidenced by risk factors of excessive blood loss during delivery, reduced intake, inadequate replacement, nausea, vomiting, increased urine output, and insensible losses.*

---

*A risk diagnosis is not evidenced by signs and symptoms, as the problem has not occurred; rather, nursing interventions are directed at prevention.

acute Pain/impaired Comfort may be related to tissue trauma and edema, muscle contractions, bladder fullness, and physical or psychological exhaustion, possibly evidenced by reports of cramping (afterpains), self-focusing, alteration in muscle tone, distraction behaviors, and changes in vital signs.
impaired urinary Elimination may be related to hormonal effects (fluid shifts, continued elevation in renal plasma flow), mechanical trauma, tissue edema, and effects of medication and anesthesia, possibly evidenced by frequency, dysuria, urgency, incontinence, or retention.
Constipation may be related to decreased muscle tone associated with diastasis recti, prenatal effects of progesterone, dehydration, excess analgesia or anesthesia, pain (hemorrhoids, episiotomy, or perineal tenderness), prelabor diarrhea and lack of intake, possibly evidenced by frequency less than usual pattern, hard-formed stool, straining at stool, decreased bowel sounds, and abdominal distention.
Insomnia may be related to pain or discomfort, intense exhilaration and excitement, anxiety, exhausting process of labor and delivery, and needs/demands of family members, possibly evidenced by verbal reports of difficulty in falling or staying asleep, dissatisfaction with sleep, lack of energy, nonrestorative sleep.
risk for impaired Attachment/Parenting is possibly evidenced by risk factors of lack of support between or from SO(s), ineffective or no role model, anxiety associated with the parental role, unrealistic expectations, presence of stressors (e.g., financial, housing, employment).*

Postpartum psychosis OB/PSY

Also refer to Depression, postpartum
ineffective Coping may be related to situational/maturational crisis, inadequate level of confidence in ability to cope, inadequate level of perception of control, possibly evidenced by inability to meet basic needs, inability to problem-solve, sleep pattern disturbance, poor concentration.
risk for other-directed Violence is possibly evidenced by risk factors of mood swings, increased anxiety, despondency, hopelessness, psychotic symptomatology.*

P

Post-traumatic stress disorder PSY

Post-Trauma Syndrome related to having experienced a traumatic life event, possibly evidenced by reexperiencing the event, somatic reactions, psychic or emotional numbness, altered lifestyle, impaired sleep, self-destructive behaviors, difficulty with interpersonal relationships, development of phobia, poor impulse control/irritability, and explosiveness.
risk for other-directed Violence is possibly evidenced by risk factors of startle reaction, an intrusive memory causing a sudden acting out of a feeling as if the event were occurring, use of alcohol or other drugs to ward off painful effects and produce psychic numbing, breaking through the rage that has been walled off, response to intense anxiety or panic state, and loss of control.*
ineffective Coping may be related to personal vulnerability, inadequate support systems, unrealistic perceptions, unmet expectations, over-

*A risk diagnosis is not evidenced by signs and symptoms, as the problem has not occurred; rather, nursing interventions are directed at prevention.

whelming threat to self, and multiple stressors repeated over a period of time, possibly evidenced by verbalization of inability to cope or difficulty asking for help, muscular tension, headaches, chronic worry, and emotional tension.

complicated Grieving may be related to actual or perceived object loss (loss of self as seen before the traumatic incident occurred, as well as other losses incurred in/after the incident), loss of physiopsychosocial well-being, thwarted grieving response to a loss, and lack of resolution of previous grieving responses, possibly evidenced by verbal expression of distress at loss, anger, sadness, labile affect; alterations in eating habits, sleep/dream patterns, libido; reliving of past experiences, expression of guilt, and alterations in concentration.

interrupted Family Processes may be related to situational crisis, failure to master developmental transitions, possibly evidenced by expressions of confusion about what to do and that family is having difficulty coping; family system not meeting physical, emotional, or spiritual needs of its members; not adapting to change or dealing with traumatic experience constructively; and ineffective family decision-making process.

Pregnancy (prenatal period) 1st trimester OB/CH

risk for imbalanced Nutrition: less than body requirements is possibly evidenced by risk factors of changes in appetite, insufficient intake (nausea, vomiting, inadequate financial resources and nutritional knowledge), meeting increased metabolic demands (increased thyroid activity associated with the growth of fetal and maternal tissues).*

impaired Comfort may be related to hormonal influences, physical changes, possibly evidenced by verbal reports (nausea, breast changes, leg cramps, hemorrhoids, nasal stuffiness), alteration in muscle tone, inability to relax.

risk for disturbed Maternal-Fetal Dyad is possibly evidenced by risk factors of environmental and hereditary factors, problems of maternal well-being (e.g., malnutrition, substance use).*

[maximally compensated] Cardiac Output may be related to increased fluid volume and maximal cardiac effort, hormonal effects of progesterone and relaxin (places the client at risk for hypertension and/or circulatory failure), and changes in peripheral resistance (afterload), possibly evidenced by variations in BP and pulse, syncopal episodes, presence of pathological edema.

readiness for enhanced family Coping is possibly evidenced by movement toward health-promoting and enriching lifestyle, choosing experiences that optimize pregnancy experience and wellness.

risk for Constipation is possibly evidenced by risk factors of changes in dietary and fluid intake, smooth muscle relaxation, decreased peristalsis, and effects of medications (e.g., iron).*

Fatigue/Insomnia may be related to increased carbohydrate metabolism, altered body chemistry, increased energy requirements to perform ADLs, discomfort, anxiety, inactivity, possibly evidenced by reports of overwhelming lack of energy, inability to maintain usual routines, difficulty falling asleep, dissatisfaction with sleep, decreased quality of life.

P

*A risk diagnosis is not evidenced by signs and symptoms, as the problem has not occurred; rather, nursing interventions are directed at prevention.

risk for ineffective Role Performance is possibly evidenced by risk factors of maturational crisis, developmental level, history of maladaptive coping, absence of support systems.*

deficient Knowledge [Learning Need] regarding normal physiological/psychological changes and self-care needs may be related to lack of information or recall, and misinterpretation of normal physiological and psychological changes and their impact on the client/family, possibly evidenced by questions, statements of concern, misconceptions, and inaccurate follow-through of instructions, development of preventable complications.

Pregnancy (prenatal period) 2nd trimester OB/CH

Also refer to Pregnancy (prenatal period) 1st trimester

disturbed Body Image is possibly evidenced by risk factors of perception of biophysical changes, response of others.*

ineffective Breathing Pattern may be related to impingement of the diaphragm by enlarging uterus, possibly evidenced by reports of shortness of breath, dyspnea, and changes in respiratory depth.

risk for [decompensated] Cardiac Output is possibly evidenced by risk factors of increased circulatory demand, changes in preload (decreased venous return) and afterload (increased peripheral vascular resistance), and ventricular hypertrophy.*

risk for excess Fluid Volume is possibly evidenced by risk factors of changes in regulatory mechanisms, sodium and water retention.*

Sexual Dysfunction may be related to conflict regarding changes in sexual desire and expectations, fear of physical injury to woman or fetus, possibly evidenced by reported difficulties, limitations, or changes in sexual behaviors or activities.

Pregnancy (prenatal period) 3rd trimester OB/CH

Also refer to Pregnancy (prenatal period) 1st trimester; Pregnancy (prenatal period) 2nd trimester

deficient Knowledge [Learning Need] regarding preparation for labor and delivery, infant care may be related to lack of exposure or experience, misinterpretations of information, possibly evidenced by request for information, statement of concerns, misconceptions.

impaired urinary Elimination may be related to uterine enlargement, increased abdominal pressure, fluctuation of renal blood flow, and GFR, possibly evidenced by urinary frequency, urgency, dependent edema.

risk for ineffective Coping/compromised family Coping are possibly evidenced by risk factors of situational or maturational crisis, personal vulnerability, unrealistic perceptions, absent or insufficient support systems.*

risk for disturbed Maternal-Fetal Dyad is possibly evidenced by risk factors of presence of hypertension, infection, substance use or abuse, altered immune system, abnormal blood profile, tissue hypoxia, premature rupture of membranes.*

Pregnancy, adolescent OB/CH

Also refer to Pregnancy (prenatal period) 1st trimester; Pregnancy (prenatal period) 2nd trimester; Pregnancy (prenatal period) 3rd trimester

*A risk diagnosis is not evidenced by signs and symptoms, as the problem has not occurred; rather, nursing interventions are directed at prevention.

P

interrupted Family Processes may be related to situational or developmental transition (economic, change in roles, gain of a family member), possibly evidenced by family expressing confusion about what to do, unable to meet physical, emotional, or spiritual needs of the members; family inability to adapt to change or to deal with traumatic experience constructively, does not demonstrate respect for individuality and autonomy of its members, ineffective family decision-making process, and inappropriate boundary maintenance.

Social Isolation may be related to alterations in physical appearance, perceived unacceptable social behavior, restricted social sphere, stage of adolescence, and interference with accomplishing developmental tasks, possibly evidenced by expressions of feelings of aloneness, rejection, or difference from others; uncommunicative, withdrawn, no eye contact, seeking to be alone, unacceptable behavior, and absence of supportive SO(s).

situational low Self-Esteem/chronic low Self-Esteem may be related to situational or maturational crisis, biophysical changes, and fear of failure at life events, absence of support systems, possibly evidenced by self-negating verbalizations, expressions of shame, guilt, fear of rejection or reaction of other, hypersensitivity to criticism, and lack of follow-through or nonparticipation in prenatal care.

deficient Knowledge [Learning Need] regarding pregnancy, developmental or individual needs, future expectations may be related to lack of exposure, information misinterpretation, unfamiliarity with information resources, lack of interest in learning, possibly evidenced by questions, statement of concern, misconception, sense of vulnerability, denial of reality, inaccurate follow-through of instruction, and development of preventable complications.

risk for impaired Parenting is possibly evidenced by risk factors of young parental age, insufficient cognitive readiness for parenting; unplanned pregnancy, stressors, low self-esteem, social isolation, or insufficient family cohesiveness.*

P

Pregnancy, high-risk **OB/CH**

Also refer to Pregnancy (prenatal period) 1st trimester; Pregnancy (prenatal period) 2nd trimester; Pregnancy (prenatal period) 3rd trimester

Anxiety [specify level] may be related to situational crisis, threat of maternal or fetal death (perceived or actual), interpersonal transmission and contagion, possibly evidenced by increased tension, apprehension, feelings of inadequacy, somatic complaints, difficulty sleeping.

deficient Knowledge [Learning Need] regarding high-risk situation/preterm labor may be related to lack of exposure to or misinterpretation of information, unfamiliarity with individual risks and own role in risk prevention and management, possibly evidenced by request for information, statement of concerns, misconceptions, inaccurate follow-through of instructions.

risk for maternal Injury is possibly evidenced by risk factors of preexisting medical conditions, complications of pregnancy.*

risk for Activity Intolerance is possibly evidenced by risk factors of presence of circulatory or respiratory problems, uterine irritability.*

---

*A risk diagnosis is not evidenced by signs and symptoms, as the problem has not occurred; rather, nursing interventions are directed at prevention.

risk for ineffective Health Management is possibly evidenced by risk factors of client value system, health beliefs and cultural influences, issues of control, presence of anxiety, complexity of therapeutic regimen, economic difficulties, perceived susceptibility.*

Pregnancy-induced hypertension (preeclampsia) **OB/CH**

Also refer to Eclampsia

deficient Fluid Volume may be related to a plasma protein loss, decreasing plasma colloid osmotic pressure allowing fluid shifts out of vascular compartment, possibly evidenced by edema formation, sudden weight gain, hemoconcentration, nausea, vomiting, epigastric pain, headaches, visual changes, decreased urine output.

decreased Cardiac Output may be related to hypovolemia/decreased venous return, increased SVR, possibly evidenced by variations in BP and hemodynamic readings, edema, shortness of breath, change in mental status.

risk for disturbed Maternal-Fetal Dyad is possibly evidenced by risk factors of vasospasm of spiral arteries and relative hypovolemia.*

deficient Knowledge [Learning Need] regarding pathophysiology of condition, therapy, self-care and nutritional needs, and potential complications may be related to lack of information or recall, misinterpretation, possibly evidenced by statements of concern, questions, misconceptions, inaccurate follow-through of instructions, or development of preventable complications.

Premenstrual dysphoric disorder **GYN/PSY**

acute Pain/chronic Pain may be related to cyclic changes in female hormones affecting other systems (e.g., vascular congestion or spasms), vitamin deficiency, fluid retention, possibly evidenced by increased tension, apprehension, jitteriness, verbal reports, distraction behaviors, somatic complaints, self-focusing, physical and social withdrawal.

excess Fluid Volume may be related to abnormal alterations of hormonal levels, possibly evidenced by edema formation, weight gain, and periodic changes in emotional status, irritability.

[moderate to panic] Anxiety may be related to cyclic changes in female hormones affecting other systems, possibly evidenced by feelings of inability to cope or loss of control, depersonalization, increased tension, apprehension, jitteriness, somatic complaints, and impaired functioning.

ineffective Coping may be related to personal vulnerability, threat to self-concept, multiple stressors, possibly evidenced by reports inability to cope, inadequate problem-solving, sleep pattern disturbance.

deficient Knowledge [Learning Need] regarding pathophysiology of condition and self-care/treatment needs may be related to lack of information, misinterpretation, possibly evidenced by statements of concern, questions, misconceptions, and continuation of condition, exacerbating symptoms.

Premenstrual tension syndrome (PMS) **GYN/CH**

Refer to Premenstrual dysphoric disorder

*A risk diagnosis is not evidenced by signs and symptoms, as the problem has not occurred; rather, nursing interventions are directed at prevention.

Pressure ulcer or sore **CH**

Also refer to Ulcer, decubitus

ineffective peripheral Tissue Perfusion may be related to reduced or interrupted blood flow, possibly evidenced by presence of inflamed, necrotic lesion.

deficient Knowledge [Learning Need] regarding cause/prevention of condition and potential complications may be related to lack of information, misinterpretation, possibly evidenced by statements of concern, questions, misconceptions, and inaccurate follow-through of instructions.

Preterm labor **OB/CH**

Refer to Labor, preterm

Prostatectomy **MS**

impaired urinary Elimination may be related to mechanical obstruction (blood clots, edema, trauma, surgical procedure, pressure or irritation of catheter and balloon) and loss of bladder tone, possibly evidenced by dysuria, frequency, dribbling, incontinence, retention, bladder fullness, suprapubic discomfort.

risk for deficient Fluid Volume/risk for Bleeding are possibly evidenced by risk factors of trauma to highly vascular area with excessive vascular losses, restricted intake, postobstructive diuresis.*

acute Pain may be related to irritation of bladder mucosa and tissue trauma or edema, possibly evidenced by verbal reports (bladder spasms), distraction behaviors, self-focus, and changes in vital signs.

disturbed Body Image may be related to perceived threat of altered body or sexual function, possibly evidenced by preoccupation with change or loss, negative feelings about body, and statements of concern regarding functioning.

CH

risk for Sexual Dysfunction is possibly evidenced by risk factors of situational crisis (incontinence, leakage of urine after catheter removal, involvement of genital area) and threat to self-concept or change in health status.*

Pruritus **CH**

acute Pain/impaired Comfort may be related to cutaneous hyperesthesia and inflammation, possibly evidenced by verbal reports, distraction behaviors, and self-focus.

risk for impaired Skin Integrity is possibly evidenced by risk factors of mechanical trauma (scratching) and development of vesicles or bullae that may rupture.*

Psoriasis **CH**

impaired Skin Integrity may be related to increased epidermal cell proliferation and absence of normal protective skin layers, possibly evidenced by scaling papules and plaques.

disturbed Body Image may be related to cosmetically unsightly skin lesions, possibly evidenced by hiding affected body part, negative

*A risk diagnosis is not evidenced by signs and symptoms, as the problem has not occurred; rather, nursing interventions are directed at prevention.

feelings about body, feelings of helplessness, and change in social involvement.

Pulmonary edema **MS**

impaired Gas Exchange may be related to alveolar-capillary membrane changes (fluid collection or shifts into interstitial space or alveoli), possibly evidenced by dyspnea, restlessness, irritability, abnormal rate/depth of respirations, lethargy, confusion.

[moderate to severe] Anxiety may be related to change in health status, threat of death, interpersonal transmission possibly evidenced by expressed concerns, distress, apprehension, extraneous movement.

risk for impaired spontaneous Ventilation is possibly evidenced by risk factors of respiratory muscle fatigue, problems with secretion management.*

Pulmonary edema, high-altitude **MS**

Refer to High-altitude pulmonary edema (HAPE)

Pulmonary embolus **MS**

ineffective Breathing Pattern may be related to tracheobronchial obstruction (inflammation, copious secretions, or active bleeding), decreased lung expansion, inflammatory process, possibly evidenced by changes in depth and/or rate of respiration, dyspnea, use of accessory muscles, altered chest excursion, abnormal breath sounds (crackles, wheezes), and cough (with or without sputum production).

impaired Gas Exchange may be related to ventilation-perfusion imbalance, alveolar-capillary membrane changes (atelectasis, airway or alveolar collapse, pulmonary edema or effusion, excessive secretions or active bleeding), possibly evidenced by profound dyspnea, restlessness, apprehension, somnolence, cyanosis, and changes in ABGs or pulse oximetry (hypoxemia and hypercapnia).

Fear/Anxiety [specify level] may be related to severe dyspnea and inability to breathe normally, perceived threat of death, threat to or change in health status, physiological response to hypoxemia and acidosis, and concern regarding unknown outcome of situation, possibly evidenced by restlessness, irritability, withdrawal or attack behavior, sympathetic stimulation (cardiovascular excitation, pupil dilation, sweating, vomiting, diarrhea), crying, voice quivering, and impending sense of doom.

Pulmonary hypertension **CH/MS**

impaired Gas Exchange may be related to changes in alveolar membrane, increased pulmonary vascular resistance, possibly evidenced by dyspnea, irritability, decreased mental acuity, somnolence, abnormal ABGs.

decreased Cardiac Output may be related to increased pulmonary vascular resistance, decreased blood return to left side of heart, possibly evidenced by increased heart rate, dyspnea, fatigue.

Activity Intolerance may be related to imbalance between O_2 supply and demand, possibly evidenced by reports of weakness, fatigue, abnormal vital signs with activity.

*A risk diagnosis is not evidenced by signs and symptoms, as the problem has not occurred; rather, nursing interventions are directed at prevention.

Anxiety may be related to change in health status, stress, threat to self-concept, possibly evidenced by expressed concerns, uncertainty, awareness of physiological symptoms, diminished productivity or ability to problem-solve.

Purpura, idiopathic thrombocytopenic **CH**

ineffective Protection may be related to abnormal blood profile, drug therapy (corticosteroids or immunosuppressive agents), possibly evidenced by altered clotting, fatigue, deficient immunity.

Activity Intolerance may be related to decreased O_2-carrying capacity/imbalance between O_2 supply and demand, possibly evidenced by reports of fatigue, weakness.

deficient Knowledge [Learning Need] regarding therapy choices, outcomes, and self-care needs may be related to lack of information/misinterpretation, possibly evidenced by statements of concern, questions, and misconceptions.

Pyelonephritis **MS**

acute Pain may be related to acute inflammation of renal tissues, possibly evidenced by verbal reports, guarding/distraction behaviors, self-focus, and changes in vital signs.

Hyperthermia may be related to inflammatory process and increased metabolic rate, possibly evidenced by increase in body temperature; warm, flushed skin; tachycardia; and chills.

impaired urinary Elimination may be related to inflammation or irritation of bladder mucosa, possibly evidenced by dysuria, urgency, and frequency.

deficient Knowledge [Learning Need] regarding therapy needs and prevention may be related to lack of information, misinterpretation, possibly evidenced by statements of concern, questions, misconceptions, and recurrence of condition.

Quadriplegia **MS/CH**

Also refer to Paraplegia

ineffective Breathing Pattern may be related to neuromuscular impairment of innervation of diaphragm—lesions at or above C5, complete or mixed loss of intercostal muscle function, reflex abdominal spasms, gastric distention, possibly evidenced by decreased respiratory depth, dyspnea, cyanosis, and abnormal ABGs.

risk for Trauma [additional spinal injury] is possibly evidenced by risk factors of temporary weakness or instability of spinal column.*

Grieving may be related to perceived loss of self, anticipated alterations in lifestyle and expectations, and limitation of future options or choices, possibly evidenced by expressions of distress, anger, sorrow, choked feelings, and changes in eating habits, sleep, communication patterns.

[total] Self-Care Deficit related to neuromuscular impairment, evidenced by inability to perform self-care tasks.

bowel Incontinence/Constipation may be related to disruption of nerve innervation, perceptual impairment, changes in dietary and fluid intake, change in activity level, side effects of medication possibly evidenced by inability to evacuate bowel voluntarily; increased ab-

*A risk diagnosis is not evidenced by signs and symptoms, as the problem has not occurred; rather, nursing interventions are directed at prevention.

dominal pressure or distention; dry, hard-formed stool; change in bowel sounds.

impaired bed Mobility/impaired wheelchair Mobility may be related to loss of muscle function and control possibly evidenced by inability to reposition self, impaired ability to operate wheelchair.

risk for Autonomic Dysreflexia is possibly evidenced by risk factors of altered nerve function (spinal cord injury at T6 or above), bladder, bowel, or skin stimulation (tactile, pain, thermal).*

impaired Home Maintenance may be related to permanent effects of injury, inadequate or absent support systems and finances, and lack of familiarity with resources, possibly evidenced by expressions of difficulties, requests for information and assistance, outstanding debts or financial crisis, and lack of necessary aids and equipment.

Rape **CH**

deficient Knowledge [Learning Need] regarding required medical and legal procedures, prophylactic treatment for individual concerns (STDs, pregnancy), community resources and supports may be related to lack of information, possibly evidenced by statements of concern, questions, misconceptions, and exacerbation of symptoms.

Rape-Trauma Syndrome related to actual or attempted sexual penetration without consent, possibly evidenced by wide range of emotional reactions, including anxiety, fear, anger, embarrassment, and multisystem physical complaints.

impaired Tissue Integrity is possibly evidenced by risk factors of forceful sexual penetration and trauma to fragile tissues.*

PSY

ineffective Coping may be related to personal vulnerability, unmet expectations, unrealistic perceptions, inadequate support systems or coping methods, multiple stressors repeated over time, overwhelming threat to self, possibly evidenced by verbalizations of inability to cope or difficulty asking for help, muscular tension, headaches, emotional tension, chronic worry.

Sexual Dysfunction may be related to biopsychosocial alteration of sexuality (stress of post-trauma response), vulnerability, loss of sexual desire, impaired relationship with SO, possibly evidenced by alteration in achieving sexual satisfaction, change in interest in self or others, preoccupation with self.

Raynaud's phenomenon **CH**

acute Pain/chronic Pain may be related to vasospasm or altered perfusion of affected tissues, ischemia or destruction of tissues, possibly evidenced by verbal reports, guarding of affected parts, self-focusing, and restlessness.

ineffective peripheral Tissue Perfusion may be related to periodic reduction of arterial blood flow to affected areas, possibly evidenced by pallor, cyanosis, coolness, numbness, paresthesia, slow healing of lesions.

deficient Knowledge [Learning Need] regarding pathophysiology of condition, potential for complications, therapy and self-care needs may be related to lack of information, misinterpretation, possibly

*A risk diagnosis is not evidenced by signs and symptoms, as the problem has not occurred; rather, nursing interventions are directed at prevention.

evidenced by statements of concern, questions, and misconceptions; development of preventable complications.

Reflex sympathetic dystrophy (RSD) **CH**
Refer to Complex regional pain syndrome

Regional enteritis **CH**
Refer to Crohn's disease

Renal failure, acute (Kidney injury, acute) **MS**
excess Fluid Volume may be related to compromised regulatory mechanisms—decreased kidney function, possibly evidenced by weight gain, edema or anasarca, intake greater than output, venous congestion, changes in BP and CVP, and altered electrolyte levels, decreased Hb and Hct; pulmonary congestion on x-ray.
risk for imbalanced Nutrition: less than body requirements is possibly evidenced by risk factors of inability to ingest or digest adequate nutrients—anorexia, nausea, vomiting, ulcerations of oral mucosa, and increased metabolic needs; protein catabolism, therapeutic dietary restrictions.*
risk for Infection is possibly evidenced by risk factors of depression of immunological defenses, invasive procedures and devices, changes in dietary intake, malnutrition.*
risk for acute Confusion is possibly evidenced by risk factors of accumulation of toxic waste products and altered cerebral perfusion.*

Renal failure, chronic **CH/MS**
Also refer to Dialysis, general
risk for decreased Cardiac Output is possibly evidenced by risk factors of fluid imbalances affecting circulating volume, myocardial workload, SVR; alterations in rate, rhythm, cardiac conduction—electrolyte imbalances, hypoxia; accumulation of toxins—urea; soft tissue calcification—deposits of calcium phosphate.*
risk for Bleeding is possibly evidenced by risk factors of abnormal blood profile—suppressed erythropoietin production or secretion, decreased RBC production and survival, altered clotting factors; increased capillary fragility.*
risk for acute Confusion is possibly evidenced by risk factors of electrolyte imbalance, increased BUN/creatinine, azotemia.
risk for impaired Skin Integrity is possibly evidenced by risk factors of altered metabolic state and circulation (anemia with tissue ischemia), altered sensation (peripheral neuropathy), decreased skin turgor, reduced activity or immobility, accumulation of toxins in the skin.*
risk for impaired oral Mucous Membrane is possibly evidenced by risk factors of decreased or lack of salivation, fluid restrictions, chemical irritation, conversion of urea in saliva to ammonia.*

Renal transplantation **MS**
risk for excess Fluid Volume is possibly evidenced by risk factors of compromised regulatory mechanism (implantation of new kidney requiring adjustment period for optimal functioning).*

*A risk diagnosis is not evidenced by signs and symptoms, as the problem has not occurred; rather, nursing interventions are directed at prevention.

R

disturbed Body Image may be related to failure and subsequent replacement of body part and medication-induced changes in appearance, possibly evidenced by preoccupation with loss or change, negative feelings about body, and focus on past strength or function.
Fear may be related to potential for transplant rejection or failure and threat of death, possibly evidenced by increased tension, apprehension, concentration on source, and verbalizations of concern.
risk for Infection is possibly evidenced by risk factors of broken skin, traumatized tissue, stasis of body fluids, immunosuppression, invasive procedures, nutritional deficits, and chronic disease.*

CH

risk for ineffective Coping/risk for compromised family Coping is possibly evidenced by risk factors of situational crises, family disorganization and role changes, prolonged disease exhausting supportive capacity of SO(s)/family, therapeutic restrictions, long-term therapy needs.*

Respiratory distress syndrome, acute **MS**

ineffective Airway Clearance may be related to loss of ciliary action, increased amount and viscosity of secretions, and increased airway resistance, possibly evidenced by presence of dyspnea, changes in depth and rate of respiration, use of accessory muscles for breathing, wheezes and crackles, cough with or without sputum production.
impaired Gas Exchange may be related to changes in pulmonary capillary permeability with edema formation, alveolar hypoventilation and collapse, with intrapulmonary shunting, possibly evidenced by tachypnea, use of accessory muscles, cyanosis, hypoxia per ABGs or oximetry, anxiety, and changes in mentation.
risk for deficient Fluid Volume is possibly evidenced by risk factors of active loss from diuretic use and restricted intake.*
risk for decreased Cardiac Output is possibly evidenced by risk factors of alteration in preload (hypovolemia, vascular pooling, diuretic therapy, and increased intrathoracic pressure, use of ventilator and positive end-expiratory pressure [PEEP]).*
Anxiety [specify level]/Fear may be related to physiological factors (effects of hypoxemia), situational crisis, change in health status and threat of death possibly evidenced by increased tension, apprehension, restlessness, focus on self, and sympathetic stimulation.
risk for [barotrauma] Injury is possibly evidenced by risk factor of increased airway pressure associated with mechanical ventilation (PEEP).*

Respiratory distress syndrome (premature infant) **PED**

Also refer to Neonatal, premature newborn
impaired Gas Exchange may be related to alveolar-capillary membrane changes (inadequate surfactant levels), altered O_2 supply (tracheobronchial obstruction, atelectasis), altered blood flow (immaturity of pulmonary arteriole musculature), altered O_2-carrying capacity of blood (anemia), and cold stress, possibly evidenced by tachypnea,

*A risk diagnosis is not evidenced by signs and symptoms, as the problem has not occurred; rather, nursing interventions are directed at prevention.

use of accessory muscles—retractions, expiratory grunting, pallor, or cyanosis, abnormal ABGs, and tachycardia.

impaired spontaneous Ventilation may be related to respiratory muscle fatigue and metabolic factors, possibly evidenced by dyspnea, increased metabolic rate, restlessness, use of accessory muscles, and abnormal ABGs.

risk for Infection is possibly evidenced by risk factors of inadequate primary defenses (decreased ciliary action, stasis of body fluids, traumatized tissues), inadequate secondary defenses (deficiency of neutrophils and specific immunoglobulins), invasive procedures, and malnutrition (absence of nutrient stores, increased metabolic demands).*

risk for ineffective Gastrointestinal Perfusion possibly evidenced by risk factors of persistent fetal circulation and exchange problems.*

risk for impaired Attachment is possibly evidenced by risk factors of premature or ill infant who is unable to effectively initiate parental contact (altered behavioral organization), separation, physical barriers, anxiety associated with the parental role and demands of infant.*

Respiratory syncytial virus (RSV) **PED**

impaired Gas Exchange may be related to inflammation of airways, ventilation perfusion imbalance, apnea, possibly evidenced by dyspnea, abnormal arterial blood gases/hypoxia.

ineffective Airway Clearance may be related to infection, retained secretions, exudate in the alveoli, possibly evidenced by dyspnea, adventitious breath sounds, ineffective cough.

risk for deficient Fluid Volume is possibly evidenced by risk factors of increased insensible losses (fever, diaphoresis), decreased oral intake.*

Retinal detachment **CH**

[disturbed visual Sensory Perception] related to decreased sensory reception, possibly evidenced by visual distortions, decreased visual field, and changes in visual acuity.

deficient Knowledge [Learning Need] regarding therapy, prognosis, and self-care needs may be related to lack of information or misconceptions, possibly evidenced by statements of concern and questions.

risk for impaired Home Maintenance is possibly evidenced by risk factors of visual limitations, activity restrictions.*

Reye's syndrome **PED**

deficient Fluid Volume may be related to failure of regulatory mechanism (diabetes insipidus), excessive gastric losses (pernicious vomiting), and altered intake, possibly evidenced by increased/dilute urine output, sudden weight loss, decreased venous filling, dry mucous membranes, decreased skin turgor, hypotension, and tachycardia.

ineffective cerebral Tissue Perfusion may be related to diminished arterial or venous blood flow and hypovolemia, possibly evidenced by memory loss, altered consciousness, and restlessness or agitation.

---

*A risk diagnosis is not evidenced by signs and symptoms, as the problem has not occurred; rather, nursing interventions are directed at prevention.

risk for Trauma is possibly evidenced by risk factors of generalized weakness, reduced coordination, and cognitive deficits.*

ineffective Breathing Pattern may be related to decreased energy and fatigue, cognitive impairment, tracheobronchial obstruction, and inflammatory process (aspiration pneumonia), possibly evidenced by tachypnea, abnormal ABGs, cough, and use of accessory muscles.

Rheumatic fever — PED

acute Pain may be related to migratory inflammation of joints, possibly evidenced by verbal reports, guarding or distraction behaviors, self-focus, and changes in vital signs.

Hyperthermia may be related to inflammatory process, hypermetabolic state, possibly evidenced by increased body temperature; warm, flushed skin; and tachycardia.

Activity Intolerance may be related to generalized weakness, joint pain, medical restrictions, and bedrest, possibly evidenced by reports of fatigue, exertional discomfort, and abnormal heart rate in response to activity.

risk for decreased Cardiac Output is possibly evidenced by risk factors of altered contractility.*

Rickets (osteomalacia) — PED

risk for disproportionate Growth and/or delayed Development is possibly evidenced by risk factors of chronic illness, economically disadvantaged, malnutrition, and prematurity.

deficient Knowledge [Learning Need] regarding cause, pathophysiology, therapy needs, and prevention may be related to lack of information, possibly evidenced by statements of concern, questions, misconceptions, and inaccurate follow-through of instructions.

Ringworm, tinea — CH

Also refer to Athlete's Foot

impaired Skin Integrity may be related to fungal infection of the dermis, possibly evidenced by disruption of skin surfaces—presence of lesions.

deficient Knowledge [Learning Need] regarding infectious nature, therapy, and self-care needs may be related to lack of information, misinformation, possibly evidenced by statements of concern, questions, and recurrence or spread.

Rubella — PED/CH

acute Pain/impaired Comfort may be related to inflammatory effects of viral infection and presence of desquamating rash, possibly evidenced by verbal reports, distraction behaviors, restlessness.

deficient Knowledge [Learning Need] regarding contagious nature, possible complications, and self-care needs may be related to lack of information, misinterpretations, possibly evidenced by statements of concern, questions, and inaccurate follow-through of instructions.

Scabies — CH

impaired Skin Integrity may be related to presence of invasive parasites and development of pruritus, possibly evidenced by disruption of skin surface and inflammation.

---

*A risk diagnosis is not evidenced by signs and symptoms, as the problem has not occurred; rather, nursing interventions are directed at prevention.

S

deficient Knowledge [Learning Need] regarding communicable nature, possible complications, therapy, and self-care needs may be related to lack of information, misinterpretation, possibly evidenced by questions and statements of concern about spread to others.

Scarlet fever **PED**

Hyperthermia may be related to effects of circulating toxins, possibly evidenced by increased body temperature; warm, flushed skin; and tachycardia.

acute Pain/impaired Comfort may be related to inflammation of mucous membranes and effects of circulating toxins (malaise, fever), possibly evidenced by verbal reports, distraction behaviors, guarding (decreased swallowing), and self-focus.

risk for deficient Fluid Volume is possibly evidenced by risk factors of hypermetabolic state (hyperthermia) and reduced intake.*

Schizophrenia (schizophrenic disorders) **PSY/CH**

[disturbed Sensory Perception (specify)] may be related to biochemical/electrolyte imbalance, psychological stress, possibly evidenced by disorientation to space/time, hallucinations, change in behavior pattern.

impaired verbal Communication may be related to altered perceptions, alteration in self-concept, psychological barriers (e.g., psychosis), possibly evidenced by inappropriate verbalizations, difficulty in comprehending usual communication pattern, difficulty in use of facial expressions.

Social Isolation may be related to alterations in mental status, mistrust of others, delusional thinking, unacceptable social behaviors, inadequate personal resources, and inability to engage in satisfying personal relationships, possibly evidenced by difficulty in establishing relationships with others, dull affect, uncommunicative or withdrawn behavior, seeking to be alone, inadequate or absent significant purpose in life, and expression of feelings of rejection.

ineffective Health Maintenance/impaired Home Maintenance may be related to impaired cognitive or emotional functioning, altered ability to make deliberate and thoughtful judgments, altered communication, and lack or inappropriate use of material resources, possibly evidenced by inability to take responsibility for meeting basic health practices in any or all functional areas and demonstrated lack of adaptive behaviors to internal or external environmental changes, disorderly surroundings, accumulation of dirt and unwashed clothes, repeated hygienic disorders.

risk for self-directed Violence/risk for other-directed Violence is possibly evidenced by risk factors of disturbances of thinking or feeling (depression, paranoia, suicidal ideation), lack of development of trust and appropriate interpersonal relationships, catatonic or manic excitement, toxic reactions to drugs (alcohol).*

ineffective Coping may be related to personal vulnerability, inadequate support system(s), unrealistic perceptions, inadequate coping methods, and disintegration of thought processes, possibly evidenced by impaired judgment, cognition, and perception; diminished problem-solving or decision-making capacities; poor self-concept; chronic an-

*A risk diagnosis is not evidenced by signs and symptoms, as the problem has not occurred; rather, nursing interventions are directed at prevention.

S

xiety; depression; inability to perform role expectations; and alteration in social participation.

interrupted Family Processes/disabled family Coping may be related to ambivalent family system or relationships, change of roles, and difficulty of family member in coping effectively with client's maladaptive behaviors, possibly evidenced by deterioration in family functioning, ineffective family decision-making process, difficulty relating to each other, client's expressions of despair at family's lack of reaction or involvement, neglectful relationships with client, extreme distortion regarding client's health problem including denial about its existence or severity, or prolonged overconcern.

Self-Care Deficit [specify] may be related to perceptual and cognitive impairment, immobility (withdrawal, isolation, and decreased psychomotor activity), and side effects of psychotropic medications, possibly evidenced by inability or difficulty in areas of feeding self, keeping body clean, dressing appropriately, toileting self, and/or changes in bowel or bladder elimination.

Sciatica — CH

acute Pain/chronic Pain may be related to peripheral nerve root compression, possibly evidenced by verbal reports, guarding or distraction behaviors, and self-focus.

impaired physical Mobility may be related to neurological pain and muscular involvement, possibly evidenced by reluctance to attempt movement and decreased muscle strength and mass.

Scleroderma — CH

Also refer to Lupus erythematosus, systemic (SLE)

impaired physical Mobility may be related to musculoskeletal impairment and associated pain, possibly evidenced by decreased strength, decreased range of motion, and reluctance to attempt movement.

ineffective Tissue Perfusion [specify] may be related to reduced arterial blood flow (arteriolar vasoconstriction), possibly evidenced by changes in skin temperature and color, ulcer formation, and changes in organ function (cardiopulmonary, gastrointestinal, renal).

imbalanced Nutrition: less than body requirements may be related to inability to ingest, digest, or absorb adequate nutrients (sclerosis of the tissues rendering mouth immobile, decreased peristalsis of esophagus or small intestine, atrophy of smooth muscle of colon), possibly evidenced by weight loss, decreased intake, and reported or observed difficulty swallowing.

risk-prone Health Behavior may be related to disability requiring change in lifestyle, inadequate support systems, assault to self-concept, and altered locus of control, possibly evidenced by verbalization of nonacceptance of health status change and lack of movement toward independence or future-oriented thinking.

disturbed Body Image may be related to skin changes with induration, atrophy, and fibrosis, loss of hair, and skin and muscle contractures, possibly evidenced by verbalization of negative feelings about body, focus on past strength or function or appearance, fear of rejection or reaction by others, hiding body part, and change in social involvement.

Scoliosis — PED

disturbed Body Image may be related to altered body structure, use of therapeutic device(s), and activity restrictions, possibly evidenced by negative feelings about body, change in social involvement, and preoccupation with situation or refusal to acknowledge problem.

deficient Knowledge [Learning Need] regarding pathophysiology of condition, therapy needs, and possible outcomes may be related to lack of information, misinterpretation, possibly evidenced by statements of concern, questions, misconceptions, and inaccurate follow-through of instructions.

risk-prone Health Behavior may be related to lack of comprehension of long-term consequences of behavior, possibly evidenced by failure to take action, minimized health status change, and evidence of failure to improve.

Seizure disorder CH

deficient Knowledge [Learning Need] regarding condition and medication control may be related to lack of information, misinterpretations, scarce financial resources, possibly evidenced by questions, statements of concern, misconceptions, incorrect use of anticonvulsant medication, recurrent episodes or uncontrolled seizures.

chronic low Self-Esteem/disturbed Personal Identity may be related to stigma associated with condition, perception of being out of control or helpless, possibly evidenced by verbalization about changed lifestyle, fear of rejection, negative feelings about "brain" or self, change in usual pattern of responsibility, denial of problem resulting in lack of follow-through, or nonparticipation in therapy.

impaired Social Interaction may be related to unpredictable nature of condition and self-concept disturbance, possibly evidenced by decreased self-assurance, verbalization of concern, discomfort in social situations, inability to receive or communicate a satisfying sense of belonging or caring, and withdrawal from social contacts and activities.

risk for Trauma/risk for Suffocation are possibly evidenced by risk factors of weakness, balancing difficulties, cognitive limitations, altered consciousness, loss of large or small muscle coordination (during seizure).*

Sepsis MS

Also refer to Sepsis, puerperal

risk for deficient Fluid Volume is possibly evidenced by risk factors of marked increase in vascular compartment, massive vasodilation, capillary permeability, vascular shifts to interstitial space, and reduced intake.*

risk for decreased Cardiac Output is possibly evidenced by risk factors of decreased preload—venous return and circulating volume; altered afterload—increased SVR; negative inotropic effects of hypoxia, complement activation, and lysosomal hydrolase.*

risk for impaired Gas Exchange is possibly evidenced by risk factors of effects of endotoxins on the respiratory center in the medulla—hyperventilation and respiratory alkalosis; hypoventilation; changes in vascular resistance, alveolar-capillary membrane changes—increased capillary permeability leading to pulmonary congestion; in-

*A risk diagnosis is not evidenced by signs and symptoms, as the problem has not occurred; rather, nursing interventions are directed at prevention.

terference with oxygen delivery and utilization in the tissues—endotoxin-induced damage to the cells and capillaries.*

risk for Shock is possibly evidenced by risk factors of infection/sepsis, hypovolemia—fluid shifts/third spacing; hypotension, hypoxemia.*

Sepsis, puerperal **OB**

Also refer to Sepsis

risk for Infection [spread/septic shock] is possibly evidenced by risk factors of presence of infection, broken skin, and/or traumatized tissues; rupture of amniotic membranes; high vascularity of involved area; stasis of body fluids; invasive procedures, and/or increased environmental exposure; chronic disease (e.g., diabetes, anemia, malnutrition)' altered immune response; and untoward effect of medications (e.g., opportunistic or secondary infection).*

Hyperthermia may be related to inflammatory process, hypermetabolic state, dehydration, effect of circulating endotoxins on the hypothalamus, possibly evidenced by increase in body temperature; warm, flushed skin; increased respiratory rate; and tachycardia.

risk for impaired Attachment is possibly evidenced by risk factors of interruption in bonding process, physical illness, perceived threat to own survival.*

risk for ineffective peripheral Tissue Perfusion is possibly evidenced by risk factors of interruption or reduction of blood flow (presence of infectious thrombi).*

Serum sickness **CH**

acute Pain may be related to inflammation of the joints and skin eruptions, possibly evidenced by verbal reports, guarding or distraction behaviors, and self-focus.

deficient Knowledge [Learning Need] regarding nature of condition, treatment needs, potential complications, and prevention of recurrence may be related to lack of information, misinterpretation, possibly evidenced by statements of concern, questions, misconceptions, and inaccurate follow-through of instructions.

Sexually transmitted infection (STI) **GYN/CH**

risk for Infection [transmission] is possibly evidenced by risk factors of contagious nature of infecting agent and insufficient knowledge to avoid exposure to or transmission of pathogens.*

impaired Skin/Tissue Integrity may be related to invasion of or irritation by pathogenic organism(s), possibly evidenced by disruptions of skin or tissues and inflammation of mucous membranes.

deficient Knowledge [Learning Need] regarding condition, prognosis/complications, therapy needs, and transmission may be related to lack of information, misinterpretation, lack of interest in learning, possibly evidenced by statements of concern, questions, misconceptions; inaccurate follow-through of instructions; and development of preventable complications.

Shock **MS**

Also refer to Shock, cardiogenic; Shock, hypovolemic/hemorrhagic

ineffective Tissue Perfusion [specify] may be related to changes in circulating volume and/or vascular tone, possibly evidenced by changes

S

*A risk diagnosis is not evidenced by signs and symptoms, as the problem has not occurred; rather, nursing interventions are directed at prevention.

in skin color and temperature and pulse pressure, reduced BP, changes in mentation, and decreased urinary output.

Anxiety [specify level] may be related to change in health status and threat of death, possibly evidenced by increased tension, apprehension, sympathetic stimulation, restlessness, and expressions of concern.

Shock, cardiogenic **MS**

Also refer to Shock

decreased Cardiac Output may be related to structural damage, decreased myocardial contractility, and presence of dysrhythmias, possibly evidenced by ECG changes, variations in hemodynamic readings, jugular vein distention, cold or clammy skin, diminished peripheral pulses, and decreased urinary output.

risk for impaired Gas Exchange is possibly evidenced by risk factors of ventilation perfusion imbalance, alveolar-capillary membrane changes.*

Shock, hypovolemic/hemorrhagic **MS**

Also refer to Shock

deficient Fluid Volume may be related to excessive vascular loss, inadequate intake or replacement, possibly evidenced by hypotension, tachycardia, decreased pulse volume and pressure, change in mentation, and decreased, concentrated urine.

Shock, septic **MS**

Refer to Sepsis

Sick sinus syndrome **MS**

Also refer to Dysrhythmia, cardiac

decreased Cardiac Output may be related to alterations in rate, rhythm, and electrical conduction, possibly evidenced by ECG evidence of dysrhythmias, reports of palpitations or weakness, changes in mentation or consciousness, and syncope.

risk for Trauma is possibly evidenced by risk factors of changes in cerebral perfusion with altered consciousness, loss of balance.*

SLE **CH**

Refer to Lupus erythematosus, systemic (SLE)

Smallpox **MS**

risk for Infection [spread] is possibly evidenced by risk factors of contagious nature of organism, inadequate acquired immunity, presence of chronic disease, immunosuppression.*

deficient Fluid Volume may be related to hypermetabolic state, decreased intake (pharyngeal lesions, nausea), increased losses (vomiting), fluid shifts from vascular bed, possibly evidenced by reports of thirst, decreased BP, venous filling and urinary output, dry mucous membranes, decreased skin turgor, change in mental state, elevated Hct.

impaired Tissue Integrity may be related to immunological deficit, possibly evidenced by disruption of skin surface, cornea, mucous membranes.

*A risk diagnosis is not evidenced by signs and symptoms, as the problem has not occurred; rather, nursing interventions are directed at prevention.

Anxiety [specify level]/Fear may be related to threat of death, interpersonal transmission and contagion, separation from support system, possibly evidenced by expressed concerns, apprehension, restlessness, focus on self.

CH

interrupted Family Processes may be related to temporary family disorganization, situational crisis, change in health status of family member, possibly evidenced by changes in satisfaction with family, stress-reduction behaviors, mutual support, expression of isolation from community resources.

ineffective community Coping may be related to man-made disaster (bioterrorism), inadequate resources for problem-solving, possibly evidenced by deficits of community participation, high illness rate, excessive community conflicts, expressed vulnerability or powerlessness.

Snow blindness **CH**

[disturbed visual Sensory Perception] may be related to altered status of sense organ (irritation of the conjunctiva, hyperemia), possibly evidenced by intolerance to light (photophobia) and decreased or loss of visual acuity.

acute Pain may be related to irritation and vascular congestion of the conjunctiva, possibly evidenced by verbal reports, guarding or distraction behaviors, and self-focus.

Anxiety [specify level] may be related to situational crisis and threat to or change in health status, possibly evidenced by increased tension, apprehension, uncertainty, worry, restlessness, and focus on self.

Somatoform disorders **PSY**

ineffective Coping may be related to severe level of anxiety that is repressed, personal vulnerability, unmet dependency needs, fixation in earlier level of development, retarded ego development, and inadequate coping skills, possibly evidenced by verbalized inability to cope or problem-solve, high illness rate, multiple somatic complaints of several years' duration, decreased functioning in social and occupational settings, narcissistic tendencies with total focus on self and physical symptoms, demanding behaviors, history of "doctor shopping," and refusal to attend therapeutic activities.

chronic Pain may be related to severe level of repressed anxiety, low self-concept, unmet dependency needs, history of self or loved one having experienced a serious illness, possibly evidenced by verbal reports of severe or prolonged pain, guarded movement or protective behaviors, facial mask of pain, fear of re-injury, altered ability to continue previous activities, social withdrawal, demands for therapy or medication.

[disturbed Sensory Perception (specify)] may be related to psychological stress (narrowed perceptual fields, expression of stress as physical problems), poor quality of sleep, presence of chronic pain, possibly evidenced by reported change in voluntary motor or sensory function (paralysis, anosmia, aphonia, deafness, blindness, loss of touch or pain sensation), *la belle indifférence* (lack of concern over functional loss).

impaired Social Interaction may be related to inability to engage in satisfying personal relationships, preoccupation with self and physical symptoms, altered state of wellness, chronic pain, and rejection

S

by others, possibly evidenced by preoccupation with own thoughts, sad or dull affect, absence of supportive SO(s), uncommunicative or withdrawn behavior, lack of eye contact, and seeking to be alone.

Spinal cord injury (SCI) **MS/CH**

Refer to Paraplegia; Quadriplegia

Sprain of ankle or foot **CH**

acute Pain may be related to trauma to and swelling in joint, possibly evidenced by verbal reports, guarding or distraction behaviors, self-focusing, and changes in vital signs.

impaired Walking may be related to musculoskeletal injury, pain, and therapeutic restrictions, possibly evidenced by reluctance to attempt movement, inability to move about environment easily.

Stapedectomy **MS**

risk for Trauma is possibly evidenced by risk factors of increased middle ear pressure with displacement of prosthesis and balancing difficulties, dizziness.*

risk for Infection is possibly evidenced by risk factors of surgically traumatized tissue, invasive procedures, and environmental exposure to upper respiratory infections.*

acute Pain may be related to surgical trauma, edema formation, and presence of packing, possibly evidenced by verbal reports, guarding or distraction behaviors, and self-focus.

STI **CH**

Refer to Sexually transmitted infection (STI)

Stimulant abuse **CH**

Also refer to Cocaine hydrochloride poisoning, acute; Substance dependence/abuse rehabilitation

imbalanced Nutrition: less than body requirements may be related to anorexia, insufficient or inappropriate use of financial resources, possibly evidenced by reported inadequate intake, weight loss or less than normal weight gain, lack of interest in food, poor muscle tone, signs or laboratory evidence of vitamin deficiencies.

risk for Infection is possibly evidenced by risk factors of injection techniques, impurities of drugs, localized trauma or nasal septum damage, malnutrition, altered immune state.*

Insomnia may be related to CNS sensory alterations, psychological stress possibly evidenced by constant alertness, racing thoughts preventing rest, denial of need to sleep, reported inability to stay awake, initial insomnia then hypersomnia.

PSY

Fear/Anxiety [specify] may be related to paranoid delusions associated with stimulant use possibly evidenced by feelings or beliefs that others are conspiring against or are about to attack or kill client.

ineffective Coping may be related to personal vulnerability, negative role modeling, inadequate support systems; ineffective or inadequate coping skills with substitution of drug, possibly evidenced by use of harmful substance despite evidence of undesirable consequences.

---

*A risk diagnosis is not evidenced by signs and symptoms, as the problem has not occurred; rather, nursing interventions are directed at prevention.

[disturbed Sensory Perception (specify)] may be related to exogenous chemical, altered sensory reception, transmission, or integration (hallucination), altered status of sense organs, possibly evidenced by responding to internal stimuli from hallucinatory experiences, bizarre thinking, anxiety or panic changes in sensory acuity (sense of smell/taste).

Substance dependence/abuse rehabilitation **PSY/CH**
(following acute detoxification)

ineffective Denial may be related to threat of unpleasant reality, lack of emotional support from others, overwhelming stress, possibly evidenced by lack of acceptance that drug use is causing the present situation, delay in seeking or refusal of healthcare attention to the detriment of health, use of manipulation to avoid responsibility for self, projection of blame or responsibility for problems.

ineffective Coping may be related to personal vulnerability, negative role modeling, inadequate support systems, previous ineffective or inadequate coping skills with substitution of drug(s), possibly evidenced by impaired adaptive behavior and problem-solving skills, decreased ability to handle stress of illness or hospitalization, financial affairs in disarray, employment or school difficulties—losing time on job or not maintaining steady employment, poor work or school performances, on-the-job injuries, verbalization of inability to cope or ask for help.

Powerlessness may be related to substance addiction with or without periods of abstinence, episodic compulsive indulgence, attempts at recovery, and lifestyle of helplessness, possibly evidenced by ineffective recovery attempts, statements of inability to stop behavior, requests for help, constantly thinking about drug and/or obtaining drug, alteration in personal, occupational, and social life.

imbalanced Nutrition: less than body requirements may be related to insufficient dietary intake to meet metabolic needs for psychological, physiological, or economic reasons, possibly evidenced by weight less than normal for height and body build; decreased subcutaneous fat or muscle mass; reported altered taste sensation; lack of interest in food; poor muscle tone; sore, inflamed buccal cavity; laboratory evidence of protein or vitamin deficiencies.

Sexual Dysfunction may be related to altered body function (neurological damage and debilitating effects of drug use), possibly evidenced by progressive interference with sexual functioning; in men, a significant degree of testicular atrophy, gynecomastia, impotence, or decreased sperm counts; in women, loss of body hair, thin, soft skin, spider angiomas, amenorrhea, and increase in miscarriages.

dysfunctional Family Processes may be related to abuse and history of alcoholism or drug use, inadequate coping skills, lack of problem-solving skills, genetic predisposition or biochemical influences, possibly evidenced by feelings of anger, frustration, or responsibility for alcoholic's behavior; suppressed rage, shame, embarrassment, repressed emotions, guilt, vulnerability, disturbed family dynamics or deterioration in family relationships, family denial or rationalization, closed communication systems, triangulating family relationships, manipulation, blaming, enabling to maintain substance use, inability to accept or receive help.

OB

risk for fetal Injury is possibly evidenced by risk factors of drug or alcohol use, exposure to teratogens.*

deficient Knowledge [Learning Need] regarding condition, effects on pregnancy, prognosis, treatment needs may be related to lack or misinterpretation of information, lack of recall, cognitive limitations, interference with learning, possibly evidenced by statements of concern, questions, misconceptions, inaccurate follow-through of instructions, development of preventable complications, continued use despite complications.

compromised family Coping/disabled family Coping may be related to codependency issues, situational crisis of pregnancy and drug abuse, family disorganization, exhausted supportive capacity of family members possibly evidenced by denial or belief that all problems are due to substance use, financial difficulties, severely dysfunctional family, codependent behaviors.

Surgery, general **MS**

Also refer to Postoperative recovery period

deficient Knowledge [Learning Need] regarding surgical procedure, expectations, postoperative routines, therapy, and self-care needs may be related to lack of information or recall, misinterpretation, possibly evidenced by statements of concern, questions, and misconceptions.

Anxiety [specify level]/Fear may be related to situational crisis, unfamiliarity with environment, change in health status, threat of death and separation from usual support systems, possibly evidenced by increased tension, apprehension, decreased self-assurance, fear of unspecific consequences, focus on self, sympathetic stimulation, and restlessness.

risk for perioperative Positioning Injury is possibly evidenced by risk factors of disorientation, sensory and perceptual disturbances due to anesthesia, immobilization, musculoskeletal impairments, obesity, emaciation, edema.*

risk for Injury is possibly evidenced by risk factors of wrong client, procedure, site, implants, equipment or materials; interactive conditions between individual and environment; external environment—physical design, structure of environment, exposure to equipment, instrumentation, positioning, use of pharmaceutical agents; internal environment—tissue hypoxia, abnormal blood profile or altered clotting factors, broken skin.*

risk for Infection is possibly evidenced by risk factors of broken skin, traumatized tissues, stasis of body fluids, presence of pathogens or contaminants, environmental exposure, invasive procedures.*

risk for imbalanced Body Temperature is possibly evidenced by risk factors of exposure to cool environment, use of medications, anesthetic agents; extremes of age, weight; dehydration.*

ineffective Breathing Pattern may be related to chemically induced muscular relaxation, perception or cognitive impairment, decreased lung expansion, energy; tracheobronchial obstruction.

risk for deficient Fluid Volume is possibly evidenced by risk factors of preoperative fluid deprivation, nausea, blood loss, and excessive gas-

*A risk diagnosis is not evidenced by signs and symptoms, as the problem has not occurred; rather, nursing interventions are directed at prevention.

trointestinal losses (vomiting or gastric suction), extremes of age and weight.*

Synovitis (knee) **CH**

acute Pain may be related to inflammation of synovial membrane of the joint with effusion, possibly evidenced by verbal reports, guarding or distraction behaviors, self-focus, and changes in vital signs.

impaired Walking may be related to pain and decreased strength of joint, possibly evidenced by reluctance to attempt movement, inability to move about environment as desired.

Syphilis, congenital **PED**

Also refer to Sexually transmitted infection (STI)

acute Pain may be related to inflammatory process, edema formation, and development of skin lesions, possibly evidenced by irritability or crying that may be increased with movement of extremities and changes in vital signs.

impaired Skin/Tissue Integrity may be related to exposure to pathogens during vaginal delivery, possibly evidenced by disruption of skin surfaces and rhinitis.

risk for disproportionate Growth/delayed Development are possibly evidenced by risk factors of congenital disorder, malnutrition, seizure disorder.*

deficient Knowledge [Learning Need] regarding pathophysiology of condition, transmissibility, therapy needs, expected outcomes, and potential complications may be related to caretaker/parental lack of information, misinterpretation, possibly evidenced by statements of concern, questions, and misconceptions.

Syringomyelia **MS**

[disturbed Sensory Perception (specify)] may be related to altered sensory perception (neurological lesion), possibly evidenced by change in usual response to stimuli and motor incoordination.

Anxiety [specify level]/Fear may be related to change in health status, threat of change in role functioning and socioeconomic status, and threat to self-concept, possibly evidenced by increased tension, apprehension, uncertainty, focus on self, and expressed concerns.

impaired physical Mobility may be related to neuromuscular and sensory impairment, possibly evidenced by decreased muscle strength, control, and mass; and impaired coordination.

Self-Care Deficit [specify] may be related to neuromuscular and sensory impairments, possibly evidenced by statement of inability to perform care tasks.

T

Tay-Sachs disease **PED**

risk for delayed Development is possibly evidenced by risk factors of genetic disorder, seizure disorder, visual/hearing impairment.*

[disturbed visual Sensory Perception] may be related to neurological deterioration of optic nerve, possibly evidenced by loss of visual acuity.

CH

[family] Grieving may be related to expected eventual loss of infant/child, possibly evidenced by expressions of distress, denial, guilt,

*A risk diagnosis is not evidenced by signs and symptoms, as the problem has not occurred; rather, nursing interventions are directed at prevention.

anger, and sorrow; choked feelings; changes in sleep and eating habits; and altered libido.

[family] Powerlessness may be related to absence of therapeutic interventions for progressive and fatal disease, possibly evidenced by verbal expressions of having no control over situation or outcome and depression over physical and mental deterioration.

risk for Spiritual Distress is possibly evidenced by risk factors of challenged belief and value system by presence of fatal condition with racial or religious connotations and intense suffering.*

compromised family Coping may be related to situational crisis, temporary preoccupation with managing emotional conflicts and personal suffering, family disorganization, and prolonged and progressive nature of disease, possibly evidenced by preoccupations with personal reactions, expressed concern about reactions of other family members, inadequate support of one another, and altered communication patterns.

Thrombophlebitis **CH/MS/OB**

ineffective peripheral Tissue Perfusion may be related to interruption of venous blood flow, venous stasis, possibly evidenced by changes in skin color and temperature over affected area, development of edema, pain, diminished peripheral pulses, slow capillary refill.

acute Pain/impaired Comfort may be related to vascular inflammation and irritation, edema formation, accumulation of lactic acid, possibly evidenced by verbal reports, guarding or distraction behaviors, restlessness, and self-focus.

risk for impaired physical Mobility is possibly evidenced by risk factors of pain and discomfort and restrictive therapies or safety precautions.*

deficient Knowledge [Learning Need] regarding pathophysiology of condition, therapy/self-care needs, and risk of embolization may be related to lack of information, misinterpretation, possibly evidenced by statements of concern, questions, inaccurate follow-through of instructions, and development of preventable complications.

Thrombosis, venous **MS**

Refer to Thrombophlebitis

Thrush **CH**

impaired oral Mucous Membrane may be related to presence of infection as evidenced by white patches or plaques, oral discomfort, mucosal irritation, bleeding.

Thyroidectomy **MS**

Also refer to Hyperthyroidism; Hypoparathyroidism; Hypothyroidism

risk for ineffective Airway Clearance is possibly evidenced by risk factors of tracheal obstruction—edema, hematoma formation, laryngeal spasms.*

impaired verbal Communication may be related to tissue edema, pain or discomfort, and vocal cord injury or laryngeal nerve damage, possibly evidenced by impaired articulation, does not or cannot speak, and use of nonverbal cues and gestures.

*A risk diagnosis is not evidenced by signs and symptoms, as the problem has not occurred; rather, nursing interventions are directed at prevention.

T

risk for Injury [tetany] is possibly evidenced by risk factors of chemical imbalance—hypocalcemia, increased release of thyroid hormones; excessive CNS stimulation.*

risk for [head/neck] Trauma is possibly evidenced by risk factors of loss of muscle control and support, and position of suture line.*

acute Pain may be related to presence of surgical incision and manipulation of tissues and muscles, postoperative edema, possibly evidenced by verbal reports, guarding or distraction behaviors, narrowed focus, and changes in vital signs.

Thyrotoxicosis — MS

Also refer to Hyperthyroidism

risk for decreased Cardiac Output is possibly evidenced by risk factors of uncontrolled hypermetabolic state increasing cardiac workload, changes in venous return and SVR, and alterations in rate, rhythm, and electrical conduction.*

Anxiety [specify level] may be related to physiological factors or CNS stimulation—hypermetabolic state and pseudocatecholamine effect of thyroid hormones; possibly evidenced by increased feelings of apprehension, shakiness, loss of control, panic, changes in cognition, distortion of environmental stimuli, extraneous movements, restlessness, and tremors.

deficient Knowledge [Learning Needs] regarding condition, treatment needs, and potential for complications or crisis situation may be related to lack of information or recall, misinterpretation, possibly evidenced by statements of concern, questions, and misconceptions, and inaccurate follow-through of instructions.

TIA — CH

Refer to Transient ischemic attack

Tic douloureux — CH

Refer to Neuralgia, trigeminal

Tonsillectomy — PED/MS

Anxiety [specify level]/Fear may be related to separation from supportive others, unfamiliar surroundings, and perceived threat of injury or abandonment, possibly evidenced by crying, apprehension, trembling, and sympathetic stimulation (pupil dilation, increased heart rate).

risk for ineffective Airway Clearance is possibly evidenced by risk factors of sedation, collection of secretions and blood in oropharynx, and vomiting.*

risk for deficient Fluid Volume is possibly evidenced by risk factors of operative trauma to highly vascular site, hemorrhage.*

acute Pain may be related to physical trauma to oronasopharynx, presence of packing, possibly evidenced by restlessness, crying, and facial mask of pain.

Tonsillitis — PED

acute Pain may be related to inflammation of tonsils and effects of circulating toxins, possibly evidenced by verbal reports, guarding or

---

*A risk diagnosis is not evidenced by signs and symptoms, as the problem has not occurred; rather, nursing interventions are directed at prevention.

distraction behaviors, reluctance or refusal to swallow, self-focus, and changes in vital signs.

Hyperthermia may be related to presence of inflammatory process, hypermetabolic state and dehydration, possibly evidenced by increased body temperature; warm, flushed skin; and tachycardia.

deficient Knowledge [Learning Need] regarding cause, transmission, treatment needs, and potential complications may be related to lack of information, misinterpretation, possibly evidenced by statements of concern, questions, inaccurate follow-through of instructions, and recurrence of condition.

Total joint replacement **MS**

Also refer to Surgery, general

risk for Infection is possibly evidenced by risk factors of inadequate primary defenses (broken skin, exposure of joint), inadequate secondary defenses, or immunosuppression (long-term corticosteroid use); invasive procedures; surgical manipulation; implantation of foreign body; and decreased mobility.*

impaired physical Mobility may be related to pain and discomfort, musculoskeletal impairment, and surgery and restrictive therapies, possibly evidenced by reluctance to attempt movement, difficulty purposefully moving within the physical environment, reports of pain or discomfort on movement, limited range of motion, and decreased muscle strength and control.

risk for ineffective peripheral Tissue Perfusion possibly evidenced by risk factors of reduced arterial or venous blood flow, direct trauma to blood vessels, tissue edema, improper location or dislocation of prosthesis, and hypovolemia.*

acute Pain may be related to physical agents (traumatized tissues, surgical intervention, degeneration of joints, muscle spasms) and psychological factors (anxiety, advanced age), possibly evidenced by verbal reports, guarding or distraction behaviors, self-focus, and changes in vital signs.

risk for Constipation is possibly evidenced by risk factors of insufficient physical activity, decreased mobility, weakness, insufficient fiber or fluid intake, dehydration, poor eating habits, decreased gastrointestinal motility, effects of medications—anesthesia, opiate analgesics; environmental changes; inadequate toileting.*

Toxemia of pregnancy **OB**

Refer to Pregnancy-induced hypertension

Toxic shock syndrome **MS**

Also refer to Septicemia

Hyperthermia may be related to inflammatory process, hypermetabolic state and dehydration, possibly evidenced by increased body temperature; warm, flushed skin; and tachycardia.

deficient Fluid Volume may be related to increased gastric losses (diarrhea, vomiting), fever and hypermetabolic state, and decreased intake, possibly evidenced by dry mucous membranes; increased pulse; hypotension; delayed venous filling; decreased, concentrated urine; and hemoconcentration.

---

*A risk diagnosis is not evidenced by signs and symptoms, as the problem has not occurred; rather, nursing interventions are directed at prevention.

acute Pain may be related to inflammatory process, effects of circulating toxins, and skin disruptions, possibly evidenced by verbal reports, guarding or distraction behaviors, self-focus, and changes in vital signs.

impaired Skin /Tissue Integrity may be related to effects of circulating toxins and dehydration, possibly evidenced by development of desquamating rash, hyperemia, and inflammation of mucous membranes.

Traction **MS**

Also refer to Casts; Fractures

acute Pain may be related to direct trauma to tissue/bone, muscle spasms, movement of bone fragments, edema, injury to soft tissue, traction or immobility device, anxiety, possibly evidenced by verbal reports, guarding or distraction behaviors, self-focus, alteration in muscle tone, and changes in vital signs.

impaired physical Mobility may be related to neuromuscular and skeletal impairment, pain, psychological immobility, and therapeutic restrictions of movement, possibly evidenced by limited range of motion, inability to move purposefully in environment, reluctance to attempt movement, and decreased muscle strength and control.

risk for Infection is possibly evidenced by risk factors of invasive procedures—including insertion of foreign body through skin and bone, presence of traumatized tissue, and reduced activity with stasis of body fluids.*

deficient Diversional Activity may be related to length of hospitalization or therapeutic intervention and environmental lack of usual activity, possibly evidenced by statements of boredom, restlessness, and irritability.

Transfusion reaction, blood **MS**

Also refer to Anaphylaxis

risk for imbalanced Body Temperature is possibly evidenced by risk factors of infusion of cold blood products, systemic response to toxins.*

Anxiety [specify level] may be related to change in health status and threat of death, exposure to toxins, possibly evidenced by increased tension, apprehension, sympathetic stimulation, restlessness, and expressions of concern.

risk for Injury is possibly evidenced by risk factor of immunological response (adverse effect).*

T

Transient ischemic attack (TIA) **CH**

ineffective cerebral Tissue Perfusion may be related to interruption of blood flow (e.g., vasospasm), possibly evidenced by altered mental status, behavioral changes, language deficit, change in motor or sensory response.

Anxiety [specify level]/Fear may be related to change in health status, threat to self-concept, situational crisis, interpersonal contagion, possibly evidenced by expressed concerns, apprehension, restlessness, irritability.

*A risk diagnosis is not evidenced by signs and symptoms, as the problem has not occurred; rather, nursing interventions are directed at prevention.

risk for ineffective Denial is possibly evidenced by risk factors of change in health status requiring change in lifestyle, fear of consequences, lack of motivation.*

Transplantation, recipient **MS**

Anxiety/Fear may be related to unconscious conflict about essential values/beliefs, situational crisis, threat of death (organ rejection), unfamiliarity with environmental experience, possibly evidenced by reports apprehension/increased tension, uncertainty, worried, insomnia, increased vital signs.

risk for Infection is possibly evidenced by risk factors of medically chronic disease, induced immunosuppression, suppressed inflammatory response, invasive procedures, broken skin/traumatized tissues.*

(Refer to specific conditions relative to compromise of failure of individual transplanted organs, e.g., Renal failure, acute; Heart Failure, chronic; Pancreatitis.)

CH

ineffective Coping/compromised family Coping may be related to situational crisis, high degree of threat, uncertainty, family disorganization or role changes, prolonged disease exhausting supportive capacity of family/SO, possibly evidenced by reports of inability to cope, sleep pattern disturbance, fatigue, poor concentration, protective behaviors disproportionate to client's needs, SO describes preoccupation with personal reaction.

ineffective Protection may be related to treatment regimen/ pharmaceutical agents or compromised immune system, possibly evidenced by weakness, maladaptive stress response.*

readiness for enhanced Health Management possibly evidenced by expressed desire to manage treatment/prevent sequelae, no unexpected acceleration of illness symptoms.

risk for ineffective Health Management is possibly evidenced by risk factors of complexity of therapeutic regimen and healthcare system, economic difficulties, family patterns of healthcare.*

Traumatic brain injury (TBI) **CH**

ineffective cerebral Tissue Perfusion may be related to interruption of blood flow—hemorrhage, hematoma, cerebral edema (localized or generalized response to injury, metabolic alterations, drug or alcohol overdose), decreased systemic BP—hypovolemia, cardiac dysrhythmias; hypoxia, possibly evidenced by altered level of consciousness, memory loss, changes in motor or sensory responses, restlessness, changes in vital signs.

risk for decreased intracranial Adaptive Capacity is possibly evidenced by risk factors of brain injuries, systemic hypotension with intracranial hypertension.*

risk for ineffective Breathing Pattern is possibly evidenced by risk factors of neuromuscular dysfunction—injury to respiratory center of brain; perception or cognitive impairment, tracheobronchial obstruction.*

[disturbed Sensory Perception (specify)] may be related to altered sensory reception, transmission and/or integration—neurological trauma or deficit, possibly evidenced by disorientation to time, place,

*A risk diagnosis is not evidenced by signs and symptoms, as the problem has not occurred; rather, nursing interventions are directed at prevention.

person; change in usual response to stimuli, motor incoordination, altered communication patterns, visual or auditory distortions, altered thought processes or bizarre thinking, exaggerated emotional responses, change in behavior pattern.

risk for Infection is possibly evidenced by risk factors of traumatized tissues, broken skin, invasive procedures, decreased ciliary action, stasis of body fluids, nutritional deficits, suppressed inflammatory response—steroid use, altered integrity of closed system—cerebrospinal fluid leak.*

risk for imbalanced Nutrition: less than body requirements is possibly evidenced by risk factors of altered ability to ingest nutrients—decreased level of consciousness; weakness of muscles for chewing or swallowing; hypermetabolic state.*

CH

impaired physical Mobility may be related to perceptual or cognitive impairment; decreased strength and endurance; restrictive therapies or safety precautions possibly evidenced by inability to purposefully move within physical environment—bed mobility, transfer, ambulation; impaired coordination; limited range of motion; decreased muscle strength or control.

risk for impaired Memory/chronic Confusion is possibly evidenced by risk factors of head injury, neurological disturbances.

interrupted Family Processes may be related to situational transition and crisis, uncertainty about ultimate outcome, expectations possibly evidenced by difficulty adapting to change or dealing with traumatic experience constructively, family not meeting needs of all members, difficulty accepting or receiving help appropriately, inability to express or to accept feelings of members.

Self-Care Deficit [specify] may be related to neuromuscular or musculoskeletal impairment, weakness, pain, perceptual or cognitive impairment, possibly evidenced by inability to perform desired or appropriate ADLs.

Trichinosis **CH**

acute Pain may be related to parasitic invasion of muscle tissues, edema of upper eyelids, small localized hemorrhages, and development of urticaria, possibly evidenced by verbal reports, guarding or distraction behaviors (restlessness), and changes in vital signs.

deficient Fluid Volume may be related to hypermetabolic state (fever, diaphoresis), excessive gastric losses (vomiting, diarrhea), and decreased intake (difficulty swallowing), possibly evidenced by dry mucous membranes; decreased skin turgor; hypotension; decreased venous filling; decreased, concentrated urine; and hemoconcentration.

ineffective Breathing Pattern may be related to myositis of the diaphragm and intercostal muscles, possibly evidenced by resulting changes in respiratory depth, tachypnea, dyspnea, and abnormal ABGs.

deficient Knowledge [Learning Need] regarding cause and prevention of condition, therapy needs, and possible complications may be re-

*A risk diagnosis is not evidenced by signs and symptoms, as the problem has not occurred; rather, nursing interventions are directed at prevention.

lated to lack of information, misinterpretation, possibly evidenced by statements of concern, questions, and misconceptions.

Tuberculosis (pulmonary) **CH**

risk for Infection [spread/reactivation] is possibly evidenced by risk factors of inadequate primary defenses (decreased ciliary action and stasis of secretions, tissue destruction with extension of infection), lowered resistance, suppressed inflammatory response, malnutrition, environmental exposure, insufficient knowledge to avoid exposure to pathogens, or inadequate therapeutic intervention.*

ineffective Airway Clearance may be related to thick, viscous, or bloody secretions; fatigue with poor cough effort, and tracheal or pharyngeal edema, possibly evidenced by abnormal respiratory rate, rhythm, and depth; adventitious breath sounds (rhonchi, wheezes), stridor, and dyspnea.

risk for impaired Gas Exchange is possibly evidenced by risk factors of decrease in effective lung surface, atelectasis, destruction of alveolar-capillary membrane, bronchial edema, thick, viscous secretions.*

Activity Intolerance may be related to imbalance between O_2 supply and demand, possibly evidenced by reports of fatigue, weakness, and exertional dyspnea.

imbalanced Nutrition: less than body requirements may be related to inability to ingest adequate nutrients (anorexia, effects of drug therapy, fatigue, insufficient financial resources), possibly evidenced by weight loss, reported lack of interest in food/altered taste sensation, and poor muscle tone.

risk for ineffective Health Management is possibly evidenced by risk factors of complexity of therapeutic regimen, economic difficulties, family patterns of healthcare, perceived seriousness or benefits (especially during remission), side effects of therapy.*

Tympanoplasty **MS**

Refer to Stapedectomy

Typhus (tick-borne/Rocky Mountain spotted fever) **CH/MS**

Hyperthermia may be related to generalized inflammatory process (vasculitis), possibly evidenced by increased body temperature; warm, flushed skin; and tachycardia.

acute Pain may be related to generalized vasculitis and edema formation, possibly evidenced by verbal reports, guarding or distraction behaviors, self-focus, and changes in vital signs.

ineffective Tissue Perfusion (specify) may be related to reduction or interruption of blood flow (generalized vasculitis, thrombi formation), possibly evidenced by reports of headache or abdominal pain, changes in mentation, and areas of peripheral ulceration or necrosis.

Ulcer, decubitus **CH/MS**

impaired Skin /Tissue Integrity may be related to altered circulation, nutritional deficit, fluid imbalance, impaired physical mobility, irri-

*A risk diagnosis is not evidenced by signs and symptoms, as the problem has not occurred; rather, nursing interventions are directed at prevention.

tation of body excretions or secretions, and sensory impairments, evidenced by tissue damage or destruction.

acute Pain may be related to destruction of protective skin layers and exposure of nerves, possibly evidenced by verbal reports, distraction behaviors, and self-focus.

risk for Infection is possibly evidenced by risk factors of broken or traumatized tissue, increased environmental exposure, and nutritional deficits.*

Ulcer, peptic (acute) MS/CH

risk for Shock is possibly evidenced by risk factors of hypovolemia, hypotension.*

Anxiety/Fear may be related to change in health status and threat of death, possibly evidenced by increased tension, restlessness, irritability, fearfulness, trembling, tachycardia, diaphoresis, lack of eye contact, focus on self, verbalization of concerns, withdrawal, and panic or attack behavior.

acute Pain may be related to caustic irritation and destruction of gastric tissues, reflex muscle spasms in stomach wall possibly evidenced by verbal reports, distraction behaviors, self-focus, and changes in vital signs.

deficient Knowledge [Learning Need] regarding condition, therapy and self-care needs, and potential complications may be related to lack of information, recall, misinterpretation, possibly evidenced by statements of concern, questions, misconceptions; inaccurate follow-through of instructions; and development of preventable complications or recurrence of condition.

Ulcer, venous stasis CH

impaired Skin /Tissue Integrity may be related to altered venous circulation, edema formation, inflammation, decreased sensation, possibly evidenced by destruction of skin layers, invasion of body structures.

ineffective peripheral Tissue Perfusion may be related to interruption of venous flow—small vessel vasoconstrictive reflex, possibly evidenced by skin discoloration, edema formation, altered sensation, delayed healing.

Unconsciousness MS

Refer to Coma

U

Urinary diversion MS/CH

risk for impaired Skin Integrity is possibly evidenced by risk factors of absence of sphincter at stoma, character and flow of urine from stoma, reaction to product or chemicals, and improperly fitting appliance or removal of adhesive.*

disturbed Body Image related factors may include biophysical factors (presence of stoma, loss of control of urine flow), and psychosocial factors (altered body structure, disease process and associated treatment regimen, such as cancer), possibly evidenced by verbalization of change in body image, fear of rejection or reaction of others,

*A risk diagnosis is not evidenced by signs and symptoms, as the problem has not occurred; rather, nursing interventions are directed at prevention.

negative feelings about body, not touching or looking at stoma, refusal to participate in care.

acute Pain may be related to physical factors (disruption of skin or tissues, presence of incisions and drains), biological factors (activity of disease process, such as cancer, trauma), and psychological factors (fear, anxiety), possibly evidenced by verbal reports, self-focusing, guarding or distraction behaviors, restlessness, and changes in vital signs.

impaired urinary Elimination may be related to surgical diversion, tissue trauma, and postoperative edema, possibly evidenced by loss of continence, changes in amount and character of urine, and urinary retention.

Urolithiasis — MS/CH

Refer to Calculi, urinary

Uterine bleeding, dysfunctional — GYN/MS

Anxiety [specify level] may be related to perceived change in health status and unknown etiology, possibly evidenced by apprehension, uncertainty, fear of unspecified consequences, expressed concerns, and focus on self.

Activity Intolerance may be related to imbalance between O_2 supply and demand/decreased O_2-carrying capacity of blood (anemia), possibly evidenced by reports of fatigue or weakness.

Uterus, rupture of, in pregnancy — OB

deficient Fluid Volume may be related to excessive vascular losses, possibly evidenced by hypotension, increased pulse rate, decreased venous filling, and decreased urine output.

decreased Cardiac Output may be related to decreased preload (hypovolemia), possibly evidenced by cold, clammy skin; decreased peripheral pulses; variations in hemodynamic readings; tachycardia; and cyanosis.

acute Pain may be related to tissue trauma and irritation of accumulating blood, possibly evidenced by verbal reports, guarding or distraction behaviors, self-focus, and changes in vital signs.

Anxiety [specify level] may be related to threat of death of self or fetus, interpersonal contagion, physiological response (release of catecholamines), possibly evidenced by fearful, scared affect, sympathetic stimulation, stated fear of unspecified consequences, and expressed concerns.

Vaginismus — GYN/CH

acute Pain may be related to muscle spasm and hyperesthesia of the nerve supply to vaginal mucous membrane, possibly evidenced by verbal reports, distraction behaviors, and self-focus.

Sexual Dysfunction may be related to physical and/or psychological alteration in function (severe spasms of vaginal muscles), possibly evidenced by verbalization of problem, inability to achieve desired satisfaction, and alteration in relationship with SO.

Vaginitis — GYN/CH

impaired Tissue Integrity may be related to irritation and inflammation and mechanical trauma (scratching) of sensitive tissues, possibly evidenced by damaged or destroyed tissue, presence of lesions.

acute Pain may be related to localized inflammation and tissue trauma, possibly evidenced by verbal reports, distraction behaviors, and self-focus.
deficient Knowledge [Learning Need] regarding hygienic and therapy needs and sexual behaviors and transmission of infection may be related to lack of information, misinterpretation, possibly evidenced by statements of concern, questions, and misconceptions.

VAP (ventilator-acquired pneumonia) **MS**
Refer to Bronchopneumonia

Varices, esophageal **MS**
Also refer to Ulcer, peptic (acute)
risk for deficient Fluid Volume/risk for Bleeding are possibly evidenced by risk factors of presence of varices, reduced intake, and gastric losses (vomiting), vascular loss.*
Anxiety [specify level]/Fear may be related to change in health status and threat of death, possibly evidenced by increased tension, apprehension, sympathetic stimulation, restlessness, focus on self, and expressed concerns.

Varicose veins **CH**
chronic Pain may be related to venous insufficiency and stasis, possibly evidenced by verbal reports.
disturbed Body Image may be related to change in structure (presence of enlarged, discolored tortuous superficial leg veins), possibly evidenced by hiding affected parts and negative feelings about body.
impaired Skin/Tissue Integrity are possibly evidenced by risk factors of altered circulation, venous stasis, and edema formation.*

Venereal disease **CH**
Refer to Sexually transmitted infection (STI)

Ventricular fibrillation **MS**
Also refer to Dysrhythmias
decreased Cardiac Output may be related to altered electrical conduction and reduced myocardial contractility, possibly evidenced by absence of measurable cardiac output, loss of consciousness, no palpable pulses.

Ventricular tachycardia **MS**
Also refer to Dysrhythmias
risk for decreased Cardiac Output is possibly evidenced by risk factors of alteration in heart rhythm, altered contractility.*

West Nile fever **CH/MS**
Hyperthermia may be related to infectious process, possibly evidenced by elevated body temperature, skin flushed and warm to touch, tachycardia, increased respiratory rate.
acute Pain may be related to infectious process and circulating toxins, possibly evidenced by reports of headache, myalgia, eye pain, abdominal discomfort.

*A risk diagnosis is not evidenced by signs and symptoms, as the problem has not occurred; rather, nursing interventions are directed at prevention.

risk for deficient Fluid Volume is possibly evidenced by risk factors of hypermetabolic state, decreased intake, anorexia, nausea, losses from normal routes (vomiting, diarrhea).*

risk for impaired Skin Integrity is possibly evidenced by risk factors of hyperthermia, decreased fluid intake, alterations in skin turgor, bedrest, circulating toxins.*

Wilms' tumor **PED**

Also refer to Cancer; Chemotherapy

Anxiety/Fear may be related to change in environment and interaction patterns with family members and threat of death with family transmission and contagion of concerns, possibly evidenced by fearful or scared affect, distress, crying, insomnia, and sympathetic stimulation.

risk for Injury is possibly evidenced by risk factors of nature of tumor (vascular, mushy with very thin covering) with increased danger of metastasis when manipulated.*

interrupted Family Processes may be related to situational crisis of life-threatening illness, possibly evidenced by a family system that has difficulty meeting physical, emotional, and spiritual needs of its members, and inability to deal with traumatic experience effectively.

deficient Diversional Activity may be related to environmental lack of age-appropriate activity (including activity restrictions) and length of hospitalization and treatment, possibly evidenced by restlessness, crying, lethargy, and acting-out behavior.

Wound, gunshot **MS**

(Depends on site and speed/character of bullet.)

risk for deficient Fluid Volume is possibly evidenced by risk factors of excessive vascular losses, altered intake or restrictions.*

acute Pain may be related to destruction of tissue (including organ and musculoskeletal), surgical repair, and therapeutic interventions, possibly evidenced by verbal reports, guarding or distraction behaviors, self-focus, and changes in vital signs.

impaired Tissue Integrity may be related to mechanical factors (yaw of projectile and muzzle blast), possibly evidenced by damaged or destroyed tissue.

risk for Infection is possibly evidenced by risk factors of tissue destruction and increased environmental exposure, invasive procedures, and decreased Hb.*

CH

risk for Post-Trauma Syndrome is possibly evidenced by risk factors of nature of incident (catastrophic accident, assault, suicide attempt) and possibly injury or death of other(s) involved.*

W

*A risk diagnosis is not evidenced by signs and symptoms, as the problem has not occurred; rather, nursing interventions are directed at prevention.

APPENDIX 1

Tools for Choosing Nursing Diagnoses

The client assessment is the foundation on which identification of individual needs, responses, and problems are based. To facilitate the steps of assessment and diagnosis in the nursing process, an assessment tool (Section 1) has been constructed using a nursing focus instead of the medical approach of "review of systems." This has the advantage of identifying and validating nursing diagnoses (NDs) as opposed to medical diagnoses. To achieve this nursing focus, we have grouped the NANDA International (NANDA-I) NDs into related categories titled Diagnostic Divisions (Section 2) that reflect a blending of theories, primarily Maslow's Hierarchy of Needs and a self-care philosophy. These divisions serve as the framework or outline for data collection and clustering that focuses attention on the nurse's phenomena of concern—the human responses to health and illness—and directs the nurse to the most likely corresponding NDs.

SECTION 1

Adult Medical/Surgical Assessment Tool

General Information

Name: ________ ❑ Age: ________ ❑ DOB: ________
Gender: ________ Race: ________
Admission: Date: ______ ❑ Time: ______ ❑ From: ______
Reason for this visit (primary concern): ________
Cultural concerns (relating to healthcare decisions, religious concerns, pain, childbirth, family involvement, communication, etc.): ________
Source of information: ___ ❑ Reliability (1 to 4 with 4 = very reliable): ________

Activity/Rest

Subjective (Reports)

Occupation: ______ ❑ Able to participate in usual activities/hobbies: ________
Leisure time/diversional activities: ________
Ambulatory: ________ ❑ Gait (describe): ________
Activity level (sedentary to very active): ______ ❑ Regular exercise/type: ________
Muscle mass/tone/strength (e.g., normal, increased, decreased):
History of problems/limitations imposed by condition (e.g., immobility, cannot transfer, weakness, breathlessness): ______
Feelings (e.g., exhaustion, restlessness, cannot concentrate, dissatisfaction): ________
Developmental factors (e.g., delayed/age appropriate): ______
Sleep: Hours: ________ ❑ Naps: ________
Insomnia: ______ ❑ related to: ______ ❑ Difficulty falling asleep: ________
Difficulty staying asleep: ___ ❑ Rested on awakening: ___
❑ Excessive grogginess: ________
Bedtime rituals: ________
Relaxation techniques: ________
Sleeps on more than one pillow: ________
Oxygen use (type): ________ When used: ________
Medications or herbals for/affecting sleep: ________

Objective (Exhibits)

Observed response to activity: Heart rate: ________
Rhythm (reg/irreg): ___ ❑ Blood pressure: ___ ❑ Respiration rate: ________ ❑ Pulse oximetry: ________

Mental status (i.e., cognitive impairment, withdrawn/lethargic): ____________________

Muscle mass/tone: ______ ❑ Posture (e.g., normal, stooped, curved spine): ____________________
Tremors: ____________ ❑ Location: ______
ROM: ____________________
Strength: ____________ ❑ Deformity: ______
Uses mobility aid (list): ____________________

Circulation

Subjective (Reports)

History of/treatment for (date): High blood pressure: ______
Brain injury: ____________ ❑ Stroke: ______
Heart problems/surgery: ____________________
Palpitations: ____________ ❑ Syncope: ______
Cough/hemoptysis: ________ ❑ Blood clots: ______
Bleeding tendencies/episodes: ________ ❑ Pain in legs w/ activity: ____________________
Extremities: Numbness: ____________________
❑ (location): ____________________
Tingling: ____________ ❑ (location): ______
Slow healing/describe: ____________________
Change in frequency/amount of urine: ______
History of spinal cord injury/dysreflexia episodes: ______
Medications/herbals: ____________________

Objective (Exhibits)

Color (e.g., pale, cyanotic, jaundiced, mottled, ruddy): ______
Skin: ____________________
Mucous membranes: __________ ❑ Lips: ______
Nailbeds: ____________ ❑ Conjunctiva: ______
Sclera: ____________________
Skin moisture: (e.g., dry, diaphoretic): ______
BP: Lying: **R** ______ **L** ______ ❑ Sitting: **R** ______ **L** ______
Standing: **R** ______ **L** ______ ❑ Pulse pressure: ______
Auscultatory gap: ____________________
Pulses (palpated 1–4 strength): Carotid: ____ ❑ Temporal: ____ Jugular: ____ ❑ Radial: ____ ❑ Femoral: ______
Popliteal: ____ ❑ Post-tibial: ____ ❑ Dorsalis pedis: ____
Cardiac (palpation): Thrill: ________ ❑ Heaves: ______
Heart sounds (auscultation): Rate: ______ ❑ Rhythm: ______
Quality: ____________ ❑ Friction rub: ______
Murmur (describe location/sounds): ______
Vascular bruit (location): ____________________
Jugular vein distention: ____________________
Breath sounds (location/describe): ______
Extremities: Temperature: ________ ❑ Color: ______
Capillary refill (1–3 sec): ____________________
____________ ❑ Varicosities (location): ______

Nail abnormalities: ______________________
Edema (location/severity +1–+4): ______________
Distribution/quality of hair: ______________
Trophic skin changes: ______________

Ego Integrity

Subjective (Reports)

Relationship status: ______________
Expression of concerns (e.g., financial, lifestyle, role changes); recent tour(s) of combat duty:
____
Stress factors: ______________
Usual ways of handling stress: ______________
Expression of feelings: Anger: ______ ❑ Anxiety: ______
Fear: ______ ❑ Grief: ______
Helplessness: ______ ❑ Hopelessness: ______
Powerlessness: ______
Cultural factors/ethnic ties: ______________
Religious affiliation: ______ ❑ Active/practicing: ______
Practices prayer/meditation: ______________
Religious/spiritual concerns: ___ ❑ Desires clergy visit: ___
Expression of sense of connectedness/harmony with self and others: ______________
Medications/herbals: ______________

Objective (Exhibits)

Emotional status (check those that apply): ❑ Calm: ______
❑ Anxious: ____ ❑ Angry: ____ ❑ Withdrawn: ____
❑ Fearful: ____ ❑ Irritable: ____ ❑ Restive: ____
❑ Euphoric: ______________
Observed body language: ______________
Observed physiological responses (e.g., palpitations, crying, change in voice quality/volume): ______________

Elimination

Subjective (Reports)

Usual bowel elimination pattern: ____ ❑ Character of stool (e.g., hard, soft, liquid): ____ ❑ Stool color (e.g., brown, black, yellow, clay colored, tarry): ______
Date of last BM and character of stool: ______________
History of bleeding: ______ ❑ Hemorrhoids/fistula: ______
Constipation acute: ______ ❑ or chronic: ______
Diarrhea: acute: ______ ❑ or chronic: ______
Bowel incontinence: ______________
Laxative: ______ ❑ how often: ______
Enema/suppository: ______ ❑ how often: ______
Usual voiding pattern and character of urine: ______________
Difficulty voiding: Urgency: ______________

Frequency: ______
Retention: ___ ❑ Bladder spasms: ___ ❑ Burning: ___
Urinary incontinence (type/time of day usually occurs): ___
History of kidney/bladder disease: ______
Diuretic use: ______ ❑ Herbals: ______

Objective (Exhibits)
Abdomen (palpation): Soft/firm: ______
Tenderness/pain (quadrant location): ______
Distention: ______ ❑ Palpable mass/location: ______
Size/girth: ______
Abdomen (auscultation): Bowel sounds (location/type): ___
Costovertebral angle tenderness: ______
Bladder palpable: ______ ❑ Overflow voiding: ______
Rectal sphincter tone (describe): ______
Hemorrhoids/fistulas: Stool in rectum: Impaction: ______
❑ Occult blood (+ or −): ______
Presence/use of catheter or continence devices: ______
Ostomy appliances (describe appliance and location): ______

Food/Fluid

Subjective (Reports)
Usual diet (type): ______
Calorie/carbohydrate/protein/fat intake (g/day): ______ ❑ # of meals daily: ___ ❑ Snacks (number/time consumed): ___
Dietary pattern/content:
B: ______ L: ______ D: ______
Snacks: ______
Last meal consumed/content: ______
Food preferences: ______
Food allergies/intolerances: ______
Cultural or religious food preparation concerns/prohibitions: ___
___Usual appetite: ______ ❑ Change in appetite: ______
Usual weight: ______
Unexpected/undesired weight loss or gain: ______
Nausea/vomiting: ______ ❑ related to: ______ ❑ Heartburn/indigestion: ___ ❑ related to: ___ ❑ relieved by: ___
Chewing/swallowing problems: ______
Gag/swallow reflex present: ______
Facial injury or surgery: ______
Stroke/other neurological deficit: ______
Teeth: Normal: ______ ❑ Dentures (full/partial): ______
Loose/absent teeth/poor dental care: ______
Sore mouth/gums: ______
Diabetes: ______ ❑ Controlled with diet/pills/insulin: ______
Vitamin/food supplements: ______
Medications/herbals: ______

Objective (Exhibits)

Current weight: ____ ❑ Height: ____ ❑ Body build: ____ ❑ Body fat %: ____

Skin turgor (e.g., firm, supple, dehydrated): ____ ❑ Mucous membranes (moist/dry): ____

Edema: Generalized: ____ ❑ Dependent: ____ ❑ Feet/ankles: ____ ❑ Periorbital: ____ ❑ Abdominal/ascites: ____

Jugular vein distention: ____

Breath sounds (auscultate)/location: Faint/distant: ____
Crackles: ____
Wheezes: ____

Condition of teeth/gums: ____

Appearance of tongue: ____
Mucous membranes: ____

Abdomen: Bowel sounds (quadrant location/type): ____
Hernia/masses: ____

Urine S/A or Chemstix: ____

Serum glucose (Glucometer): ____

Hygiene

Subjective (Reports)

Ability to carry out activities of daily living: Independent/dependent (level 1 = no assistance needed to 4 = completely dependent):

Mobility: ____ ❑ Assistance needed (describe): ____
Assistance provided by: ____
Equipment/prosthetic devices required: ____

Feeding: ____ ❑ Can prepare food: ____
Can feed self/use eating utensils: ____
Equipment/prosthetic devices required: ____

Hygiene: ____ ❑ Get supplies: ____
Wash body or body parts: ____
Can regulate bath water temperature: ____
Get in and out alone: ____
Preferred time of personal care/bath: ____

Dressing: ____ ❑ Can select clothing and dress self: ____
Needs assistance with (describe): ____
Equipment/prosthetic devices required: ____

Toileting: ____ ❑ Can get to toilet or commode alone: ____
Needs assistance with (describe): ____

Objective (Exhibits)

General appearance: Manner of dress: ____
Grooming/personal habits: ____ ❑ Condition of hair/scalp: ____ ❑ Body odor: ____
Presence of vermin (e.g., lice, scabies): ____

Neurosensory

Subjective (Reports)

History of brain injury, trauma, stroke (residual effects): ____
____
Fainting spells/dizziness: ____
Headaches (location/type/frequency): ____
Tingling/numbness/weakness (location): ____
Seizures: ____ ❑ History or new-onset seizures: ____
Type (e.g., grand mal, partial): ____
Frequency: ____ ❑ Aura: ____ ❑ Postictal state: ____
How controlled: ____
Vision: Loss or changes in vision: ____
Date last exam: ____ ❑ Glaucoma: ____
Cataract: ____ ❑ Eye surgery (type/date): ____
Hearing: Loss or change: ____ ❑ Sudden or gradual: ____
Date last exam: ____
Sense of smell (changes): ____
Sense of taste (changes): ____ ❑ Epistaxis: ____
Other: ____

Objective (Exhibits)

Mental status: (note duration of change): ____
Oriented: Person: ____ ❑ Place: ____ ❑ Time: ____
Situation: ____
Check all that apply: ❑ Alert: ____ ❑ Drowsy: ____
❑ Lethargic: ____ ❑ Stuporous: ____ ❑ Comatose: ____
❑ Cooperative: ____ ❑ Agitated/Restless: ____
❑ Combative: ____
❑ Follows commands: ____
Delusions (describe): ____ ❑ Hallucinations (describe): ____
Affect (describe): ____ ❑ Speech: ____
Memory: Recent: ____ ❑ Remote: ____
Pupil shape: ____ ❑ Size/reaction: R/L: ____
Facial droop: ____ ❑ Swallowing: ____
Handgrasp/release: R: ____ L: ____
Coordination: ____ ❑ Balance: ____
Walking: ____ Sitting: ____ Standing: ____
Deep tendon reflexes (present/absent/location): ____
Tremors: ____ ❑ Paralysis (R/L): ____
Posturing: ____
Wears glasses: ____ ❑ Contacts: ____ ❑ Hearing aids: ____

Pain/Discomfort

Subjective (Reports)

Primary focus: Location: ____
Intensity (use pain scale or pictures): ____
Quality (e.g., stabbing, aching, burning): ____
Radiation: ____ ❑ Duration: ____

Frequency: ______
Precipitating factors: ______
Relieving factors (including nonpharmaceuticals/therapies): ______
Associated symptoms (e.g., nausea, sleep problems, crying): ______ Effect on daily activities: ______
Relationships: ___ ❑ Job: ___ ❑ Enjoyment of life: ___
Additional pain focus/describe: ______
Medications: ______ ❑ Herbals: ______

Objective (Exhibits)

Facial grimacing: ___ ❑ Guarding affected area: ___
Emotional response (e.g., crying, withdrawal, anger): ______
Narrowed focus: ______
Vital sign changes (acute pain): BP: ___ ❑ Pulse: ___
Respirations: ______

Respiration

Subjective (Reports)

Dyspnea/related to: ______
Precipitating factors: ______
Relieving factors: ______
Airway clearance (e.g., spontaneous/device): ______
Cough/describe (e.g., hard, persistent, croupy): ______
Produces sputum (describe color/character): ______
Requires suctioning: ______
History of (year): Bronchitis: ___ ❑ Asthma: ___
Emphysema: ___ ❑ Tuberculosis: ___
Recurrent pneumonia: ______
Exposure to noxious fumes/allergens, infectious agents/diseases, poisons/pesticides: ______
Smoker: ___ ❑ Packs/day: ___ ❑ # of years: ___
Use of respiratory aids: ______
Oxygen (type/frequency): ______
Medications/herbals: ______

Objective (Exhibits)

Respirations (spontaneous/assisted): ___ ❑ Rate: ___
Depth: ______
Chest excursion (e.g., equal/unequal): ______
Use of accessory muscles: ______
Nasal flaring: ___ ❑ Fremitus: ___
Breath sounds (presence/absence; crackle, wheezes): ______
Egophony: ______
Skin/mucous membrane color (e.g., pale, cyanotic): ______
Clubbing of fingers: ______
Sputum characteristics: ______
Mentation (e.g., calm, anxious, restless): ______
Pulse oximetry: ______

Safety

Subjective (Reports)

Allergies/sensitivity (medications, foods, environment, latex, iodine): ____
Type of reaction: ____
Exposure to infectious diseases (e.g., measles, influenza, pink eye): ____
Exposure to pollution, toxins, poisons/pesticides, radiation (describe reactions): ____
Geographic areas lived in/visited: ____
Immunization history: Tetanus: ____ ❑ Pneumonia: ____
Influenza: ____ ❑ MMR: ____ ❑ Polio: ____
❑ Hepatitis: ____
HPV: ____
Altered/suppressed immune system (list cause): ____
History of sexually transmitted disease (date/type): ____
Testing: ____
High-risk behaviors: ____
Blood transfusion/number: ____ ❑ Date: ____
Reaction (describe): ____
Uses seat belt regularly: ____ ❑ Bike helmets: ____
Other safety devices: ____
Workplace safety/health issues (describe): ____
Currently working: ____
Rate working conditions (e.g., safety, noise, heating, water, ventilation): ____
History of injuries: (e.g. fall, vehicle crash, blast, gunshot, electrical, chemical) ____
Fractures/dislocations: ____
Arthritis/unstable joints: ____ joint replacement surgeries (type/date): ____
Back problems: ____
Skin problems (e.g., rashes, lesions, moles, breast lumps, enlarged nodes)/describe: ____
Delayed healing (describe): ____
Cognitive limitations (e.g., disorientation, confusion): ____
Sensory limitations (e.g., impaired vision/hearing, detecting heat/cold, taste, smell, touch): ____
Prostheses (type/date acquired): ____ ❑ Ambulatory devices: ____ Violence (episodes or tendencies): ____

Objective (Exhibits)

Body temperature/method (e.g., **o**ral, **r**ectal, **t**ympanic): ____
Skin integrity (e.g., scars, rashes, lacerations, ulcerations, bruises, blisters, burns [degree/%], drainage)/mark location on diagram below:
Musculoskeletal: General strength: ____
Muscle tone: ____ ❑ Gait: ____
ROM: ____ ❑ Paresthesia/paralysis: ____

Results of testing (e.g., cultures, immune function, TB, hepatitis): ______

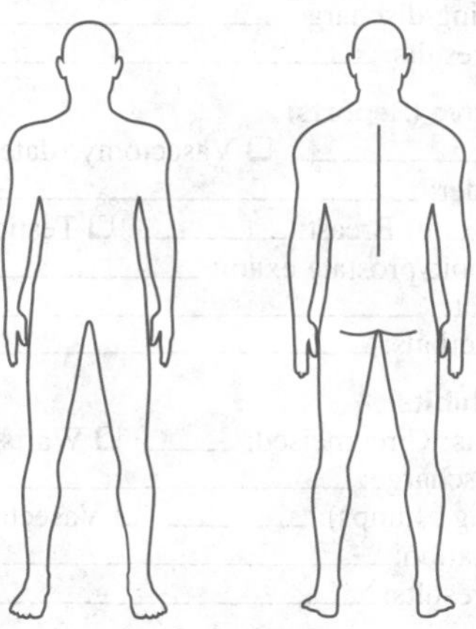

Sexuality [Component of Social Interaction]

Subjective (Reports)

Sexually active: ______ ❑ Birth control method: ______
Use of condoms: ______
Sexual concerns/difficulties (e.g., pain, relationship, role problems): ______
______
Recent change in frequency/interest: ______

Female: Subjective (Reports)

Menstruation: Age at menarche: ______
Length of cycle: ______ ❑ Duration: ______
Number of pads/tampons used/day: ______
Last menstrual period: ___ ❑ Bleeding between periods: ___
Reproductive: Infertility concerns: ______
Type of therapy: ______
Pregnant now: ______ ❑ Para: ______ ❑ Gravida: ______
Due date: ______
Menopause: Last period: ______
Hysterectomy (type/date): ______
Problem with: Hot flashes: ______ ❑ Other: ______
Vaginal lubrication: ______ ❑ Vaginal discharge: ______
Hormonal therapies: ______
Osteoporosis medications: ______
Breasts: Practices breast self-exam: ______
Last mammogram, biopsy, or surgery date: ______
Last Pap smear: ______ ❑ Results: ______

SAMPLE ASSESSMENT TOOL

Objective (Exhibits)
Breast examination: __________
Genitalia: Warts/lesions: __________
Vaginal bleeding/discharge: __________
STI type/test results: __________

Male: Subjective (Reports)
Circumcised: _____ ❑ Vasectomy (date): _____
Prostate disorder: __________
Practice self-exam: Breast: _____ ❑ Testicles: _____
Last proctoscopic/prostate exam: __________
Last PSA/date: __________
Medications/herbals: __________

Objective (Exhibits)
Genitalia: Penis: Circumcised: _____ ❑ Warts/lesions: _____
Bleeding/discharge: __________
Testicles (e.g., lumps): _____ ❑ Vasectomy: _____
Breast examination: __________
STI type/test results: __________

Social Interactions

Subjective (Reports)
Relationship status (check): ❑ Single: _____ ❑ Married: _____
❑ Living with partner: _____ ❑ Divorced: _____
❑ Widowed: _____ Years in relationship: _____
❑ Perceptionof relationship: _____ Concerns/stresses: _____
Role within family structure: __________
Number/age of children: __________
Perception of relationship with family members: _____
Extended family: _____ ❑ Other support person(s): _____
Ethnic/cultural affiliations: __________
Strength of ethnic identity: __________
Lives in ethnic community: __________
Feelings of (describe): Mistrust: __________
Rejection: _____ ❑ Unhappiness: _____
Loneliness/isolation: __________
Problems related to illness/condition: __________
Problems with communication (e.g., speech, another language, brain injury): __________
Use of speech/communication aids (list): _____
Is interpreter needed: __________
Primary language: __________
Genogram: Diagram on separate page

Objective (Exhibits)
Communication/speech: Clear: _____ ❑ Slurred: _____
Incomprehensible: _____ ❑ Aphasic: _____
Unusual speech pattern/impairment: _____
Laryngectomy present: __________

Verbal/nonverbal communication with family/significant other (SO): ______
Family interaction (behavioral) pattern: ______
______

Teaching/Learning

Subjective (Reports)

Communication: Dominant language (specify): ______
Second language: ______ ❑ Literate (reading/writing): ______
Education level: ______
Learning disabilities (specify): ______
Cognitive limitations: ______
Culture/ethnicity: Where born: ______
If immigrant, how long in this country: ______
Health and illness beliefs/practices/customs: ______
Which family member makes healthcare decisions/is spokesperson for client: ______
Presence of Advance Directives: ______ ❑ Code status: Durable Medical Power of Attorney: ______ ❑ Designee: ______
Health goals: ______
Current health problem: Client understanding of problem: ______
Special healthcare concerns (e.g., impact of religious/cultural practices): ______
Familial risk factors (indicate relationship): ______
Diabetes: ______ ❑ Thyroid (specify): ______
Tuberculosis: ______ ❑ Heart disease: ______
Stroke: ______ ❑ Hypertension: ______
Epilepsy/seizures: ______ ❑ Kidney disease: ______
Cancer: ______ ❑ Mental illness: ______
Depression: ______ ❑ Other: ______
Prescribed medications: ______
Drug: ______ ❑ Dose: ______
Times (circle last dose): ______
Take regularly: ______ ❑ Purpose: ______
Side effects/problems: ______
Nonprescription drugs/frequency: OTC drugs: ______
Vitamins: ______ ❑ Herbals: ______
Street drugs: ______
Alcohol (amount/frequency): ______
Tobacco: ______ ❑ Smokeless tobacco: ______
Admitting diagnosis per provider: ______
Reason for hospitalization per client: ______
History of current problem: ______
Expectations of this hospitalization: ______
Will admission cause any lifestyle changes (describe): ______
Previous illnesses and/or hospitalizations/surgeries: ______
Evidence of failure to improve: ______
Last complete physical exam: ______

Discharge Plan Considerations

Projected length of stay (days or hours): ____________

Anticipated date of discharge: ____________

Date information obtained: ____________

Resources available: Persons: ____________

Financial: ________ ❑ Community supports: ________

Groups: ____________

Areas that may require alteration/assistance:

Food preparation: ________ ❑ Shopping: ________

Transportation: ________ ❑ Ambulation: ________

Medication/IV therapy: ____________

Treatments: ____________

Wound care: ____________

Supplies/DME: ____________

Self-care (specify): ____________

Homemaker/maintenance (specify): ____________

Socialization: ____________

Physical layout of home (specify): ____________

Anticipated changes in living situation after discharge: ________

Living facility other than home (specify): ________

Referrals (date/source/services): Social services: ________

Rehab services: ________ ❑ Dietary: ________

Home care/hospice: ________ ❑ Resp/O_2: ________

Equipment: ____________

Supplies: ____________

Other: ____________

SECTION 2

Diagnostic Divisions: Nursing Diagnoses Organized According to a Nursing Focus

After data are collected and areas of concern or need are identified, the nurse is directed to the Diagnostic Divisions to review the list of NDs that fall within the individual categories. This will assist the nurse in choosing the specific diagnostic label to accurately describe the data. Then, with the addition of etiology or related/risk factors and signs and symptoms or cues (defining characteristics) when present, the client diagnostic statement emerges.

ACTIVITY/REST—Ability to engage in necessary or desired activities of life (work and leisure) and to obtain adequate sleep or rest

Activity Intolerance
Activity Intolerance, risk for
Activity Planning, ineffective
Activity Planning, risk for ineffective
Disuse Syndrome, risk for
Diversional Activity, deficient
Fatigue
Insomnia
Lifestyle, sedentary
Mobility, impaired wheelchair
Sitting, impaired
Sleep, readiness for enhanced
Sleep deprivation
Sleep Pattern, disturbed
Standing, impaired
Transfer Ability, impaired
Walking, impaired

CIRCULATION—Ability to transport oxygen and nutrients necessary to meet cellular needs

Adaptive Capacity, decreased intracranial
Autonomic Dysreflexia
Autonomic Dysreflexia, risk for
Bleeding, risk for
Cardiac Output, decreased
Cardiac Output, risk for decreased
Cardiovascular Function, risk for impaired

Gastrointestinal Perfusion, risk for ineffective
Renal Perfusion, risk for ineffective
Shock, risk for
Tissue Perfusion, ineffective peripheral
Tissue Perfusion, risk for decreased cardiac
Tissue Perfusion, risk for ineffective cerebral
Tissue Perfusion, risk for ineffective peripheral

EGO INTEGRITY—Ability to develop and use skills and behaviors to integrate and manage life experiences*

Anxiety [specify level]
Body Image, disturbed
Coping, defensive
Coping, ineffective
Coping, readiness for enhanced
Death Anxiety
Decision-Making, readiness for enhanced
Emancipated Decision-Making, readiness for enhanced
Emancipated Decision-Making, impaired
Emancipated Decision-Making, risk for impaired
Decisional Conflict
Denial, ineffective
Emotional Control, labile
Fear
Grieving
Grieving, complicated
Grieving, risk for complicated
Hope, readiness for enhanced
Hopelessness
Human Dignity, risk for compromised
Impulse Control, ineffective
Mood Regulation, impaired
Moral Distress
Personal Identity, disturbed
Personal Identity, risk for disturbed
Post-Trauma Syndrome [specify stage]
Post-Trauma Syndrome, risk for
Power, readiness for enhanced
Powerlessness
Powerlessness, risk for
Rape-Trauma Syndrome
Relationship, ineffective
Relationship, readiness for enhanced
Relationship, risk for ineffective
Religiosity, impaired
Religiosity, readiness for enhanced
Religiosity, risk for impaired
Relocation Stress Syndrome
Relocation Stress Syndrome, risk for
Resilience, impaired

Resilience, readiness for enhanced
Resilience, risk for impaired
Self-Concept, readiness for enhanced
Self-Esteem, chronic low
Self-Esteem, risk for chronic low
Self-Esteem, situational low
Self-Esteem, risk for situational low
Sorrow, chronic
Spiritual distress
Spiritual distress, risk for
Spiritual Well-Being, readiness for enhanced

ELIMINATION—Ability to excrete waste products*

Constipation
Constipation, chronic functional
Constipation, risk for chronic functional
Constipation, perceived
Constipation, risk for
Diarrhea
Elimination, impaired urinary
Elimination, readiness for enhanced urinary
Gastrointestinal Motility, dysfunctional
Gastrointestinal Motility, risk for dysfunctional
Incontinence, bowel
Incontinence, functional urinary
Incontinence, overflow urinary
Incontinence, reflex urinary
Incontinence, risk for urge urinary
Incontinence, stress urinary
Incontinence, urge urinary
Urinary Retention [acute/chronic]

FOOD/FLUID—Ability to maintain intake of and utilize nutrients and liquids to meet physiological needs*

Blood Glucose Level, risk for unstable
Breast Milk, insufficient
Breastfeeding, ineffective
Breastfeeding, interrupted
Breastfeeding, readiness for enhanced
Dentition, impaired
Electrolyte Imbalance, risk for
Feeding Pattern, ineffective infant
Fluid Balance, readiness for enhanced
[Fluid Volume, deficient hyper/hypotonic]
Fluid Volume, deficient [isotonic]
Fluid Volume, excess
Fluid Volume, risk for deficient
Fluid Volume, risk for imbalanced
Frail Elderly Syndrome
Frail Elderly Syndrome, risk for

Liver Function, risk for impaired
Mucous Membrane, impaired oral
Mucous Membrane, risk for impaired oral
Nausea
Nutrition: less than body requirements, imbalanced
Nutrition, readiness for enhanced
Obesity
Overweight
Overweight, risk for
Swallowing, impaired

HYGIENE—Ability to perform activities of daily living

Self-Care, readiness for enhanced
Self-Care Deficit, bathing
Self-Care Deficit, dressing
Self-Care Deficit, feeding
Self-Care Deficit, toileting
Self-Neglect

NEUROSENSORY—Ability to perceive, integrate, and respond to internal and external cues

Behavior, disorganized infant
Behavior, readiness for enhanced organized infant
Behavior, risk for disorganized infant
Confusion, acute
Confusion, risk for acute
Confusion, chronic
Dysfunction, risk for peripheral neurovascular
Memory, impaired
[Sensory Perception, disturbed (specify: visual, auditory, kinesthetic, gustatory, tactile, olfactory)]
Stress overload
Unilateral Neglect

PAIN/DISCOMFORT—Ability to control internal and external environment to maintain comfort

Comfort, impaired
Comfort, readiness for enhanced
Pain, acute
Pain, chronic
Pain, labor
Pain Syndrome, chronic

RESPIRATION—Ability to provide and use oxygen to meet physiological needs

Airway Clearance, ineffective
Aspiration, risk for
Breathing Pattern, ineffective
Gas Exchange, impaired
Ventilation, impaired spontaneous

Ventilatory Weaning Response, dysfunctional

SAFETY—Ability to provide safe, growth-promoting environment

Allergy Response, risk for
Body Temperature, risk for imbalanced
Contamination
Contamination, risk for
Dry Eye, risk for
Falls, risk for
Health Maintenance, ineffective
Home Maintenance, impaired
Hyperthermia
Hypothermia
Hypothermia, risk for
Hypothermia, risk for perioperative
Infection, risk for
Injury, risk for
Injury, risk for corneal
Injury, risk for urinary tract
Jaundice, neonatal
Jaundice, risk for neonatal
Latex Allergy Response
Latex Allergy Response, risk for
Maternal-Fetal Dyad, risk for disturbed
Mobility, impaired bed
Mobility, impaired physical
Poisoning, risk for
Positioning Injury, risk for perioperative
Protection, ineffective
Reaction to Iodinated Contrast Media, risk for adverse
Self-Mutilation
Self-Mutilation, risk for
Skin Integrity, impaired
Skin Integrity, risk for impaired
Sudden Infant Death Syndrome, risk for
Suffocation, risk for
Suicide, risk for
Surgical Recovery, delayed
Surgical Recovery, risk for delayed
Thermal Injury, risk for
Thermoregulation, ineffective
Tissue Integrity, impaired
Tissue Integrity, risk for impaired
Trauma, risk for
Trauma, risk for vascular
Violence, risk for other-directed
Violence, risk for self-directed
Wandering [specify sporadic or continual]

SEXUALITY—[Component of Ego Integrity and Social Interaction] Ability to meet requirements/characteristics of male/female roles*

Childbearing Process, ineffective
Childbearing Process, readiness for enhanced
Childbearing Process, risk for ineffective
Sexual Dysfunction
Sexuality Pattern, ineffective

SOCIAL INTERACTION—Ability to establish and maintain relationships*

Attachment, risk for impaired
Communication, impaired verbal
Communication, readiness for enhanced
Coping, compromised family
Coping, disabled family
Coping, ineffective community
Coping, readiness for enhanced community
Coping, readiness for enhanced family
Family Processes, dysfunctional
Family Processes, interrupted
Family Processes, readiness for enhanced
Loneliness, risk for
Parenting, impaired
Parenting, readiness for enhanced
Parenting, risk for impaired
Role Conflict, parental
Role Performance, ineffective
Role Strain, caregiver
Role Strain, risk for caregiver
Social Interaction, impaired
Social Isolation

TEACHING/LEARNING—Ability to incorporate and use information to achieve healthy lifestyle/optimal wellness*

Development, risk for delayed
Growth, risk for disproportionate
Health, deficient community
Health Maintenance, ineffective
Health Management, ineffective
Health Management, ineffective family
Health Management, readiness for enhanced
Knowledge, deficient [Learning Need (specify)]
Knowledge, readiness for enhanced
Noncompliance [ineffective Adherence] [specify]

---

*Information that appears in brackets has been added by authors to clarify and enhance the use of NDs.

APPENDIX 2

In Section 1, a sample plan of care formulated on data collected with the nursing model assessment tool is provided. Individualized client diagnostic statements and desired client outcomes (with timelines added to reflect anticipated length of stay and individual client and nurse expectations) were identified, and interventions were chosen based on concerns or needs identified by the client and nurse during data collection, as well as by physician orders. Although not normally included in a written plan of care, rationales are included in this sample for the purpose of explaining or clarifying the choice of interventions to enhance the nurse's learning.

Another way to conceptualize the client's care needs is to create a Mind or Concept Map (Section 2). This technique was developed to help visualize the linkages between various client symptoms, interventions, or problems as they impact each other. The parts that are great about traditional care plans (problem-solving and categorizing) are retained, but the linear or columnar nature of the plan is changed to a design that uses the whole brain—a design that brings left-brain, linear problem-solving thinking together with the freewheeling, interconnected, creative right brain. Joining mind mapping and care planning enables the nurse to create a holistic view of a client, strengthening critical thinking skills and facilitating the creative process of planning client care.

SECTION 1

Client Situation and Prototype Plan of Care

Client Situation

Mr. R. S., a client with type 2 diabetes (noninsulin dependent) for 10 years, presented to his physician's office with a non-healing ulcer of 3 weeks' duration on his left foot. Screening studies done in the doctor's office revealed blood glucose of 356/fingerstick and urine Chemstix of 2%. Because of distance from medical provider and lack of local community services, he is admitted to the hospital.

Admitting Physician's Orders

Culture/sensitivity and Gram stain of foot ulcer
Random blood glucose on admission and fingerstick BG qid
CBC, electrolytes, serum lipid profile, glycosylated Hb in a.m.
Chest x-ray and ECG in a.m.
DiaBeta 10 mg, PO bid
Glucophage 500 mg, PO daily to start—will increase gradually
Humulin N 10 units SC q a.m.. Begin insulin instruction for postdischarge self-care if necessary
Dicloxacillin 500 mg PO q6h, start after culture obtained
Darvocet-N 100 mg PO q4h prn pain
Diet—2,400 calories, three meals with two snacks
Consult with dietitian
Up in chair ad lib with feet elevated
Foot cradle for bed
Irrigate lesion L foot with NS tid, cover with sterile dressing
Vital signs qid

Client Assessment Database

Name: R. S. Informant: client
Reliability (Scale 1 to 4): 3
Age: 75 DOB: 5/3/39 Race: Caucasian Gender: M
Adm. date: 4/28/2015 Time: 7 p.m. From: home

Activity/Rest

Subjective (Reports)

Occupation: farmer
Usual activities/hobbies: reading, playing cards. "Don't have time to do much. Anyway, I'm too tired most of the time to do anything after the chores."

Limitations imposed by illness: "Have to watch what I order if I eat out."
Sleep: Hours: 6 to 8 hr/night Naps: no Aids: no
Insomnia: "Not unless I drink coffee after supper."
Usually feels rested when awakens at 4:30 a.m.

Objective (Exhibits)

Observed response to activity: limps, favors L foot when walking
Mental status: alert/active
Neuromuscular assessment: Muscle mass/tone: bilaterally equal/firm Posture: erect
ROM: full Strength: equal 4 extremities/(favors L foot currently)

Circulation

Subjective (Reports)

History of slow healing: lesion L foot, 3 weeks' duration
Extremities: Numbness/tingling: "My feet feel cold and tingly like sharp pins poking the bottom of my feet when I walk the quarter mile to the mailbox."
Cough/character of sputum: occ./white
Change in frequency/amount of urine: yes/voiding more lately

Objective (Exhibits)

Peripheral pulses: radials 3+; popliteal, dorsalis, post-tibial/pedal, all 1+
BP: R: Lying: 146/90 Sitting: 140/86 Standing: 138/90
L: Lying: 142/88 Sitting: 138/88 Standing: 138/84
Pulse: Apical: 86 Radial: 86 Quality: strong
Rhythm: regular
Chest auscultation: few wheezes clear with cough, no murmurs/rubs
Jugular vein distention: 0
Extremities:
Temperature: feet cool bilaterally/legs warm
Color: Skin: legs pale
Capillary refill: slow both feet (approx. 4 sec)
Homans' sign: 0
Varicosities: few enlarged superficial veins on both calves
Nails: toenails thickened, yellow, brittle
Distribution and quality of hair: coarse hair to midcalf; none on ankles/toes

Color:

General: ruddy face/arms
Mucous membranes/lips: pink
Nailbeds: pink
Conjunctiva and sclera: white

Ego Integrity

Subjective (Reports)

Report of stress factors: "Normal farmer's problems: weather, pests, bankers, etc."
Ways of handling stress: "I get busy with the chores and talk things over with my livestock. They listen pretty good."
Financial concerns: Medicare only and needs to hire someone to do chores while here
Relationship status: married
Cultural factors: rural/agrarian, eastern European descent, "American," no ethnic ties
Religion: Protestant/practicing
Lifestyle: middle class/self-sufficient farmer
Recent changes: no
Feelings: "I'm in control of most things, except the weather and this diabetes now."
Concerned about possible therapy change "from pills to shots."

Objective (Exhibits)

Emotional status: generally calm, appears frustrated at times
Observed physiological response(s): occasionally sighs deeply/frowns, fidgeting with coin, shoulders tense/shrugs shoulders, throws up hands

Elimination

Subjective (Reports)

Usual bowel pattern: almost every p.m.
Last BM: last night Character of stool: firm/brown
Bleeding: 0 Hemorrhoids: 0 Constipation: occ.
Laxative used: hot prune juice on occ.
Urinary: no problems Character of urine: pale yellow

Objective (Exhibits)

Abdomen tender: no Soft/firm: soft Palpable mass: 0
Bowel sounds: active all 4 quads

Food/Fluid

Subjective (Reports)

Usual diet (type): 2,400 calorie (occ. "cheats" with dessert; "My wife watches it pretty closely.")
No. of meals daily: 3/1 snack
Dietary pattern:

B: fruit juice/toast/ham/decaf coffee
L: meat/potatoes/veg/fruit/milk
D: $\frac{1}{2}$ meat sandwich/soup/fruit/decaf coffee
Snack: milk/crackers at HS. Usual beverage: skim milk, 2 to 3 cups decaf coffee, drinks "lots of water"—several quarts

Last meal/intake: Dinner: $\frac{1}{2}$ roast beef sandwich, vegetable soup, pear with cheese, decaf coffee
Loss of appetite: "Never, but lately I don't feel as hungry as usual."
Nausea/vomiting: 0 Food allergies: none
Heartburn/food intolerance: cabbage causes gas, coffee after supper causes heartburn
Mastication/swallowing problems: 0
Dentures: partial upper plate—fits well
Usual weight: 175 lb Recent changes: has lost about 6 lb this month
Diuretic therapy: no

Objective (Exhibits)

Wt: 169 lb Ht: 5 ft 10 in. Build: stocky
Skin turgor: good/leathery Mucous membranes: moist
Condition of teeth/gums: good, no irritation/bleeding noted
Appearance of tongue: midline, pink
Mucous membranes: pink, intact

Breath sounds: few wheezes cleared with cough
Bowel sounds: active all 4 quads
Urine Chemstix: 2% Fingerstick: 356 (Dr. office) 450 random BG on adm

Hygiene

Subjective (Reports)

Activities of daily living: independent in all areas
Preferred time of bath: p.m.

Objective (Exhibits)

General appearance: clean-shaven, short-cut hair; hands rough and dry; skin on feet dry, cracked, and scaly
Scalp and eyebrows: scaly white patches
No body odor

Neurosensory

Subjective (Reports)

Headache: "Occasionally behind my eyes when I worry too much."
Tingling/numbness: feet, 4 or 5 times/week (as noted)
Eyes: Vision loss, farsighted, "Seems a little blurry now." Examination: 2 yr ago
Ears: Hearing loss R: "Some." L: no (has not been tested)
Nose: Epistaxis: 0 Sense of smell: "No problem."

Objective (Exhibits)

Mental status: alert, oriented to person, place, time, situation
Affect: concerned   Memory: Remote/recent: clear and intact
Speech: clear/coherent, appropriate
Pupil reaction: PERRLA/small
Glasses: reading   Hearing aid: no
Handgrip/release: strong/equal

Pain/Discomfort

Subjective (Reports)

Primary focus: Location: medial aspect, L heel
Intensity (0 to 10): 4 to 5   Quality: dull ache with occ. sharp stabbing sensation
Frequency/duration: "Seems like all the time."
Radiation: no
Precipitating factors: shoes, walking
How relieved: ASA, not helping
Other complaints: sometimes has back pain following chores/heavy lifting, relieved by ASA/liniment rubdown

Objective (Exhibits)

Facial grimacing: when lesion border palpated
Guarding affected area: pulls foot away
Narrowed focus: no
Emotional response: tense, irritated

Respiration

Subjective (Reports)

Dyspnea: 0   Cough: occ. morning cough, white sputum
Emphysema: 0   Bronchitis: 0   Asthma: 0   Tuberculosis: 0
Smoker: filters Pk/day: $\frac{1}{2}$ No. yr: 50+
Use of respiratory aids: 0

Objective (Exhibits)

Respiratory rate: 22   Depth: good   Symmetry: equal, bilateral
Auscultation: few wheezes, clear with cough
Cyanosis: 0   Clubbing of fingers: 0
Sputum characteristics: none to observe
Mentation/restlessness: alert/oriented/relaxed

Safety

Subjective (Reports)

Allergies: 0   Blood transfusions: 0
Sexually transmitted disease: 0
Wears seat belt
Fractures/dislocations: L clavicle, 1960s, fell getting off tractor
Arthritis/unstable joints: "Some in my knees."

Back problems: occ. lower back pain
Vision impaired: requires glasses for reading
Hearing impaired: slightly (R), compensates by turning "good ear" toward speaker
Immunizations: current flu/pneumonia 3 yr ago/tetanus maybe 8 yr ago

Objective (Exhibits)

Temperature: 99.4°F (37.4°C) Tympanic
Skin integrity: impaired L foot Scars: R inguinal, surgical
Rashes: 0 Bruises: 0 Lacerations: 0 Blisters: 0
Ulcerations: medial aspect L heel, 2.5 cm diameter, approx. 3 mm deep, wound edges inflamed, draining small amount cream-color/pink-tinged matter, slight musty odor noted
Strength (general): equal all extremities Muscle tone: firm
ROM: good Gait: favors L foot Paresthesia/paralysis: tingling, prickly sensation in feet after walking $\frac{1}{4}$ mile

Sexuality: Male

Subjective (Reports)

Sexually active: yes Use of condoms: no (monogamous)
Recent changes in frequency/interest: "I've been too tired lately."
Penile discharge: 0 Prostate disorder: 0 Vasectomy: 0
Last proctoscopic examination: 2 yr ago Prostate examination: 1 yr ago
Practice self-examination: Breasts/testicles: no
Problems/complaints: "I don't have any problems, but you'd have to ask my wife if there are any complaints."

Objective (Exhibits)

Examination: Breasts: no masses Testicles: deferred
Prostate: deferred

Social Interactions

Subjective (Reports)

Marital status: married 45 yr Living with: wife
Report of problems: none
Extended family: 1 daughter lives in town (30 miles away); 1 daughter married with a son, living out of state
Other: several couples, he and wife play cards/socialize with 2 to 3 times/mo, church fellowship weekly
Role: works farm alone; husband/father/grandfather
Report of problems related to illness/condition: none until now
Coping behaviors: "My wife and I have always talked things out. You know the 11th commandment is 'Thou shalt not go to bed angry.'"

Objective (Exhibits)

Speech: clear, intelligible

Verbal/nonverbal communication with family/SO(s): speaks quietly with wife, looking her in the eye; relaxed posture

Family interaction patterns: wife sitting at bedside, relaxed, both reading paper, making occasional comments to each other

Teaching/Learning

Subjective (Reports)

Dominant language: English Second language: 0 Literate: yes

Education level: 2 yr college

Health and illness/beliefs/practices/customs: "I take care of the minor problems and see the doctor only when something's broken."

Presence of Advance Directives: yes—wife to bring in

Durable Medical Power of Attorney: wife

Familial risk factors/relationship:

Diabetes: maternal uncle

Tuberculosis: brother died, age 27

Heart disease: father died, age 78, heart attack

Stroke: mother died, age 81

High BP: mother

Prescribed medications:

Drug: DiaBeta Dose: 10 mg bid

Schedule: 8 a.m./6 p.m., last dose 6 p.m. today

Purpose: control diabetes

Takes medications regularly? yes

Home urine/glucose monitoring: Only using test strips, stopped some months ago when he ran out. "It was always negative, anyway, and I don't like sticking my finger."

Nonprescription (OTC) drugs: occ. ASA

Use of alcohol (amount/frequency): socially, occ. beer

Tobacco: $\frac{1}{2}$ pk/day

Admitting diagnosis (physician): hyperglycemia with nonhealing lesion L foot

Reason for hospitalization (client): "Sore on foot and the doctor is concerned about my blood sugar, and says I'm supposed to learn this finger stick test now."

History of current complaint: "Three weeks ago I got a blister on my foot from breaking in my new boots. It got sore so I lanced it, but it isn't getting any better."

Client's expectations of this hospitalization: "Clear up this infection and control my diabetes."

Other relevant illness and/or previous hospitalizations/ surgeries: 1960s, R inguinal hernia repair, tonsils age 5 or 6

Evidence of failure to improve: lesion L foot, 3 wk
Last physical examination: complete 1 yr ago, office follow-up 5 mo ago

Discharge Considerations (as of 4/28)

Anticipated discharge: 5/1/15 (3 days)
Resources: self, wife
Financial: "If this doesn't take too long to heal, we got some savings to cover things."
Community supports: diabetic support group (has not participated)
Anticipated lifestyle changes: become more involved in management of condition
Assistance needed: may require farm help for several days
Teaching: learn new medication regimen and wound care; review diet; encourage smoking cessation
Referral: Supplies: the Downtown Pharmacy or AARP
Equipment: Glucometer—AARP
Follow-up: primary care provider 1 wk after discharge to evaluate wound healing and potential need for additional changes in diabetic regimen

Plan of Care for Client with Diabetes Mellitus

Client Diagnostic Statement:

impaired Skin Integrity related to pressure, altered metabolic state, circulatory impairment, and decreased sensation, as evidenced by draining wound L foot.

Outcome: Wound Healing: Secondary Intention (NOC) Indicators: Client Will:

Be free of purulent drainage within 48 hr (4/30 1900).
Display signs of healing with wound edges clean/pink within 60 hr (5/1 0700).

ACTIONS/ INTERVENTIONS	RATIONALE
Wound Care (NIC)	
Irrigate wound with room-temperature sterile NS tid.	Cleans wound without harming delicate tissues.
Assess wound with each dressing change. Obtain wound tracing on adm and at discharge.	Provides information about effectiveness of therapy, and identifies additional needs.
Apply sterile dressing.	Keeps wound clean/minimizes cross contamination.
Use paper tape.	Adhesive tape may be abrasive to fragile tissues.
Infection Control (NIC)	
Follow wound precautions.	Use of gloves and proper handling of contaminated dressings reduces likelihood of spread of infection.
Obtain sterile specimen of wound drainage on admission.	Culture/sensitivity identifies pathogens and therapy of choice.
Administer dicloxacillin 500 mg PO q6h, starting 10 p.m..	Treatment of infection and prevention of complications.
	Food interferes with drug absorption, requiring scheduling around meals.
Observe for signs of hypersensitivity: pruritus, urticaria, rash.	Although no history of penicillin reaction, it may occur at any time.

Client Diagnostic Statement:

risk for unstable Blood Glucose Level evidenced by risk factors of lack of adherence to diabetes management and inadequate blood glucose monitoring with fingerstick 450/adm.

Outcome: Blood Glucose Level (NOC)
Indicators: Client Will:

Demonstrate correction of metabolic state as evidenced by FBS less than 120 mg/dL within 36 hr (4/30 0700).

ACTIONS/ INTERVENTIONS	RATIONALE
Hyperglycemia Management (NIC)	
Perform fingerstick BG qid.	Bedside analysis of blood glucose levels is a more timely method for monitoring effectiveness of therapy and provides direction for alteration of medications.
Administer antidiabetic medications:	Treats underlying metabolic dysfunction, reducing hyperglycemia and promoting healing.
10 U Humulin N insulin SC q a.m. after fingerstick BG;	Intermediate-acting preparation with onset of 2 to 4 hr, peaks at 6 to 12 hr, with a duration of 18 to 24 hr. Increases transport of glucose into cells and promotes the conversion of glucose to glycogen.
DiaBeta 10 mg PO bid;	Lowers blood glucose by stimulating the release of insulin from the pancreas and increasing the sensitivity to insulin at the receptor sites.
Glucophage 500 mg PO daily; note onset of side effects.	Glucophage lowers serum glucose levels by decreasing hepatic glucose production and intestinal glucose absorption and increasing sensitivity to insulin. By using in conjunction with DiaBeta, client may be able to discontinue insulin once target dosage is achieved (e.g., 2,000 mg/day). An increase of 1 tablet per week is necessary to limit side effects of diarrhea, abdominal cramping, vomiting, possibly leading to dehydration and prerenal azotemia.

ACTIONS/ INTERVENTIONS	RATIONALE
Provide diet of 2,400 cals—3 meals/2 snacks.	Proper diet decreases glucose levels/insulin needs, prevents hyperglycemic episodes, can reduce serum cholesterol levels and promote satiation.
Schedule consultation with dietitian to restructure meal plan and evaluate food choices.	Calories are unchanged on new orders but have been redistributed to 3 meals and 2 snacks. Dietary choices (e.g., increased vitamin C) may enhance healing.

Client Diagnostic Statement:

acute Pain related to physical agent (open wound L foot), as evidenced by verbal report of pain and guarding behavior.

Outcome: Pain Control (NOC) Indicators: Client Will:

Report pain is minimized/relieved within 1 hr of analgesic administration (ongoing).

Report absence or control of pain by discharge (5/1).

Outcome: Pain Disruptive Effects (NOC) Indicators: Client Will:

Ambulate normally, full weight-bearing by discharge (5/1).

ACTIONS/ INTERVENTIONS	RATIONALE
Pain Management (NIC)	
Determine pain characteristics through client's description.	Establishes baseline for assessing improvement/changes.
Place foot cradle on bed; encourage use of loose-fitting slipper when up.	Avoids direct pressure to area of injury, which could result in vasoconstriction/ increased pain.
Administer Darvocet-N 100 mg PO q4h as needed. Document effectiveness.	Provides relief of discomfort when unrelieved by other measures.

Client Diagnostic Statement:

ineffective peripheral Tissue Perfusion related to deficient knowledge of disease process/aggravating factors and diabetes mellitus as evidenced by diminished pulses, pale/cool feet; capillary refill of 4 sec; parathesia of feet "when walks $\frac{1}{4}$ mile."

Outcome: Knowledge: Diabetes Management (NOC) Indicators: Client Will:

Verbalize understanding of relationship between chronic disease (diabetes mellitus) and circulatory changes within 48 hr (4/30 1900).

Demonstrate awareness of safety factors and proper foot care within 48 hr (4/30 1900).

Maintain adequate level of hydration to maximize perfusion, as evidenced by balanced intake/output, moist skin/mucous membranes, and capillary refill less than 3 sec (ongoing).

ACTIONS/ INTERVENTIONS	RATIONALE
Circulatory Care: Arterial Insufficiency (NIC)	
Elevate feet when up in chair. Avoid long periods with feet in a dependent position.	Minimizes interruption of blood flow, reduces venous pooling.
Assess for signs of dehydration.	Glycosuria may result in dehydration with consequent reduction of circulating volume and further impairment of peripheral circulation.
Monitor intake/output. Encourage oral fluids.	
Instruct client to avoid constricting clothing/socks and ill-fitting shoes.	Compromised circulation and decreased pain sensation may precipitate or aggravate tissue breakdown.
Reinforce safety precautions regarding use of heating pads, hot water bottles, or soaks.	Heat increases metabolic demands on compromised tissues. Vascular insufficiency alters pain sensation, increasing risk of injury.
Recommend cessation of smoking.	Vascular constriction associated with smoking and diabetes impairs peripheral circulation.
Discuss complications of disease that result from vascular changes: ulceration, gangrene, muscle or bony structure changes.	Although proper control of diabetes mellitus may not prevent complications, severity of effect may be minimized. Diabetic foot complications are the leading cause of nontraumatic lower extremity amputations.

ACTIONS/ INTERVENTIONS	RATIONALE
	Note: Skin dry, cracked, scaly; feet cool; and pain when walking a distance suggest mild to moderate vascular disease (autonomic neuropathy) that can limit response to infection, impair wound healing, and increase risk of bony deformities.
Review proper foot care as outlined in teaching plan.	Altered perfusion of lower extremities may lead to serious or persistent complications at the cellular level.

Client Diagnostic Statement:

deficient Knowledge/Learning Need regarding diabetic condition related to misinterpretation of information and/or lack of recall as evidenced by inaccurate follow-through of instructions regarding home glucose monitoring and foot care and failure to recognize signs/symptoms of hyperglycemia.

Outcome: Knowledge: Diabetes Management (NOC) Indicators: Client Will:

Perform procedure for home glucose monitoring correctly within 36 hr (4/30 0700).

Verbalize basic understanding of disease process and treatment within 38 hr (4/30 0900).

Explain reasons for actions within 38 hr (4/30 0900).

Perform insulin administration correctly within 60 hr (5/1 0700).

ACTIONS/ INTERVENTIONS	RATIONALE
Teaching: Disease Process (NIC)	
Determine client's level of knowledge, priorities of learning needs, desire/need for including wife in instruction.	Establishes baseline and direction for teaching/planning. Involvement of wife, if desired, will provide additional resource for recall/understanding and may enhance client's follow through.

ACTIONS/ INTERVENTIONS	RATIONALE
Provide teaching guide, "Understanding Your Diabetes," 4/29 a.m. Show film "Living with Diabetes" 4/29 4 p.m., when wife is visiting. Include in group teaching session 4/30 a.m. Review information and obtain feedback from client/wife.	Provides different methods for accessing/reinforcing information and enhances opportunity for learning/ understanding.
Discuss factors related to altering diabetic control such as stress, illness, exercise.	Drug therapy/diet may need to be altered in response to both short-term and long-term stressors and changes in activity level.
Review signs/symptoms of hyperglycemia (e.g., fatigue, nausea, vomiting, polyuria, polydipsia). Discuss how to prevent and evaluate this situation and when to seek medical care. Have client identify appropriate interventions.	Recognition and understanding of these signs/ symptoms and timely intervention will aid client in avoiding recurrences and preventing complications.
Review and provide information about necessity for routine examination of feet and proper foot care (e.g., daily inspection for injuries, pressure areas, corns, calluses; proper nail cutting; daily washing and application of good moisturizing lotion such as Eucerin, Keri, Nivea bid). Recommend wearing loose-fitting socks and properly fitting shoes (break new shoes in gradually) and avoiding going barefoot. If foot injury/skin break occurs, wash with soap/dermal cleanser and water, cover with sterile dressing, and inspect wound and change dressing daily; report redness, swelling, or presence of drainage.	Reduces risk of tissue injury; promotes understanding and prevention of stasis ulcer formation and wound-healing difficulties.

ACTIONS/ INTERVENTIONS	RATIONALE
Teaching: Prescribed Medication (NIC)	
Instruct regarding prescribed insulin therapy:	May be a temporary treatment of hyperglycemia with infection or may be permanent replacement of oral hypoglycemic agent.
Humulin N Insulin, SC.	Intermediate-acting insulin generally lasts 18 to 24 hr, with peak effect between 6 and 12 hr.
Keep vial in current use at room temperature (if used within 30 days).	Cold insulin is poorly absorbed.
Store extra vials in refrigerator.	Refrigeration prevents wide fluctuations in temperature, prolonging the drug shelf life.
Roll bottle and invert to mix, or shake gently, avoiding bubbles.	Vigorous shaking may create foam, which can interfere with accurate dose withdrawal and may damage the insulin molecule. **Note:** New research suggests that shaking the vial may be more effective in mixing suspension. Refer to Procedure Manual.
Choice of injection sites (e.g., across lower abdomen in a Z pattern).	Provides for steady absorption of medication. Site is easily visualized and accessible by client, and a Z pattern minimizes tissue damage.
Demonstrate, then observe client drawing insulin into syringe, reading syringe markings, and administering dose. Assess for accuracy.	May require several instruction sessions and practice before client/wife feel comfortable drawing up and injecting medication.
Instruct in signs/symptoms of insulin reaction or hypoglycemia: fatigue, nausea, headache, hunger, sweating, irritability, shakiness, anxiety, or difficulty concentrating.	Knowing what to watch for and appropriate treatment such as $\frac{1}{2}$ cup of grape juice for immediate response and a snack within $\frac{1}{2}$ hr (e.g., one slice of bread with peanut butter or cheese or fruit and slice of cheese for sustained effect) may prevent or minimize complications.

ACTIONS/ INTERVENTIONS	RATIONALE
Review "Sick Day Rules" (e.g., call the doctor if too sick to eat normally or stay active) and take insulin as ordered. Keep record as noted in Sick Day Guide.	Understanding of necessary actions in the event of mild-to-severe illness promotes competent self-care and reduces risk of hyper/hypoglycemia.
Instruct client/wife in fingerstick glucose monitoring to be done qid until stable, then bid, rotating times such as FBS and before dinner or before lunch and HS. Observe return demonstrations of the procedure.	Fingerstick monitoring provides accurate and timely information regarding diabetic status. Return demonstration verifies correct learning.
Recommend client maintain record/log of fingerstick testing, antidiabetic medication, insulin dosage/site, unusual physiological response, and dietary intake. Outline desired goals of FBS 80–110, premeal 80–130.	Provides accurate record for review by caregivers for assessment of therapy effectiveness/needs.
Discuss other healthcare issues, such as smoking habits, self-monitoring for cancer (breasts/testicles), and reporting changes in general well-being.	Encourages client involvement awareness, and responsibility for own health; promotes wellness. **Note:** Smoking tends to increase client's resistance to insulin.

SECTION 2

Another Approach to Planning Client Care—Mind or Concept Mapping

Mind mapping starts in the center of the page with a representation of the main concept—the client. (This helps keep in mind that the client is the focus of the plan, not the medical diagnosis or condition.) From that central thought, other main ideas that relate to the client are added. Different concepts can be grouped together by geometric shapes, color coding, or by placement on the page. Connections and interconnections between groups of ideas are represented by the use of arrows or lines with defining phrases added that explain how the interconnected thoughts relate to one another. In this manner, many different pieces of information *about* the client can be connected directly *to* the client.

Whichever piece is chosen becomes the first layer of connections—clustered assessment data, NDs, or outcomes. For example, a map could start with NDs featured as the first "branches," each one being listed separately in some way on the map. Next, the signs and symptoms or data supporting the diagnoses could be added, or the plan could begin with the client outcomes to be achieved with connections then to NDs. When the plan is completed, there should be an ND (supported by subjective and objective assessment data), nursing interventions, desired client outcomes, and any evaluation data, all connected in a manner that shows there is a relationship between them. It is critical to understand that there is no preset order for the pieces because one cluster is not more or less important than another (or one is not "subsumed" under another). It is important, however, that those pieces within a branch be in the same order in each branch.

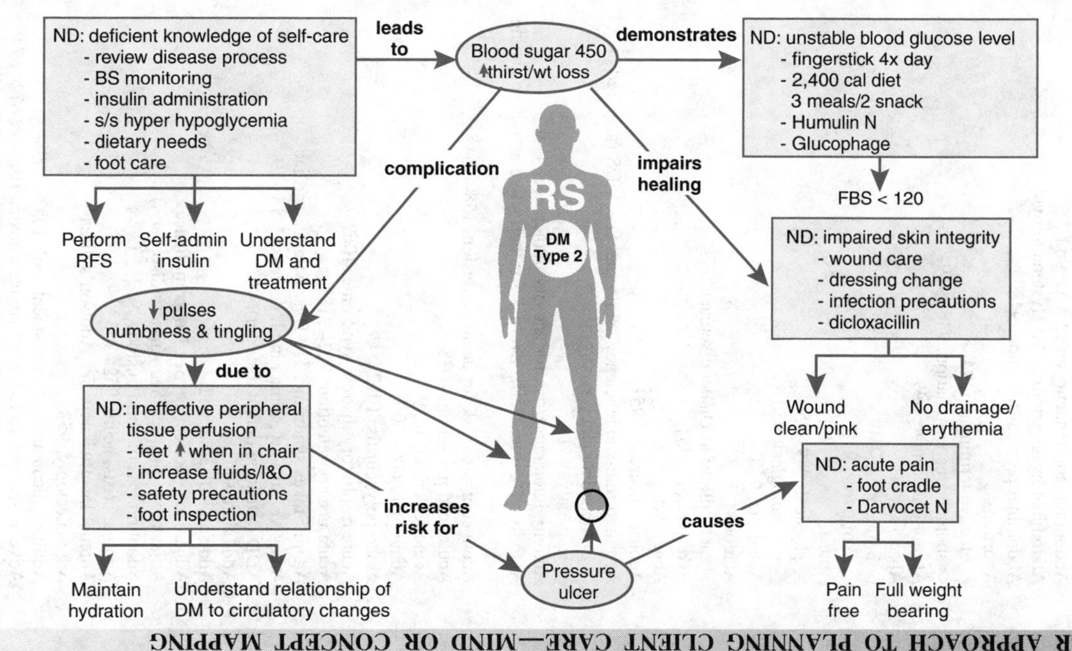
ND: deficient knowledge of self-care
- review disease process
- BS monitoring
- insulin administration
- s/s hyper hypoglycemia
- dietary needs
- foot care
leads to
Blood sugar 450
↑thirst/wt loss
demonstrates
ND: unstable blood glucose level
- fingerstick 4x day
- 2,400 cal diet
3 meals/2 snack
- Humulin N
- Glucophage
FBS < 120
complication
impairs healing
RS
DM Type 2
Perform RFS
Self-admin insulin
Understand DM and treatment
↓pulses
numbness & tingling
due to
ND: ineffective peripheral tissue perfusion
- feet ↑ when in chair
- increase fluids/I&O
- safety precautions
- foot inspection
Maintain hydration
Understand relationship of DM to circulatory changes
increases risk for
Pressure ulcer
causes
ND: impaired skin integrity
- wound care
- dressing change
- infection precautions
- dicloxacillin
Wound clean/pink
No drainage/ erythemia
ND: acute pain
- foot cradle
- Darvocet N
Pain free
Full weight bearing

Index

D

E

F

I

J

K

P

Q

R

S

T

U

V

W